Bernice A. Pescosolido · Jack K. Martin
Jane D. McLeod · Anne Rogers
Editors

Handbook of the Sociology of Health, Illness, and Healing

A Blueprint for the 21st Century

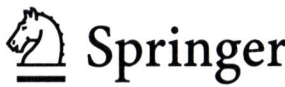

Editors
Bernice A. Pescosolido
Institute of Social Research
Indiana University
Bloomington, IN
USA
pescosol@indiana.edu

Jane D. McLeod
Institute of Social Research
Indiana University
Bloomington, IN
USA
jmcleod@indiana.edu

Jack K. Martin
Institute of Social Research
Indiana University
Bloomington, IN
USA
jkmartin@indiana.edu

Anne Rogers
University of Manchester
Manchester
UK
anne.rogers@manchester.ac.uk

ISBN 978-1-4419-7259-0   e-ISBN 978-1-4419-7261-3
DOI 10.1007/978-1-4419-7261-3
Springer New York Dordrecht Heidelberg London

© Springer Science+Business Media, LLC 2011
All rights reserved. This work may not be translated or copied in whole or in part without the written permission of the publisher (Springer Science+Business Media, LLC, 233 Spring Street, New York, NY 10013, USA), except for brief excerpts in connection with reviews or scholarly analysis. Use in connection with any form of information storage and retrieval, electronic adaptation, computer software, or by similar or dissimilar methodology now known or hereafter developed is forbidden.
The use in this publication of trade names, trademarks, service marks, and similar terms, even if they are not identified as such, is not to be taken as an expression of opinion as to whether or not they are subject to proprietary rights.

Printed on acid-free paper

Springer is part of Springer Science+Business Media (www.springer.com)

Handbook of the Sociology of Health, Illness, and Healing

Handbooks of Sociology and Social Research

Series Editor:
Howard B. Kaplan, *Texas A&M University, College Station, Texas*

HANDBOOK OF COMMUNITY MOVEMENTS AND LOCAL ORGANIZATIONS
Edited by Ram A. Cnaan (University of Pennsylvania) and Carl Milofsky (Bucknell University)

HANDBOOK ON CRIME AND DEVIANCE
Edited by Marvin J. Krohn, Alan J. Lizotte, and Gina Penly Hall (University at Albany)

HANDBOOK OF DISASTER RESEARCH
Edited by Havidán Rodríguez, Enrico L. Quarantelli, and Russell Dynes (University of Delaware)

HANDBOOK OF DRUG ABUSE PREVENTION
Theory, Science and Prevention
Edited by Zili Sloboda (University of Akron) and William J. Bukoski (National Institute on Drug Abuse)

HANDBOOK OF THE LIFE COURSE
Edited by Jeylan T. Mortimer (University of Minnesota) and Michael J. Shanahan
(University of North Carolina – Chapel Hill)

HANDBOOK OF POLITICS
Edited by Kevin T. Leicht (The University of Iowa) and J. Craig Jenkins (The Ohio State University)

HANDBOOK OF POPULATION
Edited by Dudley L. Poston (Texas A&M University) and Michael Micklin (National Institutes of Health)

HANDBOOK OF RELIGION AND SOCIAL INSTITUTIONS
Edited by Helen Rose Ebaugh (University of Houston)

HANDBOOK OF SOCIAL MOVEMENTS ACROSS DISCIPLINES
Edited by Conny Roggeband and Bert Klandermans (Vrije Universiteit, the Netherlands)

HANDBOOK OF SOCIAL PSYCHOLOGY
Edited by John Delamater (University of Wisconsin – Madison)
HANDBOOK OF SOCIOLOGICAL THEORY
Edited by Jonathan H. Turner (University of California – Riverside)

HANDBOOK OF THE SOCIOLOGY OF EDUCATION
Edited by Maureen T. Hallinan (University of Notre Dame)

HANDBOOK OF THE SOCIOLOGY OF EMOTIONS
Edited by Jan E. Stets and Jonathan H. Turner (University of California – Riverside)

HANDBOOK OF THE SOCIOLOGY OF GENDER
Edited by Janet Saltzman Chafetz (University of Houston)

HANDBOOK OF THE SOCIOLOGY OF MENTAL HEALTH
Edited by Carol S. Aneshensel (University of California – Los Angeles) and Jo C. Phelan
(Columbia University)

HANDBOOK OF THE SOCIOLOGY OF MORALITY
Edited by Steven Hitlin (University of Iowa) and Stephen Vaisey (University of California, Berkeley)

HANDBOOK OF THE SOCIOLOGY OF RACIAL AND ETHNIC RELATIONS
Edited by Hernán Vera (University of Florida) and Joe R. Feagin (Texas A&M University)
For other titles published in this series, go to www.springer.com/series/6055

Contents

Part I Rethinking Connecting Sociology's Role in Health, Illness, & Healing, From the Top Down

1 **Taking "The Promise" Seriously: Medical Sociology's Role in Health, Illness, and Healing in a Time of Social Change** 3
   Bernice A. Pescosolido

2 **Medical Sociology and Its Relationship to Other Disciplines: The Case of Mental Health and the Ambivalent Relationship Between Sociology and Psychiatry** 21
   Anne Rogers and David Pilgrim

3 **Organizing the Sociological Landscape for the Next Decades of Health and Health Care Research: The Network Episode Model III-R as Cartographic Subfield Guide** 39
   Bernice A. Pescosolido

4 **Fundamental Causality: Challenges of an Animating Concept for Medical Sociology** 67
   Jeremy Freese and Karen Lutfey

Part II Connecting Communities

5 **Learning from Other Countries: Comparing Experiences and Drawing Lessons for the United States** 85
   Mary Ruggie

6 **Health and the Social Rights of Citizenship: Integrating Welfare-State Theory and Medical Sociology** 101
   Sigrun Olafsdottir and Jason Beckfield

7 **Health Social Movements: Advancing Traditional Medical Sociology Concepts** 117
   Phil Brown, Rachel Morello-Frosch, Stephen Zavestoski,
   Laura Senier, Rebecca Gasior Altman, Elizabeth Hoover,
   Sabrina McCormick, Brian Mayer, and Crystal Adams

8 Layering Control: Medicalization, Psychopathy, and the Increasing Multi-institutional Management of Social Problems 139
Tait R. Medina and Ann McCranie

9 Community Systems Collide and Cooperate: Control of Deviance by the Legal and Mental Health Systems 159
Virginia Aldigé Hiday

Part III Connecting To Medicine: The Profession and Its Organizations

10 Medicalization and Biomedicalization Revisited: Technoscience and Transformations of Health, Illness and American Medicine 173
Adele E. Clarke and Janet Shim

11 Two Cultures: Two Ships: The Rise of a Professionalism Movement Within Modern Medicine and Medical Sociology's Disappearance from the Professionalism Debate 201
Frederic W. Hafferty and Brian Castellani

12 Medicine as a Family-Friendly Profession? 221
Ann Boulis and Jerry A. Jacobs

13 Clash of Logics, Crisis of Trust: Entering the Era of Public For-Profit Health Care? 255
Carol A. Caronna

14 Health Care Policy and Medical Sociology 271
Jennie Jacobs Kronenfeld

Part IV Connecting To the People: The Public as Patient and Powerful Force

15 The Consumer Turn in Medicalization: Future Directions with Historical Foundations 291
Anne E. Figert

16 Mundane Medicine, Therapeutic Relationships, and the Clinical Encounter: Current and Future Agendas for Sociology 309
Carl May

17 After 30 Years, Problems and Prospects in the Study of Doctor–Patient Interaction 323
John Heritage and Douglas W. Maynard

18 Enter Health Information Technology: Expanding Theories of the Doctor–Patient Relationship for the Twenty-First Century Health Care Delivery System 343
Eric R. Wright

Part V Connecting Personal & Cultural Systems

19 Culture, Race/Ethnicity and Disparities: Fleshing Out the Socio-Cultural Framework for Health Services Disparities 363
Margarita Alegría, Bernice A. Pescosolido, Sandra Williams, and Glorisa Canino

20 Health Disparities and the Black Middle Class: Overview, Empirical Findings, and Research Agenda 383
Pamela Braboy Jackson and Jason Cummings

21 Gender and Health Revisited 411
Jen'nan Ghazal Read and Bridget K. Gorman

22 Hearsay Ethnography: A Method for Learning About Responses to Health Interventions 431
Susan Cotts Watkins, Ann Swidler, and Crystal Biruk

Part VI Connecting to Dynamics: The Health and Illness Career

23 Life Course Approaches to Health, Illness and Healing 449
Eliza K. Pavalko and Andrea E. Willson

24 The Complexities of Help-Seeking: Exploring Challenges Through a Social Network Perspective 465
Normand Carpentier and Paul Bernard

Part VII Connecting the Individual and the Body

25 Bodies in Context: Potential Avenues of Inquiry for the Sociology of Chronic Illness and Disability Within a New Policy Era 483
Caroline Sanders and Anne Rogers

26 Identity and Illness 505
Kathryn J. Lively and Carrie L. Smith

27 Learning to Love Animal (Models) (or) How (Not) to Study Genes as a Social Scientist 527
Dalton Conley

28 Taking the Medical Sciences Seriously: Why and How Medical Sociology Should Incorporate Diverse Disciplinary Perspectives 543
Brea L. Perry

Index 563

Contributors

Crystal Adams
Brown University, Providence RI, USA

Margarita Alegría
Harvard Medical School/Cambridge Health Alliance, Cambridge MA, USA

Rebecca Gasior Altman
Brown University, Providence RI, USA

Jason Beckfield
Harvard University, Cambridge MA, USA

Paul Bernard
University of Montreal, Montreal QC, Canada

Crystal Biruk
University of Pennsylvania, Philadelphia PA, USA

Ann Boulis
University of Pennsylvania, Philadelphia PA, USA

Phil Brown
Brown University, Providence RI, USA

Glorisa Canino
University of Puerto Rico, San Juan PR, USA

Carol A. Caronna
Towson University, Towson MD, USA

Normand Carpentier
CSSS de Bordeaux-Cartierville-Saint-Laurent, 11822, avenue du Bois-de-Boulogne, Montréal, QC, Canada H3W 2X6

Brian Castellani
Kent State University-Ashtabula, Ashtabula OH, USA

Adele E. Clarke
University of California-San Francisco, San Francisco CA, USA

Dalton Conley
New York University, New York NY, USA

Jason Cummings
Indiana University, Bloomington IN, USA

Anne E. Figert
Department of Sociology, Loyola University Chicago, Coffey Hall 421,
1032 W. Sheridan Road, Chicago, IL 60660, USA

Jeremy Freese
Northwestern University, Evanston IL, USA

Bridget K. Gorman
Rice University, Houston TX, USA

Frederic W. Hafferty
Department of Behavioral Sciences, University of MN Medical School,
1035 University Drive, Deluth, MN 55812-2487, USA

John Heritage
University of California, Los Angeles CA, USA

Virginia Aldigé Hiday
Department of Sociology, North Carolina State University, Rm. 355, 1911 Building,
Raleigh, NC 27695-8107, USA

Elizabeth Hoover
Brown University, Providence RI, USA

Pamela Braboy Jackson
Department of Sociology, Indiana University, Ballantine 744,
Bloomington, IN 47405, USA

Jerry A. Jacobs
University of Pennsylvania, Philadelphia PA, USA

Jennie Jacobs Kronenfeld
Arizona State University, Tempe AZ, USA

Kathryn J. Lively
Dartmouth College, Hanover NH, USA

Karen Luftey
New England Research Institute, Watertown MA, USA

Jack K. Martin
Indiana University, Bloomington IN, USA

Carl May
Newcastle University, Newcastle upon Tyne, UK

Brian Mayer
University of Florida, Gainesville FL, USA

Douglas W. Maynard
University of Wisconsin, Madison WI, USA

Sabrina McCormick
Michigan State University, East Lansing MI, USA

Contributors

Ann McCranie
Indiana University, Bloomington IN, USA

Jane D. McLeod
Indiana University, Bloomington IN, USA

Tait R. Medina
Department of Sociology, Indiana University, Ballantine 744,
Bloomington, IN 47405, USA

Rachel Morello-Frosch
University of California-Berkeley, Berkeley CA, USA

Sigrun Olafsdottir
Boston University, Boston MA, USA

Eliza K. Pavalko
Indiana University, Bloomington IN, USA

Brea L. Perry
University of Kentucky, Lexington KY, USA

Bernice A. Pescosolido
Indiana University, Bloomington IN, USA

David Pilgrim
University of Central Lancashire, Lancashire, UK

Jen'nan Ghazal Read
Duke University, Durham NC, USA

Anne Rogers
University of Manchester, 5th Floor Williamson Building,
Oxford Road, Manchester M139 PL

Mary Ruggie
The John F. Kennedy School of Government, Harvard University,
Taubman 470, 79 JFK Street, Cambridge, MA 02138-5801, USA

Caroline Sanders
Primary Care, Health Sciences, University of Manchester, Williamson Bldg.,
Oxford Rd., Manchester, M13 9PL, UK

Laura Senier
University of Wisconsin-Madison, Madison WI, USA

Janet Shim
University of California-San Francisco, San Francisco CA, USA

Carrie L. Smith
Associate Professor of Sociology, Department of Sociology & Anthropology
Millersville University, P.O. Box 1002, Millersville, PA 17551-0302

Ann Swidler
University of California-Berkeley, Berkeley CA, USA

Susan Cotts Watkins
University of Pennsylvania, Philadelphia PA, USA

Sandra Williams
Cambridge Health Alliance, Somerville MA, USA

Andrea E. Willson
University of Western Ontario, London ON, Canada

Eric R. Wright
Center for Health Policy, Indiana University School of Medicine, Department of Public Health, IUPUI, 410 W. Tenth Street, HS 3119, Indianapolis, IN 46202, USA

Stephen Zaveskoski
University of San Francisco, San Francisco CA, USA

Part I
Rethinking Connecting Sociology's Role in Health, Illness, & Healing, From the Top Down

Chapter 1
Taking "The Promise" Seriously: Medical Sociology's Role in Health, Illness, and Healing in a Time of Social Change

Bernice A. Pescosolido

> "...the individual can understand his own experience and gauge his own fate only by locating himself within his period....he can know his own chances in life only by becoming aware of those of all individuals in his circumstances."
>
> C.W. Mills (1959, p. 5)

Introduction: Taking Stock of the Intellectual and Societal Landscape of Medical Sociology

In 1959, C.W. Mills published his now famous treatise on what sociology uniquely brings to understanding the world and the people in it. Every sociologist, of whatever ilk, has had at least a brush with the "sociological imagination," and nearly everyone who has taken a sociology course has encountered some version of it. As Mills argued, the link between the individual and society, between personal troubles and social issues, between biography and history, or between individual crises and institutional contradictions represents the core vision of the discipline of sociology. While reminding ourselves of the "promise" may be a bit trite, its mention raises the critical question: Why do we have to continually remind ourselves of the unique contribution that we, as sociologists, bring to understanding health, illness, and healing?

Perhaps, we remind ourselves because the sociological imagination is so complex – a multilayered perspective that ties together dynamics processes, social structures, and individual variation. While Mills (1959, p. 4) himself argued that "ordinary men...do not possess the quality of mind essential to grasp the interplay," this seems a bit overplayed. There have always been people – in the academy, in the workroom, or in the home – who have heard and understood the deafening voice of oppressive social norms drowning out opportunity. There have always been people who have noted, described, and taken advantage of changes in opportunity structures to improve their fate. And, despite modern medicine's reductionist and mechanical view of the body, which may or may not be changing, there have always been the Rudolph Virchows, the Milton and Ruth Roemers, the George Readers, and the Howard Waitzkins, alongside the majority. While the sociological perspective may find a particular challenge in the United States with its strong strain of individualism, there have always been those who have captured the hearts, sparked the intelligence, and harnessed the energy of the group as a way to overcome the existing limits of their surroundings. From the rise [and fall] of unions; to the

B.A. Pescosolido (✉)
Department of Sociology, Indiana University, 1022 E. Third Street, Bloomington, IN 47405, USA
e-mail: pescosol@indiana.edu

improvement of working conditions in toxic factory work; to the formation of professional associations in medicine, nursing and their specialties; to women's health cooperatives designed to counter the insensitivity of regular medicine, instances of confronting the status quo through affiliation and association stand as exemplars of the tacit, "on-the-ground" understanding of the sociological imagination.

I would argue, rather, that we need to be reminded of the central premises of sociology and what we bring to table precisely because we have been successful, even if quietly so. In essence, the major dilemma that we confront at present is that the "promise" is obvious, not only to ourselves, but to others. The idea that context matters has taken hold across the sociomedical sciences, the bio-medical sciences, and even the basic sciences like genetics and cognitive science (see Pescosolido 2006 for a review). Ideas of health and health care disparities (which we have called inequalities for over 100 years in sociology, and for over 50 years in the subfield of medical sociology); fundamental causes (as Link and Phelan, 1995, so eloquently labeled sociologists' baseline concern with power, stratification and social differentiation); and social networks as vectors of social and organizational influence (now renamed "Network Science") stand front and center in the concerns of the National Institutes of Health and other major scientific organizations. Whether our arguments and research findings have been persistent, robust and convincing, or whether these insights coincide with the recognition by the more reductionist sciences that even their most sophisticated approaches cannot solve the problems of the body and the mind alone, is of little consequence. When the newly appointed director of the NIH, Dr. Francis Collins, who led the Human Genome Project, announces the launching of a special program to increase attention and resources to basic behavioral and social science (November 18, 2009, www.oppnet.nih.gov) using phrases like "synergy," "vital component," and "complex factors that affect individuals, our communities and our environment," the crack in the door of mainstream biomedical science becomes just a little wider, and the seat at the table becomes just a little more possible.

Sometimes, the role of sociologists is obvious in these new declarations of important directions in science and medicine; other times, they appear as "discoveries" without much, if any, attribution. But to belabor the historical debt that contemporary health and health care researchers and policymakers may owe us is a waste of both time and energy. Sociology has a history of conceptualizing social life, making that view understandable, and having its insights and even its language absorbed as "common sense" into both academic and civil life (e.g., clique, identity, self-fulfilling prophecy, social class, disparities, networks). More to the point, Mills argued that the sociological imagination is a "task" as well as a "promise." He described that task – "to grasp history and biography and the relations between the two within society" (1959, p. 6) – through the work of major sociologists of his time as "comprehensive," "graceful," "intricate," "subtle," and "ironic." With "many-sided constructions," a focus on meaning, and a willingness to look across social institutions like polity, the economy, and the domestic sphere (1959, p. 6), Auguste Comte and others came to define sociology's aspiration as the "Queen of the Social Sciences," a phrase more commonly used now by economists or political scientists to describe their discipline. Similarly, Mills (1959) sees sociology as holding "the best statements of the full promise of the social sciences as a whole" (1959, p. 24), and I have argued elsewhere that taking sociology's view of social interactions in networks represents one promising approach to integrating the health sciences (Pescosolido 2006).

The complexities in topic, theory and methods, sometimes the object of divisions in sociology and sometimes a detriment in the "sound bite" approach to modern society, continue to be our strength, and are not always obvious to others who adopt the mantra of "context." Our research focuses on how individuals, organizations, and nations are "selected and formed, liberated and repressed, made sensitive and blunted" (Mills 1959, p. 7). We accept the unexpected, we expect latent functions of policies and actions of even those who are trying to do good, we understand that being an outsider has its advantages in understanding the world, and we embrace the notion of comparison and reject a "provincial narrowing to the interest to the Western societies" (1959, p. 12). Whenever we look at a life, a "disease," a health care system, or a nation's epidemiological profile, examining which "values are cherished yet threatened" (1959, p. 11) is inevitable. As Hung (2004) has recently documented for the SARS virus and Epstein (1996) for HIV/AIDS, the societal reactions to viral pandemics are deeply rooted in social cleavages rather than biological fact, whether this reaction unearthed the racist view of the "Yellow peril" or the homophobic view of the "Gay plague."

In sum, at this point in time, it may be more important than ever to recall our mission and accept the uneasiness which is endemic (and according to Mills, necessary) to it. The sociological imagination requires "the capacity to shift from one perspective to another – from the political to the psychological….to range from the most impersonal and remote transformations to the most intimate features of the human self – and to see the relations between the two" (1959, p. 7). Our training emphasizes this, our theories conceptualize it, and the wide variety of our research methods reflect it. We bring this self-consciousness to the problems of health, illness, and healing, and hopefully to their solutions. Which subfield of sociology, more than the sociology of health, illness, and healing, provides a critical window into making "clear the elements of contemporary uneasiness and indifference" that Mills sees as "the social scientists' foremost political and intellectual task" (1959, p. 13)? While Mills may have been premature, or flat out wrong, in his prediction that the social sciences would overthrow the dominance of the physical and biological sciences, his view was prescient regarding the rising importance of "context" in biomedical sciences (1959, p. 13) and increasing doubts about the inevitable and pristine nature of science. As those inside the "House of Medicine" itself dare to question the utility of the "gold standard" (RCT, the randomized clinical trial) versus observational studies (Concato et al. 2000), the validity of the placebo as a "control" (Leuchter et al. 2002), and the robustness of "established" genetic links (Gelernter et al. 1991), the radical critiques of the objectivity of science and the inevitability of linear progress in science have come from inside as well as outside (Gieryn 1983; Latour 1999). It is naïve to assume or even expect a reconstruction of the prestige hierarchy of the sciences, as Mills does to some extent. He forgets that institutional supports undergird that dominance, as any of us who have served on interdisciplinary review panels will attest. Yet, the idea that there may be occasional openings for concerns and approaches by social scientists was prophetic. This may be one of those unique times to work together to push not only our understandings forward, but to foster institutional social change. At the least, it is a time when social scientists, especially sociologists, need to have their voices heard; that is, to have a place at the table to guard against a crass, out-of-date, and generally poor appropriation of the social sciences' basic ideas and tools. Those of us who witnessed a wider acceptance of (even called for) social science methods such as ethnography in the 1980s and 1990s in the mental health research agenda, also witnessed the dumping of the term into one sentence of a traditional research proposal without any idea of its complexity, rigor, or even utility to expand the limited insights of clinical research. Bearman (2008, p. vi) downplays concerns that this kind of scientific diffusion may "distort the sociological project" because "the beauty of sociology as a discipline rests in its hybridity with respect to method and data" and new research concerns can become a potential "lever" for sociology to escape some of its own "hegemonic" foci.

The Task Ahead: Mapping the Landscape of Health, Illness, and Healing for the Next Decades

As Mills reminds us, the insights of sociology are both "a terrible lesson and a magnificent one." Perhaps, this is more true in medical sociology than in other areas of the discipline; maybe not. Yet, the historical and contemporary landscape of health, illness, and healing challenges medical sociologists to think about both the issues/topics that have drawn and continue to draw our attention, as well as new ones on the horizon.

The Metaphor of Cartography

Recently, Sigrun Olafsdottir and I (2009, 2010) drew from the "cultural turn" in sociology to reframe key theoretical and methodological issues in health care utilization research. We considered whether some individuals map a larger set of choices, examined if and how they differentiate between different sources of formal treatment, and questioned whether the way we ask those in our research about their experiences shapes the responses they give. This imagery of cultural landscapes and boundaries (Gieryn 1983, 1999) seems to fit the multifaceted, complex nature of health, illness, and healing in the current era. Individuals use cultural maps to make sense of the world, affecting information availability and personal understandings, as well as signaling possible appropriate action. While Gieryn's work focuses on professions, primarily scientists and the rhetorical strategies they use to establish, extend, and protect their societal authority, these ideas have broader relevance, not only for other professionals like physicians, but for the public. In particular, the concept of "boundary-work" becomes central as individuals, whatever their position, confront illness, define disease, and react to treatment options. The term "cultural mapping," targeting the terrain of choices, as well as individuals' recognition, acceptance, or rejection of them, informs us about the boundaries of their experience, and values shaping action, whether their own (as in rational choice theory) or that of others (as in labeling, social influence, and social control theories).

In essence, cultural landscapes shape individuals' everyday decisions and actions, including those of medical sociologists. The metaphor of cultural cartography allows us not only to organize our topical research agendas but also our challenges for the next generation of medical sociology. In essence, two different maps require our attention. One is a map of topographical changes in health and health care that mark out new or continued areas of inquiry; the second maps the boundaries of discipline, the joint jurisdiction of sociology with the subfield of medical sociology, and how these two symbiotically share intellectual territory.

Contextualizing and Researching Health, Medicine, Health Care, and the Biomedical Sciences: Time of Change from the Outside

There is little doubt that the essential questions of sociology and medical sociology – more specifically, of the importance of Weber's link between lifestyle (i.e., social psychological as well as social organization) and life chances – remain paramount and require our continued attention. Causes (epidemiology) and consequences (outcomes, health services research) continue to crudely, and increasingly inaccurately, define research agendas as we emphasize more dynamic processes which connect the two. Medical sociologists continue to more broadly conceive the landscape of epidemiology than do our sister subfields of medicine and public health. That is, with regard to issues of mortality and morbidity, the distribution and the determinants of disease must consider issues of professional power, social movements, contested meaning, and social construction (or its cousin specific to medical sociology, medicalization) as well as traditional risk and protective factors like genetics, biological markers, psychological trauma, or even individuals lifestyles (Brown 1995; McKinlay 1996). To understand utilization, adherence, health care system, and outcomes, we need to incorporate dynamic views, describe different response pathways, and confront changing boundaries of legitimacy regarding potential patients, healers, and formal structures of care (Pescosolido 1991, 1992).

In addition to these classic, general prescriptions, three newer but deep-seated developments call for sociological theorizing and research. Necessarily, some of these are intertwined with our classic concerns but, nevertheless, they raise new challenges.

Human Genome Project and the Larger Push for Understanding Context

Not all that new, the first phase of the project, designed to determine the sequence of base pairs in the entire human genome, began in 1990 and continued for 13 years. Yet, as Francis Collins and others have noted, we are only beginning to understand what we have and can learn both in a positive and negative sense. Sociologists have tread into that territory lightly, now starting to work their way toward the profound implications of this massive project and the larger cultural institutions that created and continue to nurture it (e.g., Phelan 2005). Perhaps, the most obvious is the potential for collaborative projects on epigenetics and on gene-environment interactions (g x e) (i.e., how environmental conditions which include society not only trigger or suppress genetic predispositions but, in fact, change the genome itself; Szyf 2009). While complicated, this may not be the most challenging. It was a recent special issue of the *American Journal of Sociology* (Bearman 2008, p. vi) that turned an obvious research question on its head: "What can we learn about social structure and social processes, and what can we learn about our accounts about social structure and social processes, by 'thinking about genetics'?" Fleshing this out even a little raises classic sociological questions. How is the genetics agenda constructed by medicine, by insurance companies, by the public, and by science itself, to name just a few? What does this mean for the definition and behavioral implications of human health, legitimate constructions of illness by the public and the profession, shifting definitions of vulnerability, and changes in the nature and targets of prejudice and discrimination? While bioethicists and philosophers have asked and deliberated on these questions, medical sociologists bring evidence to bear on the creation, maintenance, and effects of this now dominant weltanschauung in medicine, science, and society. We have the tools to ensure that the powerful forces of society are understood, elaborated, and included in our understandings of the onset of what becomes labeled disease and disorder. We have the tools to uncover the unexpected, latent functions of this direction which, in themselves, will raise new challenges for the very institutions that placed their hopes in "the language of God" (Collins 2006).

The Mess that Is "Translational Science" and the Need for Sociological Clarity

Of the new "medical speak" that dominates discussions of future directions, the current ubiquitous term is "translation." Unfortunately, while critically targeting the lack of effective transfer across stakeholder communities, this term has confounded discussions and attempts to provide solutions. Even in a quick survey of existing documents that call for "translation," at least three meanings are evident. The *first translation* dilemma, which can be referred to as a *dissemination* problem, suggests a need for more effective ways to communicate information between scientists and "end-users." The *second translation* dilemma, an *implementation* problem (also the efficacy–effectiveness gap), suggests a need to understand how to translate science into services that result in meaningful clinical care (National Advisory Mental Health Council 2000). Finally, the *third translation* dilemma, referred to as a problem of *integration*, suggests that the insights and potential contributions of different branches of science have not been fully incorporated in efforts to either establish research agendas or to provide high quality effective care in the formal treatment sector.

Each of these suggests complicated problems, all recast as problems of "translation," for a diverse array of stakeholder communities and, to date, traditional research approaches have not offered good answers. Each calls for sociological research on a series of basic questions. First, why do providers and consumers fail to take advantage of cutting-edge science? A frequent complaint expressed by research scientists, payers, and policy makers is that cutting-edge interventions are neither adopted in day-to-day clinical work nor accepted by individuals with health problems who might benefit. Second, why do treatments that have been "proven" to work in randomized clinical trials fail to work in real world settings? A continual frustration of providers is that clinical research fails to take into account the challenges of day-to-day clinical work and does not offer a realistic understanding of the complexities and limitations of providing care. A similar frustration of consumers and advocates is that clinical research fails to take into account the complex realities of the lives of persons who fall ill, especially those with chronic and stigmatized problems. Third, why has health services research not been able to bridge the gap to allow proven clinical interventions to find application to the "real world" needs of consumers, practitioners, payers, and policy makers (Pellmar and Eisenberg 2000)? Each of these requires an understanding of "cultures" – the culture of the public, the culture of the clinic, the culture of community, and of organizations. Sociological research holds the potential to understand how cultures are shaped; how they are enacted; how they clash or coincide with one another; and how, in the end, cultural scripts facilitate, retard, or even prohibit institutional social change. Sometimes, these discussions have the reductionist tone of lack of motivation without understanding the power of institution and resource as well as the social network structures that cripple innovation. More importantly, these challenges call for a holistic approach to research in which different levels of change, as well as the individuals in them, are conceptualized as linked and intertwined, with outcomes measured through innovative quantitative approaches and mechanisms observed through in-depth qualitative observations. In no way would such studies exclude the expertise of other scientists; indeed they call for it. However, the multilayered, multimethod and connected approach inherent in medical sociology provides an overarching organizing framework that can facilitate the integration of different interdisciplinary insights (Pescosolido 2006).

The "Hundred Year's War" of American Medicine and Mechanic's Continued Call for Sociological Understandings

Ironically, exactly 100 years ago, the Flexner Report "closed the books" on the blueprint for the primary structure and power of medicine in America. The 1910 document, crafted by middle-class men with middle-class values building the new institutions of industrial society, called for the active and specific funneling of large amounts of money from the new industrial tycoons who, themselves, had other ideas about what the US health care system should look like (Pescosolido and Martin 2004). However, drawing from the recent "successes" of the "new" scientific medical schools of Germany, France, and the United Kingdom, the Flexner Report set a trajectory and the Rockefeller Foundation fiscally supported a process of mimetic isomorphism for other emergent medical institutions. America's health care system was built primarily with private funds, dominated by the allopathic physician, and supported though a fee-for-service economy (Freidson 1970; Starr 1982). The era from the Flexner report until President Nixon's proclamation of a "Health Care Crisis" in 1970 has been described by McKinlay and Marceau (2002) as the "Golden Age of Doctoring," by Clarke and her colleagues as the "Medicalization Era" (Clarke and Shim 2010), and by us, using Eliot Freidson's (1970) terms, as "The Era of Professional Dominance" (Pescosolido and Boyer 2001). Working in a primarily private health care system, physicians determined both the nature of medical care and the arrangements under which it was provided. Even with the introduction of private (and later public) insurance, the American system remained an anomaly on the global landscape. The richest country in the world, which spent more on research, technology, and care than any other, also was home to the greatest number and proportion of uninsured citizens and to standard indicators of population health that fell way below those of countries with fewer resources and less of them devoted to health.

The year 2010, 100 years after the Flexner Report, saw the initial passage of President Obama's Health Care Plan. What will result from this shift in the U.S. position on health care as right and as privilege? Will it be dramatic and devastating as some claim? Dramatic and good as others claim? Given the early capitulation to (or some would say, inclusion) of key opponents of earlier reforms, will this plan result in more patching of an essentially private system in the stranglehold of insurance and pharmaceutical companies? Will reform suffer the fate of what many of us thought/hoped would be the "second great transformation" (Stone 1999) or "construction of the second social contract" between American medicine and society (Pescosolido and Kronenfeld 1995) in the Clinton Health Reform of 1990? Or, will this "accommodation," as was the case with high physician reimbursement levels during the Medicaid/Medicare deliberations, mean that something will actually change?

The failed federal effort of the 1990s nevertheless ushered in the "Era of Managed Care" which both supporters and critics of the existing health care system feared (Pescosolido and Boyer 2001). But as Mechanic et al. (2001) documented, the introduction of managed care did little to change the amount of time that physicians and patients spent together in the examining room before that event. In fact, the amount of time that physicians spent in interaction with their patients was already minimal, reflecting a typical romantization of past social institutions rather than data on its actual operation. By 1999, health care scholars talked about the "backlash" against managed care which began as early as the mid-1990s and resulted in the weakening of many of its proposed strategies to limit choice of physicians, access to specialists, and cut costs. This "managed care lite" (Mechanic 2004) did provide a short-term control of costs which soon gave way to escalating fiscal pressure and further increases in the number of uninsured Americans. By the end of the decade, Swartz (1999) proclaimed the "death of managed care" and Vladeck (1999) announced that managed care had had its "Fifteen Minutes of Fame," warning that "Big Fix" political solutions oversell, inevitably producing negative overreactions.

What will medicine, the health care system, and population health look like as a result of reform? At what point, and how, will we see the landscape of the US as truly different? Carol Boyer and I (2001) agree that the 1970s began the "end of unquestioned dominance," but are we still "drifting" as Freidson (1970) warned, or are we reconstructing the American social contract between civil society and the "medical-industrial complex" (McKinlay 1974)? How much of our view of "change" can or cannot be backed up by real data? After all, given larger claims of the "consumer backlash" or "consumer revolution" that would change the power balance, we find little significant decrease in the public's view of the authority or expertise of physicians (Pescosolido et al. 2001). If there is a decrease in the confidence in American medicine, as Schlesinger (2002) claims, how much of this disillusionment is not exclusive to modern medicine, but rather reflects a generalized reaction to social institutions, developed in the modern, industrial era, to larger changes in contemporary society (Pescosolido and Rubin 2000). Rubin (1996) argued that the social and economic bases of modern society were "tarnished" in the early 1970s, marking a general turning point for social institutions in the face of diminished growth that had accompanied the post World War II era. To simply look at trends in the response to medicine and health care may miss the point of our general prescription to understand social life in context.

Community, professional, and the health care systems are in a state of constant change, in big and small ways, and claims of improvement or deterioration pale in comparison to actual research that contextualizes and documents societal level change (Pescosolido et al. 2010, on contentions and data on the dissipating stigma of mental illness in U.S. society). Such claims are important because they often come to have a life of their own, shaping priorities for research and treatment. But claims are research questions subject to empirical examination with social science data. Have we taken up Mills' task to bring the "comprehensive," "graceful," "intricate," and "many sided constructions" of sociology to changes in health, illness, and healing? Mechanic (1993) has repeatedly pointed out that sociologists are not well represented, doing the research on the organization of care that can provide both the subtle and dramatic, expected and ironic, impacts on the profession, the public, and health institutions. A sociological perspective, alone or integrated with others, is critical in marking and analyzing the impact on individuals, organizations, and groups of reform.

Putting Our Own House in Order: Time of Change from the Inside

There are, of course, many more important questions. At this historical moment of structural reform and reconsideration of research agendas, these appear to loom large. If medical sociologists are to attend to these or other critical issues in health, illness, and healing, a reflection on where we stand is essential. In fact, the logic of this volume was designed around the reflections of the editors, the contributors, and those who attended some of our early planning events.

Sociologists have regularly, if only occasionally, lamented our basic and internal barriers to progress – whether Lester Ward (1907) arguing that sociologists do not know enough biology to reject it or Alvin Gouldner (1970) alerting us to a brewing crisis in "Western sociology" because of a blind reliance on "objective" data (more below). Sociology weathered these critiques, changing sometimes in small ways and other times in large ways, but most often, noting the critique, integrating it in some way and to some extent in some corner of the discipline, and moving on. Sociology has survived functionalism and its dominant status attainment theory in the 1960s and 1970s, Marxism and the 1980s dominating return to historical sociology, and postmodernism's declaration that everything is virtually unknowable except through one's own personal experiences (in which Anthropology did not fare so well as a discipline; Pescosolido and Rubin 2000). Sociology is likely to both encounter and survive many more of these critiques; perhaps ironically because of the embedded Catholicism in its theory and method. While our richness lies in the breadth and inclusion, as noted above, this is also the source of confusion regarding sociology's "brand."

Decoding the Discipline and the Subfield: The Three Medical Sociologies

The looseness of our boundaries of inquiry and methods of intellectual mining is not without its costs. Recently, Pace and Middendorf (2004) argued that understanding the challenges in learning the heart of a discipline's contribution requires asking a series of questions. This "decoding of the disciplines" seems just as relevant to reflecting on the research voice we use to address our "publics" (Burawoy 2005), whether students, ourselves, our colleagues in other disciplines, providers, policy makers, or the general population. While this approach places disciplines at the center of discussions, Pace and Middendorf (2004, p. 4) note the critical but paradoxical requirement to consider the boundaries that we cross with other disciplines. Decoding first relies on the identification of "bottlenecks," those places or issues where the end goals are not being met. They argue that, too often, this part of the process is skipped in favor of trying solutions which, while well meaning, miss the mark.

Following these directions, two often simultaneous concerns appear to echo through decades of writings on the discipline and the subfield. Mills (1959) warned of the "lazy safety of specialization" (Mills 1959, p. 21). Gouldner (1970), Gans (1989), Burawoy (2005), and others have asked sociologists to be more engaged with civil society, more normative and less pristinely and scientifically aloof, and more willing to engage in activities that have a more immediate impact on the world. Bringing the two concerns of relevance and specialization to the same point on the intellectual map, Collins took up the concern of whether sociology "has lost its public impact or even its impulse to public action" (1986, p. 1336), pointing to the proliferation of specialties as the source of internal, disciplinary boundary disputes, including pushing to the fringes those sociologists who took a more applied approach. While our subfields have allowed us to make the increasingly large professional association and annual meetings feel smaller, more personal and relevant, building up an "espirit de corps" (1986, p. 1341) that facilitates the socialization of our new colleague, Collins sees the result that we "scarcely recognize the names of eminent practitioners in specialties other than our own…having become congeries of outsiders to each other" (1986, p. 1340).

Medical sociology has not been immune to these centrifugal forces, arguing to the ASA that even if not formally the case, we "own" and caretake the *Journal of Health and Social Behavior;* revel in the realization that it has the third highest impact factor among journals in the discipline following our two flagship journals, the *American Sociological Review* and the *American Journal of Sociology;* or boast about our section membership hovering around the thousand mark. From its earliest days, Strauss (1957) articulated the fuzzy distinction between a sociology OF medicine and a sociology IN medicine which evoked the basic-applied distinction. We reported on concerns among our colleagues in medical sociology (Pescosolido and Kronenfeld 1995), with Levine (1995) suggesting that such territorial disputes trickle down, in part, from the larger discipline.

Not surprisingly, the second step in decoding follows from the identification of bottlenecks. In essence, knowing the landscape is key to traversing it successfully. Because Collins (1986, p. 1355), in the end, finds "a pathological tendency to miss the point of what is happening in areas other than our own," advocates that we work in two or three specialties, sequentially or simultaneously. Because Burawoy (2005) sees two dimensions that define our work (instrumental and reflexive), he argues for the legitimacy of four "brands" of sociological work which individuals can embrace simultaneously or sequentially. In medical sociology, Levine's plea for "creative integration" draws together the insights of "structure seekers" and "meaning seekers" (Pearlin 1992). In fact, using a cartological metaphor, he called for us to become more "cognizant of the theoretical and methodological 'tributaries' that feed into the subfield that is medical sociology" (Levine 1995, p. 2). In 1995, we argued for the integration of the mainstream and the subfield (Pescosolido and Kronenfeld 1995).

The Boundary Divisions that Matter: The Three Medical Sociologies

The terrain has changed because there have been deep-seated changes in the bedrock underlying medical sociology. The sources of these tectonic shifts lie in three interconnected but altered features of institutional supports. They are: (1) The demise of medical sociology training programs; (2) The growing presence of "other" sociologists in the sociology of health, illness, and healing; and (3) The increased presence of sociologists in medicine, public health, and related fields. Each comes with its own strengths and weakness, and together, they produce major impediments in building a cumulated set of findings from and for sociology in the areas of health, illness, and healing. Two dimensions are critical – training (What do we pass on in research on health, illness, and healing?) and audience (Who do we want to talk to?).

Our House and Corner of the Map: Medical Sociology by and for Medical Sociology

Post-WWII, the NIH, and particularly the NIMH, saw the development of subfields of social science within its purview. Training programs were funded in social psychology, medical sociology, and methodology, to name only a few. The demise of these training programs at sociology departments such as Yale, Wisconsin, and Indiana Universities resulted from narrowing NIH foci away from the broad concerns with stratification, institutions, medical sociology, social psychology to disease-specific problems beginning in the 1990s. But some training programs or major training emphases have survived (Rutgers, UCSF in the School of Nursing, Brandeis, Columbia), some have arisen in their wake (Indiana, Vanderbilt; Maryland), and some have fallen away (Wisconsin, Yale, UCLA).

This does not mean that there are not major medical sociologists elsewhere training individuals, nor does it mean that individuals are not doing medical sociology-relevant dissertations or research. However, it does mean two things. First, medical sociologists trained in these programs sometimes do not have the strong connection to the mainstream of the discipline, which is an aspect of Collins' concerns. The success of our own journals and lines of research have produced a bit of insularity, pushing forward streams of research that neither draw from nor are engaged in dialog with the mainstream discussions. Whether this reflects a narrowing of the mainstream journals (see Pescosolido et al. 2007) or a narrowing of medical sociologists' interests and reference groups is immaterial. Second, it also means that the findings of medical sociology that have been built over three generations have not become part of the larger stock of knowledge of the discipline and are sometimes absent in mainstream work that would profit from its insights (see below).

The main point is that the interchange between significant, relevant contributions in medical sociology and significant, relevant contributions in the mainstream disciplines and its other subfields is not happening. This decreases the accumulation of tools in the sociological toolbox, whether practitioners of our subfield, other subfields or the mainstream of the discipline.

Our Country: Mainstream Sociology with a Focus on Health, Illness, or Healing

Mills' link between larger opportunities and challenges and individual behaviors is no less applicable to our research enterprise than it is to the phenomena we research. The availability of funding sources affects how sociologists are able to do their work; with sociology's broad focus on social institutions, health becomes a focus of those who are concerned with general forces (e.g., inequality, organizations, and communities) than with the social indictors of outcomes. That is, health and health care is only one of a number of life chances affected by larger contextual forces. Dramatic instances of unequal life chances cannot help but draw the interests of sociologists. The increase in interdisciplinary research teams and the relative "wealth" of the NIH (e.g., versus the NSF) has brought more sociologists into research that addresses health, illness, and healing. All of these developments are good for the discipline and the subfield, as well as for the accumulation of social science and insights for the medical sciences.

Again, however, this focused attention by sociologists on areas traditionally defined as medical sociology is not without its costs. Specifically, it leads to a "quibble," not necessarily an unimportant one, with this brand of research. As Jane McLeod so eloquently put it in her comments on the "Author Meets the Critics" Session at ASA in 2003, such work tends to suffer from "The Fatal Attraction Syndrome." In other words, the insights of medical sociology research are ignored and "rediscovered." Declaring the need for a sociological subfield of "social autopsy" disregards medical sociology's line of research on social epidemiology that pioneered sociology's focus on how issues of class, race, and gender shape mortality and morbidity (McLeod 2004).

This is not misrepresentation, but missed opportunity. Classic works embraced by medical sociology were penned by sociologists who did not appear to consider themselves "medical sociologists" (e.g., Erving Goffman, Everett Hughes). Rather, in contemporary research, the lack of training in and knowledge of medical sociology as a subfield yields a weaker picture of sociology's contributions to our understanding of the social forces that shape health, illness, and healing. It may suggest to those both inside and outside the subfield that the discipline of sociology is not at the cutting edge.

Abandoning Home and Country for Richer, More Powerful Neighborhoods: Medical Sociologists Packed and Gone to Medicine, Public Health, and Policy

Differences in employment opportunities, either restricted in sociology or open in schools of medicine and public health, and the greater distribution and impact of scientific journals and dissemination outlets in those fields, create a third community on the sociological landscape. These are sociologists who tend to be very well trained in medical sociology and who bring a prominence to sociological ideas in health, illness, and healing. What can be the problem here? In fact, there is no immediate issue, because both sociologists and medical sociologists "find" much of their work. However, not all of their research can be fully integrated into the discipline without their presence, literally and figuratively, in sociology venues. The problem is that, in their geographic positions outside the discipline, they will not likely train the next generation of medical sociologists. In addition, many of these sociologists are precisely the ones who focus on health care organization and policy, a topic about which David Mechanic finds the subfield relatively weak in addressing. With the demise of strong medical sociology training programs in the top ranked departments, the two problems mentioned above are magnified. If the majority of sociologists tackling issues of health care organization and reform are outside our training spheres, this will likely exacerbate the shortage of a new generation of medical sociologists pursuing these topics. Avoiding the "loss" of their expertise to schools of public health, medicine and management alone, without a parallel emphasis in the subfield, requires effort on both sides, with each valuing the contributions and venues of the other.

Triangulating the Community Map to Develop a Blueprint for the Next Decade of Research

Rethinking Communities and Landscapes

The analysis of these different locations and communities on the map of the sociology of health, illness, and healing guided our vision for this *Handbook*. It was meant to suggest, in Durkheimian fashion, that the whole of our contributions is greater than the sum of its parts. The sociology of health, illness, and healing is constituted and enriched by medical sociology, mainstream sociology, and sociological work coming out of public health, medicine, and policy analysis. Of course, the divisions are fuzzy; old divisions have been eliminated: and support for them is waning. Many who do research and teaching in these areas, cross the boundary lines easily and with grace.

For example, as Collins (1989) pointed out, in some corners of the sociological landscape, the debates over whether sociology is a "science" are futile. With "science" mistakenly equated with quantitative research, Collins contends that sociology, like other sciences, engages in the "formulation of generalized principles, organized into models of the underlying processes that generate the social world" (Collins 1989, p. 1124). Similarly, to righteously equate medical sociology only with publication in sociological journals, but not publication in the general or medical journals, is equally problematic. The problem is how, in this era of proliferating opportunities for sociologists in diverse employment positions and in a wider range of journals, can we take advantage of all of these contributions and pass them on to the next generation? Sociological knowledge can advance, as Collins (1989) notes, with a coherence of theoretical conceptions across different areas and methods of research. Critique is good, and something that sociologists are extraordinarily proficient in; but this is useful only to the purpose of moving our understanding of the world forward.

This volume is a first step, we hope, in facilitating that coherence by explicitly bringing together these three different strains of medical sociology, by bringing their authors in contact with one another, with other medical sociologists, and with the next generation of researchers. That is, we have tried to take direct account of the potential contributions from diverse vantage points on the landscape of sociology. Specifically, the editors have sought out contributions from each of the three communities of sociological research on health, illness, and healing, including making an attempt, albeit a preliminary one, to escape the surface of American medical sociology. We ignore where on the intellectual and field/subfield/disciplinary map they come from. In this way, we hope to complement the *Handbook of Medical Sociology*, now in its 6th edition, which has served since 1963 to represent the cutting edge of the subfield.

Organizing by Elevation

We organize the insights along a vertically integrated map that carries the spirit of C.W. Mills forward in acknowledging individuals and contexts. In fact, in this first section, we step back even from the map of sociology so as not to ignore two facts – other disciplines aim to understand the same phenomena as medical sociology, further complicating our task of surveying existing contributions and gathering "leads;" and the U.S. brand of medical sociology, and sociology in general, tends to take one kind of perspective that may have different contours from the uniquely salient insights brought by medical sociologists in other countries. Thus, Rogers and Pilgrim, from the University of Manchester and University of Central Lancashire, respectively, follow this introduction by demarcating our relationship to other sociomedical disciplines from the UK landscape. Most importantly, taking the case of mental health, psychiatry, and sociology, they examine how these disciplines approach the same problems, how they construct them, and whether their contributions even matter to "science." They look at boundary disputes and collaborations as they have played out in the UK, arguing that boundaries have been movable historically. Conflicts and separation followed early conversations and collaboration. Yet, they see signs of a return to more congenial shared intellectual space that stems from the movement to an integrated team approach in treatment and new substantive "identities" like health services research which situate individuals of different approaches onto common property.

Whether the world is more complex, as globalization theorists claim, or the world of sociology has embraced greater complexity than it had when Mills wrote, the next chapter outlines the Network Episode Model – Phase III as a set of multiple contexts that are considered simultaneously as we proceed. While sociologists have always acknowledged multiple contexts, the NEM separates out macro-contexts that intersect and now, can be researched simultaneously, whether through team ethnography (Burton 2007; Newman et al. 2004) or through Hierarchical Linear Modeling (Xie and Hannum 1996). We also go to and beneath the micro-foundations of macro-sociology that Collins (1981) addressed. While our focus may be on the "illness career," there are levels below the individual which have to be reckoned with if we are to get past the old nature vs. nurture dichotomies. Thus, while macro levels can match the cartographic metaphor more-or-less literally of "place," the sociological insight of vertical integration also guide us to more micro levels below the surface of the individual (e.g., their genetic inheritance). But at each level, the NEM argues that sociology must explicitly measure contextual factors and the connecting mechanisms of influence, calling for multi-method approaches which maximize the ability of empirical research to match "the promise."

This section ends with a critical assessment of the theory of fundamental causality and suggests several forward-looking research directions. Freese and Lutfey argue that the SES-health association has to be unpacked in each time and place. Yet, they also see this as insufficient because it fails to tell us why this link transcends time and place. This widespread association has to be confronted with universalities, distinctions, and tensions. Ending with a focus on future research, they point to the potential of looking both in structure and "under the skin" using the interplay of quantitative and qualitative methods and offering three considerations for medical sociology to more strongly influence health policy.

Connecting Communities

This section deals with "places" above the health care system, looking to comparisons across countries (Beckfield and Olafsdottir; Ruggie); organized individuals taking on health and health care issues in the public (Brown and colleagues), policy spheres (Ruggie), or those institutions outside medicine (Aldigé, Medina and McCranie). We start with a look across countries, the area of comparative health systems, where Ruggie argues that there may be those who remain dubious about lessons that can be learned from cross-national analyses. She aims to convince them, admirably so, by pointing to the well-known paradox that was alluded to earlier about the high spending of resources and the low level of return in the U.S. She identifies persistent barriers in aims and means that result in inequitable health care in the U.S. Ruggie outlines and documents eight lessons about health care systems that the U.S. can learn from the experience of other nations. She ends by pointing to the ubiquitous relationship between poverty and poor health, in all countries, and the final lesson which supports the role that efforts outside the health care system have in improving health outcomes. Beckfield and Olafsdottir push this further, arguing that the welfare state offers a window into understanding how societies organize their economic, political, and cultural landscape. In turn, different forms of social organization are critical to understanding the causes of health, illness, and healing, and how these reverberate through the lives of individuals and societies. They lay out types and mechanisms through politics, health institutions, and lay culture, offering a set of propositions and hypotheses that, if examined empirically, will push our understandings of macro-level factors and perhaps unearth new suggestions for social change.

Remaining with the influence of civil society, Brown and his colleagues target the increasing influence of health activists and the health social movements that they populate. Arguing that such efforts have increased in number and broadened medicine's concern to include issues of justice, poverty, and toxic work conditions, they provide theoretical and analytic concepts on relevant collective actions. The concepts they find to hold the most potential – empowerment, movement-driven medicalization and disempowerment, institutional political economy, and lay-professional relationships – connect to each of the "above the individual" NEM levels. Their ecosocial view connects communities, inequalities and disproportionate exposure to toxic conditions (e.g., environmental hazards and stressors) that translate into health disparities and that set a broader territory for the institution of medicine, as well as for medical sociology.

The final two pieces examine the role of institutions outside of medicine as they work with and against the aims of the profession, its ancillary occupations, and its organizations. Medina and McCranie reopen the classic claim that medicine "won" jurisdiction over deviance, having first "dibs" to define it as a problem of disease, eliminating the power of law or religion over societal response (Freidson 1970). Looking to the case of psychopathy, they reconsider the meaning of medicalization and the potential of thinking about "layers" of control as a better fit in the contemporary era. Ending with a call for recognizing and researching the multiplicity of institutional responsibility, this piece provides the perfect lead-in to Aldigé's summary of the insights from sociology's long but fairly sparse line of research on the intersection of legal and medical control of mental illness. Focusing on the "collision" that occurred in the wake of the civil rights movement, Aldigé details the complex sociohistorical forces that have shaped and reshaped the points of strain and support between two major institutions of social control of deviance.

Connecting to Medicine: The Profession and Its Organizations

With the dominance of the concept of medicalization (Zola 1972; Conrad 2005) and its dissemination into scientific and public life, we asked Clarke and Shim, who had offered an extension of the concept (biomedicalization; Clarke et al. 2003), to step back, review the current status of different approaches, update us on their own thinking (including addressing the critiques), and craft one possible future agenda. Entering into this assessment from the view of the sociology of science and technology, rather than pure medical sociology per se, they explore the potential for building bridges across the terrains of medical sociology, medical anthropology, medicine, and other neighboring terrains that share a concern with understanding how the boundaries of medical jurisdiction expand.

Hafferty and Castellani push past issues of medicalization and pursue medical sociology's attention to and then abandonment of interest in the profession of medicine. Ironically, they contend that after medical sociologists documented and debate the rise of the profession to dominance, the subfield (and the larger discipline) has missed the take-up by medicine itself of issues of "professionalism" in light of its acknowledgement of the role of larger contextual factors defining its work. This change reopens the call for a sociological perspective and they provide a roadmap. Part of sociology's turn away from issues of the institutional situation of medicine meant that there has been little attention to the fate of women as doctors since Lorber and Moore's (2002) pioneering 1984 study. Finally, Boulis and Jacobs give us an update on the status of women in medicine. Taking us past even the insights of their comprehensive project (2008), providing the necessary background to understand where women are in the profession, they elaborate on whether medicine's early sexist climate has changed, even if only around the edges. In the end, they conclude that progress has been slow at best; and, if and how the profession changes vis-á-vis gender has more to do with structural pressures than changing values.

The final two chapters in this section move to the organization of the health care system itself, with Caronna asking about the socio-historical logics that have shaped and continue to shape medicine in the U.S., while Kronenfeld explores the absence, for the most part, of medical sociologists in research on central policy questions relevant to health and health care. The former, as Caronna herself indicates, can illuminate the past and shape the future. By emphasizing the complex web of trust issues necessary to maintain a health care system, she guides us through the three logics of the past and asks whether we are entering a fourth, calling for more sociological research. Kronenfeld refutes the idea that policy studies belong to political science, staking sociology's claim by surveying the past meaning and emphases of health care policy-making processes and noting a lacunae of broad system level analyses.

Connecting to the People: The Public as Patient and Powerful Force

This fourth section targets individuals outside the health care system as they interact with and affect it. Figert begins this journey through the community, asking whether or not medicalization theory has underplayed the potential of lay individuals in the medicalization process. The thread of reevaluating our theoretical concepts that revolve around professional power continues, with a reconsideration of Zola, Conrad, Clarke, and Epstein but expanding consideration to a more explicit role of expertise. This includes the expertise of the lay person as well as the expertise of professionals, noting that much current discussion debates the influence of the former. Tying into the earlier chapters by Brown and colleagues, she brings up how social movements may have shifted the landscape of medicine, and she reminds us of the formality of the classic formulations in Parsons' patient role. This opens the path for May's reformulation of Parsons' "vision" of the physician–patient interaction. While recognizing that the organization of health care matters because it penetrates the clinical encounter, May targets the social relationship in the clinic as the place where their effects are mobilized and enacted. The arrival of "disease management" and "self-management" have become a routine part of "mundane medicine," the care that comes with the greater prominence of chronic illness and disease. Digging further into the encounter, Heritage and Maynard review research from process, discourse, and conversational analyses that reveal in detail how the clinical encounter proceeds, what its key turning points are, and how there has been a clear and gradual movement to greater power balance between physicians and patients. Finally, Wright acknowledges that technological advances have widened the examination room, bringing with them greater expertise but also challenges from the public. With electronic records and publically available health information technology, Wright argues that sociologists should track the ramifications of these changes on trust, confidentiality, authority, and the social dynamics of how information is collected, managed, and used by both providers and their clients.

Connecting Personal and Cultural Systems

Much of the interest in the social sciences of late stems from the concern with health disparities. Alegría and her colleagues take this on in a holistic fashion, offering a larger framework within which to develop hypotheses and measures. Drawing from the notion of cumulative disadvantage across time and levels of organization, the Social Cultural Framework for Health Care Disparities serves to guide further and more integrated studies. They set the stage for more specific concerns. Among these, areas that continue to attract research attention are race and gender. In a review of the black–white differences in health, Jackson and Cummings point to the paradox of the Black middle class. Counterintuitive to the SES-health gradient, they provide evidence that the Black middle class does not fare better in health status than the White lower class, and end by suggesting that accumulated network capital, limited by residential segregation, is ripe for future research. In a similar vein, Read and Gorman turn their attention to gender. They give an overview of what we know about male–female differences in mortality and morbidity, theories used to explain these, and three challenges that remain in the gendered profile of health – immigration, the life course, and co-morbidities between mental and physical health. To assist in future research, the final note in this section involves methods for unraveling the mechanisms that underlie many of the associations that have been documented. Pairing sociologists who come from different methodological corners of the sociological landscape, Watkins, Swidler and Biruk describe and illustrate the use of "hearsay ethnography." Relying on individuals in the communities they study to hear and record what their social network ties discuss, they show the advantages over traditional survey and ethnographic methods in gathering data on "meaning" in everyday life.

Connecting to Dynamics: The Health and Illness Career

While intimately tied to the directions we take in this volume, much of what comes before this point does not deal directly with the dynamics of health and health care outcomes and the forces that shape them. There is no better way to inject dynamics into the sociology of health, illness, and healing than to draw both inspiration and insight from the life course perspective. Pavalko and Willson do just that by reviewing what has been integrated into our research and what remains less well developed. In particular, they point to two areas that would profit from further attention – individual agency within constraints and how historical and institutional changes intersect with life trajectories.

Following in this tradition, Carpentier and Bernard take on the developments in health care utilization research that have embraced temporality, social structure, multilevel effects, and culture. Using the network metaphor, they stress complexity in theory and methods that study trajectories and lay out directions to push this approach further.

Connecting the Individual and the Body

Sanders and Rogers connect the chronic illness career to potential improvements in treatment and health care policy. Specifically, they consider how processes of disruption, uncertainty, and adaptation are at work in shaping trajectories in chronic illness and illness management. They make the transition to the individually orientated factors by coupling the forces of motivation, innovation, and social networks with the social and cultural significance of the body. Lively and Smith focus more deeply on issues of identity regarding both the public self and the private self. They explore aspects of social psychological theories of identity that have not been fully utilized in the sociology of health, illness, and healing, particularly the development of positive illness identities. Conley dives deeper into the biological aspects of the body, arguing that social science and genetics can be integrated but must be done with caution. He reviews traditional genetics approaches, expressing apprehension about the endogeneity problem inherent in many studies and the current limits in mapping gene–gene interactions. He suggests that social scientists should pair with genetic researchers in a sequence of studies that use multiple methods to first identify a genetic or social effect as truly exogenous so that we do not follow the "mining" and "fishing" approaches commonly used in genetic and epigenetic research.

Perry ends the volume where we began it – with the call for diverse disciplinary approaches, expressing a central concern for collaboration without cooptation. With an acceptance of the increasing complexity of both social and genetic factors, Perry reviews and dismisses typical approaches like the chain model and provides a primer on basic places where sociologists can start to think about how social life matters in life and death. In particular, taking advantage of "the promise" may come from medical sociologists who use developmental models with an eye to social construction.

Wrapping Up

For those who contributed to this volume, as well as for the editors, this is a start, a beginning to continuing to bring the strengths of medical sociology forward. We have many to thank for their contributions and time spent. The staff at the Indiana Consortium for Mental Health Services Research, particularly Mary Hannah, shepherded this volume through, seeing the project from the beginning to end. Howard Kaplan's determination to see a volume on Health, Illness and Healing in the Sociology series was steadfast and Teresa Krauss' patient persistence was welcome.

References

Bearman P (2008) Introduction: exploring genetics and social structure. Am J Sociol 114:v–x
Boulis AK, Jacobs JA (2008) The changing face of medicine: women doctors and the evolution of health care in America. Cornell University Press, Ithaca, NY

Brown P (1995) Naming and framing: the social construction of diagnosis and illness. J Health Soc Behav Extra Issue:34–52
Burawoy M (2005) For public sociology. Am Sociol Rev 70:4–28
Burton LM (2007) Childhood adultification in economically disadvantaged families: An ethnographic perspective. Family Relations 56:329–345
Clarke AE, Shim JK (2010) Medicalization and biomedicalization revisited: Technoscience and transformations of health, illness, and American medicine. In: Pescosolido BA, McLeod JD, Martin JK, Rogers A (eds) The sociology of health, illness, and healing: blueprint for the 21st century. Springer, New York
Clarke AE, Mamo L, Fishman JR, Shim JK, Fosket JR (2003) Biomedicalization: technoscientific transformations of health, illness, and U.S. biomedicine. Am Sociol Rev 68:161–194
Collins R (1981) On the micro-foundations of macro-sociology. Am J Sociol 86:984–1014
Collins R (1986) Is 1980s sociology in the doldrums? Am J Sociol 91:1336–1355
Collins R (1989) Sociology: pro-science or anti-science? Am Sociol Rev 53:124–139
Collins FS (2006) The language of God: a Scientist presents evidence for belief. The Free Press, New York
Concato J, Shah N, Horwitz RI (2000) Randomized, controlled trials, observational studies, and the hierarchy of research designs. N Engl J Med 342:1887–1892
Conrad P (2005) The shifting engines of medicalization. J Health Soc Behav 46:3–14
Epstein S (1996) Impure science: AIDS, activism, and the politics of knowledge. University of California Press, San Diego, CA
Freidson E (1970) Professional dominance: the social structure of medical care. Atherton Press, New York
Gans H (1989) Sociology in America: the discipline and the public: American Sociological Association 1988 Presidential Address. Am Sociol Rev 54:1–16
Gelernter J, O'Malley S, Risch N, Kranzler HR, Krystal J, Merikangas KR, Kennedy JL, Kidd KK (1991) No association between an allele at the D2 dopamine receptor gene (DRD2) and alcoholism. J Am Med Assoc 266:1801–1807
Gieryn TF (1983) Boundary-work and the demarcation of science from non-science: Strains and interests in professional ideologies of scientists. Am Sociol Rev 48:781–795
Gieryn TF (1999) Cultural boundaries of science. University of Chicago Press, Chicago, IL
Gouldner AW (1970) The coming crisis of western sociology. Equinox Books, New York
Hung Ho-fung (2004) From global pandemic to global panic: SARS and the fear of "Yellow Perils" amid the rise of China. Hong Kong J Sociol 5:29–49
Latour B (1999) Pandora's hope: essays on the reality of science studies. Harvard University Press, Cambridge, MA
Leuchter AF, Cook IA, Morgan ML (2002) Changes in brain function of depressed subjects during treatment with placebo. Am J Psychiatry 159:122–129
Levine S (1995) Time for creative integration in medical sociology. J Health Soc Behav 35:1–4
Link BG, Phelan JC (1995) Social conditions as fundamental causes of disease. J Health Soc Behav Extra Issue:80–94
Lorber, Judith and Moore, Lisa Jean (2002) Gender and the Social Construction of Illness, 2nd ed. AltaMira Press, New York.
McKinlay JB (1974) A case for refocusing upstream: the political economy of illness. In: Enelow AJ, Henderson JB (eds) Applying behavioral science to cardiovascular risk. American Heart Association, Dallas, TX
McKinlay JB (1996) Some contributions from the social system to gender inequalities in heart disease. J Health Soc Behav 37:1–26
McKinlay JB, Marceau LD (2002) The end of the golden age of doctoring. Int J Health Serv 32:379–416
McLeod JD (2004) Dissecting a social autopsy. Contemp Sociol 33:151–156
Mechanic D (1993) Social research in health and the American sociopolitical context: The changing fortunes of medical sociology. Social Science & Medicine 36:95–102
Mechanic D (2004) The rise and fall of managed care. J Health Soc Behav 45:76–86
Mechanic D, McAlpine DD, Rosenthal M (2001) Are patients' office visits with physicians getting shorter? N Engl J Med 344:198–204
Mills CW (1959) The sociological imagination. Oxford University Press, London
National Advisory Mental Health Council (2000) Translating behavioral science into action. National Advisory Mental Health Council's Behavioral Science Workgroup, Bethesda, MD
Newman KS, Fox C, Roth W, Mehta J, Harding D (2004) Rampage: the social roots of school shootings. Basic Books, Cambridge, MA
Olafsdottir S, Pescosolido BA (2009) Drawing the line: the cultural cartography of utilization recommendations for mental health problems. J Health Soc Behav 50:228–244
Pace D, Middendorf J (2004) Decoding the disciplines: helping students learn disciplinary ways of thinking, vol 98, New directions for teaching and learning. Jossey Bass, San Francisco, CA
Pearlin LI (1992) Structure and meaning in medical sociology. J Health Soc Behav 33:1–9

Pellmar TC, Eisenberg L (2000) Bridging disciplines in the brain, behavioral, and clinical sciences. A report of the board on neuroscience and behavioral health, Institute of Medicine. National Academy Press, Washington, DC

Pescosolido BA (1991) Illness careers and network ties: a conceptual model of utilization and compliance. In: Albrecht GL, Levy JA (eds) Advances in medical sociology. JAI Press, Greenwich, CT, pp 161–184

Pescosolido BA (1992) Beyond rational choice: the social dynamics of how people seek help. Am J Sociol 97:1096–1138

Pescosolido BA (2006) Of pride and prejudice: the role of sociology and social networks in integrating the health sciences. J Health Soc Behav 47:189–208

Pescosolido BA, Jack K. Martin, J. Scott Long, Tait R. Medina, Jo C. Phelan, and Bruce G. Link (2010) 'A Disease Like Any Other?' A Decade of Change in Public Reactions to Schizophrenia, Depression and Alcohol Dependence. American Journal of Psychiatry In press.

Pescosolido BA, Boyer CA (2001) The American health care system: entering the 21st century with high risks, major challenges, and great opportunities. In: Cockerham WC (ed) The Blackwell companion to medical sociology. Blackwell, Oxford, pp 180–198

Pescosolido BA, Kronenfeld J (1995) Health, illness, and healing in an uncertain era: challenges from and for medical sociology. J Health Soc Behav 35:5–33

Pescosolido BA, Martin JK (2004) Cultural authority and the sovereignty of American medicine: the role of networks, class and community. J Health Polit Policy Law 29:735–756

Pescosolido BA, Olafsdottir S (2010) The cultural turn in sociology: can it help us resolve an age-old problem in understanding decision-making for health care? Forthcoming in Sociol Forum

Pescosolido BA, Rubin BA (2000) The web of group affiliations revisited: social life, postmodernism, and sociology. Am Sociol Rev 65:52–76

Pescosolido BA, Tuch S, Martin JK (2001) The profession of medicine and the public: examining Americans' changing confidence in physician authority from the beginning of the "Health Care Crisis" to the Era of Health Care Reform. J Health Soc Behav 42:1–16

Pescosolido BA, McLeod JD, Avison WR (2007) Through the looking glass: the fortunes of the sociology of mental health. In: Avison WR, McLeod JD, Pescosolid BA (eds) Mental health, social mirror. Springer, New York, pp 3–32

Phelan JC (2005) Geneticization of deviant behavior and consequences for stigma: the case of mental illness. J Health Soc Behav 46:307–322

Rubin BA (1996) Shifts in the Social Contract. Pine Forge Press, Thousand Oaks, CA

Schlesinger M (2002) A Loss of Faith: The Sources of Reduced Political Legitimacy for the American Medical Profession. Milbank Quarterly 80:185–235

Starr P (1982) The social transformation of American medicine: the rise of a sovereign profession and the making of a vast industry. Basic Books, New York, NY

Stone D (1999) Managed care and the second great transformation. J Health Polit Policy Law 24:1213–1218

Straus R (1957) The nature and status of medical sociology. Am Sociol Rev 22:200–204

Swartz K (1999) The death of managed care as we know it. J Health Polit Policy Law 24:1201–1205

Szyf M (2009) The early life environment and the epigenome. Biochim Biophysica Acta 1790:878–887

Vladeck BC (1999) Managed care's fifteen minutes of fame. J Health Polit Policy Law 24:1207–1211

Ward L (1907) The establishment of sociology. Am J Sociol 12:581–587

Xie Yu, Hannum E (1996) Regional variation in earnings inequality in reform-era urban China. Am J Sociol 101:950–992

Zola IK (1972) Medicine as an institution of social control. Sociol Rev 20:487–504

Chapter 2
Medical Sociology and Its Relationship to Other Disciplines: The Case of Mental Health and the Ambivalent Relationship Between Sociology and Psychiatry

Anne Rogers and David Pilgrim

Introduction

Within the subfield of the sociology of health and illness, mental health is a well-established and major area of sociological inquiry and interest. This prominent interest has necessarily brought sociologists into contact with other disciplines concerned with research and practice in the area of mental illness. The most notable of these has been the discipline of psychiatry. As Norman Elias noted nearly 40 years ago, this relationship necessarily involves difference and tensions because whilst sociology and psychiatry are both dealing with human behaviour, their explanatory frameworks are different[1] and each needs to protect their professional and theoretical autonomy (Elias 1969).

At times, the relationship between psychiatry and sociology has been characterised by mutual co-operation and interest, but at others points, boundary disputes have erupted and epistemological differences about the nature of mental illness have emerged. The aims of this chapter are to examine the nature and extent to which sociology has been successful in asserting its disciplinary authority and interests in the mental health field and in doing so explore something of relationship with psychiatry as a specialty within medicine. We do this through exploring the recent history of the connexions and disputes between sociology and psychiatry mainly but not exclusively focusing on the UK. Our intention is to illuminate the nuances, interests and outcomes in knowledge and disciplinary positions that are relevant to understanding boundary disputes and collaborations between sociologists of health and healing in the area of the study of mental illness using three case examples: social psychiatry, stigma and psychoanalysis. In the final section, we explore the prospects for future collaborations with psychiatry.

Sociology and Mental Disorder

Traditionally, the topic of mental disorder has been well represented within medical sociology both in the US[2] and in the UK (although by comparison in recent time the latter has had a less prominent

---

[1] Sociology, he points out, might focus on social factors of anomie and status differentials with psychiatry even at the social end referring more to personality traits and sibling rivalries.

[2] The lineage of the symbolic interactionist wing of the Chicago School of sociology has ensured a strong emphasis on deviancy theory (Cooley 1902, Mead 1934, Goffman 1961, Becker 1963, Lemert 1967, Scheff 1966).

A. Rogers (✉)
University of Manchester, 5th Floor Williamson Building, Oxford Road, Manchester M139 PL
e-mail: anne.rogers@manchester.ac.uk

position in the UK). To talk of 'the' sociology of any topic is to suggest that the boundaries between knowledge are rigid and mutually exclusive. We begin this chapter from the premise that there is no absolute distinction between social knowledge claims produced by sociologists and that offered from outside its disciplinary boundaries. Good examples of this point are academic contributions provided from historians and philosophers and from clinical psychology and general medical practice (e.g. Richard Bentall's *Madness Explained* (2004) and Christopher Dowrick's *Beyond Depression* (2004)). These contributions from outside of sociology provide illuminating ways of exploring psychological abnormality in its social context by emphasising historical analysis and a close attention to the meaning of the personal accounts of people with mental health problems. Moreover, sociology itself relies for its legitimacy on lay expertise. Indeed, there exists a paradox that sociological models, such as ethnomethodology (Coulter 1973) and symbolic interactionism, celebrate and utilise ordinary language accounts of social life, whilst at the same time wanting to claim a privileged role for the sociological codifications or meta-accounts generated.

Another body of knowledge, psychoanalysis, outwith sociology, has also been used as a resource to temper sociological assuredness. For example, Craib (1997) examines the shift towards social constructivism 'as if it was a client presenting itself for psychoanalysis' and argues that sociology (unlike the mental health professions it critically documents) has no mandate to change the lives of others. As a result, instead of entering the 'depressive position' of that disempowerment and probable irrelevance, it manifests a grandiose manic defence, with sociology offering expert knowledge claims (discourses on discourses) on anything and everything. In our third case study below, we examine psychoanalysis as a bridging resource between psychiatry and sociology. Additionally, there is simple empirical evidence that sociology cannot claim any privileged and unique understanding of mental health matters. Below we demonstrate this when examining the history of social psychiatry. Moreover, more recently, shifts in the academy about knowledge production indicate that the disciplinary boundaries of sociology and other singular disciplines are now blurred and leaky (Gibbons et al. 1994). The richness of sociological analysis has been helped by the examination and incorporation of work in other disciplines. Sometimes, this has involved using empirical findings of their studies to build up an argument, and at others, it has applied a sociological approach to their production. It is common for sociologists to co-author work with collaborators from other disciplines. The outcomes then appear in non-sociological journals. Although disciplinary silos are still often jealously protected in the academy, research in an applied and broad area like mental health invariably leads to a range of interdisciplinary outcomes.

However sociological interest in mental health has not been sustained uninterrupted within sociology. At the end of the 1980s, sociological debates about mental health and psychiatry were not as salient as they had been during the 1960s and 1970s. During those earlier decades, mental illness had been subject to considerable scrutiny and was used as an exemplar in mainstream theorising on deviance and social control. The popularity of sociological work about psychiatry during that 'counter-cultural' period was also fuelled by radical critiques from some mental health professionals, who questioned their own traditional theory and practice. While a thriving sociological interest in mental health continued in North America, in Britain, the 1980s witnessed sociological interest turning more towards mainstream topics of physical and chronic illness. At the same time, the identity of sociology has in some quarters been characterised by a shift towards a post-modern orthodoxy in social theory. Post-modern theorising has brought distinct advantages to the subdiscipline, and Pescosolido and Rubin (2000) suggest that a major contribution of this perspective is capturing rapid social change and the uncertainty that characterises contemporary social life. However, such a perspective has tended to problematise empirical knowledge claims (thus undermining empirical sociology) and the post-modern turn has brought with it a distinctive bias against realism, critical or otherwise. Instead of lay accounts offering insights into something of the reality of material social relations, they have now been offered up exclusively as 'representations' or aspects of this or that 'discourse'.

A further bit of empirical evidence of the disruption in sociological authority has been the incursion of new disciplinary forms, such as gender and cultural studies and applied social studies. The association of these applied disciplines with a-theoretical and social administrative accounts, for example in health services research, also provokes sociological wariness. Disciplines (and sociology is no exception here) jealously guard their boundaries and want to claim esoteric expertise. In this light, Strong (1979) pointed out the dangers three decades ago of 'sociological imperialism'. Similarly, Hammersley (1999) has claimed that sociology is no more than a source of specialised factual knowledge about the world, with quite a limited practical value. However, it is also the case that sociological self-doubt in the face of blind medical confidence may not offer the healthiest solution to the problem of sociological imperialism identified by Strong. Below we point out this trend when discussing psychiatric claims of privileged knowledge about stigma. Before that, we will consider the relationship between sociology and social psychiatry.

Case Study One: Social Psychiatry

Since 1970, the relationship between psychiatry and sociology could be described as distant and often hostile. They have become 'incommensurate games' (Fenton and Charsley 2000). However, prior to this time, practitioners in the two disciplines were often active collaborators. Here, we trace the rise and fall of that interdisciplinary synergy.

The Heyday of Collaboration

In nineteenth century, medical epidemiology (social medicine) sociology found a significant practical role. Indeed, the roots of medical sociology can be traced to social medicine (Rosen 1979). However, it was not until the middle of the twentieth century that mutual sympathy between environmentally orientated social psychiatrists and sociologists emerged fully.

Around the Second World War, an environmentalist period was ushered in which was characterised by a strong alliance with sociology and was given expression in the pursuance of a common agenda. Social scientists, including sociologists, were active members of academic departments of psychiatry (Klerman 1989). In its Durkheimian form, sociology presented itself as an objective project, whose purpose was to study social problems and produce knowledge to further social policy objectives. This chimed with the goals of socially orientated psychiatrists.

Eventually, an interdisciplinary collaboration was to emerge and 'social psychiatry' was formalised. This was characterised by notable collaborations of psychiatrists with both clinical psychologists (Falloon and Fadden 1993) and psychiatric social workers in the UK (Goldberg and Huxley 1992). Some of its methodological leaders were even sociologists (Brown and Harris 1978). Social psychiatry has been closely associated with a bio-psychosocial model of mental illness; an inclusive anti-reductionist approach, with a wide potential appeal to both patients and mental health workers (Engel 1980; Pilgrim 2002).

The collaborative period was in both the UK and USA particularly influenced by the human ecology of the Chicago School of Sociology (Pilgrim and Rogers 1994). In exploring the influence of poverty and deprivation, Faris and Dunham (1939) contrasted the prevalence of 'manic depressive psychosis', which appeared to be randomly distributed across the city of Chicago, with the numbers of people diagnosed with 'schizophrenia', found predominantly in poorer areas. Whereas Faris and Dunham focused on social isolation as a possible aetiological factor, Hollingshead and Redlich (1958) reflected the popular appeal of Freudian ideas, which were prevalent in the USA at that time, in their subsequent study.

This environmentalist phase of psychiatric research on inequalities in mental health began to follow those evident in mainstream public health, with a focus on social conditions and the quality of interpersonal relationships in different parts of society. A spate of influential studies identified the relationship between mental health and social class and demonstrated a consistent social patterning of mental disorders. These studies showed that rates of mental health problems were more prevalent amongst those in the 'lower' classes (Hollingshead and Redlich 1958; Srole and Langer 1962).

Consistently reported findings were that the diagnoses of 'schizophrenia' and 'personality disorder' were inversely related to social class. For so-called 'common mental health problems' (anxiety and depression), a link between social disadvantage and mental health was also established, although this appeared to be less consistent than the finding for 'schizophrenia'. The trend for 'affective psychoses' was towards greater prevalence in 'middle' and 'upper class' populations. Social class also predicted treatment type deployed by the psychiatric profession. Lower class people received drugs and ECT, whereas richer clients received versions of psychotherapy.

Given the obvious common concern for 'the social', in both medical sociology and psychiatric epidemiology after the Second World War, a trajectory was set for long-term interdisciplinary collaboration. But this failed to stabilise. The reasons for the breakdown in the relationship are complex but, for our purposes here, can be grouped into three. First, there were shifts of emphasis and theoretical preference inside sociology. Second, there were shifts inside psychiatry. Third, some of the alterations within each discipline were a function of the negative interaction of these shifts. Mutual suspicion and ambivalence occurred, which lead to a vicious circle of a declining interest in and acceptance for the other party's concerns. We now expand on these.

Theoretical Shifts in Sociology and Psychiatry

Two bonds between the disciplines had been evident in the collaborative phase – from Freud and Durkheim. With the growth in legitimacy of psychoanalysis in the 1930s and 1940s came an acceptance of 'continuum' models of psychopathology. We are 'all ill' to some degree, according to psychoanalysts. This made the lack of precise classification acceptable to those psychiatrists, who shared an over-riding commitment with their collaborating sociologists to the investigation of social conditions. The ambiguity created in Anglo-American psychiatry of psychoanalysis, and the consequent role of continuum models, defused potential tensions and cleared the way for a shared focus on the social antecedents of mental health problems. Tolerant mutuality characterised the relationship between sociology and psychiatry, as indicated here by Lawson (1989), a sociological contributor to social psychiatry:

> Psychiatry accepted that, as its disease categories were so tenuous and not generally marked by physical signs, the sociologist's concepts of impairment or disability marked by social dysfunctions could be the key to unraveling the rates of mental illness. (Lawson 1989, p. 38)

It seems that the notion of 'mental illness' remained in tact but psychiatrists were able to accept alternative views other than an illness model. Moreover, in relation to secondary and tertiary prevention, strong alliances were made with sociologists. This included research into the role of adverse and alienating conditions within mental hospitals, which demonstrably maintained and amplified pre-existing psychiatric disability – 'institutionalism' (Brown and Wing 1962).

After 1970, this reliance on a Durkheimian view in sociology and the Freudian influence on continuum models in psychiatry began to change. Sociologists (and psychologists) increasingly attacked the growth of neo-Kraepelian psychiatry, pointing to its rigid pre-occupation with categories and for confusing the map with the territory. For example, whilst psychiatrists assumed that 'schizophrenia' was a non-problematic fact, others viewed it as a codification of ordinary judgements about madness with little additional scientific value to these lay ascriptions (Coulter 1973; Bentall et al. 1988;

cf. Wing 1978). There was a similar back and forth argument between sociologists and psychiatrists in the US which centred on a challenge to the scientific and ideological validity of the concept of mental illness. Writing in the *Journal of Health and Social Behavior* in 1989, Mirowsky and Ross presented a critical analysis of the use of diagnosis as a form or categorical measurement and representation of psychological problems. This they argued represented poor science influenced by outmoded nineteenth-century thinking and acted to narrow understanding of mental health through the exclusion of the consideration of social structural and other contextual issues. On the bases of their critique, Mirowsky and Ross concluded their argument by recommending 'eliminating diagnosis from research on the nature, causes and consequences of mental, emotional and behavioural problems' (p. 11).

A riposte by a Gerald Klerman in an invited comment bemoaned the loss of the period when psychiatrists and sociologists collaborated, suggesting also that Mirowsky and Ross were overly ideologically committed to a social constructivist position, were ignoring the paradigm shift within psychiatry and re-emphasised the scientific validity of a diagnostic approach to the study of mental illness (Klerman 1989).

With psychiatric categories becoming easy targets for criticism, scepticism about the reality of mental illness sometimes reached nihilistic proportions. Earlier, radical constructivists had rejected mental illness as a total error of reasoning (a 'myth' or a 'metaphor' not a fact (Szasz 1961)). After Szasz, the radical internal critic of psychiatry, and under the sway of Foucauldian critiques of psychiatry, more and more sociologists tended to depict mental illnesses as social representations or epiphenomena produced by psychiatric activity utilising preferred reified categories (Prior 1991).

By 1980, most sociologists had neither the theoretical inclination nor the practical competence, to support social psychiatric research. Compared to an earlier era, they had become deskilled as social psychiatric collaborators. By the end of the twentieth century, possibilities for collaboration were muted because far less consideration was being given to social psychiatry. It was being contained increasingly on the margins of the medical profession (Moncrieff and Crawford 2001). The biopsychosocial model (Engel 1980), favoured by many academic psychiatrists, was being displaced by the 'decade of the brain'. Biological triumphalism was abroad in the psychiatric profession, within a self-assured 'new-Kraepelin' orthodoxy (Shorter 1998; Guze 1989; cf. Clare 1999).

Mutual agreement about the role of social factors and environment in the cause and trajectory of mental health problems evident in the earlier phase of social epidemiology gave way to discrepant views. These pitted social arguments and explanations against bio-determinism. This was most apparent in relation to the perceived utility and role of psychotropic medication. The biological aetiology of madness, confirmed in the core of the profession by the apparently dramatic impact of the phenothiazine group of drugs, was now connoted by their producers and prescribers as 'anti-psychotic' agents. For some, this terminology implied curative capability, rather than them being only symptom control adjuncts for some patients, some of the time (Moncrieff 2006).

A more critical historical analysis pointed to social forces and events which demonstrated that the 'pharmacological revolution' was, if not a total myth, a considerable uncertainty (Scull 1979). The policy of de-institutionalisation was the product of a variety of fiscal and ideological forces; these drugs had little or no impact on this policy trend (Warner 1985; Rogers and Pilgrim 2005). Social scientists in the US also pointed to similar influences particularly the central role of fiscal factors. For example, William Gronfien pointed out that Medicaid had a stronger impact than Community Mental Health Centre policies of the 1960s and 1970s and it was reimbursement schedules rather than the philosophy of community which was responsible for promoting de-institutionalisation (Gronfein 1985). However, more conservative accounts continued to depict madness as a biochemical brain disturbance, pre-determined by a genetic fault but increasingly amenable to medicinal remediation. For example, Csernansky and Grace (1998) remained committed to the 'pharmacological revolution' view. They claimed that neuroscientific research now provided us with completely unequivocal evidence of 'schizophrenia' as a genetically pre-programmed brain disease (cf. Boyle 1990).

This exemplar of the role of drugs was only one of many differences which accounts for the increasing distancing between these two disciplines. Criticisms of psychiatric theory and practice from sociologists focused on a range of other facets of mental health management. The weak construct validity of diagnostic categories; the relative absence of longitudinal studies in psychiatric epidemiology; the dominance of empiricism at the expense of theoretical development; a lack of explicit reflection on the ideological nature of psychiatric theory and practice and the 'interest' work of the drug companies in the mental health arena.

A further difference between the disciplines relates to the conceptualisation of the nature of service contact. Sociological analysis is more inclined to problematise this, whereas a psychiatric perspective tends to emphasise the inherently beneficent role of 'access' to services. As a consequence, the emphasis of psychiatric epidemiology has been on mapping the need for early intervention or on equitable service access. Services are viewed as sites of an uneven right to treatment, rather than as perhaps a potential threat to well-being and citizenship.

This has led to a pre-occupation with the epidemiological study of 'need' (i.e. numbers of identified diagnosed cases) in order to plan for 'appropriate' services, instead of inviting socio-political questions of interest to sociologists. These might include: who are these services appropriate for?; whose 'needs' are being met by mental health services? and are notions of 'access' or 'service' meaningful, when coercion is involved? Sociological interest in the new social movement of disaffected patients ensures that these types of questions are raised regularly in the sociological literature. By comparison, psychiatry limits its social policy interest to stigma and then only considers itself as part of the solution, not as part of the problem (Sayce 2000).

The distancing of sociology from psychiatry through differences in understanding of key phenomena was influenced by epistemological preferences within sociology more generally. During the 1970s, sociologists from the Marxian and Weberian traditions began to use medicine as an object of sociological understanding or to illustrate a social theory (Reid 1976). By the 1970s, medical sociologists had promoted themselves from handmaiden to 'observer status' (Illsley 1975). After 1970, sociologists increasingly saw themselves as providing a sociology of medicine. Prior to that, they had largely been content to make a sociological contribution to medicine.

Post-1970, sociology increasingly turned away from medical positivism and manifested a broad openness to other orientations. The tradition of symbolic interactionism and subsequent trends, like ethnomethodology and social constructivism, brought distance into the common ideological project of social engineering, which had previously acted to cement the enterprises of medical sociology and social psychiatry.

These theoretical shifts within sociology disrupted a prior interdisciplinary compatibility, by focusing on social phenomena being concept and context specific and by emphasising subjectivity and intersubjectivity in their field of inquiry. Meanings, not just causes, were now considered to be important – the task for sociology was increasingly descriptive and interpretive (*verstehen*) rather than explanatory (*erklaren*).

The most extreme rejection was to come from post-structuralism, especially the work of Michel Foucault, with its abandonment of causal reasoning, truth claims and confidence in an independent reality. This culminated in a focused exploration of ideas, language and 'discursive practices' and the eschewing of faith in quantitative methods, such as the survey techniques of epidemiology and the randomised controlled trial approach to testing treatment methods (including psychosocial interventions). Prior to this trend, symbolic interactionism had made a distinction between primary deviance (multi-factorially caused) and secondary deviance (socially amplified by the reactions of others).

The consequence of treating psychiatric illness with scepticism by sociologists meant that interests turned more to the social processes, which led to labelling and diagnosis, and the social consequences of psychiatric practice.

Whereas the previous relationship between psychiatry and sociology had been built on co-operation, these newer studies were explicitly critical not only of the social control role of psychiatry but also of its knowledge base (Pilgrim and Rogers 1994). Moreover, the co-operation had worked previously, largely because sociology was co-opted by medicine to help solve its problems; a convenient advantage of the empiricist legacy of Durkheim after the Second World War. By the 1980s, the sociological attack on psychiatry, and the defensive reaction it provoked, led not to a prolonged and creative debate but instead to a breakdown in interest on both sides.

The general trend of sociological criticism of psychiatry after 1970, understandably, was met with defensive counter-argument. Reactions from psychiatrists portrayed sociological critics as being part of an international oppositional movement of 'anti-psychiatry', which was setting out to denigrate and discredit their profession (Hamilton 1973; Roth 1973). This disenchantment with sociology was particularly evident from some who had previously gained much from collaboration between the disciplines (Wing 1978).

Whilst the complex field of 'anti-psychiatry' was not inhabited solely, or even mainly, by professional sociologists for more traditional psychiatrists, it was convenient to lump them under a sociological rather than psychiatric umbrella. The key high-profile 'anti-psychiatric' critics, such as Ronald Laing, David Cooper, Thomas Szasz and Franco Basaglia, were dissident members of the psychiatric profession, though their critical products were largely sociological or philosophical in character. A more recent generation of dissidents have become evident in the growth of 'critical' or 'post' psychiatry (Thomas 1997; Bracken 2003).

The technocratic approach of biomedical psychiatry was challenged by some psychiatrists, who emphasised the over-determining role of social factors in both aetiology and recovery (Warner 1985; Ross and Pam 1995) and the distorting effects of drug company interests on clinical practice (Breggin 1993; Kramer 1993; Healy 1997). This unbroken pattern of internal dissent suggests that many substantive problems about psychiatric theory and practice remain inherent and unresolved. Not only did mutual hostility culminate in sociological critics turning away from psychiatry but eventually there was even a diminishing interest in mental health as a sociological topic of inquiry. Many promising beginnings, for example in labelling theory and in the ethnographic study of psychiatric patients, petered out and were displaced by other more pressing concerns in the sociology of health and illness (Cook and Wright 1995). After 1980, sociologists still researched mental health. For example, some new work appeared on modified labelling theory (Link et al. 1989), users' views of psychiatric services (Rogers et al. 1993), problems with psychiatric nosology (Kutchins and Kirk 1997) and race and mental disorder (Nazroo 1997). However, the extent of this interest was notably less than that in the 1970s. Moreover, this work rarely attempted to re-build broken bridges with psychiatry.

A consequence of the distancing from sociology for psychiatry was that it retreated into 'methodologism' and 'quantitativism', unchecked by critical reflection with previous close collaborators of research about the use of reified diagnostic categories. Nor in the 1980s did psychiatry deal comprehensively with the philosophical attacks on its knowledge base, let alone abandon categorical reasoning as a lost cause. Instead, psychiatrists aspired to attain better construct validity. This was akin to improving the measurement of other epidemiological variables, such as hypertension (Fryers et al. 2000). At the very time when many sociologists were retreating into philosophical forms of anti-realism, within the wider trend of post-modernism noted earlier, psychiatry was marked by a 'return to medicine'.

With this professional strategy of re-medicalisation, there was an increasing interest in linking epidemiology to neuroscience and genetics (Wittchen 2000). Questions about pharmacological solutions did not lead to therapeutic pessimism and a return to the social. Instead, faith was re-stated in a biomedical approach, supported by the pharmaceutical industry producing and profiting from new agents. Thus, many in psychiatry naively took the reality of mental illness for granted and looked forward to the next breakthrough in biological treatments (the pharmacological revolution became permanent). Many in sociology abandoned reality as unknowable. A breakdown of trust and comprehension between the disciplines inevitably ensued.

Even when social psychiatry shifted (partially) from a categorical to a dimensional view of mental illness, this cleavage was sustained. For example, a number of prominent social psychiatric researchers advocated a dimensional view, in which there are gradations of psychological distress (Goldberg and Huxley 1992). This filtered down into tools such as the General Health Questionnaire (GHQ), commonly used in primary care and community population surveys. However, this dimensional view did not fully displace categorical reasoning in psychiatry. In the American Psychiatric Associations' Diagnostic and Statistical Manual (1980), categories and dimensions are preserved together and are not viewed as being incompatible.

Thus, this most recent phase in psychiatric epidemiology, since 1970, has been characterised by greater diagnostic specificity and case identification, which accord with the 'medical necessity' for intervention. This can be contrasted with the collaborative phase of research, which was more concerned with the identification of the social causes of, or dominant influences on, mental health problems. Currently, policy and practice imperatives remain firmly rooted in a concern with identifying rates of diagnosed mental illness in populations in order to provide sufficient specialist services. This has largely displaced the community and environmental focus of studies during the phase of collaboration, although in some recent studies both strands of interest can be found. Overall though, it is fair to say, in summary, that psychiatry seems to have gone full circle over a century, from eugenics to environmentalism and then back to genetic determinism and the service need it implies. This pattern can be seen in the theoretical changes in psychiatric nosology. The categories of DSM-1 were heavily influenced by both psychoanalytic theory and wartime social psychiatry (Carpenter 2000). Later shifts in DSM and the section on mental disorders in the International Classification of Diseases brought about major changes in case identification and classification. DSM-II, whilst not adhering to what may be viewed as an explicit social aetiology, nevertheless incorporated psychoanalytically influenced ideas about causal antecedents. By contrast, the specific aim of moving to DSM-III was to expunge causality from diagnosis in favour of behavioural description.

Because DSM III is generally a-theoretical with regard to aetiology, it attempts to describe comprehensively what the manifestations of the mental disorder are, and only rarely attempts to account for how the disturbances came about, unless the mechanism is included in the definition of the disorder. This approach can be said to be descriptive in that the definitions of the disorder generally consist of descriptions of the clinical features of the disorders. These patterns are described at the lowest order of inference necessary to describe the characteristic features of the disorder. (American Psychiatric Association 1980, p. 7). Although aetiology is bracketed, this induces a spurious confidence in tautological accounts. Symptoms define disorders and disorders are explained by the presence of the symptoms.

Apart from a new era of tautology, the 'a-theoretical' position about aetiology, far from signifying non-committal eclecticism had the effect (if not the intention) of eliminating confidence in social causation. Subsequent changes from DSM-III to DSM-IV represented a further elimination of patient subjectivity and their biographical and social context, in favour of an anti-holistic model of mental illness, compatible now with biological psychiatry (Mishara 1994; Wallace 1994).

This emphasis on behavioural criteria and the silencing of social causation hypotheses may signal a normative North American ideology. Carpenter (2000) argues that the trend of promoting standardised categories of normality and disorder in DSM is part of a US-inspired 'MacDonaldisation' of social and economic life. For him, DSM-IV represents 'the psychiatric equivalent of the World Trade Organisation (WTO), promoting the principles of American Universalism as objective standards that are beyond reproach' (Carpenter 2000, p. 615). Certainly, one of the consequences of this focus on measurement and 'objective' criteria has been a negation of the consideration of social context and personal experience (the routine concern of medical sociology), as a core part of the psychiatric research endeavour.

In the wake of the vicious circle of distrust described above, sociologists have become deskilled in epidemiology, and psychiatrists have become weary and defensive about philosophical attack. As a result of wholly legitimate questions about the role of their profession in society or their dubious knowledge base are pre-emptively dismissed by allusions to 'anti-psychiatry'. A blocked dialectic has occurred, so that the disciplines either do not talk or they talk past each other. Despite the multiple sources of evidence about the social origins and consequences of mental health problems, they have been weakly represented in recent health research, which has placed a greater emphasis on social inequalities in physical morbidity and mortality (Muntaner et al. 2000). In health inequality research, mental health status has been afforded central role as a mediator but has been studied less often as an outcome of social forces (Rogers and Pilgrim 2003).

One consequence of the gap of understanding between psychiatry and sociology has been the tendency for psychiatry to proceed autonomously about sociological matters. The best of example of this recently has been in the psychiatric framing of stigma.

Case Study Two: The Medicalisation of Stigma

The study of stigma by sociologists emerged was associated with classical labelling theory (Garfinkel 1956; Goffman 1963). Critiques of the theory emerged in the 1970s (Gove 1982; Jones and Cochrane 1981) and it fell out of favour for a while but it was rehabilitated, in a modified form, in the 1980s (Thoits 1985; Link et al. 1989). Labelling (or societal reaction) theory was an important departure in social science, especially in relation to mental health. It was linked to a shift from Durkheimian positivism, with its emphasis on the social causes of illness, to a neo-Weberian examination of the way in which illness was socially negotiated.

Whereas social causationism examined the aetiological role of social factors in mental illness, the study of labelling and stigma suggested that the reactions of others were important. Not only causes were now of interest but so too were the exchanges of meanings attached to illness behaviour and the sick role. Medicine traditionally singled out primary deviance (the 'push behind' of skin-encapsulated pathology), whereas sociology increasingly emphasised secondary deviance; the 'pull from the front' of the reactions of others to perceived difference.

Classical labelling theory focused on stereotyping and the rejecting actions of others but the later, modified, version of the theory emphasised the anticipated need in both parties to avoid mutual social involvement. Both versions drew attention to the demoralisation and social exclusion arising from negative ascriptions. Sociological interest in stigma, as well as modified labelling theory, has returned in recent years, suggesting that the classical work of those like Goffman retains contemporary relevance in the study of illness and disability (Link 2000; Scambler 2005).

Against this backdrop of shifts within the sociology of health, the social reform of mental health services in developed countries was leading not only to people with mental health problems becoming more numerous and visible but also to demands that their citizenship should be protected. As a consequence, both de-stigmatisation and social inclusion became progressive social policy demands for and from a range of interest groups concerned to improve the lives of those with mental health problems. By the 1990s, one of these was the psychiatric profession. This focus of interest is highlighted by an analysis of the interests involved with and expression of interest of an anti-stigma campaign led by the Royal College of Psychiatrists between 1998 and 2003.

The aims and objectives of the campaign were (cited in full) as follows.

The Stigma Campaign

- The Royal College of Psychiatrists believes that society, including the medical profession, has the potential to develop more tolerant and humane attitudes towards people with mental disorders.

- The College's 'Stigma' Campaign will aim to 'de-mythologise' those mental disorders which are currently stigmatised by mounting a wide-ranging educational campaign aimed at many different components of society, including different age groups and people from different social and ethnic backgrounds.

Campaign Objectives

- Raise awareness that mental disorders are very common and touch every family in the land at some time.
- Change attitudes so that mental disorders in general are less stigmatised.
- Demonstrate that both genetic inheritance and the environment contribute to in nearly all mental disorders.
- Show that a holistic approach to treatments is the most effective.

(Crisp A Psychiatric Bulletin 2000)

In the fifth and sixth objectives, the phrase 'more constructive working relationships' may hint at a necessity, borne of experience. (Psychiatrists may not have these already in relation to service users, their significant others or nearby mental health professionals.) The final objective concedes that psychiatry is an imprecise science and that the campaign provides an opportunity to explore 'uncertainties and challenging problems'. Finally, the summary statement rounding off the objectives listed is worth citing:

> By achieving these objectives, it is hoped that people suffering from mental disorders will be enabled optimally to contribute towards their own recovery. (Royal College of Psychiatrists 1998, p. 16)

This summary 'meta-objective' is not actually about stigma but is simply therapeutic paternalism and the hope that rates of patient non-compliance with treatment will decline. Thus, early in the document, a whole series of indicators are present about professional interests, which are separate from the commitment its authors had to the social challenge of de-stigmatisation.

In line with the discussion of the nature of mental health problems, the document from the Royal College framed the reality about mental health problems in a categorical and not in a dimensional or non-committal way. This framing is linked explicitly in the document to the history of asylum psychiatry and its claimed beneficial legacy:

> Within that setting [the asylum], medicine, and psychiatry in particular, set about the task of better differentiating the variety of mental disorders which currently finds expression in the diagnostic criteria of the International Classification of Diseases of Mental and Behavioural Disorders (ICD 10) and the American Diagnostic and Statistical Manual of Mental Disorders (DSM IV). Such classifications of mental disorders have contributed to the development of valuable treatments for many of the identified disorders (Royal College of Psychiatrists 1998, p. 13)

The axiom in the final sentence is open to challenge because the history of psychiatric treatment has tended to proceed in an ad hoc and opportunistic way. There is also little evidence that nosology has systematically and effectively guided treatment innovation. The front of the document summarises the changing minds project as a 5-year campaign to:

> ...increase public and professional understanding of mental disorders and related mental health problems; thereby to reduce the stigmatisation and discrimination against people suffering from them; and to close the gap between the differing beliefs of healthcare professionals and the public about useful mental health interventions. (Royal College of Psychiatrists 1998, p. 1)

Thus, an 'uncertainty' or 'challenging problem' (Royal College of Psychiatrists 1998, p. 7) for the profession is not about the existence of 'mental disorders' or the effectiveness of 'mental health interventions'. This lack of self-doubt is not surprising. If any medical specialty put forward policy suggestions, it is highly likely that its preferred knowledge base would be stated confidently and its therapeutic utility taken for granted.[3]

Returning to the diagnostic categories described in the campaign, these became a way of organising not clinical knowledge but sociological knowledge. Thus, the campaign does not privilege stigma but starts at the other end of the telescope – with particular diagnoses. As a result, different 'stigmas' (sic) not 'stigma' are described in the campaign document. Thus, the social process of stigmatisation is tied down to preferred clinical categories like 'depression' and 'schizophrenia'. The taking of diagnostic categories as natural givens in the campaign is what Hoff (1995) calls 'medical naturalism'. The document adheres to the view that psychiatric diagnosis or categorical reasoning is not only legitimate but that it has been linked to the incremental scientific understanding of mental illness. It is argued that diagnostic categorisation has improved treatment capability over time and ignores the opposite argument which has been made; those categories with poor conceptual and predictive validity have actually impeded our understanding of how to respond effectively to madness and distress (Mirowsky and Ross 1989; Bentall 2004).

Specific diagnostic categories of 'mental disorder' are described ('anxiety', 'depression', 'schizophrenia', 'dementia', 'drug and alcohol problems' and 'eating disorders'). The campaign used these as sections to report work. (Later, 'personality disorder' was added to create seven, not six, categories of stigma.) The website of the campaign puts different categories of mental health problem and stigma into boxes on its pages, and in this way the campaign can be seen as a vehicle to create a sense of certainty for its audience about the nature and prevalence of 'mental disorders'.

The Challenge of the Concept of Stigma for the Psychiatric Profession

Sociological work on the therapeutic impact of psychiatric labelling and treatment suggests that 'closing the gap' between lay and professional views of mental health problems is not self-evidently of value for patients. (The benefit of social regulation on behalf of the wider moral order is another matter.) For example, studies underpinning classical labelling theory, modified labelling theory and social exclusion suggest that psychiatric diagnoses and treatment may have unhelpful consequences for patients. Given this evidence, then psychiatric theory and practice may be part of the problem of stigma and social exclusion not part of the solution (Garfinkel 1956; Goffman 1961; Link et al. 1989; Skinner et al. 1995; Sayce 2000). Therefore, the preferred way of reasoning about stigma in the campaign (yoking particular forms of stigma to particular diagnoses) reflects a form of interest work for the psychiatric profession. It frames knowledge about a social phenomenon in clinical terms. Thus, conceptually, stigma becomes a form of psychiatric (not sociological) knowledge.

Classical labelling theory was held in suspicion by the psychiatric leadership of the 1970s, the predecessors of the document's authors, as part of 'anti-psychiatry' (Roth 1973; Wing 1978). Labelling theory played down the role of primary deviance and emphasised the negative impact of labelling from others, including that from psychiatrists. If psychiatry were to open its doors to a discussion of all of this sociological work, then it risks opening these old wounds. The singularly cited paper from Hayward and Bright (1997) can be viewed a buffer against this eventuality, because

---

[3] The true nature of mental health problems, according to the campaign, is contrasted with the competing and flawed views held by the general public. An explicit intention discussed under the heading of that name is to 'close the gap' between the psychiatric and lay perspectives and an explicit emphasis on the need for the profession to educate the public to accept a professional conception of mental health problems. This is pro-active attempt at what De Swaan (1990) calls 'protoprofessionalization'. While the benefits to the profession of this opportunity to promote its preferred view of reality about mental health are afforded considerable space, it is not clear what this has to do with stigma or its reversal.

it summarised and filtered a complicated sociological literature, which could then be 'cherry picked' by the College leadership for the purpose of its campaign. In doing so the social became medical.

Case Study Three: Psychoanalysis

The relationship between sociology and psychoanalysis has had a checkered history (Bocock 1976). Psychoanalysis itself is a polyvalent or open textured concept (rather like a Rorschach Card – a projective test of its own making) inviting that mixed trajectory:

- It is a wing of psychiatry but contains non-medical practitioners ('lay analysts').
- Within psychiatry, it is one bulwark against biodeterminism (the dehumanising logic of the biomedical model) but also a form of biodeterminism. Freud was a hoped-for-reductionist, who considered that ultimately human conduct would be accounted for by neuroscience.
- It is a form of biographical psychology but is mechanistic as well as existential in its method.
- It retains diagnostic reasoning – psychoanalysts have been highly influential in the development of the Diagnostic and Statistical Manual of the American Psychiatric Association (Bayer and Spitzer 1985; Wilson 1993). However, it also emphasises the hermeneutic task applied to each unique case.
- It rejects a neat separation of mental illness from normality but also retains the concept of mental illness to describe psychological difference, when arguing that 'we are all ill'.
- It is a social theory that can give comfort to both conservative and radical social forces.

The critical theorists of the Frankfurt School offered a brand of sociology by blending the views of Freud and Marx. The treatment of shellshock in the First World War was a site for this convergence, when external conditions were made manifest in symptoms but mediated by intrapsychic conflict. The intrusion of psychoanalysis into war-torn mental health work raised expectations of voluntarism in mental health services, and it challenged the eugenic assumptions of asylum psychiatry. Those breaking down in the trenches were 'England's finest blood' – officers and gentlemen and working-class volunteers (Stone 1985).

A number of writers attempted to account for the relationship between socio-economic structures and the inner lives of individuals. One example can be found in the work of Sartre (1963) when he developed his biographical progressive–regressive method. The latter aspired to understand the social context in relation to biographical accounts and biography in relation to social conditions. This existential development of humanistic Marxism competed with other elaborate discussions about the relationship between unconscious mental life and societal determinants and constraints.

Within Freud's early circle, a number of analysts took interest in using their psychological insights in order to illuminate societal processes. This set a trend for later analysts, some of whom tended to reduce social phenomena to the aggregate impact of individual psychopathology and offered social theories that were forms of psychological reductionism (e.g. Bion 1959).

However, an alternative and explicitly Marxist group of analyst competed with existentialism on one side and psychological reductionism on the other. These 'critical theorists' who were associated with the Frankfurt Institute of Social Research were led by Max Horkheimer, a German philosopher and sociologist, after 1930. The key difference between the Frankfurt School thinkers and the traditional clinical psychoanalysis was the focus of the interrelationship between psyche and society. The central importance of the interrelationships between the material environment of individuals and their cultural life and inner lives were subsequently explored by Marcuse, Adorno and Fromm (and the more marginal institute members Riech and Benjamin). The group had an explicitly emancipatory intent.

The role of this group of critical theorists in social science marginalised the notion of illness replacing it with the notion of what Fromm termed the 'pathology of normalcy'. Compatible with this the concerns of the group focused on the dialectical relationship between psyche and society through the drawing of connexions between life-negating cultural norms associated with authoritarianism and the capitalist economy and the ambiguous role of the super-ego as a source of conformity and mutuality. The latter were conceptualised as mediated by the intrapsychic mechanism of repression. Critical theory was exemplified in studies of the authoritarian personality (Adorno et al. 1950) and the mass psychology of fascism (Reich 1975) and the psychological blocks attending the transition from capitalist to socialist democracy (Fromm 1955).

An example though of the polyvalent concept of psychoanalysis is demonstrated by a range of other developments in social theory. For example, it was influential in Parson's structural functionalism as the intrapsychic factor in explaining conformity (Parsons 1964). Resonances of it can also be found in Giddens' theory of structuration (Giddens 1976). It was the basis of both left wing (Laing 1968) and right wing (Szasz 1961) 'anti-psychiatry'. It was also the conservative basis for opposing political radicalism and the Marxian developments of Reich and Marcuse (Chassegaut-Smirgel and Grunberger 1986). It was attacked by feminist social theorists (Millet 1971; Oakley 1972) but also used as a vehicle for their arguments (Mitchell 1972; Eichenbaum and Orbach 1982). Indeed, from the perspective of sociology, psychoanalysis seems to have been whatever its range of authors have wanted it to be.

Despite this highly variegated relationship between sociology and psychoanalysis, there has been regular engagement between the two bodies of knowledge. The individualism and empiricism of the latter has placed a fairly permeable boundary between psychology and psychoanalysis. Clinical psychologists have rejected it as therapeutically useless and pre-scientific (because of the un-testability of its propositions). Social psychologists have investigated their topic experimentally and avoided the hermeneutic leaps of group analysis. This gap between psychology and psychoanalysis also applies to the former and sociology. There have been seminal developments from a few social psychologists offering insights beyond that of studying small group interactions – G.H. Mead and Erving Goffman stand out in the context of this chapter. However, their legacy has been claimed largely by sociology not psychiatry or psychology.

Indeed, if we were to discount psychoanalysis as a legitimate form of psychology (as it is so contested), then only recent developments in social contructionism offer a bridge between psychology (and psychiatry) and sociology. This brings us back to the importance of the shift towards postmodern social science discussed early in the chapter, especially that inspired by French post-structuralism (e.g. Parker et al 1997; Bracken 2003; Thomas 1997).

Conclusion: Between Medical and Sociological Imperialism

This chapter has examined the relationship between sociology and psychiatry via three case studies about social psychiatry, stigma and psychoanalysis. The first highlighted the possibilities of co-operation, but these were predicated on two tendencies. On the one hand, sociology had to accept the handmaiden role in psychiatric epidemiology and, on the other, psychiatry had to concede its tenuous knowledge base and be truly open to sociological reasoning. Once sociology refused to continue in the role of subordinate and took a different epistemological turn, there was a 'return to medicine' in psychiatry, and the bridge was seriously weakened.

And once an interdisciplinary void opened up with the weakening of the project of social psychiatry and the association of sociology with 'anti-psychiatry', then this left the medical profession turning away from sociological insights. This became evident when we turned our attention to stigma. The campaign of the Royal College of Psychiatrists we described proceeded virtually without reference to sociology. Moreover, the medical profession started at the clinical not social end of the telescope.

The third case study of psychoanalysis drew attention to the multiple ways in which it could act as a bridge between psychiatry and sociology. The problem is that these multiple linkages are often internally or mutually contradictory. Nonetheless, we concluded that psychoanalysis, as a form of both psychology and psychiatry remains the one clinical discipline of regular interest to sociologists.

Mainstream academic psychology is caught between the paradigms of social science and natural science, tending to default generally to the latter. As a consequence, the distance in the academy between psychology and sociology has largely arisen from the pre-occupation of the former with empirical matters and the latter with pre-empirical and non-empirical matters (social constructs and social theory). This point is reinforced by evidence of a clear convergence between social psychology and sociology with the post-modern turn across the social sciences – social constructivism in sociology (or social constructionism) in social psychology. With the latter, there are of course cross-cultural differences. In the US Social constructivism, it did not seemingly gain such a grip on sociology and there was a greater acceptance of the legitimacy and possibilities introduced by neuro-psychiatry (Pescosolido personal communication). It appears that in the US, the introduction of a post-modern interest encouraged more of a loosening of a focus on 'status attainment' research suggesting perhaps that American sociological knowledge in the field of mental health is likely to have become a little more open and diverse rather than rejecting of psychiatric knowledge per se.

The history of the divide in a stand-off between strong advocates in each discipline which followed a heyday of early collaboration shows signs of reversing or at least tentative reversal related to two developments. One is related to changes and challenges within the psychiatric profession which has led to internal reflection and critical reflection. Starting in the 1990s, the marketisation and a more managed system in the NHS has meant that in the UK, at least the dominance of psychiatry has not been taken for granted but has resulted in a more fragmented field of mental health care (Samson 1995). An embracing of evidence-based medicine has resulted in a more critical stance towards aspects of psychiatric practice including medication[4] (Tyrer 2008). The psychiatric profession has spawned 'critical psychiatry' 'from within its own ranks.' The latter is a network of British psychiatrists who debate the reform or abolition of their own profession and adopt a critical stance derived from Foucauldian analysis and advocate the adoption of a thorough going bio-psychosocial model (Moncrieff 2006; Bracken and Thomas 2006). The common thread in the network is a willingness of its participants to concede the limits of the profession and to open up debates about how to respond in society to psychological difference. Finally, the relatively new field of health services research and other applied interdisciplinary arenas are rapidly growing which rely on both sociological and clinical talent. It is possible that within this new research environment, new synergies will be found and nurtured between sociology and medicine about the empirical and epistemological study of mental health.

---

[4] For example a *British Journal of Psychiatry* article stated that: we are reminded by Lewis and Lieberman (pp. 161–163) that the Orwellian chant of 'atypical antipsychotics good, typical antipsychotics bad' is indeed the vacant refrain of sheep-like adherents to an outdated chimera of progress.

References

Adorno TW, Frenkel-Brunswik E, Levinson DJ, Sanford RN (1950) The authoritarian personality. Harper, New York
American Psychiatric Association (1980) Diagnostic and statistical manual III. American Psychiatric Association, Washington, DC
Bayer R, Spitzer RL (1985) Neurosis, psychodynamics and DSM-III. A history of the controversy. Arch Gen Psychiatry 42:187–196
Becker HS (1963) Outsiders: studies in the sociology of deviance. Free Press, New York
Bentall RP (2004) Madness explained: psychosis and human nature. Penguin, London
Bentall RP, Jackson H, Pilgrim D (1988) Abandoning the concept of schizophrenia: some implications of validity arguments for psychological research into psychotic phenomena. Br J Clin Psychol 27:303–24
Bion WR (1959) Experiences in groups. Tavistock, London
Bocock R (1976) Freud and modern society. Thomas Nelson and Sons, London
Boyle M (1990) Schizophrenia: a scientific delusion. Routledge, London
Bracken PJ (2003) Postmodernism and psychiatry. Curr Opin Psychiatry 16(6):673–677
Bracken P, Thomas P (2006) Postpsychiatry: mental health in a postmodern world. Oxford University Press, Oxford
Breggin P (1993) Toxic psychiatry. Fontana, London
Brown GW, Harris T (1978) The social origins of depression. Tavistock, London
Brown GW, Wing JK (1962) A comparative clinical social survey of three mental hospitals. Sociol Rev Monogr 5:145–171
Carpenter M (2000) 'It's a small world' mental health policy under welfare capitalism since 1945. Sociol Health Illn 22(5):602–619
Chassegaut-Smirgel J, Grunberger B (1986) Freud or Reich? Psychoanalysis and illusion. Free Association Books, London
Clare AW (1999) Psychiatry's future: psychological medicine or biological psychiatry? J Ment Health 8(2):109–111
Cook JA, Wright ER (1995) Medical sociology and the study of severe mental illness: reflections on past accomplishments and directions for future research. J Health Soc Behav 36(5):95–114
Cooley CH (1902) Human nature and social order. Charles Scribner's Sons, New York
Coulter J (1973) Approaches to insanity. Wiley, New York
Craib I (1997) Social constructionism as social psychosis. Sociology 31(1):1–15
Crisp A (2000) Changing minds: every family in the land Psychiatric Bulletin 24:267–268
Csernansky JG, Grace AA (1998) New models of the pathophysiology of schizophrenia: editors' introduction. Schizophr Bull 24(2):185–188
De Swaan A (1990) The management of normality. Routledge, London
Dowrick C (2004) Beyond depression: a new approach to understanding and management. Oxford University Press, Oxford
Eichenbaum L, Orbach S (1982) Outside in inside out. Penguin, London
Elias N (1969) Sociology and psychiatry. In: Foulkes SH, Prince GS (eds) Psychiatry in a changing society. Tavistock, London
Engel GL (1980) The clinical application of the biopsychosocial model. Am J Psychiatry 137:535–544
Falloon I, Fadden G (1993) Integrated mental health care. Cambridge University Press, Cambridge
Faris RE, Dunham HW (1939) Mental disorders in urban areas: an ecological study of schizophrenia and other psychoses. The University of Chicago Press, Chicago, IL
Fenton S, Charsley K (2000) Epidemiology and sociology as incommensurate games: accounts from the study of health and ethnicity. Health 4(4):403–425
Fromm E (1955) The sane society. Holt, Rinehart and Winston, New York
Fryers T, Melzer D, Jenkins R (2000) Mental health inequalities report 1: a systematic literature review. Department of Health, London
Garfinkel H (1956) Conditions of successful degradation ceremonies. Am J Sociol 61:420–424
Gibbons MC, Limoges C, Nowotny H, Schwartzman S, Scott P, Trow M (1994) The new production of knowledge: the dynamics of science and research in contemporary societies. Sage, London
Giddens A (1976) New rules of the sociological method. Hutchinson, London
Goffman E (1961) Asylums: essays on the social situation of mental patients and other inmates. Anchor Books, New York
Goffman E (1963) Stigma: some notes on the management of spoiled identity. Penguin, Harmondsworth
Goldberg D, Huxley P (1992) Common mental disorders. Routledge, London
Gove WB (1982) The current status of the labelling theory of mental illness. In: Gove WB (ed) Deviance and mental illness. Sage, Beverly Hills, CA

Gronfein W (1985) Incentives and intentions in mental health policy: a comparison of the Medicaid and Community Health Programmes. J Health Soc Behav 26(3):192–206
Guze S (1989) Biological psychiatry: is there any other kind? Psychol Med 19:315–23
Hamilton M (1973) Psychology in society: end or ends. Bulletin of the British Psychological Society 26:185–189
Hammersley M (1999) Sociology, what's it for? A critique of Gouldner. Sociol Res Online 4(3):U325–U336
Hayward P, Bright J (1997) Stigma and mental illness: a review and critique. J Ment Health 6:345–354
Healy D (1997) The antidepresssant Era. Harvester, London
Hoff P (1995) Kraepelin. In: Berrios G, Porter R (eds) A history of clinical psychiatry. Athlone Press, London
Hollingshead A, Redlich RC (1958) Social class and mental illness. Wiley, New York
Illsley R (1975) Promotion to observer status. Soc Sci Med 9:63–67
Jones L, Cochrane R (1981) Stereotypes of mental illness: a test of the labelling hypothesis. Int J Soc Psychiatry 27:99–107
Klerman GL (1989) Psychiatric diagnostic categories: issues of validity and measurement, an invited comment on Mirowsky and Ross. J Health Soc Behav 30:26–30
Kramer P (1993) Listening to Prozac. Viking, New York
Kutchins H, Kirk SA (1997) Making us crazy. Free Press, New York
Laing RD (1968) The politics of experience and the bird of paradise. Penguin, Harmondsworth
Lawson A (1989) A sociological and socio-anthropological perspective. In: Williams P, Wilkinson G, Rawnsley K (eds) The scope of epidemiological psychiatry. Routledge, London
Lemert EM (1967) Human deviancy, social problems and social control. Prentice and Hall, Eglewood Cliff, NJ
Link B (2000) The stigma process: re-conceiving the definition of stigma. Paper presented at the Annual Conference of the American Public Health Association
Link B, Bruce G, Cullen FT, Struening E, Shrout P, Dohrenwend BP (1989) A modified labeling approach to mental disorders: an empirical assessment. Am Sociol Rev 54:400–23
Mead GH (1934) Mind, self and society. Chicago University Press, Chicago, IL
Millet K (1971) Sexual politics. Doubleday, New York
Mirowsky J, Ross CE (1989) Psychiatric diagnosis as reified measurement. J Health Soc Behav 30(1):11–25
Mishara AL (1994) A phenomenological critique of commonsensical assumptions in DSM III: the avoidance of the patient's subjectivity. In: Sadler JZ, Wiggins OP, Schwartz MA (eds) Perspectives on psychiatric diagnostic classification. John Hopkins University Press, Baltimore, MA
Mitchell J (1972) Psychoanalysis and feminism. Penguin, Harmondsworth
Moncrieff J (2006) The politics of psychiatric drug treatment. In: Double D (ed) Critical psychiatry: the limits of madness. Palgrave, Basingstoke
Moncrieff J, Crawford M (2001) British psychiatry in the 20th century – observations from a psychiatric journal. Soc Sci Med 53(3):349–56
Muntaner C, Eaton WW, Chamberlin CD (2000) Social inequalities in mental health: a review of concepts and underlying assumptions. Health 4(1):89–109
Nazroo J (1997) Ethnicity and mental health. Policy Studies Institute, London
Oakley A (1972) Sex gender and society. Temple Smith, London
Parker I, Georgaca E, Harper D, McLauughlin T, Stowell-Smith M (1997) Deconstructing psychopathology. Sage, London
Parsons T (1964) Social structure and personality. Collier Macmillan, London
Pescosolido BA, Rubin BA (2000) The web of group affiliations revisited: social life, postmodernism, and sociology. Am Sociol Rev 65:52–76
Pilgrim D (2002) The biopsychosocial model in Anglo-American psychiatry: past, present and future? Journal of Mental Health 11(6):585–594
Pilgrim D, Rogers A (1994) Something old, something new sociology and the organization of psychiatry. Sociology 28(2):521–538
Prior L (1991) Mind, body and behaviour: theorisations of madness and the organisation of therapy. Sociology 25(3):403–422
Reich W (1975) The mass psychology of fascism. Penguin, Harmondsworth
Reid M (1976) The development of medical sociology in Britain. Discussion Papers in Social Research. University of Glasgow
Rogers A, Pilgrim D (2003) Mental health and inequality. Palgrave, Basingstoke
Rogers A, Pilgrim D (2005) A sociology of mental health and illness, 3rd edn. Open University Press, Maidenhead
Rogers A, Pilgrim D, Lacey R (1993) Experiencing psychiatry: users' views of services. MIND/MacMillan, Basingstoke
Rosen G (1979) Madness in society. Harper, New York
Ross CA, Pam A (eds) (1995) Pseudoscience in biological psychiatry: blaming the body. Wiley, New York
Roth M (1973) Psychiatry and its critics. Br J Psychiatry 122:374

Samson C (1995) The fracturing of medical dominance in British psychiatry. Sociol Health Illn 17(2):245–68
Sartre J-P (1963) Search for a method. Knopf, New York
Sayce L (2000) From psychiatric patient to citizen: overcoming discrimination and social exclusion. Macmillan, Basingstoke
Scambler G (2005) Jigsaws, models and the sociology of stigma. J Crit Realism 5(2):273–289
Scheff TJ (1966) Being mentally Ill: a sociological theory. Chicago University Press, Chicago, IL
Scull A (1979) Museums of madness. Penguin, Harmondsworth
Shorter E (1998) A history of psychiatry: from the era of the asylum to the age of Prozac. Wiley, Chichester
Skinner LJ, Berry KK, Griffiths SE, Byers B (1995) Generalizability and specificity of the stigma associated with the mental illness label. J Community Psychol 23:3–17
Srole L, Langer TS (1962) Mental health in the metropolis: the midtown Manhattan Study. McGraw Hill, New York
Stone M (1985) Shellshock and the psychologists. In: Bynum WF, Porter R, Shepherd M (eds) The anatomy of madness. Tavistock, London
Strong P (1979) Sociological imperialism and the profession of medicine: a critical examination of the thesis of medical imperialism. Soc Sci Med 13a:199–215
Szasz TS (1961) The use of naming and the origin of the myth of mental illness. Am Psychol 16:59–65
Thoits PA (1985) Self-labeling processes in mental illness: the role of emotional deviance. Am J Sociol 91:221–49
Thomas P (1997) The dialectics of schizophrenia. Free Associations Books, London
Tyrer P (2008) Editorial. Br J Psychiatry 192:242. doi:10.1192/bjp. 192.3.242
Wallace ER (1994) Psychiatry and its nosology: an historico-philosophical overview. In: Sadler JZ, Wiggins OP, Schwartz MA (eds) Perspectives on psychiatric diagnostic classification. John Hopkins University Press, Baltimore, MA
Warner R (1985) Recovery from schizophrenia: psychiatry and political economy. Routeldge, London
Wilson M (1993) DSM-III and the transformation of American psychiatry: a history. Am J Psychiatry 150(3):399–410
Wing J (1978) Reasoning about madness. Oxford University Press, Oxford
Wittchen HU (2000) Epidemiological research in mental disorders: lessons for the next decade of research: the NAPE lecture 1999. Acta Psychiatr Scand 101(1):2–10

Chapter 3
Organizing the Sociological Landscape for the Next Decades of Health and Health Care Research: The Network Episode Model III-R as Cartographic Subfield Guide

Bernice A. Pescosolido

Introduction

The last decade has produced an extraordinary consensus in understanding health, illness, and healing. While the last 100 years of social science, and many more years for the natural sciences, was marked by greater disciplinary boundaries and specialization, these last twenty have been marked by calls for transdisciplinarity. This is not unique to medicine or to the sociomedical sciences. The centrifugal force that characterized the development of the first 100 years of empirically based research has produced schools (e.g., public health), spin-off disciplines and programs (e.g., women's studies, health services research), and subfields (e.g., medical sociology) with a solid body of rich ideas and empirical findings (Pescosolido 2006a). This period established some of the most famous dichotomies of early modern science – photons versus waves, geosynclines versus tectonic plates, nature versus nurture, the individual versus society, and culture versus structure. While some of these were eventually adjudicated and their superiority established (e.g., Geographer Wegener's theory of plate tectonics), most have reached a contemporary end point that matches what sociologists have always known: The world is intricate and messy, even if regular and patterned.

This is most elegantly stated as "Complexity Theory." In a recent issue of *Science,* political scientist Elinor Ostrom (2009, p. 11), 2009 Nobel Laureate in Economics, argued that "we must learn how to dissect and harness complexity, rather than eliminate it....This process is complicated, however, because entirely different frameworks, theories, and models are used by different disciplines to analyze their parts of the complex multilevel whole." Fig. 3.1 (from Pavalko et al. 2007) provides an illustration of this kind of complexity in medical sociology for one cohort of individuals confronting one set of problems in one place. The timeline links biography (e.g., with 6 of the 238 cases graphed here) and social history in the Vermont Longitudinal Study (VLS). The VLS stands as one of the classic studies that refuted psychiatry's initial premise that schizophrenia had an inevitable downward and degenerative course. This project on the "outcomes" for persons with severe mental illness began in 1955 when a "model program" was instituted. For each individual in Fig. 3.1, the *dashes* between *brackets* mark periods in the hospital and the blank areas in each row indicate periods outside of the hospital. The hospitalization that occurred when the patient entered the model program is indicated in *bold type*. For example, the top three cases are persons who had been hospitalized at least once prior to the model program, while the bottom three cases illustrate those who entered the model program during their first hospitalization.

B.A. Pescosolido (✉)
Department of Sociology, Indiana University, 1022 E. Third Street, Bloomington, IN 47405, USA
e-mail: pescosol@indiana.edu

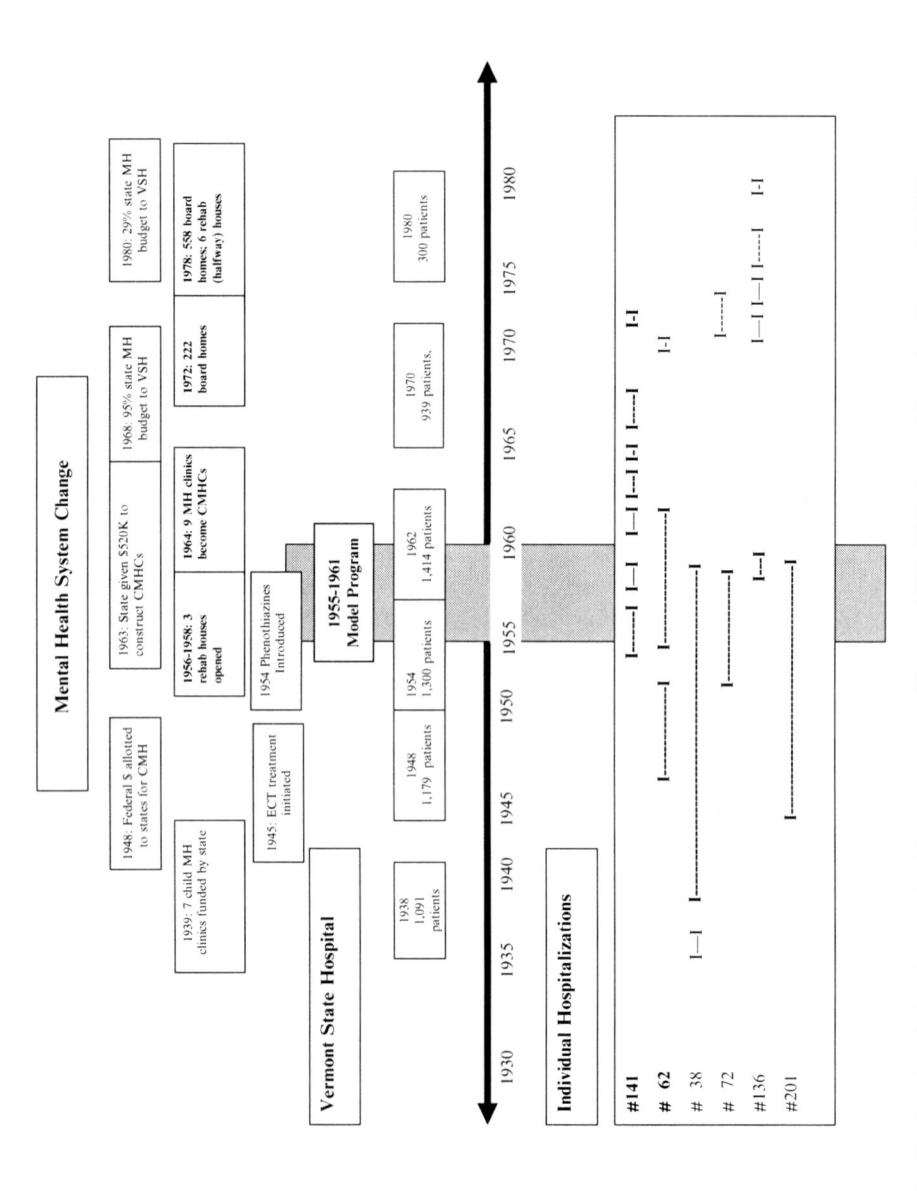

Fig. 3.1 Timeline of individual, hospital and mental health system events, Vermont 1930–1980. Adapted from Pavalko et al. (2007)

Examining the "outcomes" for individuals treated at the Vermont State Hospital (VSH) in dynamic (or more specifically, illness career) perspective requires a sophisticated understanding of individuals, illness, and contexts. The VLS included different kinds of individuals (e.g., men and women, rural and urban residents) who encountered the clinical innovation at different points in their illness careers. Furthermore, the timeline is linked to three separate sets of historical developments in the Vermont context – federal and national developments, innovations at the state government level, and the conditions/programs within VSH itself. To associate illness career outcomes with only the introduction of the new rehabilitation program in 1955 might be misleading.

In fact, individuals' hospitalization careers depended on where individuals were in their own illness career, who they were, and where their career was located in historical time. That is, across the entire span considered, the pace of earlier hospitalizations shaped the pace of later ones. Yet, patterns of hospital entry and exit differed before and after 1960. During the earlier, pre-deinstitutionalization period, social statuses were more strongly associated with the length of the initial hospitalization than were illness or community characteristics. After that point, hospital stays, overall, were shorter and more sporadic with multiple hospitalizations tending to occur in rapid succession ("the revolving door"). With the institutional reforms beginning in 1955, associations with hospital stays shifted from social to illness characteristics (Pavalko et al. 2007).

The purpose of this chapter is to address these kinds of complexities in the sociology of health, illness, and healing, further developing the Network Episode Model as an approach to contextualize epidemiological and health services research (Pescosolido 1991, 2006a; Pescosolido and Boyer 1999). The NEM represents one possible integrated, multidisciplinary framework to explicate and connect levels and dynamics. It does so through network theory using cartological imagery.[1] As set out in the Introduction to this volume, with Olafsdottir, I appropriated Gieryn's (1999) metaphor of cultural landscapes and boundaries because its theoretical flexibility and emphasis on vertical integration of contextual levels fit the dimensionality and dynamics of the multifaceted, complex nature of health, illness, and healing in the current era (Olafsdottir and Pescosolido 2009; Pescosolido and Olafsdottir 2010). As Gieryn and others from the "new" sociology of culture have argued, individuals use cultural maps to make sense of the world, affecting information availability and personal understandings as well as signaling possible and appropriate action. These maps are evoked in the community, in personal lives, and in organizations. The goal here is to further push theoretical guides by seeing networks as the lines of latitude and longitude that anchor our understandings of cultural maps. That is, the Network Episode Model (below) uses the metaphor of places, spaces, and maps to situate the levels of context "above" the individual (community, institutional, and support network systems) and the levels "below" them (individual and molecular systems).

Why Networks?

Earlier, I argued that frameworks and models which respond to the current call to integrate disciplines and subfields to address complex challenges in the cause and consequences of health and illness must fit four criteria. They must: (1) consider and articulate the full set of contextual levels documented to have impact in past empirical research; (2) offer an underlying mechanism or "engine of

---

[1] Bringing a version of complexity theory to understand health, illness, and healing brings up two sets of terms that are *au courant* and confusing – interdisciplinary and multidisciplinary. I use the former to describe research and researchers who claim to bring the expertise of many disciplines and approaches to the table; I use the latter to describe the process of researchers, each expert in their field, who come together to develop frameworks and research designs that take advantage of the interconnected strengths of each. Obvious from even this framing, my preference is for the latter.

action" that connects levels, is dynamic, and allows for a way to narrow down focal research questions; (3) employ a metaphor and analytic language familiar to both social and natural science to facilitate synergy; and (4) understand the need for and use the full range of methodological tools proven useful in the social and natural sciences (Pescosolido 2006b). But I would now add to that list: (5) provide a tangible way to engage in institutional social change, whether through formal, legal policy changes or informal, community-based activism. One fundamental utility of a social network approach is that it provides a concrete mechanism for intervention. For example, "organizational culture" and "social support" represent two social factors that have been documented in sociomedical research to be important to outcomes. As summary perceptual scales, they have been measured as totalities. Yet, perceptions of overall social climate, whether at the individual or organizational level, do not offer an intervention point. Will changing individuals' perceptions improve the situation for workers, friends, or family members? Only by understanding the social relationships that create "toxic" workplaces or "protective" homes and communities, in the social sense, we can unpack and leverage the forces of change. Even social policies and medical treatments are enacted by individuals. Sometimes innovations may be ineffective because they are poor policies and treatments; however, other times it may be the underlying human interpretation or enactment of them that cause them to be unproductive. Knowing the difference between the two is crucial.

Even earlier (Pescosolido 1992), I suggested that the network perspective was particularly apt for a sociology-based model because, despite all of our internal theoretical and methodological squabbles, one point of agreement is uncontested – social interaction stands as the basis for understanding the links between individuals and their society. This finds voice in sociological work as diverse as Goffman's (1963) early notion that stigma, of whatever type, may be an attribute known to others, but its effects materialize only in and through social relationships, to Bearman and colleagues' (Liu et al. 2010) recent contention that some significant part of the "autism epidemic" stems from lay consultations among parents in geographic proximity to one another. Most importantly, as Tilly (1984) argues, social networks create the structures so central to sociology's emphasis on inequality, meaning, and action in unpacking causes and consequences.

The emphasis on mapping the structure of social interactions has taken hold across the landscape of science. As noted above, this facilitates the acceptance and utility of a network-based model. Physicist Albert-László Barabási (2003) asserts that the increased attention to networks reflects the acknowledgement across the sciences that even the most fruitful research on single "pieces" of social and physical life cannot proceed in isolation. Networks introduce "heterogeneity into our previously homogeneous theories of populations, diseases, and societies" and "have allowed us to find generalities among seemingly different systems that, despite their disparate nature, may have similar processes of formation and/or similar forces acting on their architecture...." (Bascompte 2009, p. 419). Even some sectors of economics, which developed the most individualistic of approaches, now have turned to see "interdependencies, implemented through transnational credit and investment networks, trade relations, or supply chains that have proven difficult to predict and control" requiring "an approach that stresses the systemic complexity of economic networks and that can be used to revise and extend established paradigms in economic theory" (Schweitzer et al. 2009, p. 422).

Before these disciplinary practitioners shifted their views from particle physics or "Homo economicus," sociologists, social psychologists, anthropologists, and management scientists deliberated and mapped interconnections with graph theory, sociograms, and ego-centric network rosters. They developed new techniques or manipulated old ones to find ways to summarize network structures (see Linton Freeman's 2004 detailed history). All totaled, there was a basic stock of theories, measures, and findings which served as the foundation for the new "Network Science." Supplemented by new developments in the last 10 years, a rich set of theoretical and research tools can be appropriated for medical sociology's work.

Do We Really Need More Theories, Frameworks, and Models?

Recently, a reviewer, frustrated with the proliferation of "models" characterized "a genre of writing prominent in public health and to a lesser extent in sociology where authors review an extensive literature and propose a conceptual framework. These frameworks consist of multiple levels that all influence each other and that explain a broad range of issues related to health and health care....with the obligatory figure with multiple levels and arrows pointing up and down, left and right. You either like this kind of conceptualization or you don't. I am not a big fan...." (Anonymous reviewer, personal communication). No doubt, there is a proliferation of "models," in part, because of the looseness of our language, and, in part, as a lack of clear separation between theory and method. Harkening back to the classic statements of sociologists like Merton, Tilly, and Stinchcombe, there are differences among a framework, a theory, and a model. None of these mistake gathering together parts of one or another of these to frame an empirical analysis with "new" theorizing. A framework situates models and theories in a set of underlying assumptions and principles. By definition, it is more diffuse and less detailed than the others, offering an overarching view of what is involved and how things work. A theory is a set of interrelated propositions, while the application and tailoring of a particular framework or theory to a substantive problem can be thought of as a model (Pescosolido 1992).

While limitations in the scope of research settings often prohibit the empirical examination of the organized and integrated whole of a theory or an applied theoretical model, efforts to examine key ideas or apply them to new situations represent model adaptations, not new models (e.g., Costello et al.'s 1998 reengineering of the NEM for children). "Cherry picking" among models to justify an analyses is neither a "new" model, an "adapted" model, nor an "integrated" model; it represents a convenience and tends to result in simplistic input, throughput, and output analyses.

In the end, theoretically grounded frameworks, theories, and models do serve a useful purpose. Ostrom (2009, p. 420) makes the central point clearly:

> Without a framework to organize relevant variables identified in theories and empirical research, isolated knowledge acquired from studies of diverse resource systems in different countries by biophysical and social scientists is not likely to cumulate. A framework is thus useful in providing a common set of potentially relevant variables and their subcomponents to use in the design of data collection instruments, the conduct of fieldwork, and the analysis of findings…

Medical sociologists, like other sociologists and scientists, frame their designs, data collection, and analyses in any empirically based endeavor, whether qualitative or quantitative, in some approach. Even a crude, fairly atheoretical "risk" and "protective" factors approach offers a guide. When researchers rely on extant data, they are obliged to evaluate the match between their theoretical ideas and the potential biases and omissions in the data. Even when theoretical tools serve as the guide for new data collections, only particular propositions or hypotheses may be targeted. But when selective pieces of existing theoretical models are gathered together to provide the logical schema for an analysis under the claim that these are "new models," some backlash of the kind voiced above is justified. The proliferation of "models" rivals "kitchen sink" empiricism in eventual futility.

A first step review that includes the figure with boxes and arrows referenced above can integrate past research with some idea of how different factors operate, providing a sounding board for reaction and revision. The problem, as our anonymous reviewer points out, is that this may be insufficient without clear theoretical justification for boxes and arrows and detail on the underlying assumptions, mechanisms, and expectations. Such work tends to offer a preliminary framework or perspective, not theories or models. While sensitizing frameworks begin the process that Ostrom outlines, further theoretical work is required for empirical use.

I argue, along with Ostrom, that we need serious, collaborative work on frameworks, theories, and the tailored models that proceed from them. Rational choice models are useful because they derive from clear principles of rational choice theory (RCT) and a framework of modern economics. Prochaska's Transtheoretical Model (TTM, also called Stages of Change Model; Prochaska and

DiClemente 1982, 1984) is based in theories of motivation and cognition, and a framework of "psychological" social psychology. Labeling theory emerged from the conflict framework in sociology and produced a number of social control-oriented approaches (e.g., Donald Black's *Behavior of Law* 1976) as a provocative response to functional theory's dominance of the time.

At this point in the history of social science, there may be nothing particularly provocative about comprehensive models like the TTM, RCT, or NEM; yet, that is not their purpose or insight. At their inception, they cast and/or recast questions and called for matching methodological approaches in the hopes of providing new insight. Not surprisingly, particular approaches came from particular disciplines; and also not surprisingly, these have become more complex over time, taking account of one another's contributions and incorporating some thread of them. RCT theorists now reject originally stated or implied principles of omniscience, structural irrelevance, and total atomism, and their new "strategically rational actors" take the environment into account and engage in reflection (see Pescosolido 1992). More specifically, sociomedical models of utilization like the Health Belief Model (HBM; Rosenstock 1966) or the Sociobehavioral Model (Andersen 1968) have broadened from their original insights and become more inclusive, though continuing to privilege one set of explanatory factors over others (Pescosolido 1991).

Fleshing Out the NEM

The Network Episode Model struck a claim for the primacy of social network and social influence processes which had been either downplayed or implied in previous health care utilization theories. The NEM made no claim of originality. It drew from a wide range of macro/micro and qualitative/quantitative work in sociology and anthropology, including early dynamic, qualitative work from the 1950s (e.g., Clausen and Yarrow 1955), the 1970s (Chen 1975; Janzen 1978; Zola 1973), and the 1980s (Young 1981). These latter studies provided very textured data on the response to illness which had virtually been ignored in the wake of large survey studies, but provided a solid foundation of information on utilization. The Social Organization Strategy (SOS) framework and the NEM derived from it, then, are pristinely and proudly synthetic, drawing liberally from many insights across the discipline and across the social sciences. Like the alternative approaches described above, the SOS and the NEM privileged one explanation – social interaction – providing a fundamentally different starting point and placing different priorities on similar sets of explanatory factors already found to be useful.

Under Ostrom's exemplar, we may be able to do for health, illness, and healing what collaborative research and a wide group of colleagues have done and continue to do for "socioecological systems." Any of the above-mentioned models like the HBM or SBM from the sociomedical sciences have the potential to serve as scaffolding for medical sociology; here the NEM serves that function.

The Origins and Base of the NEM in Brief

The Network Episode Model, originally proposed in 1991, draws on a set of social network principles laid out in the SOS framework (1992; see Pescosolido 2006a for an overview of social network terms, types, and traditions). Two central features of the model were developed in this first phase – the dynamics of the illness career and the role of social networks in shaping health care outcomes.

The NEM begins with the premise that dealing with health is a phenomenon given meaning through a social process managed by the social networks that individuals have contact with in the community, the family and friend set, the treatment system, and social service agencies (including support groups, churches, and police/jails). Even social institutions that have clear structural elements can be unpacked in terms of influence by examining the social interactions that occur within their walls.

The NEM does not assume that individuals are isolated and ever-consciously rational; however, that does not translate into conceptualizing individuals as "social dopes" or "social dupes," unconscious puppets of the society in which they live (Pescosolido 1992). Rather, following Giddens (1984) and Heise (1989), the NEM sees individuals as skillful actors with a "practical consciousness" that allows them to both improvise and routinize. They shape and are shaped by the possibilities and limits of social network formation in the community, in organizations, and in historical periods.

As pragmatists with commonsense knowledge and cultural routines, individuals may seek out and/or respond to others when behavior, outside of their normal expectations, occurs (as in Parsons' 1951 list of lay evaluations of severity, prognosis, diagnosis, and well role expectations). As Parsons' noted, granting the sick role is done in the community by family, friends, neighbors, and bosses, but not by doctors, nurses, or other clinical practitioners. The latter, should it occur, constitutes entry into the patient role through professional diagnosis. That is, individuals face changes in health and illness in the course of their day-to-day lives by interacting with others who may recognize (or deny) a problem, send them to (or provide) treatment, and support, cajole, or nag them about appointments, medications, or lifestyle. Unlike Parsons, who saw these lay evaluations as guided by universally similar norms in modern society, the NEM follows the more typical sociological view (e.g., Koos 1954) which examines a constellation of sociocultural circumstances that produce different evaluations, sometimes shifting individuals into a cost–benefits analysis, as in RCT.

However, social interactions and *habitus* (as in Bourdieu 1990 and Camic 1986), not mental calculus, provide the initial sources of normative meanings and individual reactions. A *decision or choice* to act, the sole possibility under RCT, represents only one possible response path. Individuals may experience the onset of illness as a social process of *coercion* or a process of *muddling through* with large social networks playing a key role in concert with the types of nonnormative behaviors or conditions that have arisen (Pescosolido et al. 1998a). Social networks, then, can be conceptualized as the mechanism linking individuals across levels, time, and place. In fact, contacts collated across social networks comprise a pathway of care, the essence of the clinical encounter, and the most proper focus of analysis (e.g., see Heritage and Maynard 2010), replacing a focus on individuals. Indeed, while sociodemographic characteristics are not ignored, they are seen as less potent in contemporary society than they were in earlier social forms.

Of course, pathways are facilitated or constrained by both individuals beliefs (as in the Health Belief Model; Rosenstock 1966) and real/perceived access to care (as in Andersen's 1968, 1995 Sociobehavioral Model). All social science models and even medical science models, at this point, understand that such dynamic, microprocess does not operate in a vacuum. Where the NEM differs is in the contention that the entire process is dynamic, constituted, and embedded in individuals' social networks. What individuals know, how they evaluate the potential efficacy and suitability of a range of options and providers, and what they do (in what order and under which "tone") are fundamentally tied to, negotiated in, and given meaning through social interactions. Both the "structure" and the "culture" of network ties interact with each other and with the progress of the health problem (Freidson's 1970 Lay Referral System) to shape the process of responding to changes in health, thereby creating the health and illness career, long or short.

With the basic dynamic and mechanism in place, the first revision of the NEM (Phase II; Pescosolido and Boyer 1999, 2010) elaborated network systems, theorizing a more complex view of social network influences and types. The NEM-Phase II split the "social support system" into personal networks (those "outside" treatment systems) and (inter- and intraorganizational networks (those "inside" treatment/community systems).[2] This added greater specificity to the understanding of context

---

[2] From a social science point of view, these labels may seem somewhat backwards. However, these terms originated in a set of arguments designed to convince those in the medical and mental health treatment systems, who were skeptical at best, that social networks were "active ingredients" within clinics, hospitals, and programs that affected the delivery and outcomes of their manualized treatments.

and the role of formal and informal social organization. Most importantly, it allowed for theorizing about the interaction of these two systems which the NEM posits as critical to issues of diagnosis, utilization, adherence and health care outcomes. In essence, individual careers may be facilitated or impeded by the interaction of treatment and community systems which set both structures and dynamics for the behaviors and outcomes for individuals who define themselves or are defined by others as "sick."

Embracing Complexity Without Losing Utility: The NEM III-R

Since the original version of the NEM-Phase II was proposed in 1999, three things have happened.

First, as detailed in the introductory chapter to this volume and alluded to above, there has been a decided move toward transdisciplinarity, defined as the incorporation of insights across disciplines and fields to provide a fuller understanding of any particular phenomena.

Second, the most visible and prominent development in the biomedical sciences has been research surrounding the Human Genome Project. The end result of this massive research endeavor has been that both social and medical sciences have had to rethink initial narrow prejudices. On the medical side, the decoding of human DNA sequences has led to the conclusion that the "environment" matters in triggering, suppressing, and even changing genetic predispositions and structures. In both positive and negative ways, macro to micro levels of social life have been implicated in phenotypic expression (Pescosolido 2006a). Epigenetics has become a vibrant line of medical inquiry drawing research and researchers from the social sciences. Social scientists have had to reconsider their stance regarding the body and its physical limits and strengths, not just its social construction (Pescosolido et al. 2008a). As Bearman (2008) has concluded, sociologists need to consider how the prominence of genetics changes our own theorizing about the effects of social structure. This reconfiguration is currently unfolding as individuals develop new projects that require transdisciplinarity or push existing projects further (e.g., the addition of biomarkers and DNA samples to the National Longitudinal Study of Adolescent Health Study, Add Health).

Third, the attention to geography and community as the influence of "place and space" has again become more visible in research. The work of sociologists has contributed to moving these issues to the forefront of transdisciplinary considerations (see Rob Sampson, David Takeuchi, Thomas Gieryn, Sigrun Olafsdottir, and Jason Beckfield, the latter pair who have pioneered a renewed emphasis on comparative health systems, both nationally and internationally; see Olafsdottir and Beckfield, this volume). In concert with Mechanic's (2004) call for more engagement of medical sociologists in health policy and Cockerham's consistent international focus, the reconceptualization of difference by geography has moved more to the center of our concerns. Thus, the resurgence of interest in communities, the advent of GPS technology and associated data, the development of multilevel modeling, and resurgence in cross-cultural work all pointed to greater elaboration of "context" in the NEM.

In response to these directions and on the occasion of the Reeder Lecture in 2005, the NEM-Phase III was sketched out. To be fair to any and all critics, the NEM has not proceeded systematically along the lines that Ostrom recently suggested. That sketch was preliminary and more was promised (Pescosolido 2006a). Moving that promise forward is the goal of this chapter – specifically, to define the "core subsystems" (i.e., the first level) that are key to health, illness, and healing outcomes, and begin a comprehensive listing of the concepts (i.e., the second level) of the NEM. Second-level concepts bring together factors that have proven promising in existing research. Individual researchers can select from them, propose new ways to think about and measure them (i.e., the third level), and add to the list. As Ostrom (2009, p. 420) notes, "The choice of relevant second or deeper levels of variables for analysis (from the large set of variables at multiple levels) depends on the particular questions under study….and the spatial and temporal scales of analysis."

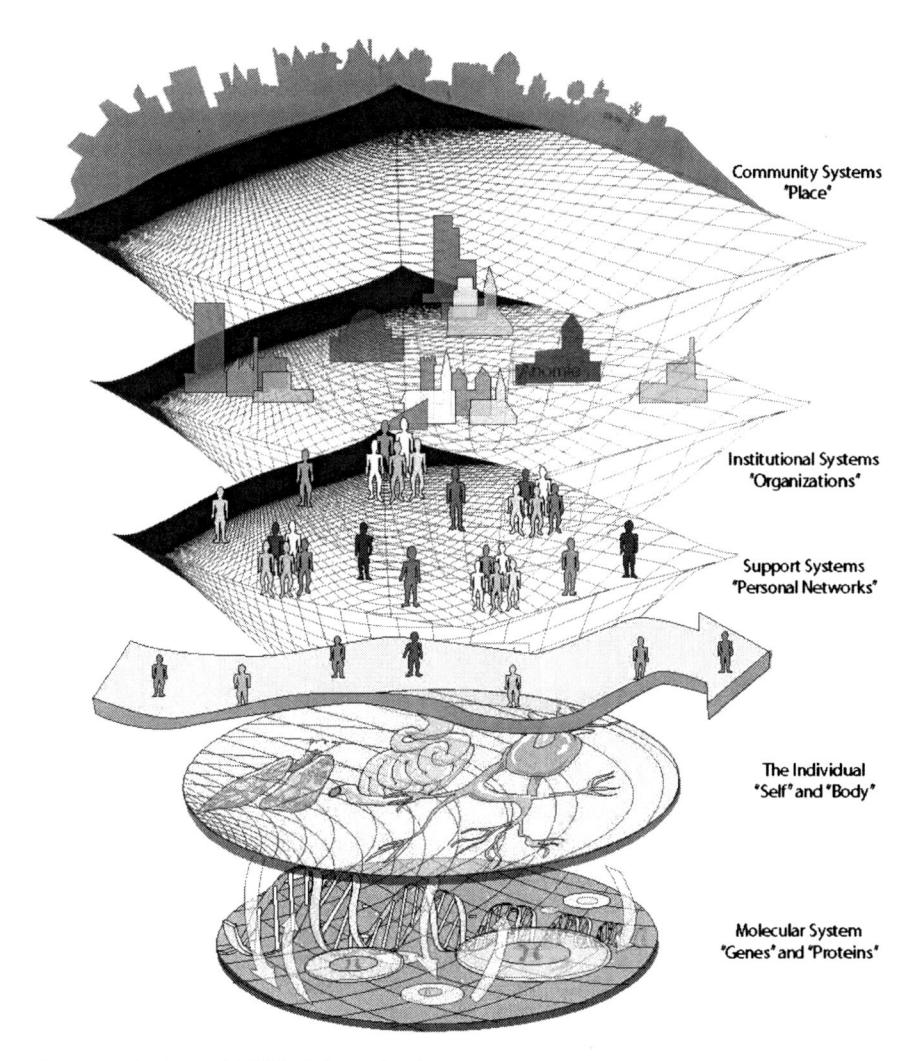

3 Organizing the Sociological Landscape for the Next Decades of Health

Fig. 3.2 Network episode model III-R, Primary level subsystems

The further development of the NEM requires an adaptation of and revision from its initial presentation (Pescosolido 2006a). As depicted in Fig. 3.2, the NEM III-R has the same five core systems as the NEM-Phase III – the community or "place," institutions or "organizations," the support system or "personal networks," the individual or "self" and "body," and the molecular system or "genes" and "proteins." The focus is on the dynamics of what happens to individuals in their health and illness careers (the arrow). These careers can trace lifelong patterns or simply encapsulate the onset and/or response to one set of health/illness problems. This is a key change in this third-phase of the NEM. Though initially developed as a utilization model, the NEM, backed by a wealth of evidence on the relevance and operation of social network ties *as an underlying cause* of health and illness (see review in Pescosolido and Levy 2002), has an expanded scope – as an organizing model potentially useful for social epidemiology as well as health services research. In that sense, the NEM started from the less-populated corners of medical sociology. As Bury (1991, p. 451) noted, sociologists "tend to be more interested in problems than in people's responses to tackling them."

This distinction, between epidemiology and health services research, in the sociomedical sciences has always been an artificial, even if pragmatically useful, one. In many cases, onset and response are intertwined even as we tend to ignore the interconnections because of subfield boundaries. In fact, much epidemiological data rely on an "official" label of disease that becomes known only because a diagnosis or death certificate determination has been made by a physician or other medical personnel (e.g., McKinlay 1995 on heart disease; Pescosolido and Mendelsohn 1986 on suicide). As indicated earlier, some pathways may not be initiated at the focal individual's request (e.g., employment or sports physicals; involuntary commitment); nevertheless, they involve the use of allopathic health services. Thus, identifying "cases" for many epidemiological studies is dependent on the lay recognition that something is wrong and on a response pathway that ends up in the formal health care system.[3] That said, it will be no surprise that more theoretical effort will need to go into the NEM's epidemiological side since what follows will draw heavily from "consequences" rather than "causes" research within medical sociology, and will rely on substantive areas where this approach has been most readily adopted (i.e., mental health and illness; substance abuse, chronic illness, infectious disease).

A major goal of this chapter is to take the first step in moving the NEM III-R forward toward a complex approach. To do so, three issues are critical to theorizing the health, illness, and health care career: (1) defining dynamic processes and outcomes; (2) defining the central forces that shape pathways to illness/disease (epidemiology) and treatment (use of health services); and (3) conceptualizing the complexity of cross-level influences.

Defining Dynamics in the Health and Illness Career: The Core Target of the NEM III-R

The undulating arrow in Fig. 3.2 is designed to make clear that the production of many illnesses, particularly complex chronic ones, as well as the response to them is embedded in a dynamic process with outcomes at each point potentially conditioned by earlier ones. Table 3.1 provides an initial set of Level 2 variables for the health and illness career. The focus is on key role "entrances" and

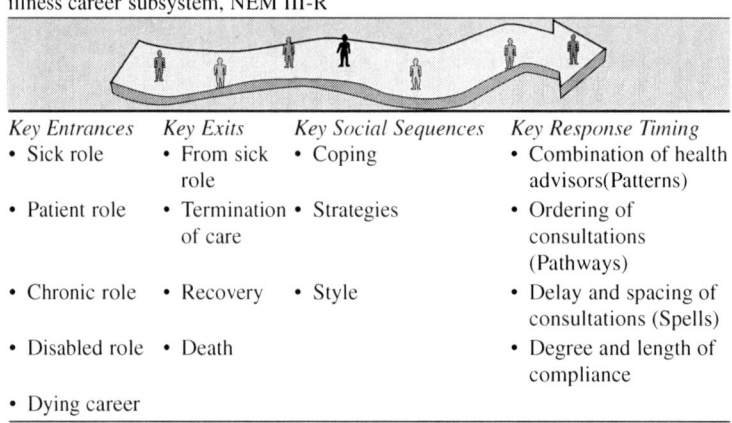

Table 3.1 Relevant network concepts in the secondary level – health and illness career subsystem, NEM III-R

Key Entrances	Key Exits	Key Social Sequences	Key Response Timing
• Sick role	• From sick role	• Coping	• Combination of health advisors (Patterns)
• Patient role	• Termination of care	• Strategies	• Ordering of consultations (Pathways)
• Chronic role	• Recovery	• Style	• Delay and spacing of consultations (Spells)
• Disabled role	• Death		• Degree and length of compliance
• Dying career			

---

[3] In population studies that have developed sophisticated tools (e.g., the CIDI in the National Comorbidity Studies; Kessler et al. 1998) to measure population-based prevalence rather than rely on institutional data, this is not the case. Yet the effort that goes into establishing prevalence has generally meant little remaining time for a health services component or even a sophisticated social network component for etiological analyses.

"exists," as "punctuation points" in the social process of illness, as well as on patterns, pathways, and trajectories. Key social sequences include a cognitive stream (coping), a action stream (strategy), and an affective stream (style; Bury 1991). Given its affinity to life course perspective, the NEM III-R targets timing and spacing (when the transitions occur); duration (time to complete a transition); and order (the sequencing of role changes; Elder 1978). The NEM III-R provides the freedom to isolate the decision to seek out a physician, for example, but it requires some understanding of when this occurs in relation to previous choices (Elder's 1978 "multiphased decision process"). It embraces the examination of "research-discovered need" (e.g., as in the National Comorbidity Studies) and looks at the network forces that translate that into various response patterns. In sum, these findings both came from and support the first descriptive hypothesis of the NEM III-R.

Unlike early stage models, events do not have to occur in a particular sequence. Rather, research can map "a flexible set of points which can be transversed over again, going backward and forward" (Twaddle and Hessler 1987). For example, an individual whose claim of illness has been rejected by the social network (i.e., barred entry to the sick role) can still proceed to the decision to seek out formal advice (i.e., attempt entry into the patient role). As noted above, an individual's illness career may begin at the point of physical examinations required by various social institutions (e.g., school sports physicals, employment or insurance exams, mandatory college vaccinations).

Understanding different pathways and sequences becomes a critical part of a dynamic approach to health, illness, and healing (Pescosolido 1991). Some of these steps are recognizable and researchable in and of themselves as dynamic processes: onset (the timing of physical or mental behavior or capacities); recognition (the decision that something is wrong, that is, entry into the sick role); utilization (the decision to seek care, that is, entry into patient role); health care outcomes (including the decision to follow advice of the various "providers" sought out, e.g., medication or regime adherence); and health outcomes (recovery, death, disability, stability, or chronicity). Each comprises a dynamic sequence and can be used to draw boundaries around and coordinate the research map. Alternatively, they can be strung together marking the borderlines between health and illness; and for the increasing presence of chronic and severe illnesses, tracing the emergent character of health problems and the "biographic disruption" that follows (Bury 1982).

A general advantage of the NEM over earlier models is that it neither prescribes nor proscribes the "proper" response to health problems (e.g., physician-based versus alternative medical systems). It problematizes each stage, asking that we come to understand, through the collection of empirical data on coping (cognitive), strategy (action), and style (affective), what possible patterns and sequences exist (Bury 1991). The NEM argues, in fact, that not homogenizing such different processes into simple static variables may open up understandings to critical issues in health, illness, and healing that have frustrated researchers, providers and policy makers to date. Figure 3.3, adapted from Xie et al.'s recent study (2009) of the 10-year "careers" of individuals with comorbid mental health and substance abuse disorders, provides an illustration.

In a traditional research frame, "recovery" or "outcomes" might be operationalized as a zero-one dichotomy ("successful treatment outcomes" or not). Both the heterogeneity of the patterns and the key influences of timing would likely be lost. A trajectories approach accepts such heterogeneity and enhances our ability to understand and intervene on the distal or proximal root causes. Xie and colleagues (2009, p. 804) document four patterns regarding drug use: no abstinence, early abstinence, late abstinence, and unstable abstinence. By identifying these through a latent class trajectory analysis, they suggest that different clinical approaches could be tailored to individual differences.[4] However,

---

[4] Other analyses might also be used to take advantage of these time-ordered, detailed data (e.g., examining the timing or "spells" of substance abuse, Pavalko et al. 2007).

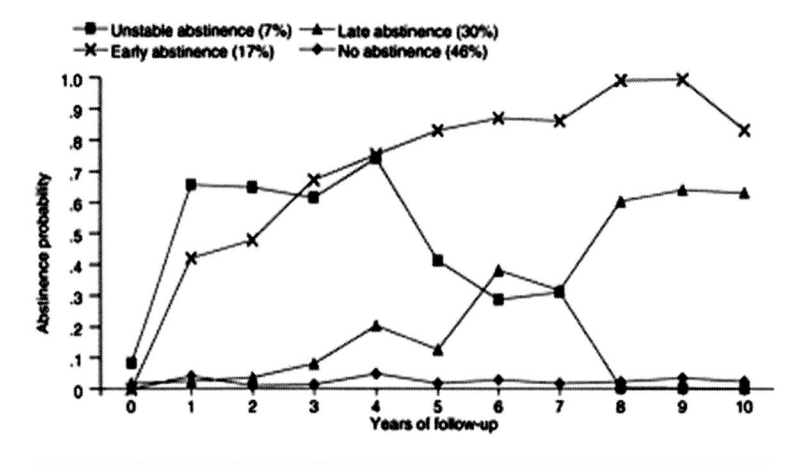

ᵃ Top: trajectories based on stage of substance abuse recovery, as defined by the Substance Abuse Treatment Scale (SATS) (possible scores range from 1 to 8, with higher scores indicating higher stages of recovery). Bottom: trajectories of abstinence

Fig. 3.3 Ten-year substance abuse outcome trajectories for 177 clients with serious mental illness and cooccurring substance use disorders. Reprinted with Permission from Xie et al. (2009)

examining complex patterns and diverse pathways has rarely been considered even when theories have long claimed that individuals may reach very similar endpoints traveling very different routes.[5]

Other work has provided findings indicating that we can, in fact, uncover both different pathways and different trajectories. In the Indianapolis Network Mental Health Study (Pescosolido et al. 1998) the Mental Health Care Utilization among Puerto Ricans Study (Pescosolido et al. 1998), and The National Survey of Access to Medical Care (Pescosolido 1992), we were able to map a set of limited pathways to care using clustering methods and multinomial logit models. More recent research has provided even greater support for dynamic approaches. Judge et al.'s (2008) narrative from 15 individuals identified three basic response patterns – withdrawal, avoiding help, and coming to terms – in confronting psychotic illness. The "Pathways to Care" Study in the UK found that 100 out of the 500 illness episodes they recorded ended up in primary care (approximating the number expected in traditional survey research). More interesting are the sequenced "containment" strategies people employed in their response to illness, "suppressing signs and symptoms, ignoring them, concealing them or attending to them....moving among the continuum from containment to an illness state" (Rogers et al. 1999, p. 106; see also Carpentier and Bernard (2010).

These patterns, types, and trajectories, in and of themselves, become the focus of explanation and a preliminary analytic charge that can be mapped onto alternative hypotheses. Regarding caregiver health problems, for example, Pavalko and Woodbury (2000) suggest both the adaptation hypothesis (i.e., stress increases and plateaus then remain stable or even improve as care giving continues) and the stress proliferation ("wear and tear") hypothesis (i.e., stress increases as the person continues to provide care). Both patterns may be in operation over time for the same individuals, or these patterns may characterize individuals in different social locations (e.g., gender. kin/non-kin) or who face different kinds of health issues (e.g., Alzheimer's, schizophrenia, cancer). Pavalko and Woodbury conclude that the body of research on caregiver health is inconsistent, in part, because they have tapped into different stages of the caregiving process.

---

[5]For example, Durkheim's classic work on suicide (1897/1951) laid out four types – altruistic, egoistic, anomic, and fatalistic – each stemming from very different social contexts in which individuals find themselves. Yet, there are few, if any, studies that separate out suicides by type or any schematics to classify suicide types.

According to Elder (1978), dynamic approaches avoid the "conventional script" flavor of other models. While a strength, this view raises addition complexities to be considered. In particular two factors, implied above, are primary. *First*, the lines of disease and disorder are fluid, indicated, for example, in mental health by the "consensus" conversations that will create the new version of the Diagnostic and Statistical Manual (DSM) of the American Psychiatric Association as well as in cancer by the continually moving line of "precancerous" changes. The processes underlying what happens in this arena can result from contagion or homophily (Christakis and Fowler 2009), parallel to the classic concerns in medical sociology with social selection versus social causation processes (e.g., Wheaton 1978). Pragmatically, however, research proceeds by cutting into intertwined dynamic processes at some point, which, as Conley (2010) argues for genetic influences, have to be carefully thought out. Claiming that research is looking to "associations" alone does not get one "off the hook" regarding issues of causality, at minimum, because such claims do not align with using statistical tools that have implicit notions of causality built into them.

Second, this problem extends to the response to the onset of symptoms. Who is considered a "medical care advisor" and what separates a network tie "consultation" for advice on what to do from one on who to see? Such individuals in contemporary US society are not limited to practitioners legitimated by the modern medical establishment (see Pescosolido 1992 for a list; also Kelner et al. 2000). Drawing from the SOS Framework, the NEM assumes that (1) all societies hold a vast reserve of people who can be and are consulted during an illness episode (i.e., Gurin et al. 1960 view that a multiplicity of resources share therapeutic functions); (2) at best, rationality is "bounded" and individual "satisfice" (Simon 1976) resulting in a series of decisions over some stretch of time that form "strategies" through successive limited comparison (Lindblom1959); and (3) through mutual exchange (or lack thereof) individuals come to attach meaning to situations and determine actions (Pescosolido 1992).

Thus, network processes can be both cause and consequence, and it is possible for network theory to provide theoretical guides and empirical strategies for both. In Puerto Rico, the "search for care" among those who recognized mental health problems produced a set of patterns which variously included family, friends, the clergy, primary care providers, and mental health specialists. Thus, the activation of network ties, themselves, created utilization patterns.

More recent work has embraced and unpacked this complexity in dynamic processes, multiple levels of influence, and social network structures. Carpentier and colleagues (2010) built on traditional narrative approach using network data to analyze the initial phases of the social processes associated with care trajectories for individuals eventually diagnosed with Alzheimer's disease. Analyzing the analysis of action sequences reported by caregivers, they defined entry into the care trajectory as the period from first recognition of dementia symptoms to the point of diagnosis. This new, intriguing research moves past earlier research that focused on caregivers' characteristics. The nature of the onset of this disease, recognition "is intimately linked to interactions not only amongst family members but also amongst friends, neighbours and health professionals" (Carpentier et al. 2010, p. 1501). They combined a focus on social networks, social dynamics, and action sequences, seeing the understanding of initial phases of care trajectories as essential to early detection and intervention, as well as understanding the course of the disease and outcomes.

The data structure from their research is reproduced, with permission, in Fig. 3.4. On the left, the caregiver's social network at the first sign of symptom manifestation (T_0) is listed. In this example, the initial network included six ties – the caregiver (CG), the ill relative (IR), and four individuals who provided the caregiver with support (labeled 1, 2, 3, and 4). The rest of the graph reveals the narrative analysis of social network dynamics. Actors are represented by lines that begin when the network tie enters into the social process and ends when they are no longer involved. Some actors provided support (individuals 1 through 4), while some did not (individuals 5 and 6). Developing over 100 codes to represent significant actions or events, Carpentier and Bernard superimposed codes on tie dynamics.

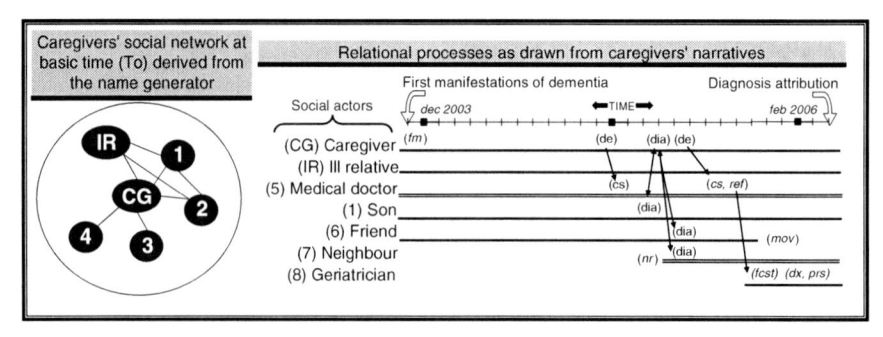

[Figure 3.4 diagram]

- (fm) First manifestation
- (de) Decision to see a doctor
- (cs) Medical consultation
- (dia) Discussion/dialogue with the son, the friend and the neighbour
- (nr) New relationship
- (ref) Referral by the doctor
- (fcst) First consultation by a team at a memory clinic
- (dx) Diagnosis of Alzheimer's disease
- (prs) Prescription
- (mov) Move of residence

Fig. 3.4 Timeline, social networks and the pathways to care data for one case at T_0 in Alzheimer's caregiver study. Reprinted with Permission from Carpentier et al. (2010)

In the end, they find five trajectories which they name by the key factor shaping them: families' past experience; watershed events; organizational effects; complex trajectories with gentle negotiations, and complex trajectories with difficult negotiations. The trajectories influence the timing of diagnosis. In Types 1, 2, and 3, diagnoses occurred earlier, within a year, while Types 4 and 5 revealed both greater complexity in social interactions coupled with later diagnosis. Analyses like these provide new insights into the dynamic processes of onset, diagnosis, and treatment, hopefully becoming more common as data collection and analytic tools improve, and as researchers embrace the inevitable complexity of health and health care outcomes.

Defining the Core Factors that Shape Illness/Disease and Treatment Pathways

Understanding a complex whole requires knowledge about specific variables and how their component parts are related (Ostrom 2009, p. 10). As Elder (1978) notes, life course models are not explanatory models. Describing patterns, pathways, and trajectories has often led to the neglect of explaining them (Hagestad and Neuganen 1985). The health and illness career represents a single life path, helping to impose order to our observations by providing "a conceptual mechanism that links individuals and their experiences to the community, lay and professional" (Freidson 1970, p. 242). The next step lies in understanding how these are shaped by both internal and external forces.

The NEM III-R, unlike other models, privileges the explanatory power of social networks. The general question is how are these theorized to work? In its most basic form, social structures can be conceptualized as a net, made up of network connections with different features topographically (see Fig. 3.5). According to Durkheim, two dimensions cut across social contexts. The dimension running from left to right in Fig. 3.5 represents integration (i.e., care and concern) with underintegration represented by sparse network ties (i.e., connections far apart) and overintegration by dense network ties (i.e., connections very close together). Another dimension, running back to forward in

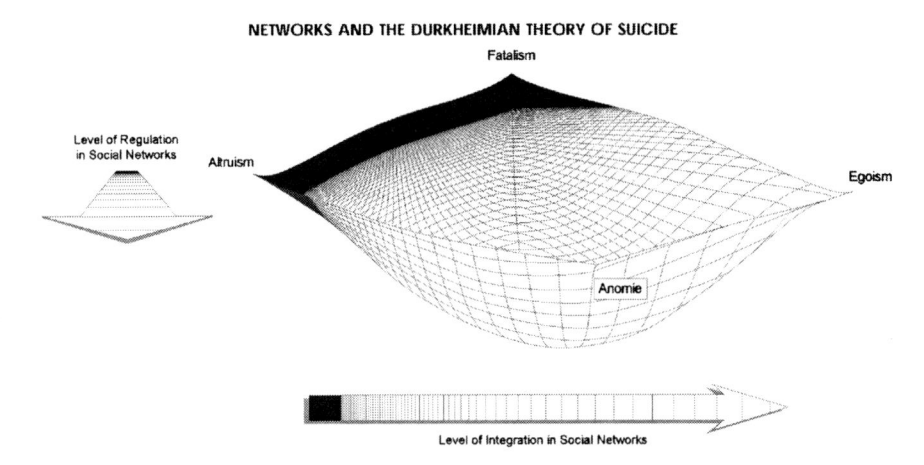

Fig. 3.5 Network translation of the Durkheimian Theory of Suicide. Reprinted with Permission from Pescosolido and Levy (2002)

Fig. 3.5, represents regulation (i.e., guidance, appraisal, pressure) and similarly runs from dense to sparse in terms of network ties. When these two are considered simultaneously, four "most dangerous locations" are defined by the poles. When individuals exist in social structures with too little integration or regulation, the social net is "loose'" or "open," and there is little in the social structure to "catch" individuals when crisis destabilizes their equilibrium. In the face of challenge, the social network ties are insufficient and individuals "fall" through the net. Thus, the absence of a modest number of network ties that provide love, care, and support *or* guidance, limits and oversight results in problems – disease, death, inadequate care, lonely neighborhoods, unmethylated genes, etc. For Durkheim, the location on the spatial network map with too little integration produced a state of egoism in the social structure, a higher "egoistic" suicide rate (at the macro level) or a greater probability of egoistic suicide (at the micro level). For similar topographical reasons, locations characterized by under-regulation also put individuals and societies at a similar level of risk, but for fundamentally different reasons. With networks that provide too little regulation, the social structure is in a state of "anomie," the individual in a state of "anomia," and the probability of suicide is high. Both locations produce "diseases of the infinite" because they provide no "grip" in the societal safety net that supports people during times of individual or community crises.

Figure 3.5 also depicts problem locations in societies which are too regulated or too integrated. Here, social networks are overbearing and the safety net closes up. There is no flexibility or "give" to the social net. When individuals, organizations, or societies face crisis, the overbearing nature of social networks produces a wall which shatters rather than supports. Like the situation of "too little," the situation of "too much" has dire consequences. Confronting challenges in the context of an over-integrated social structure produces altruistic social structures and correspondingly altruistic suicide (e.g., war heroes, saints) or on the overregulated location a fatalistic social structure with fatalistic suicides (e.g., mass cult suicides).

Research in the medical social sciences has tended to have a view of modern societies as problematic and social support as good. However, they can become "perverse utopias" (Coser and Coser1979). Even though communities that are overintegrated or overregulated are, by their very nature, not open to free observation by outsiders, we have caught occasional glimpses (e.g., People's Temple in 1978; see Pescosolido 1994 for examples and detail). Furthermore, we have tended to think in unidimensional terms. But, Umberson's wellness-regulation model (Umberson 1987; Umberson and Greer 1990) examines the link between social relationships and mortality through the monitoring and regulating functions of social networks in marriage (assumed to be "good" for health because it provides support). Marital ties produce more regulation for men with a positive effect on health, controlling for the level of integration in the marriage, which has its own positive effect. The loss of the marital bond increases negative health behaviors for everyone, but particularly for men. Men "profit" in marriage, to use Durkheim's terms, at least in part by the regularity with which their wives cajole, coerce, or demand that their husbands engage in healthy behavior.

Thus, the "safety net" is made up of the two most important and general dimensions of "societies," in Simmel's sense of social circles – integration and regulation – with a general curvilinear prediction surface.[6] That is, Fig. 3.5 looks like safety net on purpose. The middle (or lowest point) which in a safety net has the greatest supportive bounce is where social networks are optimal (i.e., moderate on both dimensions). Like a safety net, it is the best place to "land," and predictions would be for better health. As individual social actors fall on places on the net that are "higher" (i.e., more extreme values or amounts), the predictions are more grave for health, illness, and healing. Perhaps what is most crucial to understand about the net is that it does not depict what any one individual "has." Rather it depicts the theoretical space on which an individual's networks can exist. Individual social actors, because of the networks they "have," stand on or over a particular spot on the net. This spot describes or summarizes their networks and, as a result, is accompanied by a prediction regarding outcomes.

This conceptualization allows us to move away from the general tendency to think of social structures as fixed. The net is fixed because it is a theoretical projection; however, what can change, and often does dramatically in the face of health and health care crises, is where social actors stand on the net. Movement across the landscape of the net represents a dynamic that also has predictive implications for dynamics across the illness career. At the initial phase of the illness career, individuals may wish to provide support; however as a situation evolves into a lengthy chronic one, ties (particularly those at the periphery) may "chain off" in response to caregiver burden, other responsibilities, or lack of reciprocity in the relationship.

This predictive surface can be useful for understanding the complexities and potential impact of social structures. As such, only the levels "above" the individual are depicted in this way in Fig. 3.2. And, while Barabási (2003) claims that *all* networks have a similar structure (basically core-periphery), there is insufficient theoretical or empirical work to support the claim that the response surface of brain networks (Sporns et al. 2004) or protein transport systems at the molecular level would take on the same predictions as in Fig. 3.5. Thus, while it might be the case that gaps or excess in the number of neural networks, for example, may signal problems, no research yet suggests common dimensions that may define the predictive space. Thus, the NEM III-R simply represents levels below the individual as involving networks and linking to other levels through network connections.

The NEM III-R Core Subsystem: The Community

As listed in Table 3.2, Panel A, this level of social structure taps into a range of possible geographic contexts – the global system (Alderson and Beckfield 2004); regions (e.g., the EU); nation states; relevant within-nation units (states, departments, counties, parishes); communities (Christakis and Fowler 2009); and neighborhoods (natural or administratively smaller units such as Census blocks, Liu et al. 2010; Mazumder et al. 2010). "Place-based contacts" have been

---

[6]Durkheim's use of the term "society," or even "societies," weakens the power of sociological explanations (Tilly 1984, pp. 27–28; Pescosolido 1994). If we replace "society" with "network," this idea becomes less ambiguous. Each context into which an individual social actor is connected represents a network that can offer the "constant interchange of ideas and feelings, something like mutual moral support" that Durkheim (1951, p. 210) discusses.

Table 3.2 Relevant network concepts in the secondary level – NEM III-R

Panel A: Community core subsystem

Key communities	Key network structures	Key network contents	Key network dynamics
• Global	• In and out degrees	• Collective effervescence	• Diffusion
• National	• Centrality	• Relevant cultural beliefs	• Shifting alliances, beliefs, and structures
• Regional	• Multiplexity	• Social and economic resources	• Duration
• Political divisions (states, departments, parishes)			• Changing overall forms
• Community			
• Neighborhood			

Panel B: Institution and organization core subsystem

Key institutions and organization	Key treatment network structures	Key network content	Key network dynamics	Key network functions
• Treatment system	• Position in inter-organizational networks	• Cultural climate	• Shifting resource patterns	• Information
• Civic and religious organizations	• Intra-organizational structure	• Collective effervescence	• Diffusion	• Advice
• Professional organizations	• Multiplexity			• Regulation
				• Expressive or emotional support
				• Material or practical support

Panel C: Personal networks core subsystem

Key network domains	Key network structures	Key network content	Key network functions
• Family	• Size	• Beliefs	• Information
• Friends	• Density	• Attitudes	• Advice
• Work	• Duration	• Cultural "toolboxes"	• Regulation
• Voluntary organization	• Reciprocity		• Expressive or Emotional support
	• Strength of tie		• Material or practical support
	• Multiplexity		• Appraisal

Panel D: Individual core subsystem

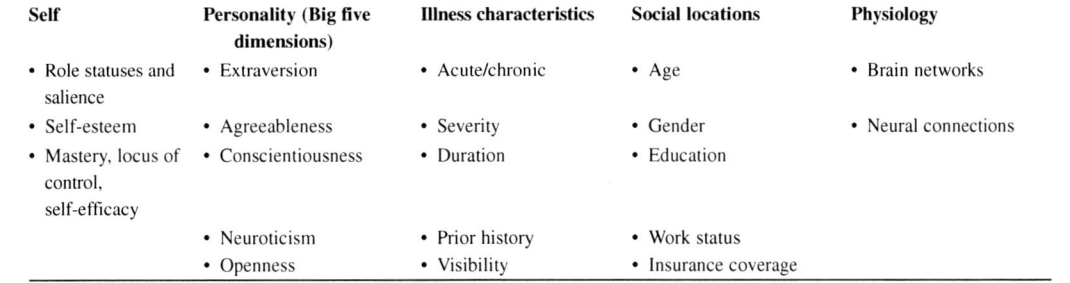

Self	Personality (Big five dimensions)	Illness characteristics	Social locations	Physiology
• Role statuses and salience	• Extraversion	• Acute/chronic	• Age	• Brain networks
• Self-esteem	• Agreeableness	• Severity	• Gender	• Neural connections
• Mastery, locus of control, self-efficacy	• Conscientiousness	• Duration	• Education	
	• Neuroticism	• Prior history	• Work status	
	• Openness	• Visibility	• Insurance coverage	

shown to shape tuberculosis transmission (Klovdahl et al. 2002) and suicide (Pescosolido and Georgianna 1989). Penner (2008) points out that there is considerable variation in genetic differences internationally, a finding not easily explained by biological theories, but that suggests the importance of geographic contexts.

At this level, while actual social network data on ties are often (but not always) unavailable, proxies are available. The critical point is to map the available data onto predictions about the key network structures, contents, and dynamics outlined with only basic exemplars in Table 3.2, Panel A. For example, the divorce profile of a county or city reveals something about the weakness of the social safety net in general. It may also hint at the opportunity, or lack thereof, for individuals to find other people with similar experiences with whom to commiserate or with whom to form new ties and expectations (in the spirit of Gibbs' theory of status integration [Gibbs and Martin 1964; 1974]). Religion, as another example, is often thought to be a protective structure; and, in much medical sociology research, it has been found to be so. But Durkheim reminded us that different religions can have different amounts of regulation and integration, and contemporary research in the U.S. has debated the protective power of religion, particularly Catholicism and Protestantism (Brashears 2010; Breault 1986; Pescosolido and Georgianna 1989).

So, we have evidence that place matters. Further, it contextualizes influences at other levels. In the above example about the religious profiles of "communities," the more interesting question lies in whether the same religion has the same protective influence across contexts. While areas that have a large number of Jewish "adherents" are associated with a lower suicide rate in the northeast; it is not the case in the south (Pescosolido 1990). The effects of religious affiliation appear to be more pronounced in regions of traditional historical strength where the opportunity to construct and maintain strong ties comes from the solid infrastructure grounding of the community, and also in urban or other high-population-density areas where the sheer likelihood of locating coreligionists is greater.

The Core Subsystem of the NEM III-R: Institutional Systems

Three important types of institutional systems (indicated in Table 3.2, Panel B) are central: to the NEM III-R: (1) the focal organizations, in this case, those primarily in the health care system; (2) professional and advocacy organizations directly related to the social construction of and resource availability for health care generally and medically defined problems specifically; and (3) civic organizations which help to shape the social environments and individuals connections to it. As Tilly (1984) argued, network interactions produce systematic structures and contents (or cultures) and sometimes become crystallized into organizations and institutions that, in turn, affect social interactions.

Regarding treatment organizations, networks theoretically tie components of the physician–patient relationship, the therapeutic alliance, notions of organizational culture and climate, and system integration. That is, in the treatment organizational field, six basic sets of relationships exist: (1) between individuals and providers, (2) among providers in each organization, (3) between providers and the lay community, (4) between providers and the set of organizations that constitute the "service system," (5) among organizations in the organizational field, and (6) between providers and the administrative structure representatives within the treatment and larger political systems (Pescosolido 1996). In most situations, social networks are not "treatment" per se, but they shape the likelihood that both individuals and providers will subscribe to treatment regimens, comply with them, search for alternative approaches, and facilitate transition to the community. The kinds of social networks that exist in treatment settings create a climate of care, affect the work of medical providers, and shape reactions of individuals in treatment (Pescosolido and Boyer1999; Pescosolido et al. 1995). In turn, organizational climate affects family involvement

(Wright 1997; Wright et al. 2003) and connections to community-based resources, both of which influence outcomes. For example, treatment programs that better coordinate psychiatric and drug treatment with housing programs reduce the cycle of incarceration, homelessness, and treatment disruptions for vulnerable populations (Copeland et al. 2009). These ties to other organizations in the social service system and even to civic and religious organizations have been linked to better outcomes. More importantly, such ties can reduce health disparities. Children from families with relatively low levels of human and financial capital fare better with respect to health status when their mothers are more active participants in community organization (Nobles and Frankenberg 2009).

In fact, Fallot (1993) has argued that various theories and models of case management in mental health, for example, can be understood as distinct cultures that represent divergent images of the individual person and the world in which people live. That is, central to each class of case management models lies an image and, more importantly, a blueprint of whether and how to link individuals with three structures in the community most relevant to their success – the treatment system, the social service system, and the lay community. Models differ in significant ways with regard to both the extensiveness and types of ties that are created with and around individuals in each of these spheres. Community-based care models, compared with long-term institutional care models, hold a different view of the important structural elements of "community" and the potential of individuals with serious mental illness is to "recover" or "survive" in the community (Pescosolido et al. 1995).

The Core Subsystem of the NEM III-R: The Support System: Personal Networks

Personal networks represent the most easily understood and well-researched arena that connects social networks to health, illness, disease, and health care outcomes (Berkman and Glass 2000). Strong social ties have been found to mitigate against negative health outcomes but also to be the vectors of health risk, morbidity, and mortality (tuberculosis, Klovdahl et al. 2002; obesity, Christakis and Fowler 2007). At the most basic level, Cornwell and Waite (2009) note that, in a wide variety of ways and for a range of problems, research has identified that social isolation poses health risks. They find that living alone, having a small social network, infrequent participation in social activities, and feelings of loneliness tap into social disconnectedness and social isolation, each of which is independently associated with lower levels of self-rated health among older Americans.

The idea behind social network ties and health, and how they work regarding health and health care, at least in part, is now well accepted across the landscape of the biomedical and sociobehavioral sciences. According to Rogers et al. (1999, p. 112) "It is thought that social networks not only buffer the experience of stress which reduces the need for help, but they may also provide emotional support, material aid, services and information, so precluding the necessity of professional assistance. Also, networks also transmit norms and values about help-seeking. Most important… is the way in which social networks act as screening and referral agents to professional services." For example, the interaction between high life stress exposure and low social support was consistently linked to increased rates of health service utilization (Counte and Glandon 1991). Among psychiatric outpatients, less cohesive network structures were associated with a longer time frame for initiating treatment because the absence of social ties delayed problem recognition (Carpentier and White 2002).

However, what seems like inconsistent effects of social networks can be clarified through four tenants embedded in the NEM and reflected in Table 3.2, Panel C. First, as predicted by Durkheim in Fig. 3.5, more is not better. Falci and McNeely (2009) document that adolescents with *either* too large or too small a network have higher levels of depressive symptoms. Riley and Eckenrode (1986) caution that larger networks are more likely to have more interpersonal problems, also suggesting that networks can be too large. Second, the influence of social networks may differ for individuals in different social locations. In Falci and McNeeley's study, depression among girls only occurred at low levels of network cohesion. For boys, the negative mental health effects of over-integration occurred only at high levels of network cohesion. Similarly, Artis (1997) found an interaction between network structure and how adults perceive and react to depression. That is, opposite sex dyads were more accepting of behaviors "outside the norm" than were network members in same sex dyads. Third, many different conceptualizations exist under the umbrella of "social ties"; accumulated knowledge is far from clear; and, as a result, the research is scattered in its specific conclusions while providing general support that social ties matter (Nobles and Frankenberg 2009; Pescosolido 2006). Rarely is more than one dimension of social networks explored. As a recent exception, Song and Lin (2009) document that social capital contributes to health in ways that are beyond and distinct from the contribution of social support. Fourth, as Freidson (1970) long ago theorized, and as the NEM incorporated from its beginnings, networks are not, in and of themselves, predictive. While the greater substance of personal networks can determine the amount of influence (i.e., the "push"), only the cultural norms held in them can determine the trajectory (i.e., for or away from health or the formal health care system). Thus, if they are the "friends and supporters of psychotherapy" that Kadushin (1966) described among the urban upper and middles classes in New York City, we can expect greater use of the private mental health system, However, if they are the strong and plentiful family ties of individuals who recognize mental health problems in Puerto Rico, then the use of the formal system is likely to be low. Each network structure provides a rich, deep, and consistent "united front" to individuals with mental health issues; they hold substantial sources of daily resources and influence; and the cultural content of those networks pushes individuals in opposite directions regarding the use of services (Pescosolido et al. 1998b).

The Core Subsystem of the NEM III-R: The Individual: Self and Body

At the individual level, Table 3.2 (Panel D) displays a complex range of factors derived from different disciplines. Some of these are clearly outside of sociology's purview (e.g., brain networks, Sporns 2004) or skirt at the edges of our subfield of social psychology (e.g., the "Big Five" personality traits). Suffice it to say, at this point, that we can expect these to matter, in and of themselves, but they remain for our sister social sciences to explore. However, the NEM III-R's expectation that, within this level, these factors will interact with social forces that sociologists traditionally examine, calls for collaboration. For example, the single best predictor of the use of mental health services is the need for care. However, the relationship between need for treatment and the use of services by those in need is far from perfect. Even the nature of the illness itself shapes psychosocial reactions routinely associated with service use. In mental illness, positive symptoms appear to influence hope and self-esteem, mediating internalized stigma and increasing social avoidance and avoidance coping (Yanos et al. 2008).

The proposition that the "self" is a social product, defined and developed through social interactions, lies directly in our intellectual territory (Stryker 1980; Lively and Smith 2010). Across the health and illness career, we can expect social networks to support or discourage identity shifts (at the social psychological or cognitive levels) that can reframe and reinforce the view of (1) a medical problem as real and chronic *or* ignorable and temporary (e.g., the low adherence rates of hypertensive drugs), (2) symptom relief *or* doctor's orders as the appropriate marker for discontinuing medication (e.g., compliance problems with all of the most common antibiotics), and 3) social costs (i.e., stigma) *or* medical costs (i.e., need) as the important determinant of illness behavior (e.g., Day et al. 2005; Rosenfield 1997).

Finally, while perhaps only hinting at other social factors (e.g., cultural norms), research has repeatedly shown how social location matters at various contextual levels. For example, Kandula et al. (2009) find that, among Asian-American men, higher levels of perceived neighborhood cohesion were associated with lower odds of smoking. But the effects are complex. As Schnittker and colleagues (2005) note, even opposing sides seem to take for granted that African-Americans are more averse to using health care and more skeptical of effectiveness. But in their research, as well as in Snowden et al.'s (2009) work using the National Survey of American Life and National Comorbidity Study-Replication (NCS-R), the reluctance to use and actual use of mental health services did not fit the stereotypical predictions. For example, while American and Caribbean blacks reported higher odds than whites of having psychiatric hospitalization, this was not the case for foreign-born Caribbean blacks (Snowden et al. 2009).

The Core Subsystem of the NEM III-R: The Molecular System: Genes and Proteins

This level is the one least familiar to sociologists. My focus here is neither to lay out the basics nor to suggest within-level research since both are done better by others (see Conley 2010 or Perry 2010). Thus, Table 3.2 has no panel corresponding to this level. All of my attention lies *across* levels, in how social factors interact with the genome, with protein signaling mechanisms, and with other molecular processes. The goal here is to recall and reinforce Bearman's (2008) recent insights on the relationship of sociological investigations to epigenetic issues.

Bearman claims that our concerns about collaboration on genetic issues are based on three suspicions – all untenable. The focus on genetics neither legitimates the status quo, recalls the eugenics movement of the early twentieth century, nor undermines the "sociological project." Rather, he argues the opposite: "The obvious fact is that genetic expression can only reveal itself through social structural change" (p. v). It is, for example, the case that obesity can only occur in a society with food surpluses; alcohol abuse disorders can only occur where alcohol is allowed. The point is, looking at genetics "reveals" the complex role of the family in obesity, where it can predispose individuals to health problems (Martin 2008), and in alcohol disorders, where strong family support virtually washes away the enhanced risk arising from genetic endowment (Pescosolido et al. 2008). *That* social factors matter is no longer contested; rather, *how* they matter and in what ways they matter lies at the heart of the sociological contribution to the new generation of transdisciplinarity research on health, illness, and healing. And, in the end, as both Bearman (2008) and Martin (2008) remind us, sociological research engaged at this level is likely to reveal more and different insights about the power of social forces, social structures, and social interactions.

Conceptualizing Cross-level Influences: Thinking in Fractal Terms

With all of these levels of social structure (and the many levels noted within each level in Table 3.2), how can the NEM and sociology resolve or even assist us in thinking through the potential complexity of social structure? When sociologists draw from Durkheim's theory, the most adaptable reference is geographic – states, nations, communities that can be characterized as having some degree of integration and regulation (Table 3.2, Panel A). This image is clear simply by referencing the bulk of sociological and social science research on suicide which analyzes geographically based suicide rates, even when looking at time trends. However, this research has been done at cross-national,

national, and regional levels. Furthermore, community-based social networks are not the only examples of over-regulated social structures. On a much smaller scale, there have been scores of sensational descriptions of perverse or severely "dysfunctional" family structures (e.g., Lundgren's schismatic Mormon sect in West Virginia and Ohio) as well as endless media reports of sexual abuse and incest in families, daycare centers, or other social organizations which depend on secrecy and excessive regulation (Pescosolido 1994). Figure 3.2 provides an overall view, while Table 3.2 addresses the more complex and refined types and valences of resources that come from the complexity of social network ties (Wellman and Wortley 1990).

This raises a question about contextual levels. Where does this "net" exist? How can personal networks be context and, at the same time, operate in a larger cultural context that, itself, is a social network structure that can facilitate or inhibit acceptance of general cultural norms and beliefs (White et al. 1976)? The answer may lie in coupling Simmel's (1955) original notion that individuals shape and are shaped by their interaction in several "social circles" that have their own structure with Abbott's (2001) claim that social processes and structures are, in essence, fractal structures.[7]

In Simmel's conceptualization (Fig. 3.6), the individuality and identity of individuals in modern society result from their position at the intersection of social circles (white "dot" in Fig. 3.6). Compared with premodern societies that could be described by totally nested, concentric social circles, the greater freedoms in contemporary society allow for "individuation" (see Pescosolido and Rubin 2000 for more detail). Figure 3.6, in essence, is a picture of the individual in society with a view from

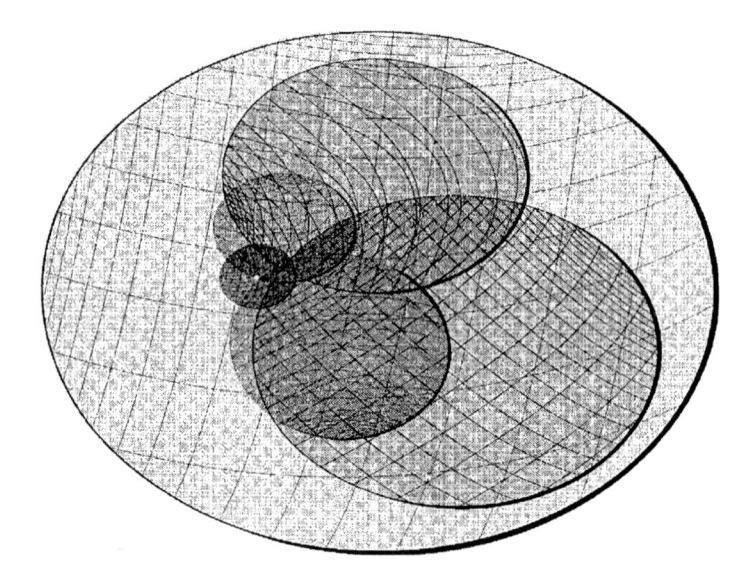

Fig. 3.6 Graphical interpretation of Simmel's network conceptualization of the dominant social structural form in modern society. Reprinted with Permission from Pescosolido and Rubin (2000)

---

[7] I also considered whether the net, itself, could be conceived of as a two-dimensional cantor set which mathematically describes structures that become either more "loose" from the center (e.g., spider web) or more "tight" from the center (an inverse cantor set). After much discussion with colleagues, the net when split along a plane diagonally cutting through the net would result in half fitting the usual notion of a cantor set, and the other half, an inverse cantor set. In fact, the Durkheimian net provided in Figure 3.2 could not be drawn using traditional mathematical algorithms. After many attempts in graphic programs to match the theoretical conceptualization, only an artist could provide the representation. Thus, I rejected the idea of a cantor set because it neither image exactly nor did it provide a parsimonious explication for the theory. I would like to thank Andy Abbott, Brea Perry, Alex Capshew, and Mary Hannah for their contributions to this discussion.

"above." Individuals not only belong to different families, workplaces, churches, and counties, for example; but also, within each network, stand in a particular position in that network.

What Abbott's (2001) translation of the image of fractals from mathematics to social structures and processes does for this conceptualization is to bring together Durkehim's idea of the predictive net with Simmel's notion of the multiplicity of social circles. Fractals, as conceptualized in mathematics, are complex but self-similar geometric shapes that play out at various levels and scales (e.g., reflecting a square mirror into a square mirror). The idea that social networks exist on a similar structural plane which recurs in finer and finer levels fits with analogies of nested boxes from sociology (Goffman's 1974 frame analysis) to public health (Susser and Susser's 1996 Chinese boxes) to the real world (Russian Matryoshka dolls).

In this case, each net contains many smaller nets within it. The predictive surface for social structures looks the same in large and small scale; in this case, at every contextual level, even as the predictive surface, itself, is too complicated to be described by traditional Euclidian geometry. Of course, as we move from macro to micro levels, the scale of the net is reduced. But used metaphorically, the image in the NEM III-R fits the design paradigm's "m principle" – similar object within similar object – or the fractal notion of infinite recursion. Furthermore, the image of Russian Matryoshka doll, similar in shape but often depicted with quite different "faces" (e.g., different Russian/Soviet leaders), may capture and/or align with different cultural values, beliefs, permitting a theoretical flexibility too often missing from mathematically oriented network analyses.

Because social circles have elevation (unlike Fig. 3.6) defined by the level of social structure, the appropriate, the earlier image of the NEM-Phase III (Pescosolido 2006) is too simplistic. For example, the "community" is broadly depicted here but social research has focused on natural neighborhoods, census blocks, counties, regions, nations, and global structures. So, for example, there may be regional variations in stigma (e.g., the US South reporting greater prejudice toward persons with mental illness; Martin et al. 2007) but they exist in a country that, itself, has a particular profile in the global landscape of stigma (Pescosolido et al. 2008). Similarly, at the institutional level, not only do individuals belong to or access resources at many institutions but each organization has a network structure (Barley 1989) and is embedded in an interorganizational network (e.g., the "service system" Morrissey et al. 2002). At the individual level, there are different "domains" that may make up the personal network system – for instance, the "important matters" network, the "health matters" network, and the "mommy" network (Perry 2009). The theoretical result is both simple and complex. Fractals allow us to conceptualize different levels of *social structure* as having similar topographic qualities (i.e., infinite recursion), but adopting this view requires us to explicitly take on the definition of the contextual levels with which our research is concerned in any one study.

However, for any particular social actor, even this depiction takes on greater complexity because as Fig. 3.6 shows, individuals are unlikely to fall at exactly the same point on each level of the net. The depiction of an individual in context has to consider dimensionality within levels, elevation across contextual levels, and the individual's relative position on each net simultaneously. Because the key for an individual social actor (no matter whether persons, organizations, or societies) is *where* they find themselves on the networked landscape of the *relevant* contextual levels. In their own personal support systems, an individual falls on some particular place on the net that facilitates or blocks entry to formal care; they may receive treatment in a place within an organization that has a particular network configuration (see Coser 1962 on differential integration in medical and surgical wards). In turn, that organization holds a particular position in the health care system that may or may not have ties to other important organizations (e.g., shelters, nursing homes, rehab centers), and the health care system itself is embedded in a particular national and even international system of power and tangible resources.

Of course, this level of complexity is not necessary to the vast majority of studies. But, understanding this kind of multilevel embedding does two things: (1) it reminds us that the findings of even our most individually targeted analyses need to be tempered by considering the larger contexts in which the research was done; and (2) it facilitates complex thinking about multi-level hypotheses concerning the reinforcing or cancelling resilience or fragility of their "social safety net." This view permits and encourages us to see network structures as having the potential to be structurally reinforcing or opposing across levels in opposition to other network structures.

Summary: Looking Forward

The NEM calls for a reconsideration and reformulation of the way that we conceptualize many of the phenomena we study as medical sociologists beyond directly privileging the role of structured social interactions as a primary driver. The translation of Durkheim's classic theory into a contemporary, cartographic network scheme allows us to think in more multidimensional, dynamic, and holistic terms about social factors in health. Health problems and responses to them are embedded in social contexts that can be, at least partly, understood through the social ties that individuals have with each other in families, workplaces, and neighborhoods. While integrative and regulative functions may occur together, they do not always do so. Network structures create the potential to provide members with integrative and regulative benefits. These functions can exist together or out of balance, affecting the ability of individuals and communities to face crises. And across levels, an individual's position on one level of a safety net may be reinforced or cancelled out by their position on another. Furthermore, as networks change, the place that individuals, organizations, and societies find themselves on the network map also change, reconfiguring the potential influence of social factors in health, illness, and healing. Finally, because individual actors live in a multiplicity of social circles, Abbott's image of fractal structures provides a way to think through the complexity of social contexts, guiding which ones to consider and which to eliminate from our research designs. Adding elevation to Simmel's notion of the intersection of social circles, fractals allow for a view of complex, multilevel embedding in social networks.

In the end, the NEM ends where it started – as one potential approach to develop complexity theory in the sociomedical sciences. The dynamic, network approach does not invalidate the more standard approaches; it complements them but pushes them further and together. For example, Carpentier and Bernard (2010) found, on average, that it took 2 years from perceived onset to diagnosis. This is typically what has been found in caregiver research; however, they show that this average hides the "more efficient" pathways that some kinds of networks produce. Similarly, Rogers et al. (1999) found that illness behaviors could occur over shorter or longer periods, depending on previous experience embedded in the network (e.g., a mother recognizing symptoms previously seen in an older child). Finally, it appears that more severe problems tend to result in more complicated, indirect pathways rather than direct ones (e.g., Pescosolido et al. 1996). These new directions draw from the NEM and its focus on complexity in understanding health, illness, disease, and health care outcomes; yet, they are only the first steps in embracing the wealth of accumulated (and sometime contradictory) knowledge developed over the last 100 years in this research area and confronting the limits that those approaches encountered. The NEM III-R is designed to help draw the blueprint and lay the foundations for the next generation of the sociology of health, illness, and healing.

References

Abbott A (2001) Chaos of disciplines. University of Chicago Press, Chicago, IL
Alderson AS, Beckfield J (2004) Power and position in the World City System. Am J Sociol 109:811–851
Andersen R (1968) A behavioral model of families' use of health services. Center for Administration Studies, University of Chicago, Chicago

Andersen R (1995) Revisiting the behavioral model and access to medical care: does it matter? J Health Soc Behav 36:1–10
Artis JE (1997) Gendered perceptions of dependency in discussions of mental illness. J Health Soc Behav 38(4):387–402
Barabási A-L (2003) Linked: how everything is connected to everything else and what it means. Plume, New York
Barley SR (1989) The alignment of technology and structure through roles and networks. Ithaca NY, Cornell University, p 57
Bascompte J (2009) Disentangling the web of life. Science 325:416–419
Bearman P (2008) Introduction: exploring genetics and social structure. Am J Sociol 114:v–x
Berkman LF, Glass T (2000) Social integration, social networks, social support and health. In: Berkman LF, Kawachi I (eds) Social epidemiology. Oxford University Press, New York
Black DW (1976) The behavior of law. Academic, New York
Bourdieu P (1990) Structures, habitus, practices. In: Bourdieu P (ed) The logic of practice. Stanford University Press, Stanford, CA, pp 52–79
Brashears ME (2010) Anomia and the sacred canopy: testing a network theory. Soc Networks 32:187–198
Breault KD (1986) Suicide in America: a test of Durkheim's theory of religious and family integration, 1933–1980. Am J Sociol 92:628–656
Bury M (1982) Chronic illness as biographical disruption. Sociol Health Illn 4:167–182
Bury M (1991) The sociology of chronic illness: a review of research and prospects. Sociol Health Illn 13:451–468
Camic C (1986) The matter of habit. Am J Sociol 91:1039–1087
Carpentier N, Bernard P (2010) The complexities of help-seeking: exploring challenges through a social network perspective. In: Pescosolido BA, McLeod JD, Martin JK, Rogers A (eds) The handbook of the sociology of health, illness, & healing: blueprint for the 21st century. Springer, New York
Carpentier N, Bernard P, Grenier A, Guberman N (2010) Using the life course perspective to study the entry into the illness trajectory: the perspective of caregivers of people with Alzheimer's disease. Soc Sci Med 70:1501–1508
Carpentier N, White D (2002) Cohesion of the primary social network and sustained service use before the first psychiatric hospitalization. J Behav Health Serv Res 29(4):404–418
Chen PCY (1975) Medical systems in Malaysia: cultural bases and differential use. Soc Sci Med 9:171–180
Christakis NA, Fowler JH (2007) The spread of obesity in a large social network over 32 years. N Engl J Med 357(4):370–379
Christakis NA, Fowler JH (2009) Connected: the surprising power of our social networks and how they shape our lives. Little Brown, New York
Clausen JA, Yarrow MR (1955) Pathways to the mental hospital. J Soc Issues 11:25–32
Conley D (2010) Learning to love animal (models) (or) how (not) to study genes as a social Scientist. In: Pescosolido BA, McLeod JD, Martin JK, Rogers A (eds) Handbook of the sociology of health, illness, and healing: blueprint for the 21st century. Springer, New York
Copeland LA, Miller AL, Welsh DE, McCarthy JF, Zeber JE, Kilbourne AM (2009) Clinical and demographic factors associated with homelessness and incarceration among VA patients with bipolar disorder. Am J Public Health 99:871–877
Cornwell EY, Waite LJ (2009) Social disconnectedness, perceived isolation, and health among older adults. J Health Soc Behav 50:31–48
Coser RL (1962) Life in the ward. Michigan State University Press, East Lansing, MI
Coser RL, Coser LA (1979) Jonestown as Perverse Utopia. Dissent 26:158–263
Costello EJ, Pescosolido BA, Angold A, Burns BJ (1998) A family network-based model of access to child mental health services. In: Morrissey JP (ed) Social networks and mental illness, vol 9, Research in community and mental health. JAI Press, Stamford CT, pp 165–190
Counte MA, Glandon GL (1991) Elderly stressful life events, coping resources and health outcomes. In: Humphrey JH (ed) Human stress: current selected research, vol 5. AMS, New York
Day JC, Bentall RP, Roberts C, Randall F, Rogers A, Cattell D, Healy D, Rae P, Power C (2005) Attitudes toward antipsychotic medication: the impact of clinical variables and relationships with health professionals. Arch Gen Psychiatry 62:717–724
Durkheim E (1951[1897]) Suicide. Free Press, New York
Elder GH Jr (1978) Family and the life course. In: Haveven TK (ed) Transitions: the life course in historical perspective. Academic, New York, pp 16–61
Falci C, McNeely C (2009) Too many friends: social integration, network cohesion and adolescent depressive symptoms. Soc Forces 87(4):2031–2061
Fallot RD (1993) The cultures of case management: an exploration of assumptive worlds. In: Harris M, Bergman H (eds) Case management for mentally ill patients: theory and practice. Harwood Academic Publishers, New York
Freeman LC (2004) the development of social network analysis: a study in the sociology of science. Empirical Press, Vancouver, BC
Freidson E (1970) Profession of medicine: a study of the sociology of applied knowledge. Dodd, Mead, New York

Gibbs JP, Martin WT (1964) Status integration and suicide. University of Oregon Press, Eugene, OR

Gibbs JP, Martin WT (1974) A problem in testing the theory of status integration. Soc Forces 53:332–339

Giddens A (1984) The constitution of society: outline of the theory of structuration. Polity Press, Cambridge

Gieryn TF (1999) Cultural boundaries of science. University of Chicago Press, Chicago, IL

Goffman E (1963) Stigma: notes on the management of spoiled identity. Prentice-Hall, Englewood Cliffs, NJ

Goffman E (1974) Frame analysis: an essay on the organization of experience. Harvard University Press, Cambridge, MA

Gurin G, Veroff J, Feld S (1960) Americans view their mental health: a nationwide survey. Basic Books, New York

Hagestad GO, Neugarten BL (1985) Age and the life course. In: Binstock RH, Shanas E (eds) Handbook of aging and the social sciences. VanNostrand Reinhold, New York, pp 35–61

Heise DR (1989) Modeling event structures. J Mathl Sociol 14:139–169

Heritage J, Maynard DW (2010) After 30 years, problems and prospects in the study of doctor-patient interaction. In: Pescosolido BA, McLeod JD, Martin JK, Rogers A (eds) The handbook of the sociology of health, illness, and healing: blueprint for the 21st century. New York, Springer

Janzen JM (1978) The quest for therapy in Lower Zaire. University of California Press, Berkeley, CA

Judge AM, Estroff SE, Perkins DO, Penn DL (2008) Recognizing and to responding to early psychosis: a qualitative analysis of individual narratives. Psychiatr Serv 59:96–99

Kadushin C (1966) The friends and supporters of psychotherapy: on social circles in urban life. Am Sociol Rev 31:786

Kandula NR, Wen M, Jacobs EA, Lauderdale DS (2009) Association between neighborhood context and smoking prevalence among Asian Americans. Am J Public Health 99(5):885–92

Kelner M, Wellman B, Saks M, Pescosolido BA (2000) Complementary and alternative medicine: challenge and change. Harwood Academic Publishers, Amsterdam

Kessler RC, Wittchen H-U, Abelson JM, McGonable K, Schwarz N, Kendler KS, Knäuper B, Zhao S (1998) Methodological studies of the Composite International Diagnostic Interview (CIDI) in the U.S. National Comorbidity Survey (NCS). Int J Methods Psychiatr Res 7(1):33–55

Klovdahl AS, Graviss EA, Musser JM (2002) Infectious disease control: combining molecular biological and network methods. In: Levy JA, Pescosolido BA (eds) Social networks and health, vol 8, Advances in medical sociology. JAI, New York, pp 73–100

Koos EL (1954) The health of Regionville: what the people thought and did about it. Columbia University Press, New York

Lindblom C (1959) The science of muddling through. Public Adm Rev 19:79–88

Liu, Ka-Yuet, Marissa King, and Peter S. Bearman (2010) Social influence and the autism epidemic. American Journal of Sociology 115:1387–1434

Lively KJ, Smith C (2010) Identity and Illness. In: Pescosolido BA, McLeod JD, Martin JK, Rogers A (eds) Handbook of the sociology of health, illness, and healing: blueprint for the 21st century. Springer, New York

Martin JK, Pescosolido BA, Olafsdottir S, McLeod JD (2007) The construction of fear: modeling Americans' preferences for social distance from children and adolescents with mental health problems. J Health Soc Behav 48:50–67

Martin MA (2008) The intergenerational correlation in weight: how genetic resemblance reveals the social role of families. Am J Sociol 114(S1):S67–S105

Mazumdar S, King M, Zerubavel N, Bearman P (2010) The spatial structure of autism in California, 1993–2001. Health Place 16:539–546

McKinlay JB (1995) Bringing the social system back. In: An essay on the epidemiological imagination. New England Research Institute, Boston, MA

Mechanic D (2004) The rise and fall of managed care. J Health Soc Behav 45:76–86

Morrissey JP, Calloway MO, Thakur N, Cocozza J, Steadman HJ, Dennis D (2002) Integration of service systems for homeless persons with serious mental illness through the ACCESS program. Access to community care and effective services and supports. Psychiatr Serv 53:949–957

Nobles J, Frankenberg E (2009) Mothers' community participation and child health. J Health Soc Behav 50(1):16–30

Olafsdottir S, Pescosolido BA (2009) Drawing the line: the cultural cartography of utilization recommendations for mental health problems. J Health Soc Behav 50:228–244

Ostrom E (2009) A general framework for analyzing sustainability of social-ecological systems. Science 325:419–422

Parsons T (1951) The social system: the major exposition of the author's conceptual scheme for the analysis of the dynamics of the social system. Free Press, New York, NY

Pavalko EK, Harding CM, Pescosolido BA (2007) Mental illness careers in an era of change. Soc Probl 54:504–522

Pavalko EK, Woodbury S (2000) Social roles as process: caregiving careers and women's health. J Health Soc Behav 41:91–105

Penner AM (2008) Gender differences in extreme mathematical achievement: An international perspective on biological and social factors. Am J Sociol 114:S138–S170

Perry B (2010) Taking the medical sciences seriously: why and how medical sociology should incorporate diverse disciplinary perspectives. In: Pescosolido BA, McLeod JD, Martin JK, Rogers A (eds) The handbook of the sociology of health, illness, and healing: blueprint for the 21st century. Springer, New York

Perry BL, Pescosolido BA (Forthcoming) Children, stigma and mental health. In: Pilgrim D, Rogers A, Pescosolido BA (eds) The handbook of mental health and mental disorder. Sage, Thousand Oaks, CA

Perry BL (2009) The ripple effect: social network dynamics, social location, and strategies of interaction in mental illness careers. Dissertation, Department of Sociology, Indiana University

Pescosolido BA (1990) The social context of religious integration and suicide: pursuing the network explanation. Sociol Q 31:337–357

Pescosolido BA (1991) Illness careers and network ties: a conceptual model of utilization and compliance. In: Albrecht GL, Levy JA (eds) Advances in medical sociology. JAI Press, CT, pp 161–184

Pescosolido BA (1992) Beyond rational choice: the social dynamics of how people seek help. Am J Sociol 97:1096–1138

Pescosolido BA (1994) Bringing Durkheim into the 21st century: a social network approach to unresolved issues in the study of suicide. In: Lester D (ed) Emile Durkheim: le suicide – 100 years later. The Charles Press, Philadelphia, PA, pp 264–295

Pescosolido BA (1996) Bringing the "community" into utilization models: How social networks link individuals to changing systems of care. In: Kronenfeld J (ed) Research in the sociology of health care, vol 13. JAI Press, Greenwich, CT, pp 171–198

Pescosolido BA (2006a) Of pride and prejudice: the role of sociology and social networks in integrating the health sciences. J Health Soc Behav 47:189–208

Pescosolido BA (2006b) The sociology of social networks. In: Bryant CD, Peck DL (eds) The handbook of 21st century sociology. Sage Publications, Thousand Oaks, CA, pp 208–217

Pescosolido BA, Boyer CA (1999) How do people come to use mental health services? Current knowledge and changing perspectives. In: Horwitz AV, Scheid TL (eds) A handbook for the study of mental health: social contexts, theories, and systems. Cambridge University Press, New York, pp 392–411

Pescosolido BA, Boyer CA (2010) Understanding the context and dynamic social processes of mental health treatment. In: Horwitz AV, Scheid TL (eds) A handbook for the study of mental health: social contexts, theories, and systems. Cambridge University Press, New York, pp 420–438

Pescosolido BA, Wright ER, Sullivan WP (1995) Communities of care: a theoretical perspective on care management models in mental health. In: Albrecht G (ed) Advances in medical sociology, vol 6. JAI Press, Greenwich, CT, pp 37–80

Pescosolido BA, Brooks-Gardner C, Lubell KM (1998a) How people get into mental health services: stories of choice, coercion and 'muddling through' from 'first-timers'. Soc Sci Med 46:275–286

Pescosolido BA, Georgianna S (1989) Durkheim, religion, and suicide: toward a network theory of suicide. Am Sociol Rev 54:33–48

Pescosolido BA, Levy JA (2002) The role of social networks in health, illness, disease and healing: the accepting present, the forgotten past, and the dangerous potential for a complacent future. Soc Networks Health 8:3–25

Pescosolido BA, Mendelsohn R (1986) Social causation or social construction? An investigation into the social organization of suicide rates. Am Sociol Rev 51:80–101

Pescosolido BA, Olafsdottir S (2010) The cultural turn in sociology: can it help us resolve an age-old problem in understanding decision-making for health care? Sociol Forum

Pescosolido BA, Rubin BA (2000) The web of group affiliations revisited: Social life, postmodernism, and sociology. Am Sociol Rev 65:52–76

Pescosolido BA, Wright ER, Alegria M, Vera M (1998b) Social networks and patterns of use among the poor with mental health problems in Puerto Rico. Med Care 36:1057–1072

Pescosolido BA, Olafsdottir S, Martin JK, Long JS (2008a) Cross-cultural issues on the stigma of mental illness. In: Arboleda-Florez J, Sartorius N (eds) Understanding the stigma of mental illness: theory and interventions. Wiley, London, pp 19–35

Pescosolido BA, Martin JK, McLeod JD, Perry BL, Olafsdottir S, Pescosolido FJ (2008b) Public understanding of child MH: National stigma study-children. Brown Univ Child Adolesc Behav Lett 24:3–4

Prochaska JO, DiClemente CC (1982) Trans-theoretical therapy – toward a more integrative model of change. Psychotherapy Theory, Res Prac 19(3):276–288

Prochaska JO, DiClemente CC (1984) The transtheoretical approach: crossing traditional boundaries of therapy. Dow Jones-Irwin, Homewood, IL

Riley D, Eckenrode J (1986) Social ties: costs and benefits within different subgroups. J Pers Soc Psychol 51:770–778

Rogers A, Hassell K, Nicolaas G (1999) Demanding patients? analysing the use of primary care. Open University Press, Philadelphia, PA

Rosenfield S (1997) Labeling mental illness: the effects of received services and perceived stigma on life satisfaction. Am Sociol Rev 62:660–672

Rosenstock IM (1966) Why people use health services. Milbank Meml Fund Q 44:94–106

Schnittker J, Pescosolido BA, Croghan TW (2005) Are African Americans really less willing to use health care? Soc Probl 52(2):255–271

Schweitzer F, Fagiolo G, Sornette D, Vega-Redondo F, Vespignani A, White DR (2009) Economic networks: the new challenges. Science 325:422–425

Simmel G (1955) Conflict and the web of group affiliations. Free Press, New York, Translated by K. J. Wolff and R. Bendix

Simon H (1976) Administrative behavior. The Free Press, New York

Snowden LR, Hastings JF, Alvidrez J (2009) Overrepresentation of black Americans in psychiatric inpatient care. Psychiatr Serv 60:779–785

Song L, Lin N (2009) Social capital and health inequality: evidence from Taiwan. J Health Soc Behav 50(2):149–163

Sporns O, Chialvo D, Kaiser M, Hilgetag CC (2004) Organization, development and function of complex brain networks. Trends Cogn Sci 8:418–425

Stryker S (1980) Symbolic interactionism. Benjamin, Menlo Park, CA

Susser M, Susser E (1996) Choosing a future for epidemiology: II. From black box to Chinese boxes and eco-epidemiology. Am J Public Health 86:674–677

Tilly C (1984) Big structures, large processes, huge comparisons. Russell Sage, New York

Twaddle AC, Hessler RM (1987) A sociology of health. Allyn & Bacon, London

Umberson DA (1987) Family status and health behavior: social control as a dimension of social integration. J Health Soc Behav 28:306–319

Umberson DA, Greer M (1990) Social relationships and health behavior: the wellness regulation model. In: Annual Meeting of the American Sociological Association. Washington, DC

Wellman B, Wortley S (1990) Different strokes from different folks: community ties and social support. Am J Sociol 96:558–588

Wheaton B (1978) The sociogenesis of psychological disorder: reexamining the causal issues with longitudinal data. Am Sociol Rev 43:383–403

White HC, Boorman SA, Brieger RL (1976) Social structure from multiple networks. I. Blockmodels of roles and positions. Am J Sociol 88:135–160

Wright ER (1997) The impact of organizational factors on mental health professionals' involvement with families. Psychiatr Serv 48:921–927

Wright ER, Linde B, Rau NL et al (2003) The effect of organizational climate on the clinical care of patients with mental health problems. J Emerg Nurs 29(4):314–321

Xie H, McHugo GJ, Drake RE (2009) Subtypes of clients with serious mental illness and co-occurring disorders: latent-class trajectory analysis. Psychiatr Serv 60:804–811

Yanos PT, Roe D, Markus K, Lysaker PH (2008) Pathways between internalized stigma and outcomes related to recovery in schizophrenia spectrum disorders. Psychiatr Serv 59:1437–1442

Young JC (1981) Medical choices in a Mexican village. Rutgers University Press, New Brunswick, NJ

Zola IK (1973) Pathways to the doctor – from person to patient. Soc Sci Med 7:677–689

Chapter 4
Fundamental Causality: Challenges of an Animating Concept for Medical Sociology

Jeremy Freese and Karen Lutfey

Arguably, the most important problem at the intersection of sociology and epidemiology is how to understand the pervasive positive relationship between various indicators of social position (hereafter, socioeconomic status or SES) and health. The lower status people are, the sooner they die, and the worse health they have while alive. Negative associations between SES and health overall have been found in almost every place and time for which data permit adequate study, implying that the generalization has held even as the prevalence of particular causes of ill-health and death have varied (see reviews in Marmot 2004; Link and Phelan 1995; Deaton 2002; House et al. 1990). In addition, data suggest that the negative association between at least some indicators of SES and some indicators of health may be increasing in some populations, including the United States (Duncan 1996; Lauderdale 2001; Preston and Elo 1995; Steenland et al. 2004; Krieger et al. 2008). Meara et al. (2008) found that while life expectancy had increased 1.6 years between 1990 and 2000 among those who had attended college, it had not increased at all over this same period among those who had not. While various caveats can be raised, none should detract from appreciating that socioeconomic disparities in health in studied populations overwhelmingly are pervasive and profound.

The obvious scientific question about this inverse relationship between SES and health is "Why?," but two distinct "Why?" questions exist. First, for any population in which an association between SES and health exists, we can ask why that association exists, there and then. Even if we have complete knowledge of the causal mechanisms responsible for the association within one population, however, that knowledge cannot, by itself, explain why the association extends to other times and places in which the causes of ill-health and mortality differ considerably. Therefore, a second question is why the association persists across populations even as the specific threats to population health change.

Toward addressing the latter, there has been considerable enthusiasm in medical sociology for the proposition that SES is a "fundamental cause" of health. Notwithstanding the contributions of significant precursors (e.g., House et al. 1990; Lieberson 1985), the most prominent and sustained exposition of "fundamental causality" has been by Link and Phelan (1995, 1996, 2000, 2002, 2005); Link et al. 1998; Link 2008; Phelan et al. 2004; Phelan and Link 2005). Although they have articulated the details somewhat differently in different papers, Link and Phelan's argument consistently emphasizes the intersection of information and resource inequalities for understanding the enduring SES–health relationship.

J. Freese (✉)
Department of Sociology, Northwestern University, 1810 Chicago Ave., Rm. 211, Evanston, IL 60208, USA
e-mail: jfreese@northwestern.edu

To understand their position in brief, consider the following sentence from an article by Sankar et al (2004, p. 2985) in *JAMA*:

> Disparities in health status have increased in the United States in the last 50 years despite remarkable advances in our ability to prevent, diagnose, and treat disease.

This sentence places two stylized facts about the recent history of population health in an *ironic* relationship to one another: we know more about how to protect health, and yet inequalities in health outcomes have increased. By contrast, the fundamental cause concept replaces the ironic connection with a causal one – that disparities in health status have increased in the United States in the last 50 years *in significant part because of* remarkable advances in our ability to prevent, diagnose, and treat disease. In other words, work on SES as a fundamental cause of health emphasizes the differential distribution of control over disease and its implications for the resulting distribution of health outcomes. Scientific and technological advances increase health opportunity and those with higher SES benefit more from that opportunity than do others. The fundamental causality literature thereby offers the possibility of a general logic by which the pervasive and enduring character of disparities may be understood as well as the logic for expecting when such disparities would increase or decrease. In doing so, the literature contributes to a greater theoretical understanding of health inequalities than is afforded by studies of specific causes, outcomes, or interventions.

"Fundamental causality" as a concept has informed a wide range of studies in the last decade. As valuable as this work has been, we think that medical sociology and social epidemiology going forward would benefit from increased appreciation of some distinctions and tensions regarding fundamental causality, as these may help animate future inquiry. Accordingly, we attempt to develop a forward-looking articulation of fundamental causality and health disparities from a friendly but critical explication of previously published arguments on this topic. We begin by providing a systematic exposition of Link and Phelan's arguments about fundamental causality as both conceptual and theoretical contributions; then we consider opportunities for possible synergy among different social science research methods; and finally we consider some implications for policy. Our goal, emphatically, is *constructive*: we seek to provide a theoretical clarification and elaboration which we believe suggests ultimately that the concept of "fundamental causality" may be even more "fundamental" to the sociological agenda for understanding health than has been so far recognized.

Fundamental Causality as a Concept

Proclaiming that "SES is a *fundamental* cause of health" is not especially interesting if it means only that "SES is a cause of health" or even that "SES is an important and enduring cause of health." Instead, the adjective "fundamental" must add something specific and meaningful, making "fundamental causality" a particular type of causal relation. One should then be able to articulate the meaning of fundamental causality abstractly, without needing to invoke either "SES" or "health." Although Link and Phelan have not articulated fundamental causality in such abstract terms, we believe that our formulation in this section is compatible with their reasoning. Briefly articulating "fundamental causality" as a *concept* will also help highlight the distinction between *whether* SES is a fundamental cause of health and any particular explanation of *why* SES is a fundamental cause of health.

First, for X to be a fundamental cause of Y, X has to be a cause of Y. Saying that SES is a fundamental cause of health implies that if individuals' SES had been different, then their subsequent "life chances" for health outcomes would be different. If the correlation between SES and health was entirely due to poor health causing lower SES, SES would not be a cause of health, much less a fundamental one. Likewise, if the correlation between SES and health was entirely due to some third variable causing both, such as the unlikely theory that "intelligence" is largely responsible for the apparent causal relationship between SES and health, then SES would not be a cause of health (Gottfredson 2004; Link et al. 2008; Cutler and Lleras-Muney Forth coming).

For X to be a fundamental cause of Y, X must have diverse immediate consequences and Y diverse immediate causes. The many consequences of SES-related resources may influence the many causes of health through a large and complicated series of paths, each of which can be called a *mechanism*. For example, Adler and Newman (2002, p. 66) write, "Low-SES peoples also experience greater residential crowding and noise…Noise exposure has been linked to… hypertension among adults." If correct, SES differences cause housing differences, which cause noise exposure differences, which cause blood pressure differences, which presumably then cause some increased mortality risk from cardiovascular disease. Even if the ultimate effect is only very slight, this would still be one mechanism linking SES to health. That X has diverse consequences and Y has diverse causes raises the possibility of *massively multiple mechanisms*, a very large number of distinct, specific ways that X and Y are causally connected.

"Fundamental causality" is more compelling as a distinct type of cause if one also stipulates that no single intervening variable accounts for the bulk of the enduring relationship between two variables. For example, if pervasive racial disparities in health were entirely explained by the effects of race on SES and of SES on health, then we would say that race is not itself a fundamental cause of health, but SES (perhaps) would be. Similarly, if the reason SES affected health was dominantly that SES was associated with "stress" and "stress" had various implications for health, then we would see less point to asserting that SES itself was a fundamental cause of health as opposed to just calling attention to the dominant mediating role of stress.

X is not a fundamental cause of Y if there are massively multiple causal mechanisms linking X and Y but they largely cancel each other out. If having higher SES is good for health in many ways, there could still be no association if higher SES was also bad for health in many ways. Instead, then, a fundamental cause relationship implies a *systematic asymmetry* by which the mechanisms overwhelmingly imply an influence of X on Y in one direction rather than the reverse. There may be ways that higher SES is detrimental to health (see, e.g., the discussion of *status pursuit* by Lutfey and Freese 2005, p. 1365), but these must be much weaker in their ultimate consequence than the ways that higher SES promotes health.[1]

The sine qua non of the fundamental cause claim is that this asymmetry in mechanisms is systematically produced, such that, when new mechanisms emerge, they can be expected, more often than not, to preserve the underlying relationship. This distinguishes fundamental causes from other distal causes, because it implies an ultimate limitation to any attempt to "explain" the influence of a fundamental cause solely by reduction to proximate causes. Instead, one must explain also what would warrant the predictive claim that new mechanisms will tend to preserve the relationship between X and Y. We have elsewhere called this a *metamechanism*: an abstract mechanism that explains the generation of multiple concrete mechanisms that reproduce a particular relationship in different places and different times (Lutfey and Freese 2005). The metamechanism provides what we term a *durable narrative* to why the SES–health relationship should be robust to changes in health threats and treatments – an explanation of why a similar association would be observed in diverse sociohistorical contexts. In our view, the existence of a durable narrative is what makes fundamental causes "fundamental."

---

[1] Some have asserted that gender can also be considered a fundamental cause of health (Graham 2004, p. 112). Surely, it is easy to see many pathways between gender inequalities and health outcomes. However, the greater longevity of the socially disadvantaged group (women) makes us wish for a more detailed explication of the understanding of the fundamental cause concept that yields the assertion that, by simple analogy to SES or race, we can think of gender as a fundamental cause of health.

Regardless of the terminology used, the fundamental cause claim implies not just that mechanisms connecting SES and health typically result in an inverse relationship between the two, but that there are systemic, articulatable reasons why this is so. It is not sufficient, for example, to note the existence of enduring "contextual" features like neighborhood differences, but rather this must be linked to explanation of why wealthier neighborhoods should be, in general, more health-promoting than poorer ones. Systemic explanation is why the fundamental cause concept applied to health can be taken as a challenge to the relentless focus on "risk factors" in epidemiology. *A complete articulation of specific proximate mechanisms of inequality is not a full explanation if it misses an incisive explanation of the mechanisms themselves – incisive in that it makes sense of a diverse set of mechanisms, offers predictive insight into why the population distribution of disease will be surprisingly robust to changes in the causes of ill-health, and calls attention to the possibility of more encompassing interventions.* The notion of fundamental causes allows findings about specific causes and specific disease outcomes to be understood cumulatively in the context of more diffuse, encompassing constructs like socio-economic status and health.

Fundamental Causality as a Theory

In articulating their arguments about fundamental causality, Link and Phelan have been engaged primarily with alternatives to the idea that SES is a fundamental cause of health – for example, the assertion that the health gradient is mostly attributable to health causing SES or to stress and other psychophysiological consequences of social hierarchies (Marmot 2004). As useful as this has been, engagement with the issue of whether SES is a fundamental cause of health has resulted in some blurring of theoretical claims about why SES is a fundamental cause of health. Additionally, the primary explanatory concepts are diffuse, and this diffuseness has both virtues and limitations. For future work on health using the notion of fundamental causality to develop most fruitfully, we think distinctions on both these fronts need to be clearer.

Differences in Means

Why do changes in the proximate determinants of health result in new mechanisms that sustain the inverse SES–health relationship in much the same way that the old ones did? Link and Phelan have offered several concise theoretical statements on this question. Consider:

> Socioeconomic status operates as a 'fundamental cause' of disease by allowing people with high socioeconomic status to use broadly serviceable resources, such as knowledge, money, and power, to avoid risks and to minimize the consequences of disease once it occurs. (Link and Phelan 1996, p. 599)

> SES disparities in mortality arise because people of higher SES use flexible resources to avoid risk and adopt protective strategies. (Phelan and Link 2005, p. 30)

> [P]eople with superior resources can use those resources to garner health advantages. (Link and Phelan 2002, p. 732)

> [N]ew mechanisms arise because persons higher in SES enjoy a wide range of resources – including money, knowledge, prestige, power, and beneficial social connections – that they can utilize for their advantage. (Link and Phelan 2005, p. 73)

These statements articulate an elegant metamechanism for the pervasiveness of health disparities. Using words like "utilize," "use," "avoid," and "strategies," Link and Phelan direct attention to the role of individual purposive action, or what they call "health-directed human agency" (Link and Phelan 2002, p. 732). More specifically, they posit SES differences in the *means* of achieving health goals as being the crucial difference by which the fundamental relationship between SES and health is preserved.

If years of health could be bought at auction, presumably the rich would buy more (Goldman and Lakdawalla 2005). If the resources identified with SES confer advantage for actors realizing their preferences for health, then we would expect those with higher SES to have better health. Medical advances have increased the opportunity for health-related agency to yield fruit, thereby allowing differences in access and action to manifest themselves as differences in health outcomes. In principle, the existence of purposive actors with differential means to achieving a broadly valued end is *sufficient* to predict the existence disparate outcomes, but that implies nothing about the true extent to which purposive action with different means actually leads to observed disparities.

The Ambiguity of "Resources"

As the statements by Link and Phelan above make clear, the workhorse construct for their theorizing about means has been "resources." "Resource" implies agency, a potentiality that can be drawn upon toward furthering ends. In Link and Phelan's formulation, traditional indicators of social standing – namely education, wealth, and occupation – yield heterogeneous resources that purposive actors can use to benefit their health. Material resources like money can be used to secure access to items or services that protect health. Social resources like interpersonal relationships can be used to draw upon to receive access to quality health information or access to providers. Cognitive resources allow individuals to better understand how their actions influence health, to better utilize information sources to protect health, and to better exploit available technologies.

Of these, material resources are most prototypic, but numerous lines of evidence suggest that the importance of specific material resource differences for health disparities may be easily overstated. Increases in population wealth bear an uncertain relationship to population health once state- and institution-level public health changes are taken into account, calling into question how much individuals help their own health by becoming wealthier (Cutler et al. 2006). Various studies by economists have estimated little short- or medium-run gains to individual health from exogenous increases in income (Smith 2007). This creates the possibility for an unfortunate shell game in how researchers think and talk about health disparities: "SES" most immediately evokes income, but education differences are more consequential for health in the United States; "resources" most immediately evokes money, but nonmonetary differences are more important (see Mirowsky and Ross 2003 regarding the "money fallacy"). Deaton (2002, p. 14, 21) goes so far as to call SES "unhelpful" and "useless for thinking about policy" for health disparities because of its vagueness. More pressing for fundamental causality as a theory of health disparity, however, is the question of how far the notion of differences in the agentic use of resources can be stretched and still be useful for explaining the enduring character of disparities.

As elegant as differences in means is as a metamechanism, many of the specific mechanisms invoked by Link and Phelan's arguments and examples do not involve differences in means. They cite health-promoting behaviors whose costs are minimal and for which information about benefits have widely diffused (e.g., "wearing seat belts" [Link and Phelan 2005, p. 74]). They also invoke SES-related circumstances that have implications for health but are not necessarily the result of any personally health-directed effort (e.g., "living in neighborhoods where garbage is picked up often," "having children who bring home useful health information" [Link and Phelan 2000, p. 41, 2002, p. 30, 2005, p. 74]).

The result is a dilemma. On the one hand, purposive action with different means is a clear metamechanism and offers a coherent theoretical narrative of why SES is enduringly related to health, but also stretches the concept of "resources" to where it fits uneasily at best. We do not regard wearing seat belts as an example of how SES produces differentials in "access to a broad range of circumstances" that promote health (Link and Phelan 2005, p. 74), because there is little reason to think the SES gradient in seat belt usage in the United States has much to do either with "access" to seatbelts (they are legally required in all cars in the United States) or with information about their benefits. On the other hand, when less purposive language is used, arguments may seem to lose the semantic content of a theory altogether. When Phelan and Link (2005, p. 27) state elsewhere that people of higher SES benefit from new health innovations because they can better "harness the benefit" of those innovations, it is unclear what verbs like "harness" mean beyond just saying that people of higher SES benefit more because they benefit more. To be sure, all these examples underscore the distinction between Link and Phelan's position and social selection or stress-centered theories of health disparities. But a theory focused on health-related human agency does not provide a satisfactory explanation of how the fundamental relationship between SES and health is preserved, and this reveals important opportunities for both future theoretical development and empirical research.

Complements to Means

As we have argued, differences in means provide one durable narrative of health disparities, but differences in means among purposive agents do not account for all the cited ways that SES causes health. One way forward is to posit additional metamechanisms of the SES–health relationship that are distinct from differences in means. The relative importance of different metamechanisms in a population is an empirical matter, and one relevant for policy interventions to lower disparities. To this end, we outline three additional metamechanisms here: SES differences in (1) spillovers, (2) habitus, and (3) the ways that social institutions process individuals. In articulating these, we hope also to further clarify the difference between identifying ways that resources may affect health and developing a more comprehensive theory of the pervasive and enduring character of health disparities.

Spillovers. Individuals are embedded in social relations in which other people also value their health, and the actions of other people have consequences that accrue differently to people of different social positions. As a result, we might expect that even among high- and low-status individuals who do not especially care about their health, higher SES individuals will have better health because they gain more spillover benefits from the purposive actions of others in their social networks. For example, a business executive who cares less than the average person about her health may still realize health benefits from her choices of job, neighborhood, and social networks, despite none of those choices purposely "utilizing" resources or enacting "strategies" to improve health.

Link and Phelan provide examples of "contextual" effects as support for their position, but they do not articulate a durable narrative for why a decision to live in the most expensive neighborhood one can afford carries health benefits even though the decision itself need not be motivated by any health concerns. Neighborhoods connect individuals to others, many of whom do care, and the differential means by which these others act for their own health – vigilance about local environmental hazards, for instance, or caring about the quality of nearby health services – can have positive spillovers for others to whom they are connected. More generally, such spillovers most affect those to whom one is socially close (e.g., neighbors, family, friends), and social distance is lower for individuals of similar SES. As a result, new knowledge about health confers disproportionate benefit to high-SES individuals independent of the exercise of their own agency.

We suggest that spillovers provide an important route for connecting findings about social network effects to the idea of health as a fundamental cause. Christakis and Fowler (2007, 2008) provide evidence that both becoming obese and smoking may be influenced by having a friend who has done the same. If so, then becoming obese or smoking have differing social costs depending on social ties as a result of earlier behavior by others. If SES is correlated with social ties, then spillovers provide a metamechanism by which network diffusion can preserve a fundamental relationship between SES and health.

In the same way, spillovers may also help understand the relationship between fundamental causality and proffered mechanisms like lower SES individuals being exposed to "more advertising for tobacco and alcohol" (Adler and Newman 2002, p. 69). If advertisers of particular unhealthy products target low-SES populations more than other market groups, it seems not likely due to sinister corporate executives being especially eager to damage those at the bottom of the social ladder. More plausible to us is that such advertising is responsive to reasonably accurate estimates of profit opportunity. As a consequence, the health-related agency of others to whom one is tied in advertising markets influences the advertising one receives. Again, this is not an example of "using" or "utilizing" resources to "garner health advantages," as the advantage is gained without individuals themselves doing anything health-directed at all.

Habitus. In consumer theory, if two people buy different quantities of a good, this might be explained by their having different means, but another immediate possibility is that the person who bought more wanted more. The analogy to health is to posit that while everyone might prefer being healthy to being unhealthy, some people may exhibit a stronger and more consistent preference for future good health than others. The idea that differential preferences might have anything to do with health disparities might seem virtually unspeakable in sociological and public health discourses about unequal health outcomes, given how readily it might be construed as "blaming the victim" (Mirowsky and Ross 2003; Klinenberg 2006). Worse, given the current political dominance of narrow neoliberal doctrines about individual sovereignty, such ideas can contribute to discourse that public health advocacy is the meddling of a "nanny state." This, in turn, provides strong incentive toward an explanatory idiom that is predominated by language of "access" to resources and of "constraints," in ways that presume that low-SES individuals share the values of their high-SES counterparts, and differences in outcomes are exclusively the result of agency thwarted.

Indeed, some contend that, as a *matter of definition*, "health disparities reflect unequal opportunities to be healthy" and that "reducing health disparities means giving disadvantaged social groups equal opportunities to be healthy" (Braveman 2006, p. 187). In this light, consider how Adler and Newman (2002, p. 69) discuss education and disparities in health behavior: "Limited education may mean less exposure to information about risk, but the same people may be locked into neighborhoods with poor recreational facilities, fewer stores selling fresh produce, and more advertising for tobacco and alcohol." Smoking and obesity are perhaps today the most prominent SES-related indicators of health behavior, and we have no current evidence that those with lower education are unaware that smoking and obesity are unhealthy (regarding smoking, see Link 2008). Facilities for recreation for low-SES individuals can surely be improved, but it is unknown how much this will reduce the SES gap in exercise. The same can be said for making healthier food more easily available (after all, the fast food outlets frequently lamented in the health inequalities literature offer healthier salads at prices competitive to their burgers). As for advertising, the SES gradient for tobacco use is greater than that for alcohol use, even though tobacco advertising is much more strictly regulated. Emphatically, we agree that equalizing access to health-promoting resources is desirable, but we think sociologists should resist any premature conclusion that SES differences in health are only or even primarily caused by lack of information and "opportunity."

Our goal here is not to draw specific conclusions about SES-based differences in health preferences, but instead to note that, while such differences are not incompatible with the fundamental cause thesis, they do prompt contemplation about the metamechanism(s) responsible. For example, massive differences in the economic quality of life in old age provide one impetus for predicting that those of higher SES might be enduringly more motivated toward maximizing length of life than those of lower SES (Deaton 2002). Similarly, the more people feel in control of their lives and are spared immediate environmental demands and interpersonal subordination, the more easily they may be able to cultivate a lifestyle of prioritizing long-term health consequences (Mirowsky and Ross 2003). Rose (2007) talks about the rise of a cultural imperative to "live one's life as a project" with respect to health, and like many cultural developments this may be firstly an elite practice that has only partly diffused down the social hierarchy (see also Aronowitz 2008, p. 7).

"Habitus" is an encompassing term used in some areas of sociology used to refer to basic dispositions of interpretation and action that reflect an actor's social position (Bourdieu 1984; Sallaz and Zavisca 2007). Differences in habitus regarding health are distinct from either differences in means or spillovers. In our view, some concept like habitus is needed to better integrate theory of SES as a fundamental cause of health with evidence that higher SES individuals better "weave together a healthy lifestyle from otherwise incoherent or diametric practices allocated by subcultural forces" (Mirowsky and Ross 2003, p. 7). Precisely a strength of sociology compared to economics has been its openness to the malleability of preferences to differential experiences and influence, and sociology going forward may be particularly well suited for finding ways of talking about health preferences that move beyond the familiar dichotomy of either asserting a lack of informed opportunity or engaging in blame.

Institutions. Both Link and Phelan's existing work and the two durable narratives discussed above – spillovers and habitus – orient to social institutions as static entities to which individuals may or may not have access and may or may not engage to their health advantage. That is, there is an implicit assumption that agency lies exclusively with the individual, and not with the institutions which may facilitate health gains. Individual-based agency narratives are perpetuated with the assumption that schools, neighborhoods, and physicians provide equitable health returns to all the individuals who come in contact with them, or at least returns that are commensurate with the "resources" put into "harnessing" health benefits. While access is certainly critical, it does not provide the full story for how institutional externalities affect health. An access narrative limits consideration of some of the more sociological aspects of institutions and how they might interact with individual actions and resources to amplify disparities. Therefore, a third durable narrative we see as implicit in existing work is the agentic, dynamic action of institutions.

Using the example of medical care, there is extensive evidence of variation in medical practice according to patient characteristics (including SES, but also gender, race, and age), physician attributes (McKinlay 1996; McKinlay et al. 2002), and healthcare systems (Arber et al. 2004), even when patient case presentation is standardized through the use of vignettes. In previous ethnographic work, we found that a multitude of factors operated from within one healthcare system to further exacerbate SES–health differentials in diabetes care, conditional on patients having access to and utilizing care (Lutfey and Freese 2005). The medical system is not a neutral conduit through which resources are exercised in the way that one might stretch a grocery budget to maximize the purchase of health foods at a store. Rather, it is a dynamic institution that may respond directly to a patient's efforts to mobilize resources for health, but may also either amplify or mitigate those same efforts. Consider again the example of the business executive who does not make health decisions her top priority. Based on the above studies, we would expect that the well-off business executive and her working class co-worker may receive differential treatment based on SES differences, despite having access to the same healthcare system, insurance, and even physician. Even though the co-worker may actively mobilize her resources to procure the best insurance she can afford, once they are both in the same system, research suggests that they are at risk of being diagnosed and managed differently.

The inclusion of institutional agency adds an important dimension to the fundamental cause story because these dynamics interact differentially with individual SES-related characteristics to affect health. Furthermore, these dynamic externalities change over time. In the case of healthcare, medical diagnosis and treatment vary according to state-of-the-art knowledge of how to mobilize scientific, technological, pharmaceutical, and policy information to improve health outcomes. In this way, the

SES–health link is not simply a matter of whether or not individuals take up public health and medical advice. Access, utilization, and adherence are moot if one's SES potential for purposive health improvement is undermined by the action of the institution and its agents. Similar dynamics apply for other institutions that have indirect connections to health but robust relationships to both SES and health, including schools, employment (Pager 2007), and the legal system (Massoglia 2008).

Fundamental Causality and Inquiry

The fundamental cause perspective provides a counterpoint to the dominant epidemiological focus on identifying highly specific risk factors for particular conditions, but its arguments also depend vitally on risk-factor research. The more we know about the causes of disease, the more we can elaborate our understanding of the causes of these causes. For many years in social epidemiology, there has been a disjuncture between highly focused studies of risk factors and studies connecting general health outcomes to broad socioeconomic conditions. The metaphor of "looking upstream" for social causes was the most common framework for thinking about connections between the two (McKinlay 1975). We are now at the point where an array of connections are being made between risk factors and social conditions, and the prospect of approaches that span from "cells to society" or "neurons to neighborhoods" no longer seem like fantastic slogans. For example, Gehlert et al. (2008) outline a series of projects on racial disparities in breast cancer inspired by a "downward causation" model that begins with basic social determinants and proceeds to allostatic load and to environmental mediation of gene expression. While current research often attends to the question of how social inequities get "under the skin," the fundamental cause perspective calls attention to the concurrent, more encompassing project of understanding how *information* gets under the skin – by emphasizing the centrality of differential returns to knowledge and control *per se* for understanding health disparities.

Conventional risk-factor epidemiology is driven mostly by within-sample comparisons. In a case-control study, ill individuals are matched with healthy controls to try to identify antecedent differences that cause disease. An important contribution of the fundamental cause perspective has been to emphasize the continued importance of quantitative research that is *explicitly comparative* across samples. Comparisons across countries, for example, allow for the possibility of seeing if the magnitudes of health inequalities are linked to broad differences in the distribution of resources or policy regimes (e.g., Beckfield 2004; Olafsdottir 2007; Mackenbach et al. 2008). Likewise, comparisons over time allow for assessment of the effects of changes in dominant threats or available treatments (e.g., Duncan 1996; Lauderdale 2001; Schnittker 2004; Krieger et al. 2008).

To date, research on fundamental causality offers little direct defense against the critique that SES is conceptually too vague and that research on health disparities would be better served by referring simply to the specific indicators that compose SES measures (Deaton 2002; Mirowsky and Ross 2003). There is no evidence for the possibility of a globally applicable SES construct that would allow for equalizing SES by reapportioning its different components, such that x increase in education would be consistently equivalent to y increase in income or z increase in occupational prestige for health outcomes (Warren and Hernandez 2007). Even so, SES remains useful for understanding the macrosociology of disparity and for considering intervention in broad terms. Indeed, a major appeal of the fundamental cause concept is its macrosociological focus, including its potential applicability to places and times without much formal education, where the determinants of social standing may be quite different.

As a complement to macrosocial comparison, ethnographic research allows for the possibility of explicating what fundamental cause relationships actually look like in naturalistic settings. By this, we mean that ethnographic observation affords a unique opportunity to see how the lives of individuals of differing SES implicate a massive, nonrandom set of circumstances that can be plausibly entertained as contributing, each however slightly, to large ultimate differences in health outcomes. A study of ours was based on observation of two diabetes clinics, one of which served a largely high-SES patient population and the other an overwhelmingly low-SES population (Lutfey and Freese 2005). We focused on diabetes because the strong, well-documented relationship between glucose control and long-term outcomes affords the possibility to observe – even in the relatively brief encounter of the routine clinic visits that we studied – means by which larger trajectories of long-term glucose control are connected to social circumstances (Diabetes Control and Complications Trial 1993). Regardless of the specific fates of individuals observed, ethnographic observation of their experiences and circumstances highlights potential pathways of the aggregate, probabilistic association between SES and diabetes outcomes.

Our findings were a large array of potential mechanisms operating both inside and outside the clinic, as well both internal and external to patients. Additionally, we identified several instances of what we called "compensatory inversions," in which resources were distributed disproportionately to the patients with the least need for them. For example, the clinic with higher SES patients had far superior diabetes education resources, even though there is ample reason to expect better self-education and self-management from them higher SES patients anyway. Ethnographic observation also allowed us to observe plausibly negative cases of "countervailing mechanisms" that work against higher SES patients. For example, teenage girls and even older women were known to capitalize on the weight loss side effects of uncontrolled diabetes, preferring thinness over appropriate glucose control. Going forward, we hope that comparative quantitative research and in-depth ethnography will complement one another toward the end of providing a fuller picture of the systemic relations between disadvantage and disease.

Fundamental Causality and Policy

Taking seriously the idea that SES has sustained, dynamic influences on health differentials, which transcend the individual-level risk factors commonly identified in public health and epidemiology, poses unique challenges for health policy. Although discussions of fundamental causes of health may be faulted sometimes for being vague about policy implications, one central implication is not at all vague: policies that influence social and economic inequalities are health policies and should be recognized as such. A corollary to this statement is that health disparities will exist so long as there are resource disparities, and so it may be naïve to imagine that the two can be decoupled. Such a conclusion could prompt a figurative throwing up of hands: absent a profound and permanent restructuring of social resources, there may seem no points of leverage for meaningfully reducing disparities.

The emphasis of recent work on the relatively greater importance of education than income at least provides some hope, as substantially reducing education inequalities is not quite so utopic-seeming as doing so for income inequality (Mirowsky and Ross 2003; Mechanic 2007). Beyond a more general equalization of resources, Link and Phelan (2005) discuss the most promising policy implications of a fundamental cause perspective. In summary, their arguments "point to policies that eliminate or reduce the ability to use socioeconomic advantage to gain a health advantage – either by reducing disparities in socioeconomic resources themselves, or by developing interventions that, by their nature, are more equally distributed across SES groups" (Link and Phelan 2005, p. 77). Toward this end, they highlight policies that provide benefit irrespective of individual resources or initiative, as well as policies that attend specifically to the social distribution of knowledge about disease risk and the capacity to act on that knowledge. Although we are supportive of many of the policy ideas they mention, we believe that these ideas also highlight some of the important tensions for sociologists interested in health policy.

1. *Scope of interventions independent of agency.* Two examples of public interventions cited by Link and Phelan that do not depend on voluntary action are "requiring window guards in all high-rise apartments versus advising parents to watch their children carefully" and "banning smoking in public buildings versus advising people to avoid secondhand smoke" (p. 79). Such ideas are a useful riposte, we think, for tendencies toward chronic over-optimism about interventions based purely on providing information. They also, of course, harken to a long tradition of public health triumphs like centralized sanitation and fluoridated water, which brought massive benefits to population health and, for a long while, may have had greater ultimate impact than medical developments (McKeown 1976; McKinlay and McKinlay 1977; Mirowsky and Ross 2003; cf. Timmermans and Haas 2008). Even so, another example of theirs may be especially telling: "air bags rather than seatbeats" to reduce road fatalities. Air bags deploy automatically; seat belts are typically not automatic, and a strong education gradient in seat belt use has been documented (Shinar et al. 2001). Yet, air bags actually work far better in conjunction with seatbelts than they do alone. Moreover, above the minimum standard, there is an array of airbags that can be purchased to further reduce the probability of death in a car crash. As a result, while contextual interventions can be expected to reduce disparities, they still afford opportunities for more effective use by those with the most resources and strongest preferences. While such interventions presumably still reduce disparities by raising the floor of health attainment – e.g., the driver unprotected by air bags – the extent to which that raised floor reduces disparity remains to be empirically assessed. More generally for sociologists interested in inequality and innovation, advancing technologies raise important questions about the social conditions that encourage innovations that improve prospects for the bottom of the health distribution as opposed to further expanding possibilities for those at the top.

2. *Health paternalism.* A main reason for advocating for interventions that minimize the role of individual choice in health is that, for financial and other reasons, lower SES individuals disproportionately make choices that sociologists and many others would rather they did not. At the same time, who pays for those air bags and window guards? If mandating such features is a cost passed on to the consumer by the car manufacturer or landlord, then presumably the people affected most are those who are on the margin of being able to afford a car or apartment. Even if one imagines using taxes to pay for air bags and window guards, one is still proposing a use of money that could be more directly redistributed to lower SES individuals. When we consider reducing agency as a strategy for health disparities, we confront questions both about the morality of restricting choice and about tradeoffs between health and income (Deaton 2002). Our point here is not to take any stance regarding health paternalism ourselves. We do think sociologists interested in policy should be clear that there are no free air bags, and so advocating policies involving mandates also implies thinking about tradeoffs. The issue is especially timely as mandating health insurance premiums has been one of the most controversial aspects of legislation to expand health insurance coverage in the United States. The fundamental causality perspective highlights the tension between the social value placed on individual liberties and the value placed on reducing disparity.

3. *Technology policy and health policy.* Using the example of the high costs of AIDS drugs, Link and Phelan (2005, p. 80) underscore the importance of developing interventions that are broadly accessible and affordable so as to avoid the sorts of cross-national disparities currently observed with those treatments. They also note the importance of constructing interventions that simultaneously address other potential barriers to implementation. As discussed above, we have used the phrase "compensatory inversions" to describe instances in which a health-enhancing resource is distributed disproportionately to higher SES individuals even as lower SES individuals might stand to gain more from them. We think more attention could be directed to ways that compensatory inversions are already rooted in and nourished by the current organization of our health care system. As a major example, the United States health care system makes extensive use of

high-end technological advances, which allows those who can afford it to have some of the most sophisticated treatments available. At the same time, this structure increases costs and so competes with the alternative goal of ensuring the broadest possible access.

At the same time, when considering technological development and health, we think it important for sociology not to view innovation as an innocent or ironic catalyst of disparity. Link (2008) characterizes as an important feature of a "social shaping approach" to health the need "to understand the social distribution of useful knowledge and technology." We agree and believe it important especially to give greater attention to social factors in the development of useful technology. Cross-societal health disparities provide the most transparent examples of the crucial point: consider the difference in the effort for developing treatments for malaria, which relatively few people in wealthier regions get, versus developing treatments for Alzheimer's disease, which relatively few inhabitants of poorer regions get. Private efforts to develop medical innovations are closely related to potential market returns, which in turn is predictably connected to the available resources of the affected (Kremer and Glennerster 2004). For that matter, public efforts can be expected to be associated with the capacity for political influence of particular health constituencies. Even for innovations that already exist and can be produced at relatively low marginal cost (e.g., certain drug treatments), there has been much struggle over solving the social problem of providing them for low cost while they command much higher prices in the United States.

We think medical sociology could participate more in interrogating the development of medical innovations, and also in documenting and understanding this tradeoff and the degree to which it is supported by public health policy and the expenditure of public funds on health research. Much health research defined as "groundbreaking" is directed toward optimizing the health of the optimal patient (Lutfey and Freese 2005). As Link and Phelan (2005, p. 8) put it, "When we create interventions that are expensive and difficult to distribute broadly, we create health disparities." At the same time, there is perhaps often an implicit suggestion of eventual "trickle down" to those with less material and psychological resources for treatment. One can posit that the first step of innovation is figuring out a treatment that can work under relatively ideal conditions (the higher SES condition), and then later work can bring its costs down and facilitate its diffusion (Goldman and Lakdawalla 2005; Glied and Lleras-Muney 2008). Social science has an important role to play in our understanding of how the ultimate health benefits of public expenditures on science are distributed.

4. *Institutional policy leverage.* We urge sociologists interested in health disparities to attend to the institutional settings, medical, and otherwise that mediate SES and health. Knowledge, resources, and interventions are not only distributed at the level of the individual, but also in institutional contexts. To the extent that health policy efforts focus on the former, possible routes for minimizing disparities are truncated at that level. A major contribution sociologists can make to policy efforts is an understanding of how these processes operate at institutional levels and the ways in which framing the problem as one of individual access to "good" schools, physicians, or work settings precludes an evaluation of what happens once people are in those systems. In this sense, a fundamental causes approach calls for more integration of traditional individual-level risk factor interventions with, for example, the Institute of Medicine's (2003) work on quality of care and the role of healthcare providers in contributing to disparities. However, to truly capitalize on existing sociological knowledge of a range of institutions, research on nonhealth institutions should also be included so that we might understand generic dynamics underlying health gradients and how new mechanisms may regenerate in the future. In the global context of health policy research, which predicts challenges such as the disappearance of primary care (McKinlay and Marceau 2008) and expanding pressure for the commercialization of healthcare around the world (Mackintosh and Koivusalo 2005), a policy strategy focused on individual-level interventions may be inadequately prepared to anticipate and address new mechanisms as they emerge and sustain disparities.

Conclusion

"Fundamental causality" has been one of the most fertile concepts in the recent sociology of health. We have here attempted to provide a systematic exposition of conceptual and theoretical contributions of fundamental causality to the study of SES-based health disparities, focusing especially on the highly influential work of Link and Phelan. We began by articulating fundamental causality as a type of cause, distinct from "distal," "basic," "root," "enduring," or "important" causes. We next identify four durable narratives for why SES is enduringly related to health. By explicitly developing these narratives, we hope to contribute to moving fundamental causality toward being a more clearly defined theoretical apparatus in medical sociology and health policy. We also address methodological approaches for studying fundamental causality, including quantitative studies of contemporary populations, ethnographic methods, and historical approaches. Finally, we discuss several tensions in sociological thinking about health policy that the fundamental cause concept highlights, drawing again on work from Link and Phelan (2005). In sum, the idea of fundamental causality highlights the importance of placing particularistic studies of risk factors in a larger context of history and inequality, and we anticipate the value of thinking in these terms will be ever more compelling as medical science continues to increase the leverage human beings have over their health.

References

Adler NE, Newman K (2002) Socioeconomic disparities in health: pathways and policies. Health Aff 21(2):60–76

Arber S, McKinlay JB, Adams A, Marceau LD, Link CL, O'Donnell AB (2004) Influence of patient characteristics on doctors' questioning and lifestyle advice for Coronary heart disease: a UK/US video experiment. Br J Gen Pract 54(506):673–678

Aronowitz R (2008) Framing disease: an underappreciated mechanism for the social patterning of health. Soc Sci Med 67:1–9

Beckfield J (2004) Does income inequality harm health? New cross-national evidence. J Soc Behav 45:231–248

Bourdieu P (1984) Distinction: a social critique of the judgment of taste. Harvard University Press, Cambridge, MA

Braveman P (2006) Health disparities and health equity: concepts and measurement. Annu Rev Public Health 27:167–194

Christakis NA, Fowler JH (2007) The spread of obesity in a large social network over 32 years. N Engl J Med 357:370–379

Christakis NA, Fowler JH (2008) The collective dynamics of smoking in a large social network. N Engl J Med 358:2249–2258

Cutler DM, Lleras-Muney A (Forth coming) Education and health: evaluating theories and evidence. In: House JS, Schoeni RF, Kaplan G, Pollack H (eds) The effects of social and economic policy on health. Russell Sage, New York

Cutler DM, Deaton A, Lleras-Muney A (2006) The determinants of mortality. J Econ Perspect 20(3):97–120

Deaton A (2002) Policy implications of the gradient of health and wealth. Health Aff 21(2):13–29

Duncan GJ (1996) Income dynamics and health. Int J Health Serv 26:419–444

Gehlert S, Sohmer D, Sacks T, Mininger C, McClintock M, Olopade O (2008) Targeted health disparities: a model linking upstream determinants to downstream interventions. Health Aff 27(2):339–349

Glied S, Lleras-Muney A (2008) Health inequality, education, and medical innovation. Demography 45:741–761

Goldman D, Lakdawalla DN (2005) A theory of health disparities and medical technology. Contrib Econ Anal Policy 4(1): Article 8 (http://www.bepress.com/bejeap).

Gottfredson L (2004) Intelligence: is it the epidemiologists' elusive 'fundamental cause' of social class inequalities in health? J Pers Soc Psychol 86:174–199

Graham H (2004) Social determinants and their unequal distribution: clarifying policy understandings. Milbank Q 82(1):101–124

House JS, Kessler RC, Herzog AR, Mero RP, Kinney AM, Breslow MJ (1990) Age, socioeconomic status, and health. Milbank Q 68:383–411

Institute of Medicine (2003) Unequal treatment: confronting racial and ethnic disparities in healthcare. The National Academies Press, Washington, DC
Klinenberg E (2006) Blaming the Victims: Hearsay, Labeling, and the Hazards of Quick-Hit Disaster Ethnography. American Sociological Review 71:689–698
Kremer M, Glennerster R (2004) Strong medicine: creating incentives for pharmaceutical research on neglected diseases. Princeton University Press, Princeton, NJ
Krieger N, Rehkopf DH, Chen JT, Waterman PD, Marcelli E, Kennedy M (2008) The fall and rise of US inequities in premature mortality: 1960-2002. PLoS Med 5:e46
Lauderdale D (2001) Education and survival: birth cohort, period, and age effects. Demography 38:551–561
Lieberson S (1985) Making it count: the improvement of social research and theory. University of California Press, Berkeley, CA
Link BG (2008) Epidemiological sociology and the social shaping of population health. J Health Soc Behav 49:367–384
Link BG, Phelan JC (1995) Social conditions and fundamental causes of disease. J Health Soc Behav Extra Issue:80–94
Link BG, Phelan JC (1996) Understanding sociodemographic differences in health –The role off fundamental social causes. Am J Public Health 86:471–473
Link BG, Phelan JC (2000) Evaluating the fundamental cause explanation for social disparities in health. In: Bird CE, Conrad P, Fremont AM (eds) Handbook of medical sociology. Prentice Hall, Englewood Cliffs, NJ
Link BG, Phelan JC (2002) McKeown and the idea that social conditions are the fundamental causes of disease. Am J Public Health 92(5):730–732
Link BG, Phelan JC (2005) Fundamental sources of health inequalities. In: Mechanic D, Rogut LB, Colby DC, Knickman JR (eds) Policy challenges in modern health care. Rutgers University Press, New Brunswick, NJ, pp 71–84
Link BG, Northridge ME, Phelan JC, Ganz M (1998) Social epidemiology and the fundamental cause concept: on the structuring of effective cancer screens by socioeconomic status. Milbank Q 76(3):375–402
Link BG, Phelan Jo C, Miech R, Westin EL (2008) The resources that matter: fundamental social causes of health disparities and the challenge of intelligence. J Health Soc Behav 49:72–91
Lutfey K, Freese J (2005) Toward some fundamentals of fundamental causality: socioeconomic status and health in the routine clinic visit for diabetes. Am J Sociol 110(5):1326–1372
Mackenbach JP, Stirbu I, Roskam AJ, Schaap MM, Menvielle G, Leinsalu M, Kunst AE (2008) Socioeconomic inequalities in health in 22 European countries. N Engl J Med 358:2468–2481
Mackintosh M, Koivusalo M (eds) (2005) Commercialization of health care: global and local dynamics and policy responses. [Series on social policy in a development contextg, United Nations Research Institute for Social Development]. Macmillan, New York
Marmot M (2004) The status syndrome: how social standing affects our health and longevity. Holt, New York
Massoglia M (2008) Incarceration as exposure: the prison, infectious disease, and other stress-related illness. J Health Soc Behav 49(1):56–71
McKeown T (1976) The Role of Medicine: Dream, Mirage, or Nemesis. Nuffield Provincial Hospitals Trust, London
McKinlay JB (1975) A case for refocusing upstream: the political economy of illness. In: Enelow AJ, Henderson JB (eds) Behavioral aspects of prevention. American Heart Association, Dallas, TX, pp 9–25
McKinlay JB (1996) Some contributions from the social system to gender inequalities in heart disease. J Health Soc Behav 37(1):1–26
McKinlay JB, Marceau LD (2008) When there is no doctor: reasons for the disappearance of primary care physicians in the U.S. during the early 21st century. Soc Sci Med 67:1481–1491
McKinlay JB, McKinlay SM (1977) The questionable contribution of medical measures to the decline of mortality in the United States in the twentieth century. Milbank Q 55:405–428
McKinlay JB, Lin T, Freund K, Moskowitz M (2002) The unexpected influence of physician attributes on clinical decisions: results of an experiment. J Health Soc Behav 43(1):92–106
Meara ER, Richards S, Cutler DM (2008) The gap gets bigger: changes in mortality and life expectancy, by education, 1981-2000. Health Aff 27(2):350–360
Mechanic D (2007) Population health: challenges for science and society. Milbank Q 85(3):533–559
Mirowsky J, Ross CE (2003) Education, social status, and health. Aldine de Gruyter, New York
Olafsdottir S (2007) Fundamental causes of health disparities: stratification, the welfare state, and health in the United States and Iceland. J Health Soc Behav 48:239–253
Pager D (2007) Marked: race, crime, and finding work in an era of mass incarceration. University of Chicago Press, Chicago, IL
Phelan JC, Link B (2005) Controlling disease and creating disparities: a fundamental cause perspective. J Gerontol 60B(Special Issue II):27–33

Phelan JC, Link B, Diez-Roux A, Kawachi I, Levin B (2004) Fundamental causes of social inequalities in mortality: a test of the theory. J Health Soc Behav 45:265–285

Preston SH, Elo IT (1995) Are educational differences in adult mortality increasing in the United States? J Aging Health 7:476–496

Rose N (2007) The politics of life itself: biomedicine, power, and subjectivity in the twenty-first century. Princeton University Press, Princeton, NJ

Sallaz JJ, Zavisca J (2007) Bourdieu in American sociology, 1980–2004. Annu Rev Sociol 33:21–41

Sankar P, Cho MK, Condit CM, Hunt LM, Koenig B, Marshall P, Lee SS, Spicer P (2004) Genetic research and health disparities. JAMA 291(24):2985–2989

Schnittker J (2004) Education and the changing shape of the income gradient in health. J Health Soc Behav 45:286–305

Shinar D, Schechtmana E, Compton R (2001) Self-reports of safe driving behaviors in relationship to sex, age, education and income in the U.S. adult driving population. Accid Anal Prev 33(1):111–116

Smith JP (2007) The impact of socioeconomic status on health over the life-course. J Hum Resour 42(4):739–764

Steenland K, Hu S, Walker J (2004) All-cause and cause-specific mortality by socioeconomic status among employed persons in 27 U.S. states, 1984–1997. Am J Public Health 94:1037–1042

The Diabetes Control and Complications Trial Research Group (1993) The effect of intensive treatment of diabetes on the development and progression of long-term complications in insulin-dependent diabetes mellitus. N Engl J Med 329:977–986

Timmermans S, Haas S (2008) Toward a sociology of disease. Sociol Health Illn 30:659–676

Warren JR, Hernandez EM (2007) Did socioeconomic inequalities in morbidity and mortality change in the united states over the course of the twentieth century? J Health Soc Behav 48:335–351

Part II
Connecting Communities

Chapter 5
Learning from Other Countries: Comparing Experiences and Drawing Lessons for the United States

Mary Ruggie

Are there any medical sociologists who believe in the notion of American "exceptionalism" and resist considering US healthcare policy in comparative perspective? Alternatively, are there any who question whether comparisons of seemingly vastly different settings can yield fruitful lessons for the US? This paper seeks to convince the dubious in the worlds of both academia and healthcare policymaking that a comparative lens best illuminates the successes and failures of American health care and the unique framework within which it operates. We have much to learn from the experiences of other countries, not only about healthcare policy but also about the political and social parameters and the norms and values that shape it and its outcomes. Moreover, despite apparent differences, there are important similarities between our struggles and those of other countries. Understanding how and why their efforts have succeeded or failed can inform a more fruitful direction for American endeavors.

At the same time, this paper highlights a seemingly paradoxical insight gained from comparative analysis, one that should drive future research – the US spends more than other countries on health care, has the most advanced medical technology available anywhere in the world, and yet exhibits worse health outcomes than a number of less-wealthy countries. I propose that by drawing on the experiences of other countries, we can identify a number of persistent barriers to appropriate goal setting and implementation that impede progress toward more equitable health care in the US. The discussion of these issues is oriented toward both the lessons that we can derive as well as suggestions for future research; the former appear throughout this essay, the latter are presented at the end.

Theoretical grounding for this study is based on sociological approaches to the role of the state and in particular the welfare state. The most relevant theories for analyzing healthcare policy consider relationships between state and market, public and private sector actors, and society and individuals. Applied to the empirical problem of state retrenchment in social provision, which occurred in the 1980s and 1990s, scholars have tried to determine the causes, consequences, and future of downsizing in the scope of state activities at the macro, meso, and micro levels of analysis (Allen and Pilnick 2006). Disagreements on these issues persist. Some argue that developments have followed institutional paths, resulting in little significant change in the roles of states and markets (Pierson 2000; Hacker 2004). Others argue that a transformation is occurring in which the state is allowing other social actors to perform functions previously reserved for government, and social provision is becoming harsher as a result (Gilbert 2002; Quadagno and Street 2006). Others still suggest that the state is becoming stronger, although its role is changing from provision to regulation and guidance of other actors (Ruggie 1996; Saltman 2002). It may be that there are

---

M. Ruggie (✉)
The John F. Kennedy School of Government, Harvard University, Taubman 470, 79 JFK Street, Cambridge, MA 02138-5801, USA
e-mail: mary_ruggie@harvarel.edu

different trajectories and relations in different policy areas; that is, governments may have less interest in poverty alleviation than in maintaining a healthy workforce, and its role in the former is, accordingly, less robust than in the latter. However, it is also important to note that any single policy area is deeply embedded in a broader social policy context. As research on this and related issues continues, scholars should keep sight of how developments in one social policy area affect others and how the parts interact with the whole.

The fields of health care and healthcare policy are inherently interdisciplinary. But a foray into politics and economics ought not to deter medical sociologists concerned about theoretical integrity. Ultimately, we are all in the business of advocating for more equitable and better health care; the more tools we can garner, the more persuasive will our efforts be. As the following discussion demonstrates, empirical contributions from other fields can support sociological perspectives.

Themes in Health Policy Research

Is Cost Control Best Achieved by the State or the Market?

Until recently, both American and comparative health policy research have been preoccupied by the unrelenting increase in expenditures that has plagued all countries. Studies have focused on reforms in funding, provision and management of health care systems – specifically, the introduction of market mechanisms as counterbalances to public sector growth. For the most part, these reforms have been policy-driven, geared toward reducing public expenditure and increasing efficiency in health care. They have brought more challenges than opportunities to non-state institutional actors (providers, insurers, and patients). However, insofar as marketization has been accompanied by privatization, important changes have been occurring in the relationship between the public and private sectors. Some countries have experienced a quantitative shift from public to private ownership, funding, and/or healthcare provision. Other countries have undergone a more qualitative change, with the state retaining control over some functions (primarily funding) and contracting out other functions to the private sector (primarily delivery). Cross-national policy learning sought to evaluate the effectiveness of various market-based measures adopted both in the US and abroad and to understand why so many countries were emulating what had apparently failed in the US (Ranade 1998). The main lesson, a profoundly sociological one, was that mechanisms are not simply exported; policymakers import selected measures and adapt them to national contexts. As a result, these measures performed differently. Ironically, using competition and choice, other countries have managed to control their expenditures better than the US because of the tighter regulatory framework they constructed for market forces.

Is There a Trade-Off Between Efficiency and Equality?

Recently, comparative research has turned its focus to health outcomes. Whether because costs in other countries have come under relative macro-level control (Saltman 2002)[1] or because all countries, including the US, are concerned about the persistence of certain illnesses and the rise of new

---

[1] Saltman's assertion ought not to be taken too far. European countries have contained costs better than the US, but they continue to be concerned about high health care expenditures and continue to search for methods of control.

ones; everywhere interest has turned to steering funding and provision more directly toward improvements in health. The US fares particularly poorly in international comparisons of health outcomes (Mattke et al. 2006). Not only are there significant health disparities among Americans but also our ranking on such measures as life expectancy and infant mortality is embarrassingly low. However, a question that is straining efforts to improve health outcomes in the US, where costs continue to spiral, is whether quality care and cost control are compatible. Some suspect that they are not and argue, accordingly, that if choices must be made, it is better to err on the side of increased expenditures. They claim that the high-quality health care that results yields ample returns in better health outcomes, confirming the worthy investment (Cutler 2004). The alternative is rationing, abhorrent in the American context.

This perspective misses the comparative lesson. Other countries have demonstrated that quality health care need not bankrupt the system. Moreover, elsewhere efforts to achieve economy and quality are guided by the principle of equality. These three goals – equality, efficiency, and effectiveness – are closely inter-related in the health policy frameworks of other advanced countries.[2] The US pays lip service to these goals, but persistent ideologies about the role of the state vis-à-vis the market impede progress toward them.[3] There is potential in our health care system, but there are also contradictions, tensions, and irrationalities that deter fulfillment of our potential. To resolve these problems, we need to settle on a fundamental principle underpinning the provision of health care – its status as a basic human right.

Is Health Care a Right or a Responsibility?

The main issue currently consuming American health care policy is how to cover the estimated 44 million people who are uninsured.[4] While politicians and scholars debate the feasibility of single-payer systems versus employer and individual mandates as appropriate means to a necessary end, they forget the overarching value that empowers any funding system and, in fact, reduces the significance of the differences among them. Were American politicians to recognize health care as a social right based on citizenship (Marshall 1949), as all other advanced societies do, they would acknowledge at the same time that government has primary responsibility for assuring universal access. This understanding would be a major rather than an incremental step for American policymakers, insofar as the concept of social rights goes beyond the minimal, negative, civil, and political rights enshrined in the American constitution and sustained by American capitalism.

Politicians are hesitant to embrace the idea of health care as a social right because of the expanded government role entailed. However, opinion polls show that the majority of Americans not only believe that government has a central role to play in this and related health care functions but also express willingness to pay more taxes as long as those taxes are used for universal healthcare coverage (Toner and Elder 2007).[5] Furthermore, two of the most powerful opponents of universal coverage in the past, the American Medical Association and the insurance industry, now support it. Arguably,

---

[2] Examples here will be drawn from the experiences of Canada, Britain, and Germany.

[3] In explaining President Bush's threatened veto of an expansion of the State Children's Health Insurance Program, a former advisor said the President's objections are "philosophical and ideological. [An expansion] would move the nation toward a single payer system with rationing and price controls" (Pear 2007).

[4] In 2007 the Census Bureau revised the figure downward by two million. The data do not distinguish insured and under-insured.

[5] Also, polls conducted by the Kaiser Family Foundation find that Americans rank health care second only to Iraq as the issue they most want presidential candidates to talk about, and coverage for the uninsured ranks higher than costs as an issue they would like to see more focus on (http://www.kff.org/kaiserpolls/upload/7655.pdf).

democracy in the US is reflected more at the local than the national level; witness those states (albeit few in number) that are considering legislation establishing health care as a right.

Lessons on Social Values and Ideologies

The themes that dominate comparative research lend themselves to specific lessons. The thoughts presented below are suggestive only; validating these lessons and directing them toward improving American health care will require further research and argumentation.

Public and Private Funding and Control

1. Countries with universal access to health care have found that the role of government is best suited (that is, better than the market) to eliminating financial barriers to access but less well suited to delivering healthcare services. This does not necessarily mean that government has to become the main financier of health care; there is considerable variation across advanced countries in the public–private contribution to financing. But, within the framework of government as the payer of last resort, if not the first, private funding of health care in other countries more effectively contributes to the overall economic health than private funding in the US. Even though the private share of total health care expenditure in the US is relatively large – 55%, compared to, say, 30% in Canada – it is decreasing. Public expenditure, on the other hand, is increasing because of the inefficiencies and ineffectiveness of our health care system. For instance, the aggregate data mask significant government assistance and private sector ineptness. Consider, for example, that government subsidization of employer-sponsored health insurance is over $200 billion per year (Selden and Gray 2006). Were this and similar covert public subsidies included in the calculations, the public share of total expenditures would be closer to 60%. Another hidden cost in our complex and fragmented employer-based insurance system, one borne primarily by people who are insured, is administration. It is estimated to absorb nearly one-third of health care expenditures in the US, exceeding comparable expenditures in other countries by at least 10–15%. Considering that administrative expenditures in the Medicare program are approximately 3%, we can understand why so many Americans advocate a single-payer system of universal coverage, such as Canada's.

Although formally a single-payer system, the financial arrangements between the provincial and federal governments in Canada resemble more closely our Medicaid program (of health care for the poor). In return for its share of overall spending, the federal government in Canada sets certain requirements for provincial administration. Provinces in turn enlist the services of independent physicians and hospitals, paying them according to negotiated schedules and budgets. The regulations that govern federal–provincial and provincial–provider relations specify principles more than practices – public administration, comprehensive and universal coverage, and accessibility. Similar to what occurs in our Medicare program (for the elderly and disabled), the Canadian healthcare system prohibits private insurance from covering services offered in the public program. Nevertheless, the majority of Canadians have private insurance, because the public program does not cover outpatient prescriptions, something that was not considered "medically necessary" when the program became fully instituted in 1966. The shift in public–private expenditures noted above reflects the growing role of pharmaceuticals in health care.

None of this should sound alien to Americans. The principles of the Canadian healthcare system already exist in the American Medicaid program and in parts of Medicare as well. We already have the experience of shared national-state funding, national guidelines for state administration, and public regulations restricting the role of private insurers and providers. With more of the same, we could approximate the Canadian system. This expansion would require adjustments, but not radical structural change.

Lesson #1: One lesson we can derive from the case of Canada concerns the role of the public sector, which is the only actor capable of furthering the public interest in health care. As Canada demonstrates, a fairly equitable system can be based on a minimum level of provision for everyone, leaving the private sector to act as a supplement.

Lesson #2: For the sake of equality and systematic organization, the federal government is better situated than provincial/state governments to set an overall framework of principles for healthcare provision, leaving decentralized levels to work out details and oversee delivery. The most important principle is equality in access to necessary medical services. The example of Germany following immediately reinforces this lesson.

2. The dominance of employer-based insurance in the US reflects both the historical position of employers as well as a visceral disdain of "socialized medicine" on the part of both policymakers and providers. There is considerable agreement among economists that inefficiencies abound in our employer-based system (Pauly 2006). Moreover, employers are no longer interested in playing the prominent role they have been given. Their disenchantment is reflected in the various types of cost-shifting they are engaging in, placing more of the burden for health care directly on workers.

Another country where employers play an important role in health care is Germany. The main funding for Germany's health care system comes from workers and employers. Each worker's paycheck is deducted by 7% of income, a sum that is matched by employers.[6] In Germany, contributions are mandatory for all workers, except those in high-income brackets (about 10% of the population).[7] Hence, the German system is a form of social insurance, closer to Part A of our Medicare program than our employer-based system. But unlike the German system, workers in the US pay twice – for their current (if they can) as well as their future coverage. It is an oddity that only payments for the future are mandatory in the US (except in the state of Massachusetts). This contradiction may have a rational element, insofar as health care costs are higher in old age and the only way to make sure people contribute is to require them to do so. It is also irrational, however, when one considers the fact that health care costs in old age could be lower were the health care needs of non-elders x properly attended. Witness the high cost of caring for those who were previously uninsured once they become eligible for Medicare (McWilliams et al. 2007).

Lesson #3: We already have mandatory social insurance in the US. Expanding Medicare (especially by lowering the age of eligibility) would put us more in line with the German system as far as funding is concerned. This expansion would require adjustments, but not radical structural change.

The role of the federal government in organizing the German health care system used to be minimal, involving the issuance of broad guidelines for the system as a whole. The German government basically allowed the thousands of sickness funds, which are similar to non-profit insurance companies, to administer the system on behalf of workers and employers. This is not too unlike what occurs in the US Medicare program, where the federal government sets guidelines for local, non-profit fiscal intermediaries to use when paying providers. Although there is some variation among these local Medicare payments, they pale in comparison to what occurs in the private insurance sector. But the German healthcare system recently underwent a transformation that carries an important lesson for the US. Because of the fragmentation and inequalities that resulted from its multiple payer system,

---

[6]The proportion of salary that workers in the US contribute to private insurance varies from a low of about 2% to well over 7%. Note too that under the new individual mandate in Massachusetts, some previously uninsured individuals who do not qualify for state assistance will have to pay more than 7% of their income for private coverage.

[7]It took several decades for the government to fold into the system unemployed people, students, and others who were not members of employment-based sickness funds.

the federal government in Germany began to streamline the number of sickness funds and limit their budgetary discretion. The government now controls over 90% of sickness fund expenditures.

Lesson #4: Allowing employers to control health care is neither just nor sensible. Making employer-based insurance the social insurance system that it implicitly is would create more systematization and coordination. Although this type of organization favors the regulatory powers of government, it is also opportune to shift a measure of control over the details of supervision and implementation to non-governmental agencies whose profits are regulated.[8]

Regulating the Market

American health policy makers worry that a stronger government role inhibits freedom of choice for consumers and the ability of competitive markets to coordinate supply and demand. Comparative experiences demonstrate that this fear is unfounded when governments act in the public interest. Even health care systems that are highly regulated by the state have allowed market forces to do what they do best (re-allocate supply according to consumer preferences), but they also make sure that the adverse consequences (creating inequalities based on ability to pay) are avoided. It is now more commonly accepted among both researchers and policymakers in other countries that the roles of states and markets are complementary and that market competition is more effective when properly guided by state regulation. Specifically, other countries have learned that the state is best suited to setting macro-level goals for micro-level market mechanisms of action. How hospitals in Britain's National Health Service (NHS) function is a case in point.

Starting under Conservative Prime Minister Margaret Thatcher and continuing under Labour Prime Minister Tony Blair, the British government has been allowing hospitals that meet fiscal and quality standards to become Trusts. Hospital Trusts are semi-autonomous agencies. They have to operate within certain broad strictures – for instance, hospital Trusts cannot sell their assets without NHS permission and they must re-invest profits in their enterprises. Within these criteria of accountability, hospital Trusts can control how they spend their funds. So that they provide what purchasers want, the NHS permits hospital Trusts to compete with one another for contracts with local authorities.[9] Although price is a competitive factor, so too is quality. One of the most severe problems with quality in British hospitals has been wait times for elective surgeries. Through competition in this internal market, wait times have improved significantly (Le Grand 2006). In addition, the NHS has set explicit government targets for wait times that both guide hospitals in their planning and provide incentives for them to improve. Hospital Trusts can contract with private surgery clinics if need be, deciding the terms of these contracts on their own, as long as they conform to NHS rules. In this way hospital Trusts can expand in accordance with their ability to re-invest profits. Canada has a similar form of funding hospitals (global budgets with decentralized decision making).

The organizing idea behind the funding of hospital Trusts in Britain approximates the hospital payment system in the US Medicare program. In the 1980s Medicare adopted a type of global budgeting system based on diagnostic-related groups (DRGs). DRGs set expenditure limits on hospital services for specific categories of disorders but did nothing more to guide hospitals as they struggled to maintain quality health care. The DRGs achieved part of what they set out to do. By imposing some discipline on hospital activities, the rate of increase in Medicare Part A expenditures has consistently been lower than increases in privately-reimbursed hospital expenditures.[10] But hospital

---

[8] Both Canada and Germany have for-profit insurers but regulations in both are much tighter than in the US.

[9] Primary Care Trusts (PCTs) now control 80% of NHS expenditures. They contract with General Practitioners and hospitals to meet the needs of their constituents.

[10] Most hospitals responded to the DRGs by reducing lengths of hospital stays and by various forms of cost shifting, including the development of more outpatient services and day surgeries.

payments under Medicare Part A have continued to increase along with the number of procedures performed. One reason is that, unlike in the British hospital Trusts, there are no hospital-level limits on the volume of activity, only on the unit payment for treating a disease category. Nor do the DRGs include competition as an additional method of cost control. The comparison with hospital Trusts in Britain demonstrates that the American DRGs are too narrowly focused on unit costs alone; they assume a market response but they provide little direction for it. Confirming policy-makers concerns, this example of government intervention does indeed constrain the market and reduce its potential. But the fault lies with the nature not the fact of government intervention. It seems that the US has much to learn about how government can be more effective in meeting its goals through more expansive goal-setting.

Lesson #5: Competition can be based on quality and overall cost control, not just unit price. Profits should be regulated and re-invested in healthcare improvements.

The US health care system remains heavily tilted toward market-driven principles of organization and relatively weak government regulation. Examples like the DRGs hint at the possibility of change, however, at least with regard to government's willingness to intervene. In addition, the US government's contribution to overall funding is by necessity increasing, and will likely continue to do so if public opinion has any impact. Comparative experiences clearly demonstrate that it is in the best interests of the health care system as a whole that the government deliberately engages in the regulation of the private sector to avoid, above all, the inequitable and inefficient consequences of multiple private sources of funding. But government could do much more to guide private sector actors. A similar lesson emerges from comparative experiences with other dimensions of the delivery of health care.

Lessons on Authority and Power in Decision Making

Health care providers, behaving as private actors, once possessed sole discretion over medical decisions. Cloaked in the mantle of professional autonomy, physicians in particular have also held to strict confidentiality regarding their judgments. As in other areas of contemporary society, hierarchies in medicine are giving way to alternative structures of authority and control. Other social actors in both the public and private sectors are now more involved in weighing the details of health care. Whether because of the growing awareness that some of the causes of health disparities occur in the delivery system, or because of the growing realization that health care resources are limited and must be spent more wisely, the state as the representative of the public interest as well as non-government payers of health care are asking providers for more information about their procedures and pressing them to change their behaviors. In addition, whether because people are better educated than in the past, or because new sources of information have enhanced health literacy, patients are becoming stronger advocates of their health care needs. The sections below demonstrate that, despite other differences, health care providers in the US and other countries are moving toward more open and inclusive methods of decision making.

Rewarding and Guiding Providers

Physicians everywhere place a particularly high value on professional autonomy. American physicians have surpassed others in financial autonomy – until recently, that is, with the rise of managed care. Ironically, American physicians have had less clinical autonomy than physicians in other countries where the state plays a stronger but broader regulatory role. Part of the problem has been the "paradox of liberal intervention" – because the US government hesitates to intervene, when it does, either the result is less than intended or there are unintended consequences, both of which require more intervention (Ruggie 1996). Micromanagement is an unfortunate outcome. In the American setting clinical autonomy is checked primarily through the reimbursement system. However, more explicit methods of control are also being developed. They are constraining physicians and other providers as private actors but they are also enhancing health care as a public good.

Wherever physicians are paid on a fee-for-service basis, the health care they provide tends to reflect the payment they receive (Wynia et al. 2003; Reschovsky et al. 2006). This is not to say that physicians necessarily discriminate according to payment, although some may. It does suggest, however, that fee-for-service physicians tend to adopt a *modus vivendi* of "take two aspirin and see me again tomorrow." Most fee-for-service reimbursement systems have by now developed prospective fee schedules that try to capture the resources physicians typically use for specific services; the Medicare Fee Schedule is an example. As with the DRGs, however, this and similar fee schedules do little to contain the overall volume of physician activity. Incongruous as it may seem, the Medicare Fee Schedule was paying more for poor quality health care that required repeat visits than for efficient and effective health care that could be delivered in fewer visits, regardless of patients' severity of illness (Milgate and Cheng 2006). Capitation payment systems, which many managed care organizations (MCOs) employ, are better at discouraging such inefficiency. Salary systems, which are common in academic medical centers and hospitals, are even better because they can be used to reward productive physicians.[11] Other countries developed volume controls on fee-for-service physician reimbursements year ago and can offer useful lessons. However, the main lesson here already exists within American borders – fee-for-service payment needs volume control, capitation and salary payments work better to control both costs and related inefficiencies.

Following the lead of a few innovative private health plans, both the Medicare and Medicaid programs are experimenting with a controversial corrective to their fee schedules, based on the market principle of monetary incentives to change behavior. Pay for performance (P4P) seeks to reward physicians and other providers for achieving positive health outcomes, such as a reduction in the blood sugar levels of diabetics.[12] Unlike the DRGs, however, P4P measures specify the kind of care physicians ought to provide; they rely on preventive services, in which American physicians are not well trained. One criticism of P4P, therefore, is that its measures are oriented as much to procedures as to outcomes. But this shortcoming may be temporary, awaiting the institutionalization of preventive care. P4P has also been criticized for paying physicians more to provide the kind of care they should already be providing and for encouraging them to do more, which will increase rather than reduce Medicare expenditures. This criticism may be shortsighted. Studies have shown that prevention can delay if not avert the need for hospitalization; the medical literature is replete with examples. So P4P may be paying physicians to do more now in the expectation that they and the health care system will be able to do less later. P4P is still in its infancy and there are many problems that need to be addressed (McMahon et al. 2007).Whether or not it survives the test of time, it has been motivating important changes. If nothing else, the collection of data enabling providers and policy-makers to better focus on healthcare processes and outcomes may be worth the effort.

Implicit in P4P, but not always well integrated with it, are clinical practice guidelines (CPGs). In general, CPGs are a separate component of the effort to influence clinical behavior in the US. The Institute of Medicine (1990, p. 29) defines CPGs as "systematically developed statements to assist practitioner and patient decisions about appropriate care for specific clinical circumstances." While

---

[11] Each of these three main forms of compensation also contain perverse incentives – fee for service may reward the provision of inappropriate services, capitation may reward the denial of appropriate services, and salary may undermine productivity (Robinson 2001).

[12] The Centers for Medicare and Medicaid Services have developed comparable measures for hospitals, home health agencies, end-stage renal dialysis centers, and Medicare Advantage Plans, which are provided by managed care organizations.

CPGs may be "systematically developed" by the organizations which create them, a major problem in the US is that there are too many organizations involved in their creation. Government agencies, medical organizations, health plans, and for-profit consultants have developed different CPGs for the same medical procedures. The proliferation of these guidelines, the lack of standardization among them, and their inconsistent use are emblematic of the fragmentation and complexity that afflict American health care.

As the practice of medicine becomes more evidence-based, physicians have become more willing to consult CPGs. The peculiarities of defensive medicine in the US also encourage their use. As long as physicians can prove that they followed legitimate and formal procedures, they may be relieved from individual liability. However, because physicians frequently contract with multiple health plans, they are often unsure about which set of guidelines to follow (Ayres and Griffith 2007). Although the use of CPGs is voluntary in private fee-for-service practice, MCOs and hospitals are more likely to use them and to monitor their use. CPGs represent an intrusion on professional autonomy, to be sure. It is noteworthy, however, that younger physicians, already more inclined toward practice environments that are collaborative and rely on information technology, readily accept CPGs (O'Malley et al. 2007).

Only a few countries, such as Britain, have experimented with P4P types of incentives to influence clinician behavior. Since most physicians in Britain work in some sort of collective setting, the incentives pertain to the group as much as the individual practitioner, offsetting many of the complaints incurred in the US. Most countries are using CPGs to achieve better health outcomes; some have gone much further than the US in systematizing and therefore deriving value from them.

The best example comes from Britain, which has emerged as an international leader in this and related fields, primarily because of its comprehensive and integrated programs and the transparency of its processes. The most important agency in Britain's effort to improve efficiency and effectiveness in health care is the National Institute for Clinical Excellence (NICE), which functions under the auspices of the Department of Health. Established in 1999 NICE is charged with conducting reviews of certain existing and new health technologies (drugs, devices, and diagnostic tools), determining whether and how these should be used in the NHS, and developing appropriate CPGs to advise healthcare professionals (Rawlins 2004). Although NICE is a government agency, it commissions independent (and unpaid) advisory bodies, drawn from the NHS and academia, to conduct systematic reviews. It also conducts public hearings and consultations, and examines the feedback from all stakeholders, including manufacturers and patients, before reaching final decisions. The Department of Health occasionally instructs NICE to project the national cost of implementing guidelines throughout the NHS, especially when a proposed guideline is likely to have significant budgetary impact. Additionally, cost templates are developed to help Primary Care Trusts (PCTs), the main purchasers in the NHS, make realistic projections on how a new guideline will impact local resource allocation. Even guidelines that do not undergo this costing process are evaluated in terms of their overall cost effectiveness.

Because the NHS is a unitary system, all physicians are expected to use the guidelines issued by NICE. PCTs monitor their use by general practitioners and hospitals monitor specialists. The NHS has invested huge sums of money in information technology, an area where the US lags, to ease the transition to evidence-based medicine. Standardized CPGs are also the bedrock of performance awards. Americans may balk at the overarching power of the state implied in this example. Efforts to decentralize the NHS are indeed less visible in standard-setting than in implementation. Nevertheless, the consistency of care that results from the use of CPGs in Britain has raised the country's standing in international comparisons of health outcomes.

Lesson #6: A government agency is needed to assess the clinical efficacy of the many technologies now available to healthcare providers, to decide which work best, and to develop appropriate clinical guidelines. Standardization in these efforts is needed to reduce healthcare inequalities and improve health outcomes.

Rationing

Undoubtedly the greatest fear that everyone – policymakers, providers, and patients alike – harbors about government imposition of cost control and regulation of the private sector is the inevitability of rationing. The question we should be asking about rationing is not whether it occurs – it does occur, everywhere – but what its rationale is. In the US, most rationing is market-based, implicit, and hidden. It enters when patients have no or inadequate insurance coverage, when insurers deny coverage for specific treatments, when patients or providers refrain from purchasing products because the price is too high, or providers refrain from delivering services because the cost is too high relative to the reimbursement. Rationing also arises when the supply of healthcare products or providers is lower than the demand, whether that demand is ongoing or the result of an emergency. Although governments everywhere can and do increase supply, eventually they must confront the limits inherent in provision.

The state of Oregon has been a pioneer in the effort to develop medical and cost-effectiveness criteria to guide the use of health care resources (Oberlander 2007). Oregon's plan for rationing in its Medicaid program was the result of admirable grassroots organization and consensus building. But because it was so controversial the Department of Health and Human Services demanded that it be scaled back, considerably. Other efforts in the US to develop rational criteria for the allocation of health care resources exist more on paper than in reality. For example, the Centers for Medicare and Medicaid Services (CMS) commission the Agency for Health Care Research and Quality to evaluate selected technologies. These evaluations focus on the clinical effectiveness of each product; they do not compare products so they cannot indicate whether a new product will improve health care. Nor do technology assessments in the US include cost-effectiveness considerations.

Contrast the American approach to what we see in Britain where NICE incorporates cost effectiveness in its technology assessments and compares the cost effectiveness of different technologies to determine which ones the NHS should use. Although NICE refrains from explicit cut-off values, technologies costing over $45,900 per quality-adjusted-life-year are generally not considered cost effective and are less likely to be adopted (Pearson and Rawlins 2005). Once NICE determines that the NHS should adopt a technology and produces guidelines on how it should be used, PCTs must provide funding within three months.

Canada is working on a different approach to rationalize the use of limited health care resources. Physicians, researchers, and various levels of government are collaborating to reduce wait times for elective surgeries. In some provinces individual doctors were managing their own wait lists, often in conflict with hospitals, which had separate lists and criteria. This confusion exacerbated unconscionably long waits. To improve the situation, the Western Canada Wait List Project is developing "valid, reliable, practical, and clinically transparent measures" of urgency in order to prioritize wait times for selected procedures (Western Canada Wait List Project 2005, p. i). Based on the research and feedback from clinicians, patients, and the broader public, priority scores were developed and are now being tested for hip and knee replacement, cataract surgery, general surgery, magnetic resonance imaging, and children's mental health. Other provinces are conducting similar projects. Ontario, for instance, has implemented a system of surgical wait times for heart disease and cancer. Federalism in Canada encourages considerable learning through the sharing of information across the provinces.

Restricting the use of health care resources in cases where the benefits are dubious and effectiveness is low and channeling them instead to cases where they will decidedly improve health advances overall health outcomes. As we have seen, the US prefers to reward private actors to achieve this goal. It remains to be seen whether American methods can reorient norms and values and bring about lasting social change. Other countries have instead harnessed the authority of the public sector to institutionalize a new vision of what health care is all about. Their attention is focused on goals to which the choice of means is subservient.

Lesson #7: Rationing is a reality that must be confronted. Transparent criteria are preferable to the implicit processes that currently prevail in the US.

Primary Care

The growing concern about health outcomes has increased interest in primary care, which is an essential route to good health. Compared to other countries, the US continues to regard specialized care oriented toward curing disease more highly than primary care, prevention, and the management of chronic illness. Despite a growing interest among younger physicians in primary care several years ago, poor reimbursement created disincentives and resulted in a decline in physicians choosing and remaining in primary care fields in the US. Physicians, especially those working on a fee-for-service basis, continue to find that the time required to engage in preventive care is insufficiently appreciated and rewarded (Ayres and Griffith 2007). We can see the consequence in a recent report by the Commonwealth Fund that ranked the US lowest among the six countries it compared on primary care measures (Davis et al. 2007).

Physicians in the US exercise considerable control over the terms of their livelihoods and the pursuit of their interests. In other countries the state has been more interventionist by, for example, limiting the number of places for certain specialties in medical school and in practice settings. And yet, the fact of state intervention does not deter people elsewhere from choosing medicine as a profession. In fact, the US is below the average among OECD countries in the proportion of practicing physicians per population. Physicians in the US are also poorly distributed across the nation. Underserved areas and populations inhabit inner cities as well as rural locales. Nurses are as, if not more important, than physicians when it comes to primary care. The US is also far from the top among OECD countries when it comes to the proportion of practicing nurses per population as well as the ratio of nurses to physicians.

Nevertheless, change is discernible in the US if one looks hard enough. Rather than turn to what other countries are doing when it comes to primary care, we might examine instances of innovation in the US. They are occurring in organizations that decades ago held the promise of instituting primary care, as implied in the term health maintenance, but lost their way during the 1990s because of economic pressures (Mechanic 2004). Those pressures have since motivated many MCOs to search for alternative administrative and delivery systems that have re-invigorated progress toward their original goals.

For instance, while the use of nurse practitioners (NPs) is indeed a device to control costs, it has also accompanied a renewed interest in prioritizing access to health care according to need. In MCOs that employ NPs as primary care providers, less-ill patients can more fully discuss their conditions with NPs, while physicians are reserved for more complex healthcare services. Greater use of NPs in primary care has also facilitated the development of disease management programs, a critical element in the quest for improved health outcomes for such chronic conditions as diabetes, obesity, and heart disease (Rothman et al. 2006). These programs require considerable patient self-care, which can sometimes be problematic and has raised concerns about shifting responsibility from providers to patients. This problem can be mitigated if patients are well guided and monitored and all providers are well integrated into the continuum of care (Nagelkerk et al. 2006). Sound disease management programs that encourage patient self-care and prevent overuse of the health care system, including hospitalization, can realize considerable cost savings (Starfield et al. 2005). Accordingly, some state Medicaid programs have encouraged their adoption by the private MCOs that enroll Medicaid recipients. And, recognizing the important role that patients themselves must play, some states have developed systems of incentive payments to Medicaid patients who engage in preventive self-care measures (Redmond, Solomon, Lin 2007).

For their part, physicians are learning to be part of management teams and to shed the traditional doctor-centered model of health care (Light 2000). In a transformation that has been in the offing for years, physician–patient relations are becoming more co-participatory and cooperative (Heritage and Maynard 2006). These changes in the social relations of health care invite deeper investigation of the norms and values underpinning delivery of health care and their consequences for health outcomes.

Although government is guiding the expansion of primary care, following the lead of MCOs, the benefits of this type of delivery system pertain to all social actors. Payers, whether public or private, profit from lower costs, even though they must play a stronger role in organizing the supply and demand side factors of care. Providers are playing a less central role, but their loss of power may be offset by the gains derived from partnership. Patients are being drawn more into new domains of responsibility, negotiating their interests in multi-layered contexts of autonomy and collaboration. The significance of these tensions may wither if improvements in health outcomes materialize.

Lesson #8: Primary health care lowers cost and improves health outcomes.

Conclusion

There are many reasons for the low ranking of the US in comparative health outcomes. That we still do not recognize health care as a right and many Americans lack access as a result is critical, to be sure. But there is more to the picture, both here and abroad. For, even in countries with universal access, poor people, whose health care needs are higher than their wealthier counterparts, use health care less than they should (Schoen and Doty 2004; van Doorslaer et al. 2006). Governments everywhere are trying to tackle these inequalities. In light of the larger proportion of the population in poverty in the US, most egregiously including the high level of child poverty, we have a harder uphill struggle.

The relationship between poverty and poor health is well established in the literature (Budrys 2003; Mullahy et al. 2004). While significant health care resources must be spent on such poverty-related conditions as substance abuse and poor diet, we ought not lose sight of the importance of non-health assets that could do a great deal to improve the lives of society's less fortunate. Social policies and programs in the areas of education and employment are critical to offering the opportunity for self-sufficiency and the foundations for good health.

In addition, research is demonstrating that discrimination based on race, ethnicity, age, gender, sexual orientation, religious affiliation, and so on is an independent factor related to worse health outcomes, whether it occurs in the health care system (Smedley et al. 2003; Laditka and Laditka 2006), in workplace or educational settings (Sellers et al. 2006), or in society at large. Although social discrimination is not confined to the US, it is exacerbated by the extent of disparities in access to health care, which is unique to the US (Davis et al. 2006). It is unfortunate that race and ethnicity are often taken as proxies for socioeconomic disadvantage. Although the practice demonstrates the difficulty of collecting data on race and ethnicity, including privacy concerns, the Institute of Medicine, among others, has called on healthcare providers and insurers to record all relevant information, so as to enable more focused research. Studies in these fields are inherently policy relevant, but they can easily segue into being policy-oriented as well (Gray and O'Leary 2000).

Lesson #9: Improvements in poverty reduction and in fostering human and social capital can improve health outcomes. Short-term expenditures may be large but the long-term benefits are worth the investment.

Sociologists must continue to expose the irrationalities and contradictions that confound health care in the US as well as the many inequalities it has created and exacerbates, not only in health. Such studies contribute to what leaders in our discipline, most recently William Julius Wilson (1991) and Michael Burawoy (2005), have called public sociology. Their hope is that eventually policy makers will pay attention, whether out of conscience or self-interest.

Convincing the Dubious and Shaping Policy

To topple those who may still be sitting on the fence about the value of comparative lessons, I suggest a number of areas for future research. Policymakers will also benefit from the specification that elaborated study can bring. While theoretical explanations will remain in the hands of sociologists, we ought to remember that the ability to communicate with the world outside our hallowed corridors elevates the role of public sociology.

1. We have seen that the balance between public and private sectors favors the former in Canada, Germany, and Britain. Future research should elaborate the regulatory measures that these and other countries have adopted to control the excesses of market forces while allowing competition and choice to advance the goal of efficiency. Then, to assure transportability, researchers should suggest how these measures could be instituted or approximated in the US and with what consequences.
2. All countries are struggling with the trade-off between efficiency and equality, but some have been more successful than others in achieving an acceptable balance. Researchers must continue to work on identifying the mechanisms that mediate the relationship between efficiency and equality and that enable harmonization between them.
3. The main goal of policy reform is optimum health. We have seen that this outcome need not break the bank. Researchers must demonstrate empirically that the quality measures accelerating improvements in health care also create efficiencies and reduce long-term costs.
4. More research is needed on how open and inclusive decision making evolves – wherever it occurs. Researchers should identify the features of different models. They should also attempt to situate these models in appropriate settings in the US health care system (primary care, hospitals, etc.) and demonstrate their ability to solve problems. We can expect considerable variation around common themes in best practices. Future research may demonstrate that the variations are due less to country-specific factors than to other kinds of contextual factors.
5. Future debate on the issue of rationing is inevitable and will require considerable preparatory groundwork. To enable open discussion by a well-informed public, researchers should gather examples of transparent processes of and criteria for rationing scarce healthcare resources, both in the US and other countries.
6. There are many exemplary cases of primary care in the US. Researchers should find them and demonstrate how they can be expanded across the nation.
7. We must all be engaged in developing pragmatic arguments for establishing health care as a right. Sociologists can offer a special contribution by demonstrating empirically the human and social capital benefits that would follow from universal access to equitable health care, and by suggesting corresponding responsibilities on the part of all the major actors in health care.

Bibliography

Allen D, Pilnick A (2006) The social organisation of healthcare work. Blackwell, London
Ayres CG, Griffith HM (2007) Perceived barriers to and facilitators of the implementation of priority clinical preventive services guidelines. Am J Manag Care 13(3):150–155
Budrys G (2003) Unequal health: how inequality contributes to health or illness. Roman and Littlefield Publishers, New York

Burawoy M (2005) 2004 Presidential Address: For Public Sociology. Am J Soc 70(1):4–28
Cutler DM (2004) Your money or your life. Oxford University Press, New York
Davis K et al (2006) Mirror, mirror on the wall: an update on the quality of American Health Care through the patient's lens. The Commonwealth Fund. http://www.cmwf.org/usr_doc/Davis_mirrormirror_915.pdf
Davis K et al (2007) Mirror, mirror on the wall: an international update on the comparative performance of American Health Care. The Commonwealth Fund. http://www.commonwealthfund.org/usr_doc/1027_Davis_mirror_mirror_international_update_final.pdf?section=4039
Gilbert N (2002) Transformation of the welfare state: the silent surrender of public responsibility. Oxford University Press, New York
Grand JL (2006) Debate: choice and competition in the British National Health Service. Eurohealth 12(1):1–3
Gray BH, O'Leary J (2000) The evolving relationship between medical sociology and health policy. In: Bird CE, Conrad P, Fremont AM (eds) The handbook of medical sociology. Prentice-Hall, New Jersey, pp 258–270
Hacker JS (2004) Review article: dismantling the health care state? Political institutions, public policies and the comparative politics of health reform. Br J Polit Sci 34:693–724
Heritage J, Maynard DW (2006) Problems and prospects in the study of physician-patient interaction: 30 years of research. Annu Rev Sociol 32:351–374
Institute of Medicine (1990) Clinical practice guidelines: directions for a new program. National Academies Press, Washington, D.C
Laditka JN, Laditka SB (2006) Race, ethnicity, and hospitalization for six chronic ambulatory care sensitive conditions in the US. Ethn Health 11(3):247–263
Light DW (2000) The medical profession and organizational change: from professional dominance to countervailing power. In: Bird CE, Conrad P, Fremont AM (eds) The handbook of medical sociology. Prentice-Hall, New Jersey, pp 201–216
Marshall TH (1949) Citizenship and social class. In: Marshall TH (ed) Class, citizenship, and social development. Doubleday, New York, pp 65–123
Mattke S et al (2006) Health care quality indicators project: initial indicators report. OECD health working papers, No. 22. OECD, Paris
McMahon LF Jr, Hofer TP, Hayward RA (2007) Physician-level P4P –DOA? Can quality-based payment be resuscitated? Am J Manag Care 13(5):233–236
McWilliams JM et al (2007) Use of health services by previously uninsured Medicare Beneficiaries. N Engl J Med 357(2):143–153
Mechanic D (2004) The rise and fall of managed care. J Health Soc Behav 45:76–86
Milgate K, Cheng SB (2006) Pay-for-performance: the MedPAC perspective. Health Aff 25(2):413–419
Mullahy J, Roberts S, Wolfe B (2004) Health, income, and inequality. In: Kathryn Neckerman (ed) Social inequality. Russell Sage, New York, pp 523–544
Nagelkerk J, Reick K, Meenga L (2006) Perceived barriers and effective strategies to diabetes self-management. J Adv Nurs 54(2):151–158
O'Malley AS, Pham HH, Reschovsky JD (2007) Predictors of the growing influence of clinical practice guidelines. J Gen Intern Med 22:742–748
Oberlander J (2007) Health reform interrupted: The unraveling of the Oregon Health Plan. Health Aff 26(1):96–105
Pauly M (2006) The tax subsidy to employment-based health insurance and the distribution of well being. Law Contemp Probl 69:83–92
Pear R (2007) A battle over expansion of children's insurance. The New York Times. <http://www.nytimes.com/2007/07/09/washington/09child.html?ex=1189310400&en=65b8426fe2c28fe8&ei=5070>
Pearson SD, Rawlins MD (2005) Quality, innovation, and value for money: NICE and the British health service. J Am Med Assoc 294(20):2618–2622
Pierson P (2000) Increasing returns, path dependence and the study of politics. Am Polit Sci Rev 94:251–67
Quadagno J, Street D (2006) Recent trends in US social welfare policy. Res Aging 28(3):303–316
Ranade W (ed) (1998) Markets and health care. Addison Wesley, London
Rawlins MD (2004) NICE work – Providing guidance to the British National Health Service. N Engl J Med 351(14):1383–1385
Redmond P, Solomon J (2007) Can incentives for healthy behavior improve health and hold down Medicaid costs? Center on budget and policy priorities. http://www.cbpp.org/6-1-07health.pdf
Reschovsky JD, Hadley J, Landon BE (2006) Effects of compensation methods and physician group structure on physicians' perceived incentives to alter services to patients. Health Serv Res 41(4):1200–1220
Robinson JC (2001) Theory and practice in the design of physician payment incentives. Milbank Q 79(2):149–177
Rothman RL et al (2006) Labor characteristics and program costs of a successful diabetes disease management program. Am J Manag Care 12(5):277–283

Ruggie M (1996) Realignments in the welfare state: health policy in the United States, Britain, and Canada. Columbia University Press, New York

Saltman RB (2002) The Western European experience with health care reform. http://www.euro.who.int/observatory/Studies/20021223_2

Schoen C, Doty MM (2004) Inequities in access to medical care in five countries: Findings from the 2001 Commonwealth fund international health policy survey. Health Policy 67:309–322

Selden T, Gray BM (2006) Tax subsidies for employment-related health insurance: Estimates for 2006. Health Aff 25(6):1568–1579

Sellers RM et al (2006) Racial identity matters: the relationship between racial discrimination and psychological functioning in African American adolescents. J Res Adolesc 16(2):187–216

Smedley BD, Stith AY, Nelson AR (2003) Unequal treatment: confronting racial and ethnic disparities in health care. National Academies Press, Washington, DC

Starfield B, Shi L, Macinko J (2005) Contribution of primary care to health systems and health. Milbank Q 83(3):457–502

Toner R, Elder J (2007) Most support U.S. guarantee of health care. The New York Times. http://query.nytimes.com/gst/fullpage.html?sec=health&res=9E06E7D71631F931A35750C0A9619C8B63

van Doorslaer E, Masseria C, Koolman X (2006) Inequalities in access to medical care by income in developed countries. Can Med Assoc J 174(2):177–183

Western Canada Wait List Project (2005) Moving forward: final report. http://www.wcwl.org/media/pdf/news/moving_forward/report.pdf.

Wynia MK et al (2003) Do physicians not offer useful services because of coverage restrictions? Health Affairs 22(4):190–197

Chapter 6
Health and the Social Rights of Citizenship: Integrating Welfare-State Theory and Medical Sociology

Sigrun Olafsdottir and Jason Beckfield

Social scientists have long been interested in the link between societal processes and individual outcomes. The founders of sociology were interested in how social integration affected suicide rates (Durkheim 1951 [1897]), how the social organization of labor relations impacted worker experience (Marx and Engels 1964 [1848]), how religious principles translated into individuals' work ethics (Weber 1930), how modern society impacted mental health (Simmel 1950), how mental health institutions shaped individual inmates (Goffman 1961) or how the social system impacted health care utilization (Parsons 1951). All addressed issues of health, illness, and healing in one way or another, yet medical sociologists have tended to pay less attention to the distal forces of societal-level institutions, focusing instead on the more proximate micro- and meso-level determinants of individual health.

Comparative research provides an important lens to understand variation in the relationship between society and individuals, as it illuminates how different social organization may lead to a different lived experience across contexts. While many approaches have been taken to understand variations in social organization (e.g., Anderson 1972; Hall and Soskice 2001; Lee 1982), we argue that the social organization of the welfare state is a major force shaping the economic, political, and cultural landscape that contextualizes and shapes the proximate causes of health, illness, and healing in advanced, industrialized nations. The welfare state – defined as "interventions by the state in civil society to alter social and market forces" (Orloff 1993) – sets the stage for such mechanisms as health policy preferences, social citizenship rights, logics of the "appropriate" social organization of health care, characterizations of "legitimate" or stigmatized health problems, and the social stratification of health. In short, the welfare state matters because, as a complex set of institutionalized citizenship rights, it shapes the causes and consequences of health, illness, and healing.

In this chapter, we provide an overview of the major approaches to understanding variations in health care systems and welfare states. We then consider three broad institutional domains that may connect the welfare state to health, illness, and healing within a nation: the stratification order, social policy, and national culture. We conclude by proposing a new research agenda for medical sociology that incorporates the welfare state as an economic, political, and cultural institution into current understandings of health and illness. Throughout this chapter, our goals are twofold: First, we want to consider what attention to health, illness, and healing can add to the political sociology of the welfare state. That is, we aim to make a start on the medical sociology of the welfare state. Second, we want to consider what new knowledge attention to the welfare state can add to medical sociology. That is, we want to develop a political sociology of health, illness, and healing. Our hope

S. Olafsdottir (✉)
Department of Sociology, Boston University, 96 Cummington St., Boston, MA 02215, USA
e-mail: sigrun@bu.edu

is that a better understanding of the connections between the welfare state and health[1] will help to advance inquiry into "embodiment," conceptualized as that process whereby "we literally incorporate, biologically, the world around us" (Krieger 2001, p. 668). We argue that the welfare state is an undertheorized part of that world.

Classifying Health Care Systems and Welfare States

Health care is one of the key dimensions of all modern welfare states, yet it has been relatively absent from major welfare-state theories (cf. Wilensky 2002). If, as Esping-Andersen notes, the welfare state is more than a collection of social policies and, instead, should be conceptualized as "an explicit redefinition of what the state is all about" (1999, p. 34), then the quantity and quality of the state's intervention into the market forces that shape health comprises a fundamental part of what a welfare state is. Similarly, all health care systems are embedded within a national welfare system; however, comparative health researchers often omit discussion of the welfare state, when categorizing nations based on social organization of health care. Researchers have pointed out that health care systems are converging as a consequence of similar pressures (e.g., aging populations and increased cost) faced by policymakers (Mechanic and Rochenfort 1996). However, they have simultaneously argued for the importance of local context, suggesting that national variations result in different health care systems and health outcomes. Among the factors that have been theorized to be different across nations are the orientation toward the use of professionals, availability of facilities, and the larger cultural environment (Antonovsky 1972).

Comparative health service researchers have attempted to organize nations into clusters based on the social organization of health care. One such classification was suggested by Stevens (2001) naming health care systems as the *Beveridge*, *Bismarck*, and *Semashko* health care systems after the key historical figure that created them. These systems differ by organizational configuration and by the role of three principal actors – the medical profession, the state, and the payers. The *Bismarck* model represents systems that are financed through insurance fee collected from the insured. Under this model, the role of the state is quite limited to setting and maintaining a system of contracts among patients, providers, and insurers. The provision of services is left to the profession of medicine. Countries belonging to this type include Canada, France, Germany, Japan, and the United States. Under the *Semashko* model, citizens have free universal access to health care that is controlled directly by the state. The state owns health care facilities, finances them through the state budget, and allocates services throughout the country. Nations included in this type are Bulgaria, Czech Republic, Hungary, Poland, and Russia. Finally, the *Beveridge* model provides free access to health care through publicly owned hospitals. However, complete state control of all health care facilities is absent, the medical profession has more autonomy, and physicians are allowed to opt out of the system. Countries belonging to this system are Italy, New Zealand, Spain, Sweden, and the United Kingdom (Lassey et al. 1997; Stevens 2001).

Welfare-state researchers have been equally interested in classifying welfare states into regime clusters. Esping-Andersen (1990) provides the most widely used categorizations of welfare state, dividing nations into liberal, conservative, and social-democratic welfare states. This typology is largely based on the generosity of the welfare state – specifically, the extent to which the state "decommodifies" labor by making it possible for people to maintain a standard of living outside the market – but health care spending does not receive similar attention as various benefits linked to the labor market (e.g., unemployment benefits). The liberal welfare states (e.g., Canada, the

---

[1] By health, we are referring to both physical and mental health.

United Kingdom, and the United States) are characterized by a minimum state intervention in labor market processes and the state does little to interfere with inequalities created in the market. The conservative welfare states (e.g., Germany, France, and Italy) prefer familial and charity solutions to social problems with the state serving as a safety net once those other types of solutions have failed. In addition, benefits are frequently tied to the labor market, rather than representing a universal right. Finally, the social-democratic welfare states (e.g., Denmark, Iceland, and Sweden) are most active in correcting inequalities created by the market. Benefits are universal and tied to citizenship, rather than employment status.[2]

Juxtaposing these two categorizations reveals some similarities, but also important differences. Nations like the United States are categorized coherently across the two classifications. For example, the United States does little regarding welfare and it does little about the health system – owing, arguably, to the public–private mix of health insurance provision in the U.S. (Hacker 2002; cf. Ruggie 1992). Countries like the United Kingdom pose more of a problem. It is classified as a liberal welfare state, with a high reliance on the market, yet the *Beveridge* system originated there, and in fact, the United Kingdom was one of the first nations to establish a national health care system in 1919 (Lassey et al. 1997). These differences may result from a general tendency to overlook or downplay health when conceptualizing welfare states (cf. Hacker 2002). Especially within the neo-Marxist tradition, there is a natural emphasis on the economy and the conditions of labor in identifying the "new social risks" such as unemployment, low-wage labor, income insecurity, and skill formation that shape welfare states in the postindustrial era (Esping-Andersen 1999, p. 146; Taylor-Gooby 2004). Current scholarship moves toward health in identifying population aging and declines in fertility as aspects of the "crisis" of the welfare state, but these are typically conceptualized as placing additional fiscal burdens on the welfare state, rather than as health inequalities or health policies that are constitutive of what it means to be a welfare state (Brady et al. 2005; Castles 2004; Huber and Stephens 2001).

Goodwin (1997) provides one of the few attempts to link welfare-state classification and health care systems in his conceptualization of the three worlds of mental health policy. As Esping-Andersen, he divides nations into the liberal regime, conservative regime, and social-democratic regime. Within the liberal regime, mental health policy is a reflection of the market and the main goal of mental health policy is to restore people in order to be able to participate in the market. Conversely, mental health policy reflects reaction and reliance on other types of organizations in the conservative regime. Finally, in the social-democratic welfare regime, mental health policy illustrates commitment to social rights. This work provides an example of a consolidation between welfare-state theories and a domain of health care services.

While these categorizations provide important insights into the overall organization of the health care system and/or the welfare system, two key tasks await researchers. First, medical sociology and welfare-state theories would benefit from a mutual discourse that attempts to integrate health care into welfare-state categorization or vice versa. Two big questions on this theme should be addressed: (a) How much overlap is there between "health regime" and welfare-state regime and (b) If welfare states can be understood through their constitutive purposes (Esping-Andersen 1990) as well as through their effects (Goodin et al. 1999), then how do the politics and policy of health reinforce or revise our conceptualizations of welfare states? Second, these classifications tend to focus on the macro-level and provide description of the system, rather than attempt to understand how the different organizations affect the health outcomes of populations. Consequently, the question becomes, how are health, illness, and healing patterned by health regimes and welfare states? More specifically, if health is a "good" or an "asset" that is stratified in society, how does the welfare state produce and re-produce

---

[2] Welfare state researchers have suggested different categorization of nations, including classifying Australia and New Zealand as a wage-earner regime (Huber and Stephens 2001). They have also pointed out that the Esping-Andersen scheme is problematic when gender is considered (Orloff 1993; O'Connor et al. 1999).

health stratification? To date, much welfare-state research (e.g., Brady 2003, 2005; Kenworthy 1999, 2004) naturally follows in the tradition of stratification research in focusing on economic outcomes like income, poverty, and jobs (Grusky 2001), but we think there is ample opportunity for work that tackles the question of how the welfare-state structures health inequalities.

Theories of the Welfare State: What Attention to Health Adds

While theorizing cross-national differences in regimes, health policy researchers and welfare-state scholars have also developed explanations for cross-national variation in health care systems and welfare states. Research on health policy, especially English-language scholarship, focuses on explaining the "exceptionalism" (Lipset 1997) of American policy in the health domain, and explains the lack of health insurance as a citizenship right in the United States as a function of antistatist American values, an unusually weak labor movement, the racial politics of the American South, the federal structure and policy feedbacks of the American government, or the mobilization of groups with vested interests in existing health policy (Quadagno 2005). Research on the welfare state, again focusing on cross-national differences within the advanced industrial countries or "rich democracies" (Wilensky 2002), explains welfare-state formation and variation as a result of economic development, class politics, political institutions, public opinion (Brooks and Manza 2007), or institutionalized investments in human capital (Iversen 2005).

Note the resonance: both literatures, while too rarely in direct conversation with each other (cf. Quadagno 2005), highlight the strong effects of labor unions in pushing for health benefits, the independent influence of political institutions in shaping policy, and the substantial impact of actors with vested interests in health policy. For instance, the "power resources" approach to the welfare state, which argues that a combination of a strong labor movement with powerful left parties and a democratic polity produces generous welfare states that are most akin to Esping-Andersen's social-democratic regime type (Esping-Andersen 1990; Hicks 1999; Huber and Stephens 2001), clearly concurs with claims from political economists of health that the absence of a strong labor movement coupled with a labor party accounts for the absence of universal health insurance in the U.S. (Navarro 1989). Also, arguments that "veto points" in federal polities and the dynamics of policy feedbacks generate continuing divergences on welfare-state development (Pierson 1994, 2001) sound remarkably similar to arguments that foreground the same factors in explaining how efforts to institutionalize health insurance were "vetoed" at various points in the American political process over the last century (Hacker 1997; Immergut 1990; Steinmo and Watts 1995). Finally, recent arguments about the role of established public constituencies in the durability of differences among welfare states (Brooks and Manza 2007) resonate with reasoning that the mobilization of established private constituencies, or "stakeholders," blocked efforts at establishing national health insurance in the U.S. (Quadagno 2005).

It would appear that health policy should be seen as a case of welfare politics, or as a "policy domain" (Burstein 1991) of the welfare state. But we think a closer look at these three approaches also reveals areas where better integration would be fruitful. As a first example, labor- and left-centric "power resources" approach tends to take for granted that labor pushes for the state to do more across policy domains, but attention to health policy can lead to a better understanding of when, how, and why the labor movement might favor efforts in one domain over another. Such research could generate synthetic accounts that would explore how politics and policy within the health domain spill over into other domains, and modify the very politics of social policy outside the health domain (thus building on both the power-resources and political–institutional approaches). Second, while the political–institutional approach itself highlights the federal structure of the American welfare state, attention to varying health inequalities and their connections to policy differences across the 50 U.S.

states would help to reveal the mechanisms whereby political institutions matter. Third, comparative research in the "varieties of capitalism" (VoC) tradition (Hall and Soskice 2001) could show how the process of stakeholder mobilization varies cross-nationally and historically, and how that mobilization (be it on the part of capitalist firms or individual citizens) interfaces with political institutions. Fourth, welfare-state researchers could usefully extend Iversen's (2005) synthesis of the VoC employer-centered tradition with a focus on the formation of human capital by exploring the implications of investment in health capital as a non-asset-specific good that potentially affects the realization and formation of human capital.

Another promising line of research that would contribute to both political sociology and medical sociology is inquiry into the impact of the global political economy on health policy. For instance, the "logic of industrialism" approach to the welfare state argues that as rich democracies develop, they grow more similar because of similar demographic pressures and economic resources (Wilensky 1975, 2002) and comparative health care scholars point to the convergence of medical systems, due to similar processes (Mechanic and Rochefort 1996). Thinking about how this convergence applies to health raises several questions: Do health policies converge at the same rate and through the same processes as other policies are alleged to converge? Do health outcomes at the population level and health inequalities within populations converge with the process of development as well, or do health policy regimes condition this convergence? Although health inequalities at the global level have been described (Goesling and Firebaugh 2004), their production and possible intersection with the welfare state have only begun to be explored (Conley and Springer 2001; Macinko et al. 2004; Olafsdottir 2007). Finally, while welfare-state research has focused on economic globalization as an additional source of convergence (Brady et al 2005), macro-institutionalist approaches within sociology offer good reasons to expect health care systems to change in ways that are isomorphic to one another, through the adoption of common policy scripts created and diffused in and through international organizations (Meyer et al. 1997). Attention to the evolution of health policy and politics could shed light on this question of global or even regional convergence in the face of national institutional heterogeneity.

Institutionalizing Inequalities: The State and the Economy

The welfare state is one of the political and cultural institutions that establishes the "architecture of markets" (Fligstein 2001). It does so by institutionalizing the rules that allow for and become taken for granted by people and organizations in market exchanges. For instance, welfare states vary dramatically in the degree to which they insulate people and organizations from the pressures and instabilities of market competition: corporatist bargaining between labor and capital, and generous unemployment, sickness, and pension benefits, tend to reduce both economic inequality and poverty (Alderson and Nielsen 2002; Brady 2003, 2005; Kenworthy 1999, 2004; Moller et al. 2003). These inequalities have garnered much attention by social scientists interested in the relationship between inequality and health – much research explores how aggregate inequality at the macro-level (e.g., the Gini or Theil index) impacts population health (e.g., life expectancy or the infant mortality rate). While this work does not necessarily address the welfare state, levels of inequality are shaped by the social organization of welfare (DiPrete 2002). Some welfare states actively try to eliminate inequalities created by the market, whereas others are more inactive. Figure 6.1 shows the level of income inequality in nations belonging to different welfare regimes.[3]

---

[3] These figures are based on the Gini-Coefficient, one of the most widely used measures for income inequality. These numbers are provided by the World Bank.

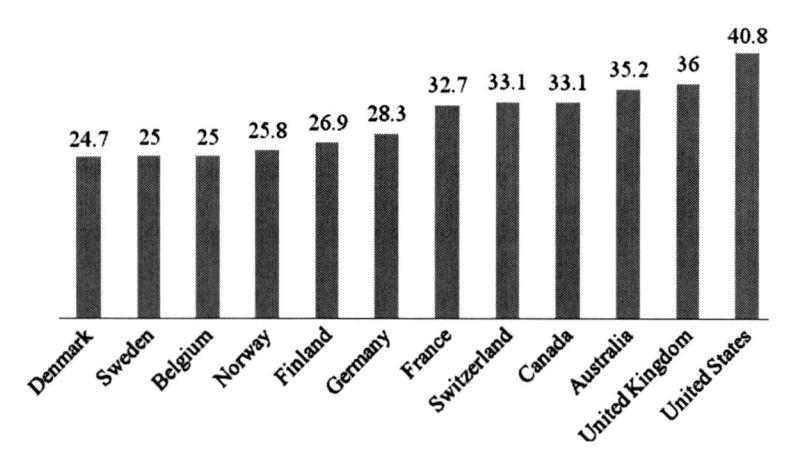

Fig. 6.1 Income inequality in 12 advanced, industrialized nations

The figure shows that nations belonging to the social-democratic regime have the lowest levels of inequality, followed by nations belonging to the conservative regime, and not surprisingly the liberal welfare states have the highest levels of income inequality. This indicates that welfare states, at least partly, shape the income distribution within a country, which has been theorized to impact the health of citizens.

Despite many agreeing that inequality is bad for health, empirical evidence for the relationship between macro-level inequality and health is mixed. Wilkinson (1996) argues that inequality is bad for health and shows that aggregate health outcomes (life expectancy and infant mortality) are better in nations that have less income inequality. He identifies social cohesion as a central mechanism, specifically that nations with lower levels of income inequality have more solidarity among citizens that then translate into better health. Supporting this, research has shown that trust in other people improves health at the aggregate and individual level (Rostila 2007). Yet, using data from more countries, along with better measures and more appropriate methods, Beckfield (2004) fails to support for the relationship between income inequality and aggregate health measures. Similarly, a review of 98 studies on this relationship concluded that there is little support for this relationship; yet suggests that income inequality may affect some health outcomes more than others (Lynch et al. 2004).

Does this mean that the way in which welfare states shape income inequality does not matter for population health? Our answer is no. The social organization of welfare impacts individuals from conception to death, making it problematic to focus on macro-level relationships at one or even several points in time. Scholars have focused on cumulative advantage as a mechanism for inequality, suggesting that a favorable position obtained by an individual or families is a resource that translates into future gains (DiPrete and Eirich 2006). Here, researchers have suggested health as one domain that is affected by such advantage, by arguing for the cumulative effect of education on health (Ross and Wu 1996) or the cumulative effect of discrimination on race differences in health (Krieger 1994). Similarly, research has also established the impact of family poverty on children's mental health trajectories (McLeod and Shanahan 1993, 1996; McLeod and Nonnemaker 2000). Considering the long-term impact of inequality, Neckerman and Torche (2007) point out that cross-sectional studies on the relationship between health and income inequality are problematic since they do not capture cumulative exposures to a disadvantageous position over a long period of time. Furthermore, the welfare state is also one of the "upstream" factors that shapes meso-level health determinants such as social networks (Berkman et al. 2000).

Welfare-state scholars have increasingly paid attention to the consequences of the welfare state, such as its role in reducing income inequality (Hicks and Swank 1992; Korpi and Palme 1998) and shaping social networks (Lee 2005). Broadly, the welfare state creates institutional arrangements that shape individual life chances (Esping-Andersen et al. 2002) and determine the impact of negative life events, such as job loss or divorce, on individual lives (DiPrete 2002; DiPrete and McManus 2000). While researchers have traditionally been more interested in other outcomes (e.g., earnings, wealth, or power) health increasingly serves as a source of stratification (Esping-Andersen et al. 2002; Ross and Bird 1994). Indeed, we think that the welfare state shapes not only the level and pattern of social inequality within a society, but also the effects of social inequality on health within and across societies.

For instance, research has shown that health inequalities based on employment and education remained stable in the Nordic countries during a period of economic recession and increased levels of unemployment, suggesting that institutional arrangements buffer against widening health inequalities caused by increased labor market inequalities (Lahelma et al. 2002). Similarly, researchers have suggested that the relatively favorable health trends in the Nordic countries can be explained by the encompassing welfare states (Kunst et al. 2005). Finally, considering the differences across regimes, a comparison of a liberal welfare state with high levels of inequality (the United States) and a social-democratic welfare state with low levels of inequality (Iceland) found that the impact of education and poverty on self-rated health was similar in the two nations. Yet, two important differences emerged. First, the more advantaged appeared to be able to translate their position into better health in the United States, possibly reflecting a health care system where citizens can pay for better health care. Second, both single and married parents had better health in Iceland, which may be related to a better support to families in Iceland than in the United States (Olafsdottir 2007).

The research that has begun to explore the relationship between the welfare state, income inequality, and health is arguably still in its infancy, as much work remains to be done that focuses on the connections between social inequality and inequalities in health (Bianchi et al. 2004; Hout 2003; Neckerman 2004). We argue for the importance of continuing this stream of theorizing and empirical research and highlight three fruitful avenues of research. First, research should consider how the welfare state creates inequality over the life-course, rather than consider the impact of income inequality at selected time-points. Second, research needs to focus more on individual-level health outcomes within and across the nation, since the differences may not lie in aggregate health outcomes, but in the quality of life citizens enjoy across welfare regimes. Third, research should focus on establishing a link between the macro-level of the welfare state and micro-level health outcomes. More specifically, it should explore whether and how specific welfare policies or provision affect various health outcomes.

The Welfare State as a Provider of Health Care

The political domain of welfare states represents what the government does as well as what it is expected to do. All welfare states provide some health care for their citizens and most provide some health care for all citizens. The United States is the notable exception, with public spending on health constituting less than half of the total health care spending (Quadagno 2004, 2005). However, the United States also spends the most on the health care of all nations in the world, although the health care spending may do more to increase health inequalities than decrease them. In fact, the United States has among the least favorable health outcomes at the aggregate level (Pampel 2001) and patients stay shorter times in hospitals in the United States than in other industrialized nations (Anderson and Poullier 1999). Conversely, hospital expenditure per day is most expensive in the United States, and physicians have substantially higher income (Anderson and Poullier 1999).

Much of the research on government involvement in health care has focused on public attitudes toward health care, which is important since it indicates the pressures policymakers face within a nation, which then impacts welfare priorities (Brooks and Manza 2006, 2007). Researchers have defined four main dimensions of welfare-state attitudes, the function of the welfare state (what it should do), the financing of the welfare state, the means of the welfare state (institutions, programs, and actors), and the intended and unintended consequences of the welfare state (Andreß and Heien 2001). Hayes and Vanden Heuvel´s (1996) five-nation study finds Britons, Italians, and Australians more supportive than Americans and West Germans of increases in government spending on health care. They suggest that these variations may be explained by the differing degree of government involvement in health care, that is the nature, breadth, and generosity of existing programs. Research has also shown that the impact of individual-level factors varies across countries. For example, in 1985, women were more supportive of health care spending in West Germany, Italy, and Australia but not in the United States and Great Britain. Similarly, those with more education are less likely to want spending more on health care in West Germany and Italy, but not in the United States, Great Britain, and Australia (Hayes and VandenHeuvel 1996).

When the public evaluates the health care system across welfare regimes, research has shown that the poor do not give worse evaluations based on the type of welfare state they live in, however, those who are better off evaluate the performance of the health care system more negatively in many countries, and whether an individual lives in a country classified as a welfare leader rather than a laggard impacts public opinion (Pescosolido et al. 1985). Finally, research has shown that public attitudes not only cluster around the historical organization of health care, but also relate to the current economic and demographic realities. Individuals living in countries that adopted the NHS or Centralized model of health care are more supportive of government involvement in health care than those living under the Insurance model.[4] However, citizens in countries that currently spend more on health care and have a greater burden of chronic illness are less supportive (Kikuzawa et al. 2008).

Research on the welfare state as a provider of health care suggests three avenues for future research. First, while current research describes differences across national context, more work should focus on why these differences exist between nations and how they relate to the social organization of health care and the welfare state. Second, while much is known about the differences in social organization of health care, spending on health care, performance of health care, or aggregate health outcomes, less is known about how these differences at the macro-level impact individual-level health outcomes. Consequently, research should pay attention to the way in which these factors shape individual health. Third, public attitudes provide an important insight into the pressures policymakers face when formulating national health policies. Yet, more work needs to focus on how public expectations shape actual health care policy, as well as focusing on the relationships between public attitudes, policymaking, and policy domains (on path dependency, see Pierson 1994, 1996; on the relationship between the health policy domain and other policy domains, see Giaimo 2001).

The Welfare State as Reflecting and Shaping National Culture

Responses to health and illness are embedded within the cultural context. Research on the role of social networks in utilization illustrates that it is the cultural content of the networks that matters, rather than the structure of the network (Pescosolido 1991, 1992). Similarly, Furedi argues (2006, p. 17) that "people's perception of health and illness is shaped by the particular account that their culture offers about how they are expected to cope with life and about the nature of the human potential." While multiple factors in society can provide "culture," we argue that the social organization of the welfare state provides the overarching national culture that citizens have come to expect. It defines

---

[4] NHS refers to Beveridge, Centralized to Semashko, and Insurance to Bismarck.

whether everyone is entitled to benefits when encountered with a negative life event, whether there is stigma associated with receiving benefits, and who is entitled to what kind of health service. More specifically, it sets the stage for what citizens have come to expect regarding the relationship between the state, the market, and medicine.

Studies on the U.S. welfare state have generally lacked attention to the role of culture regarding policy development (Amenta et al. 2001), but researchers increasingly argue for the importance of incorporating the cultural aspects of the welfare state (Burstein 1991; Campbell 2002). One attempt to understand the role of culture in the development of U.S. social policy has been through the theorizing of cultural categories of worth that define some individuals more worthy of government assistance than others (Katz 1986, 1989; Patterson 1994). These categories create boundaries between groups in a society and reflect the taken-for-granted assumptions citizens have about who should be assisted and who should not be assisted. Scholars have only recently begun to explore how these categories were constructed in the U.S., specifically focusing on guaranteed income policy (Steensland 2006). We agree with Steensland (2006) that it would be fruitful to explore this further in the area of health policy, and argue further that health provides an excellent case to examine cultural categories of worth in a comparative perspective. While most outcomes are deeply embedded within the institutional arrangements of a society (e.g., the structure of the labor market or education system), health can be considered as a "universal" good. Of course, issues of health, illness, and healing are culturally bound (Angel and Thoits 1991; Kleinman 1988), yet the loss of health is something that can happen to anyone.[5] Consequently, which individuals and groups are viewed as worthy of different types assistance when encountered with illness (e.g., universal benefits, mental health care, sickness benefits) provides insights into the broader ideology of the welfare state. We argue that the exploration of cultural categories of worth, as they relate to issues of health, illness, and healing, would be a fruitful research direction for welfare-state scholars and medical sociologists alike.

Scant research has focused on how culture shapes issues of health, illness, and healing across welfare states. Yet, a discourse analysis of national media across three welfare states reveals strong welfare-state patterns in response to mental health problems[6] (Olafsdottir 2010). In the United States, a liberal welfare state with minimum state interference, the media attributes mental illness to individual causes and does not consider the state as a key actor responding to mental health problems. Rather individuals with mental illness are viewed as a "bad" part of society that often belong in prison. Contrast this with the discourse in Iceland, a social-democratic country with a strong commitment to the welfare state. Here, individuals experiencing mental health problems are viewed as an integral part of society, and it is the responsibility of the state to provide solutions. The discourse in Germany, a conservative welfare state with reliance on the family and charities, is less clear. It appears that the German media discourse on mental health problems is embedded within its unique historical trajectory of World War II and the Nazi Period. The main concern is to avoid mistakes of the past (Olafsdottir 2007). Similarly, research has shown that public stigma toward mental illness may be related to broader societal factors and possibly the social organization of the welfare state. For example, a comparison of five European nations reveals that levels of stigma are lowest in Iceland, the nation with the most encompassing welfare state (Pescosolido et al. 2008).

Comparative health care researchers have pointed out that the taken-for-granted assumptions about the relationship between the state, medicine, and patients, play a role in how and when individuals use health services. For example, the German health care system (and welfare state)

---

[5]It may of course be more likely to happen to some individuals, as compared to others, and relates to broader inequalities (e.g., class, race, and gender) in society. Yet, we argue that it is one of the few outcomes that can be viewed as potentially affecting all citizens, across all nations.

[6]National media discourses are an important indicator of the overarching cultural and political context and they both reflect and create public opinions and reactions toward various social problems (Gamson and Modigliani 1989).

emphasizes a "social contract" among citizens and the government (Inglehart 1991). Consequently, Germans feel entitled to health care and exercise these rights whenever they encounter a need (Cockerham 1995). Research within the U.S. has shown that utilization preferences are related to cultural toolboxes (Swidler 1986), specifically that some individuals within the U.S. may have more treatment options in their toolkit (Olafsdottir and Pescosolido 2009). While there is variation in cultural resources within a nation, the welfare state inevitably sets the stage for the overall cultural approach for when and how to seek medical attention. This underscores the importance of continuing to explore the role of culture in utilization within nations, but expanding that focus to understand how utilization preferences are embedded within different cultural norms of different welfare states.

The cultural turn in sociology (Bourdieu 1984; DiMaggio 1997; Jameson 1998) highlights the role of culture in providing information and organizational schemes to individuals. This type of culture is brought to the public through various mechanisms, including institutions, networks, and social movements (DiMaggio 1997). We argue that the social organization of welfare is a cultural institution that provides individuals with the overarching understanding of how the world works. Therefore, the task of researchers is at least twofold: First, understanding how the welfare state as a cultural institution shapes issues of health, illness, and healing within and across nations. Second, exploring whether variations in welfare state cultures impact the health and illness experiences of individuals living in different welfare states.

Toward a New Research Agenda

We argue that both political sociology and medical sociology would be advanced by seriously considering insights from one another. Figure 6.2 represents our suggested research agenda that considers the relationship between the welfare state, as an economic, political, and cultural institution and issues of health, illness, and healing. It also defines three different approaches to understanding health and illness: the social construction of health and illness, health outcomes, and responses to health problems. We argue that each of the three approaches to understanding health and illness is advanced by looking at how they are impacted by the broader economy, politics, and culture, as well as paying attention to issues of health, illness, and healing increases our understanding of the political economy.

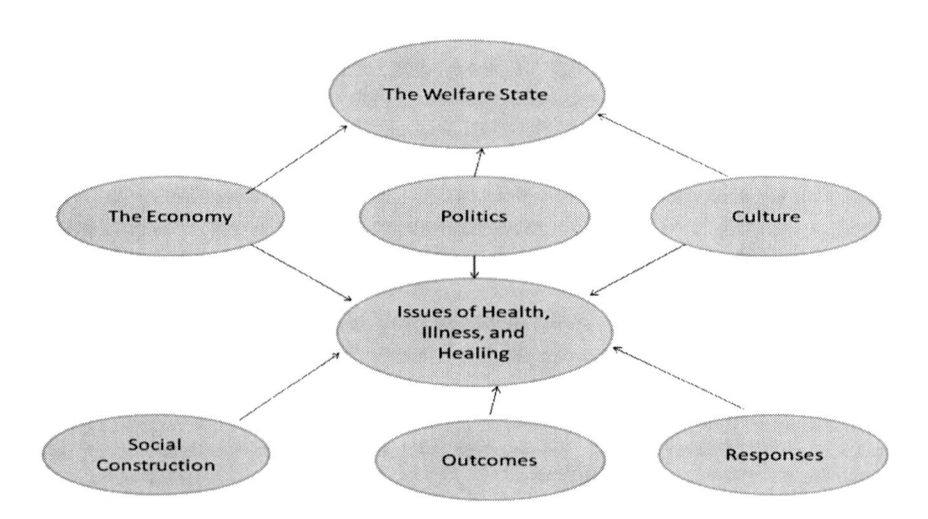

Fig. 6.2 A conceptual model of a new research agenda

Table 6.1 The welfare state, health, and health policy: Causes, mechanisms, and effects

Welfare state	Mechanisms	Health effects
Level of decommodification	Levels of inequality	Population health
Level of decommodification	Levels of inequality	Inequality in health
Level of decommodification	Logic of appropriateness	Health policy opinion
Level of decommodification	Exclusion/inclusion	Inequality in health
Level of decommodification	Exclusion/inclusion	Stigma
Health policy regime	Public opinion	Regime persistence
Health policy regime	Logic of appropriateness	Health policy opinion
Health policy regime	Public/private provision	Inequality in health
Health policy regime	Logic of attribution	Stigma
Health policy regime	Meaning of health	Experiences of illness
Health insurance	Stakeholder mobilization	Policy persistence
Health insurance	Cumulative (dis)advantage	Inequality in health

While the conceptual model shown here offers a general depiction of how the welfare state affects health through political, economic, and cultural mechanisms, we believe it is also important to suggest how attention to the welfare state can generate testable hypotheses that contribute to both political and medical sociology. We view the stratification order as the set of social mechanisms that connects the welfare state to health, illness, and healing. Crucially, the stratification order includes mechanisms that explain how changes in health and health inequalities impact the welfare state, as well as the better-known mechanisms that account for the causal effects of the welfare state on health. Below, we outline some of the overarching questions and specific hypotheses that we view as potentially generative of creative new work on the political sociology of health and the medical sociology of the welfare state by listing the causes, mechanisms, and effects that connect the welfare state to issues of health, illness, and healing.

Table 6.1 outlines three ways in which the welfare state can impact health as well as different mechanisms that link each of those to issues of health, illness, and healing. The welfare state determines decommodification within a nation, referring to the extent to which citizens are depends on the labor market for survival (Esping-Andersen 1990). We theorize about three mechanisms that link level of decommodification to health. First, it shapes level of inequality within a nation, which can impact both population health (e.g., life expectancy, infant mortality) as well as inequalities in individual-level health outcomes (e.g., rates of disease, chronic disability). Second, it defines what is viewed as an appropriate relationship between the state, the market, medicine, and citizens, which has implications for public opinions on health policy. Along these lines, it has implications for the creation of cultural categories of who is worthy of welfare-state benefits and who is not worthy. Third, it defines in-groups and out-groups in society, which contributes to both inequalities in health and the boundaries citizens draw, regarding who is stigmatized and who is not.

While we highlight the importance of reconciling welfare-state classifications and health system classifications, the welfare state undoubtedly plays a key role in deciding what kind of health policy regime exists within a nation. The overall health policy regime is theorized to have five different effects on health that are linked through five different mechanisms. First, the overarching health policy regime impacts the future directions of the social organization of health care through public opinion (Brooks and Manza 2006, 2007; Pierson 1994). Second, and related, it impacts public opinion, since it shapes what citizens have come to expect regarding the relationship between the state, the market, and medicine. Third, it affects inequalities in health, through the configuration of public versus private provision of health care. Fourth, it impacts stigma of various health problems, because it defines who is worthy of benefits and what is viewed as a legitimate health problems. Finally, it shapes lived illness experiences within a nation, because the meaning of health is linked to the overarching health policy of a nation.

The final impact of the welfare state comes through health insurance, which is theorized to have two possible health effects. First, it can impact policy persistence by defining who the main stakeholders in the health field are and what kind of claims they can make to the government. Second, it contributes to inequality in health, by shaping cumulative advantage and disadvantage over the lifecourse. While these theorized contributions, mechanisms, and health effects are not exhaustive of all the ways in which the welfare state may impact health, they do provide a starting point for research that takes insights from political sociology and medical sociology seriously.

References

Alderson AS, Nielsen F (2002) Globalization and the great U-turn: income inequality trends in 16 OECD countries. Am J Sociol 107:1244–99

Amenta E, Bonastia C, Caren N (2001) US Social Policy in Comparative and Historical Perspective: Concepts, Images, Arguments, and Research Strategies. Annu Rev Soc 27:213–234

Anderson GF, Poullier JP (1999) Health Spending, Access, and Outcomes: Trends in Industrialized Countries. Health Aff 18(3):178–192

Anderson OW (1972) *Health Care: Can there be Equity? The United States, Sweden, and England.* New York, NY: Wiley

Andreß H-J, Heien T (2001) Four Worlds of Welfare State Attitudes? A Comparison of Germany, Norway, and the United States. European Soc Rev 17(4):337–356

Angel R, Thoits PA (1987) The Impact of Culture on the Cognitive Structure of Illness. Culture, Medicine, and Psychiatry 6:465–494

Antonovsky A (1972) A Model to Explain Visits to the Doctor: With Specific Reference to the Case of Israel. J Health and Soc Behav 13(4):446–454

Beckfield J (2004) Does Income Inequality Harm Health? New Cross-national Evidence. J Health and Soc Behav 45:231–248

Berkman LF, Glass T, Brissette I, Seeman TE (2000) From social integration to health: Durkheim in the new millennium. Soc Sci Med 51:843–57

Bianchi S, Cohen PN, Raley S, Nomaguchi K (2004) Inequality in parental investment in child-rearing: expenditures, time, and health. In: Neckerman K (ed) Social inequality. Russell Sage, New York, pp 149–188

Bourdieu P (1984) *Distinction: A Social Critique of the Judgement of Taste.* Cambridge, MA: Harvard University Press

Brady D (2003) The politics of poverty: left political institutions, the welfare state and poverty. Soc Forces 82:557–588

Brady D (2005) The welfare state and relative poverty in rich western democracies, 1967–1997. Soc Forces 83:1329–1364

Brady D, Beckfield J, Seeleib-Kaiser M (2005) Economic globalization and the welfare state in affluent democracies, 1975–1998. Am Sociol Rev 70:921–48

Brooks C, Manza J (2006) Social Policy Responsiveness in Developed Democracies. Am Sociol Rev 71(3):474–494

Brooks C, Manza J (2007) Why welfare states persist: the importance of public opinion in democracies. University of Chicago Press, Chicago

Burstein P (1991) Policy domains: organization, culture, and policy outcomes. Annu Rev Sociol 17:327–350

Castles FG (2004) The future of the welfare state: crisis myths and crisis realities. Oxford University Press, Oxford

Campbell JL (2002) Ideas, Politics, and Public Policy. Annu Rev Sociol 28:21–38

Cockerham WC (1995) *Medical Sociology* (6th ed.). Englewood Cliffs, N.J.: Prentice Hall

Conley D, Springer K (2001) The welfare state and infant mortality. Am J Sociol 106:768–807

DiMaggio P (1997) Culture and Cognition. Ann Rev Sociol 23:263–287

DiPrete TA (2002) Life Course Risks, Mobility Regimes, and Mobility Consequences: A Comparison of Sweden, Germany, and the United States. Am J Sociol 108(2):267–309

DiPrete TA, Eirich GM (2006) Cumulative Advantage as a Mechanism for Inequality: A Review of Theoretical and Empirical Developments. Annu Rev Sociol 32(1):271–297

DiPrete TA, McManus PA (2000) Family Change, Employment Transitions, and the Welfare State: Household Income Dynamics in the United States and Germany. Am Sociol Rev 65(3):343–370

Durkheim E (1987/1951) Suicide: a study in sociology. The Free Press, New York, NY

Esping-Andersen G (1990) Three worlds of welfare capitalism. Princeton University Press, Princeton, NJ
Esping-Andersen G (1999) Social foundations of postindustrial economies. Oxford University Press, Oxford
Esping-Andersen G, Gallie D, Hemerijck A, Myles J (2002) *Why We Need a New Welfare State*. Oxford: Oxford University Press
Fligstein N (2001) The architecture of markets. Princeton University Press, Princeton, NJ
Furedi F (2006) The End of Professional Dominance. Society 43(6):14–18
Gamson WA, Modigliani A (1989) Media Discourse and Public Opinion on Nuclear Power: A Constructionist Approach. Am J Sociol 95(1):1–37
Giaimo Susan (2001) Who pays for health care reform? In: Pierson P (ed) The new politics of the welfare state. Oxford University Press, Oxford, pp 334–367
Goesling B, Firebaugh G (2004) The trend in international health inequality. Popul Dev Rev 30:131–146
Goffman E (1961) *Asylums: Essays on the Social Situation of Mental Patients and Other Inmates* ([1st] ed.). Garden City, N.Y.,: Anchor Books
Goodin RE, Headey B, Muffels R, Dirven H-J (1999) The real worlds of welfare capitalism. Cambridge University Press, Cambridge
Goodwin S (1997) *Comparative Mental Health Policy: From Institutional to Community Care*. London, UK: Sage Publications
Grusky David (2001) The past, present, and future of social inequality. In: Grusky D (ed) Social stratification: race, class, and gender in sociological perspective. Westview Press, Boulder, CO, pp 1–51
Hacker J (1997) The road to nowhere. Princeton University Press, Princeton
Hacker J (2002) The divided welfare state: the battle over public and private social benefits in the United States. Cambridge University Press, Cambridge
Hall PA, Soskice D (eds) (2001) Varieties of capitalism: the institutional foundations of comparative advantage. Oxford University Press, Oxford
Hayes BC, Heuvel AV (1996) Government Spending on Health Care: A Cross-National Study of Public Attitudes. J Health and Soc Policy 7:61–79
Hicks A (1999) Social democracy and welfare capitalism: a century of income security politics. Cornell University Press, Ithaca, NY
Hicks AM, Swank DH (1992) Politics, Institutions, and Welfare Spending in Industrialized Democracies, 1960–82. Am Political Sci Rev 86(3):658–674
Hout M (2003) Money and morale: what growing inequality is doing to Americans' views of themselves and others. Unpublished manuscript
Huber E, Stephens JD (2001) Development and crisis of the welfare state. The University of Chicago Press, Chicago, IL
Iglehart JK (1991) Germany's Health Care System. New England J Medicine 324(24):1750–1756
Immergut EM (1990) Institutions, Veto Points, and Policy Results: A Comparative Analysis of Health Care. J Public Policy 10(04):391–416
Iversen T (2005) Capitalism, democracy, and welfare. Cambridge University Press, Cambridge
Jameson F (1998) *The cultural turn: Selected Writings on the Postmodern, 1983–1998*. London, UK: Verso
Katz MB (1986) *In the Shadow of the Poorhouse: A Social History of Welfare in America*. New York, NY: Basic Books
Katz MB (1989) *The Undeserving Poor: From the War on Poverty to the War on Welfare*. New York, NY: Pantheon Books
Kenworthy L (1999) Do social-welfare policies reduce poverty? A cross-national assessment. Soc Forces 77:1119–1140
Kenworthy L (2004) Egalitarian capitalism: jobs, income and growth in affluent countries. Russell Sage, New York
Kikuzawa S, Olafsdottir S, Pescosolido BA (2008) Similar Pressures, Different Contexts: Public Attitudes toward Government Intervention for Health Care in 21 Nations. J Health and Soc Behav 49:385–399
Kleinman A (1988) Rethinking Psychiatry: From Cultural Category to Personal Experience. New York, NY: Free Press
Korpi W, Palme J (1998) The paradox of redistribution and strategies of equality: welfare state institutions, inequality, and poverty in the Western countries. Am Sociol Rev 63:661–688
Krieger N (1994) Epidemiology and the Web of Causation: Has Anyone Seen the Spider. Soc Sci Med 39:889–903
Krieger N (2001) Theories for social epidemiology in the 21st century: an ecosocial perspective. Int J Epidemiol 30:668–677
Kunst AE, Bos V, Lahelma E, Bartley M, Lissau I, Regidor E, et al. (2005) Trends in Socioeconomic Inequalities in Self-Assessed Health in 10 European Countries. Internat J Epidem 34(2):295–305
Lahelma E, Kivelä K, Roos E, Tuominen T, Dahl E, Diderichsen F, et al. (2002) Analysing Changes of Health Inequalities in the Nordic Welfare States. Soc Sci Med 55(4):609–625
Lassey ML, Lassey WR, Jinks MJ (1997) *Health Care Systems around the World: Characteristics, Issues, Reforms*. Upper Saddle River, NJ: Prentice Hall

Lee RPL (1982) Comparative Studies of Health Care Systems. Soc Sci Med 16:629–642
Lee C-S (2005) The social bases and outcomes of welfare states in the era of globalization and post-industrial economy. Ph.D. Dissertation, University of North Carolina
Lipset SM (1997) American exceptionalism: a double-edged sword. W.W. Norton, New York
Lynch J, Smith GD, Harper S, Hillemeier M, Ross N, Kaplan GA, et al. (2004) Is Income Inequality a Determinant of Population Health? Part 1. A Systematic Review. Milbank Quarterly 82(1):5–99
Macinko JA, Shi LY, Starfield B (2004) Wage inequality, the health system, and infant mortality in wealthy industrialized countries, 1970–1996. Soc Sci Med 58(2):279–292
Marx K, Engels F (1964) *The Communist Manifesto*. New York, NY: Washington Square Press
McLeod JD, Nonnemaker JM (2000) Poverty and Child Emotional and Behavioral Problems: Racial/Ethnic Differences in Processes and Effects. J Health Soc Behav 41(2):137–161
McLeod JD, Shanahan MJ (1993) Poverty, Parenting, and Children's Mental Health. Am Sociol Rev 58(3):351–366
McLeod JD, Shanahan MJ (1996) Trajectories of Poverty and Children's Mental Health. J Health Soc Behav 37(3):207–220
Mechanic D (1996) Comparative Medical Systems. Annu Rev Soc 22:239–270
Meyer JW, Boli J, Thomas GM, Ramirez FO (1997) World society and the nation-state. Am J Sociol 103:144–181
Moller S, Bradley D, Huber E, Nielsen F, Stephens JD (2003) Determinants of relative poverty in advanced capitalist democracies. Am Sociol Rev 68:22–51
Navarro V (1989) Why Some Countries have National Health Insurance, Others have National Health Services, and the U.S. has Neither. Soc Sci Med 28(9):887–898
Neckerman KM (ed) (2004) Social inequality. Russell Sage, New York
Neckerman KM, Torche F (2007) Inequality: Causes and Consequences. Ann Rev Sociol 33(1):335–357
Orloff A (1993) Gender and the social rights of citizenship: the comparative analysis of gender relations and welfare states. Am Sociol Rev 58:303–28
O'Connor JS, Orloff AS, Shaver S (1999) *States, Markets, Families: Gender, Liberalism, and Social Policy in Australia, Canada, Great Britain, and the United States*. Cambridge: Cambridge University Press
Olafsdottir S (2007) Fundamental Causes of Health Disparities: Stratification, the Welfare State, and Health in the United States and Iceland. J Health Soc Behav 48:239–253
Olafsdottir S (2010) Medicalization and Mental Health: The Critique of Medical Expansion, and a Consideration of how National States, Markets, and Citizens Matter. In D. Pilgram, A. Rogers & B. A. Pescosolido (Eds.), *Handbook of Mental Health and Mental Disorder: Perspectives from Social Science*.
Olafsdottir S, Pescosolido BA (2009) Drawing the Line: The Cultural Cartography of Utilization Recommendations for Mental Health Problems. J Health Soc Behav 50:228–244
Pampel FC (2001) The institutional context of population change: patterns of fertility and mortality across high income nations. University of Chicago Press, Chicago, IL
Parsons T (1951) *The Social System*. Glencoe, IL: Free Press
Patterson JT (1994) *America's Struggle against Poverty in the Twentieth Century, 1900-1994* (New ed.). Cambridge, MA: Harvard University Press
Pescosolido BA (1991) Illness Careers and Network Ties: A Conceptual Model of Utilization and Compliance. In G. Albrecht (Ed.), *Advances in Medical Sociology* (Vol. 2, pp. 164–181). Greenwich: JAI Press
Pescosolido BA (1992) Beyond Rational Choice: The Social Dynamics of How People Seek Help. Am J Sociol 97:1096–1138
Pescosolido BA, Carol A, Boyer, Wai Ying Tsui (1985) Medical Care in the Welfare State: A Cross-National Study of Public Evaluations. J Health Soc Behav 26:276–297
Pescosolido BA, Olafsdottir S, Martin JK, Long JS (2008) Cross-Cultural Issues on the Stigma of Mental Illness. In J. Arboleda-Florez & N. Sartorius (Eds.), *Understanding the Stigma of Mental Illness: Theory and Interventions* (pp. 19–35). West Sussex, England: John Wiley and Sons
Pierson P (1994) Dismantling the welfare state? Reagan, Thatcher, and the politics of retrechment. Cambridge University Press, Cambridge
Pierson P (1996) The New Politics of The Welfare State. World Politics 48:143–179
Pierson P (2001) *The New Politics of the Welfare State*. Oxford England Oxford University Press
Quadagno J (2004) Why the United States has no National Health Insurance. J Health Soc Behav, 45(Extra Issue) 25–44
Quadagno JS (2005) One nation, uninsured: why the U.S. has no National Health Insurance. Oxford University Press, Oxford
Ross CE (1996) The Links Between Education and Health. Am Sociol Rev 60:719–745
Ross CE (1994) Sex Stratification and Health Lifestyle: Consequences for Men's and Women's Perceived Health. J Health Soc Behav 35:161–178

Rostila M (2007) Social Capital and Health in European Welfare Regimes: A Multilevel Approach. J European Soc Policy 17(3):223–239

Ruggie M (1992) The paradox of liberal intervention: health policy and the American welfare state. Am J Sociol 97:919–44

Simmel G (1950) *The Sociology of Georg Simmel*. Glencoe, IL: Free Press

Steensland B (2006) Cultural Categories and the American Welfare State: The Case of Guaranteed Income Policy. Am J Sociol 111(5):1273–1326

Steinmo S, Watts J (1995) It's the Institutions, Stupid! Why Comprehensive National Health Insurance Always Fails in America. J Health Politics Policy Law 20(2):329–372

Stevens F (2001) The Convergence and Divergence of Modern Health Care Systems. In W. C. Cockerham (Ed.), *The Blackwell Companion to Medical Sociology* (pp. 158–179). Malden, MA: Blackwell Publishers Inc

Swidler A (1986) Culture in Action: Symbols and Strategies. Am Sociol Rev 51(2):273–286

Taylor-Gooby P (2004) New risks, new welfare: the transformation of the European welfare state. Oxford University Press, Oxford

Weber M (1930) *The Protestant Ethic and the Spirit of Capitalism*. New York, NY: Scribner

Wilensky H (1975) The welfare state and equality: structural and ideological roots of public expenditures. University of California Press, Berkeley, CA

Wilkinson RG (1996) *Unhealthy Societies: The Afflictions of Inequality*. London, UK: Routledge

Wilensky H (2002) Rich democracies: political economy, public policy, and performance. University of California Press, Berkeley, CA

Chapter 7
Health Social Movements: Advancing Traditional Medical Sociology Concepts

Phil Brown, Rachel Morello-Frosch, Stephen Zavestoski, Laura Senier, Rebecca Gasior Altman, Elizabeth Hoover, Sabrina McCormick, Brian Mayer, and Crystal Adams

Introduction

Over the last decade, a growing number of social scientists have turned their attention to the study of activism around health issues. Health social movements (HSMs) have pressed the institution of medicine to change in dramatic ways, embracing new modes of healthcare delivery and organization. Health activists have also pushed medicine to evolve by connecting their health concerns to other substantive issues such as social and environmental justice, poverty, and occupational or environmentally induced diseases. HSMs therefore serve as an important bridge, connecting the institution of medicine to other social institutions. In similar fashion, the study of HSMs has motivated medical sociology to develop new tools and theoretical perspectives to understand these alterations in the medical landscape. Medical sociologists stand to learn a great deal about the institution of medicine by observing it as it comes into conflict with patients and activists around issues of health care delivery, science and policy, and regulatory action. This broad sweep of interests must be systematized, which is our project here.

As medical sociologists take HSMs more seriously, they are beginning to understand that theoretical and empirical work on the illness experience and medical interaction should focus not only on personal experience and dyadic encounters in the clinic, but should also explore the ways that illness experiences linked to collective action can shape healthcare institutions, medical research, and government policy. We offer a set of theoretical and analytical concepts to help organize this inquiry. Following a history and typology of HSMs, we draw on several core theoretical concepts from medical sociology to illustrate some of the opportunities for integrating and advancing research in the study of HSMs and medical sociology.

We use the environmental breast cancer movement (EBCM) as a case study throughout, while also touching on other movements. In our treatment of the EBCM and other cases, we will show how HSM scholarship stands to benefit from and can substantially extend three concepts that have been central to medical sociology: empowerment, lay-professional conflict and cooperation, and challenges to institutional political economy. For each example, we will show how medical sociology contributes to our understanding of HSMs, and how studying HSMs advances medical sociology in return. Although we use the EBCM as our primary example, these theoretical tools and approaches may easily be applied to other types of HSMs. We conclude by proposing some research questions that are ripe for further exploration.

P. Brown (✉)
Department of Sociology, Brown University, 112 George St., 201 Maxcy Hall, Providence, RI 02912, USA
e-mail: phil_brown@brown.edu

Background: The History of HSMs

HSMs have profoundly influenced the health care system and public awareness of health and illness, and played a significant historical role in pressing for social change. Organizing around health issues dates back to the Industrial Revolution, when activists within the settlement house movement and industrial hygienists focused on urban poverty and occupational health (Waitzkin 2000). In the latter part of the twentieth century, women's health activists challenged medical stereotypes of women, broadened reproductive rights, demanded expanded funding and services in many areas, pressed for changes in traditional standards of clinical care (especially in obstetric and gynecologic care and breast cancer), and changed medical research practices (Ruzek 1978; Ruzek et al. 1997; Morgen 2002). Similarly, AIDS activists secured expanded funding for research and treatment, advocated for the application of complementary and alternative treatment approaches, and engineered major shifts in the design and execution of clinical trials (Epstein 1996). Mental patients' rights activists won major victories in mental health care, including the provision of many civil rights for mental patients (who formerly had fewer rights than prisoners), winning both the right to better treatment and the right to refuse certain treatments (Brown 1984).

HSM activists have fought campaigns for a broad variety of reasons. Citizens campaigning around issues of general health access have fought against the closing of community hospitals, protested the curtailment of medical services and the institution of restrictions by insurers, and managed care organizations (Waitzkin 2001). Political organizations fighting for black and Latino rights set the stage for major shifts in health policy, as with the Black Panther Party's free health clinic program (Sze 2007) and the Young Lord's pressure for lead paint removal (Brown 2007). Self-care and alternative care activists have broadened health professionals' awareness of the capacity of laypeople to cope with their health problems independently, and have helped bring many complementary and alternative medicine approaches into routine clinical care (Goldstein 1999). Disability rights activists have garnered major advances in public policy on disability rights such as accessibility and job discrimination, while also countering stigma against people with disabilities (Shapiro 1993). Participation in HSMs is not restricted to laypeople; physicians have formed national and regional organizations to press government institutions to provide health care for the underserved, to reduce health inequalities, to implement a national health plan, and to stop the nuclear arms race (McCally et al. 2007).

HSMs link health concerns to related substantive areas, often in the realm of environmental health. Toxic waste activists brought national attention to the health hazards of chemical, radiation, and other hazards; helped to shape the development of the Superfund Program, leading to the remediation of many hazardous waste sites; and obtained regulations and bans on many toxic substances (Brown and Mikkelsen 1990; Szasz 1994). Environmental justice activists, who are centrally concerned with environmental health, have drawn attention to the links between physical health and social inequality and racism, as they call attention to needed reforms that cut across a variety of social sectors, such as housing, transportation, and economic development. This led to a presidential Executive Order requiring all federal agencies to deal with environmental inequities (a promise not well fulfilled), and generated numerous academic–community partnerships to study, address, and prevent a range of environmental health problems common in poor communities and communities of color (Bullard 1994; Shepard et al. 2002). Occupational health and safety movements have brought medical, governmental, and public attention to a wide range of ergonomic, radiation, chemical, and stress hazards in many workplaces, leading to the creation of the Occupational Safety and Health Administration and National Institute of Occupational Safety and Health and the promulgation of protective regulations (Rosner and Markowitz 1987).

In observing the challenges that HSMs pose to conventional, medicalized conceptions of health and illness, medical sociology likewise broadened its conceptual foundations to explain these phenomena. For instance, the women's health movement's focus on sexism in clinical interactions, gender differences in health outcomes, sex discrimination in the health professions, reproductive rights, obstetric care and birth practices in hospitals, alternative clinics, medical training (Morgen 2002; Ruzek et al. 1997) provided enormous amounts of subject matter for sociology. This also extended beyond women's health; because the women's health movement focused so widely on clinical interaction, it led medical sociology to highlight power differentials in all clinical interactions and to examine power relations not only in terms of gender but also to explore how race and class shape clinical encounters. The broad impact of the women's health movement put HSMs on the map as a key concern for sociologists.

The above examples demonstrate how activism around health issues has been important in social change, show the extent of social scientific research on these movements, and provide one example of how HSMs have affected medical sociology, both theoretically and empirically. With that background, we offer a way to comprehensively assess HSMs by developing a framework for their study. Here, we focus on one subset of these movements, Embodied Health Movements (EHMs) (Brown et al. 2004).

Our Approach to HSMs

We draw on Della Porta and Diani's (1999, p. 16) definition of social movements as "informal networks based on shared beliefs and solidarity which mobilize around conflictual issues and deploy frequent and varying forms of protest." We conceptualize HSMs as collective challenges to medical policy and politics, belief systems, research, and practice that include an array of formal and informal organizations, supporters, networks of cooperation, and media. These movements can be broadly understood within a three-part typology (Brown et al. 2004). *Health Access Movements* seek equitable access to health care and improved provision of health care services. These include movements for national health care reform, demands for consumers' rights to select specialists, and campaigns to extend health care access to uninsured people. *Constituency-Based Health Movements* address health inequalities based on race, ethnicity, gender, class, and/or sexuality differences. These groups argue for ameliorating disproportionate health outcomes and challenge scientific work or regulatory actions that stigmatize their members. They include the women's health movement, the gay and lesbian health movement, and the environmental justice movement. EHMs address disease, disability, or illness experience by challenging science on etiology, diagnosis, treatment, and prevention. This group of movements includes "contested illnesses," which are either unexplained by current medical knowledge or have hypothesized environmental explanations that are deemed controversial (Brown 2007). As a result, EHM groups, including the EBCM, the AIDS movement, and the tobacco control movement, organize to achieve medical recognition, treatment, and/or research. Additionally, some established EHMs may include constituents who are not ill, but who perceive themselves as vulnerable to the disease.

EHMs: Challenges to Science and Society

We focus on EHMs because their study requires drawing upon a wide breadth of medical sociology theory and concepts. Although our focus will be on empowerment, lay-professional conflict and cooperation, and challenges to institutional political economy, other medical sociology concepts relevant to the understanding of EHMs include illness experience, disease definition, challenges to professionalism, and health care system reform. As discussed below, a number of concepts from other related disciplines are also relevant to understanding EHMs.

EHMs are defined by three characteristics (Brown et al. 2004). First, they introduce the biological body to social movements in central ways, especially in terms of the embodied experience of people who have the disease or condition. An illness identity emerges first and foremost out of the biological disease process happening inside the person's body. This identity represents the intersection of social constructions of illness and the personal illness experience of a biological disease process. Furthermore, illness sufferers have a variety of medical and nonmedical options for care and treatment, yet the immediacy of their physical needs often means that they cannot avoid the health care system altogether. Thus, one unique feature of EHMs is that constituents regularly interface with the very institutions they seek to change. Most importantly, people who have a disease uniquely experience the disease process, its personal illness experience, its interpersonal effects, and its social ramifications. They therefore have a lived perspective that is unavailable to others, which also lends moral credibility to the mobilized group in the public sphere and scientific world. Yet not many sick people come to link their illness experience to the collective identity of an HSM. Theorizing how HSMs mobilize individual illness experiences into collective movement identities is just one of the many dimensions of HSMs that medical sociology is suited to develop.

Second, EHMs typically include challenges to existing medical/scientific knowledge and practice. Activists seek scientific support for their illness claims, and hence EHMs become inextricably linked to the production of scientific knowledge and to changes in research practices. We refer to this standardized model of illness held by medical and scientific consensus as the dominant epidemiological paradigm (DEP), a shared set of entrenched beliefs and practices about disease treatment and causation embedded within a network of institutions, including medicine, science, government, and the media (Brown 2007). Of course, other social movements challenge science, but what sets EHMs apart from other movements is less *that* they challenge science, but *how* they go about doing it. EHM activists often judge science based on its relevance to their intimate, firsthand knowledge of their bodies and illness. When little was known about AIDS, activists challenged the scientific enterprise to prod medicine and government to act quickly, and with adequate knowledge (Epstein 1996). Even EHMs that focus on well-understood and treatable diseases are dependent upon science. Although they may not necessarily push for more research, they typically must advocate for more resources (e.g., treatment, disability benefits) and point to scientific evidence of causation, to shift a traditional focus on treatment to prevention. Advances in HSM research have drawn extensively from science and technology studies' understanding of knowledge contestation, democratization of knowledge and civic engagement in science, and legitimation processes (Corburn 2005; Moore 2006, McCormick Forthcoming).

Third, EHMs often involve activists collaborating with scientists and health professionals in pursuing treatment, prevention, research, and expanded funding. Lay activists in EHMs strive to gain a place at the scientific table so that their personal illness experiences can help shape research design. For example, asthma activists in Boston's Alternatives for Community and Environment, who sought more data on inner city air pollution, pressed EPA and state officials to install an air monitor on the building that houses their office. This allowed them to use the data to educate and mobilize neighborhood residents, while also showing the power of their own scientific engagement in air pollution measurement (Loh and Sugarman-Brozan 2002). Even if activists do not get to participate in the research enterprise, they often realize that their movement's success will be defined in terms of scientific advances, or in terms of transformation of scientific processes, which in turn are key to securing resources to support campaigns and constituency building. Part of the dispute over science involves a disease group's dependence on medical and scientific allies to help them press for increased funding for research and to raise money to enable them to run support groups and get insurance coverage. The more scientists can testify to those needs, the stronger patients' and advocates' claims are.

Beyond Typologies

The categories of our typology are ideal types. The goals and activities of some specific movements or individual health activist organizations may span several categories. The women's health movement, for example, can be seen as a constituency-based HSM because it represents a large population with specific interests, but it also contains elements of both access HSMs (e.g., in seeking expanded clinical services for women) and embodied HSMs (e.g., in challenging assumptions about psychiatric diagnoses for premenstrual symptoms; Figert 1996). In a recent review, Epstein (2007) cautions against the fixed categorization of HSMs because there is so often overlap between categories and HSMs so often integrate actors not typically considered as part of a social movement network. To be sure, the range of organizational agendas within any movement will not always fit neatly into any specific category.

While we find the typology useful to inform a historical and categorical view, we do not intend to discuss how each of the three types operates in each of the areas we will cover, or how specific HSMs push the margins of the typology. Our focus is on EHMs generally, and in particular the EBCM, as its struggle around issues of health care delivery, science and policy, and regulatory action captures the breadth of what medical sociologists stand to learn about the institution of medicine by studying HSMs.

Cross-Pollination Between HSMS and Medical Sociology: Tools and Theories

Issues raised by HSMs engage problems that are becoming important to the field of medical sociology such as how medicine responds to market dynamics, political economic pressures, and scientific controversies. By observing these changes in policy, markets, and science, we can appreciate the overlapping influences of medical institutions and lay activism, and learn something new about illness experience, physician–patient relations, professional dominance, and the organizational structure of medicine. We examine several core concepts from medical sociology – empowerment, lay-professional interaction, and political economy – which are useful for studying HSMs.

Empowerment

Medical sociology has typically approached empowerment at the level of the individual and her or his interactions with health care systems. Going further, medical anthropologists have pointed out how "…science and medical practice … [break] down bodies-literally through surgical transformations, or metaphorically through language and daily practice-into increasingly atomized fragments" (Sharp 2000, p. 314). Scheper-Hughes and Lock (1987, p. 10) argue that physicians have claimed both the biomedical conception of disease and the patient's subjective experience of illness for the medical domain, and that as a result "the 'illness' dimension of human distress (i.e., the social relations of sickness) are (sic) being medicalized and individualized, rather than politicized and collectivized."

Studying HSMs requires us to ask how individual sick bodies become empowered to mobilize and organize at the level of social movements. How does the most personal of experiences – one's bodily experience of disease as it intersects with one's social situation – become politicized ways that allow the individual to see what he or she shares in common with a collectivity, whether social movement or other?

Our approach to answering this question has relied on the concept of a politicized collective illness identity (Brown et al. 2004). This approach borrows the concept of collective identity from social movement scholars (Poletta and Jasper 2001) and combines it with the concept of illness identity (Charmaz 1991). When individuals develop a "cognitive, moral, and emotional connection" (Poletta and Jasper 2001, p. 285) with other illness sufferers, a collective illness identity emerges. HSMs politicize the collective illness identity by focusing attention on the role of power and politics in shaping the forces that lead to disease. We argue that a politicized collective illness identity emerges through people's experiences within a DEP (discussed below and in Fig. 7.1) (Brown et al. 2001). The DEP molds the assumptions underlying the processes of disease discovery, definition, etiology, treatment, and prevention. "These beliefs include who is to blame for the disease, who is responsible for curing the disease, whether or how the sick are stigmatized, and whether key social institutions deem the disease worthy of resources for research or prevention" (Zavestoski et al. 2005, p. 261). Not all collective illness identities are politicized. Support groups, for example, might provide their members with a sense of cognitive, moral, or emotional connection. But they might not necessarily compel individuals, in a Millsian sense, to transform the individual experience of disease from a personal trouble into a social problem.

Illness identities can become politicized through a number of routes, all of which entail bumping up against, finding inadequate, and growing frustrated with the institutionalized knowledge about a disease or condition that is embedded in the DEP. But a person with a politicized illness identity

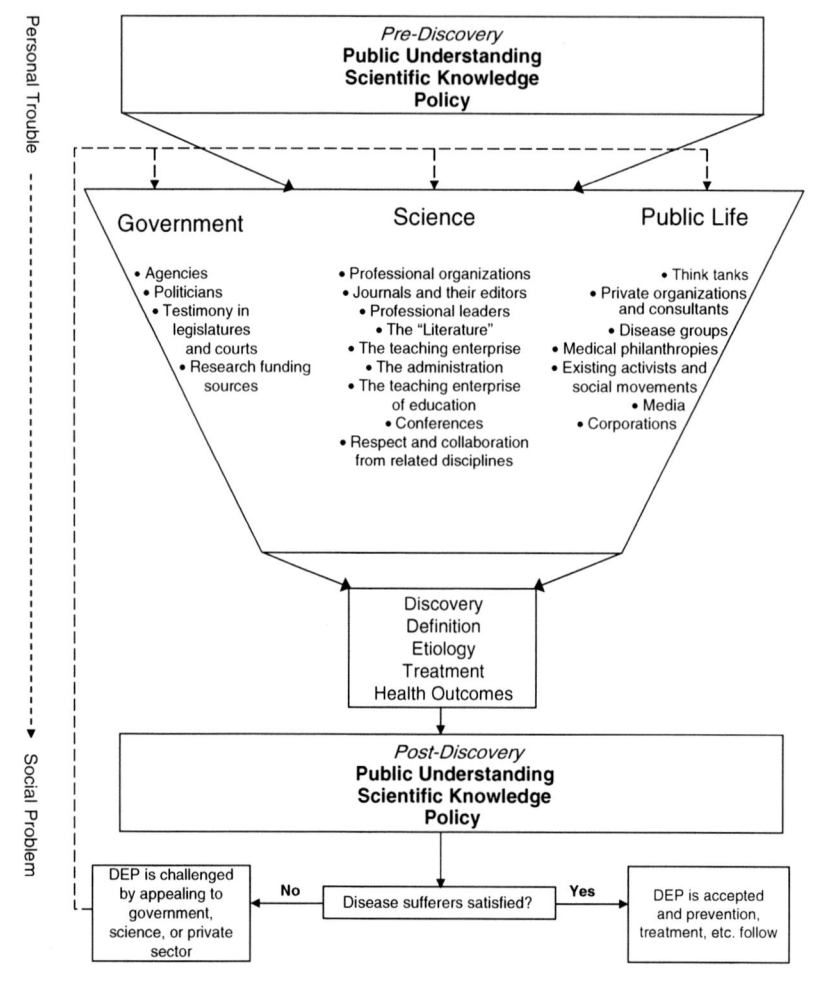

Fig. 7.1 The dominant epidemiological paradigm's process of disease discovery, definition, etiology, treatment, and outcomes

might not feel empowered to alter the DEP. Empowerment comes from the linking up of a politicized illness identity with a collective identity to form a politicized collective illness identity. Individuals with politicized illness identities might seek out a collective (e.g., a social movement organization) to join, or a group or organizational affiliation might facilitate the politicization of their collective illness identity. We observed both processes among women in the EBCM. In the former instance, women who grew increasingly frustrated with the traditional scientific and medical emphasis on genetic causes of breast cancer sought out alternative breast cancer organizations, such as organizations in the EBCM that inquired about other causes of breast cancer. In the latter instance, women with backgrounds in feminist, environmental, or other social movements prior to their breast cancer diagnosis, drew on their identification with existing social movements to frame breast cancer in new ways (e.g., in terms of a feminist critique or environmental justice narrative).

Regardless of the process by which politicized illness identities get collectivized, social movements that challenge institutionalized theories and practices about a disease depend on the politicized collective illness identity much in the way that conventional social movements depend on the collective identity of their adherents. Just as other social movements frame their causes in ways that broaden their support base, movements that form around illness turn to the families and friends of the ill, and sometimes the doctors who care for them or the scientists who study their condition, to broaden their bases of support.

Movement-Driven Medicalization and Disempowerment

Social movements are fundamentally about challenging power. If the concept of the politicized collective illness identity helps us understand how individuals become empowered to challenge dominant conceptions of disease and illness, then the concept of medicalization can help us to see where the power lies that HSMs aim to challenge. As the following discussion of medicalization suggests, there may be new sources of power that future research is able to identify and analyze more critically by looking at the targets against which HSMs organize (or the partners with which they ally).

In some instances, a movement seeks medical legitimacy for a poorly understood disease or condition, and may seek support or involvement of medical researchers or doctors. We can think about this as a case where patients, sufferers, and activists work to medicalize a particular condition. Sociology typically has focused on the role that medical professionals and social movement groups have played in bringing nonmedical issues (e.g., child abuse, alcoholism, and learning disabilities) into the realm of medical expertise, usually by redefining them as illness or disease (Conrad 2000; Conrad and Leiter 2004). In this situation, the *apolitical* collective illness identities of individuals seek to medicalize their illness experiences. For these HSMs, gaining medical legitimacy may come with significant tradeoffs; once a disease is medically recognized, the movement may become co-opted by medical institutions that exert control over treatment, research, funding, and can work to exclude alternative etiological explanations. Medicalization may also result in only a partial understanding of the problem and its root causes, by failing to support a robust program of research that critically examines social and political factors. For example, efforts by women's health advocates to establish clinics and programs for the treatment of domestic violence often de-emphasize the structural changes (e.g., pay equity, child care services) that are necessary to redress the underlying gender inequality that leads to violence. Medicalization, in other words, can be a double-edged sword for movements. In some instances, movements gain resources, broader support and legitimacy, while at the same time, they generate new opportunities for agendas to be taken over by the medical establishment in ways documented by sociologists since the 1970s (Zola 1972; Conrad 2000, 2005; Conrad and Leiter 2004; Clarke et al. 2003).

Some movements resist medicalization while others pursue it. The inherent tension between movement aims in this regard demonstrates how medicalization as a theoretical construct needs to be broadened to capture a wider variety of actors engaged in medicalization efforts. Throughout the 1970s and 1980s, medical sociologists focused on three social forces driving medicalization: the power and authority of the medical profession, the activities of social movements and interest groups, and organizational or professional activities that promulgated medicalization. Since the 1980s, the delivery of medical care has been affected by the rise of biotechnology, medical consumerism, and managed care. These factors have shifted the drivers of medicalization, so that it is now as likely to be directed by private industry, consumers, and market forces as by medical professionals (Conrad and Leiter 2004; but see Clarke et al. 2003 for an opposing view, which argues that technological advancements have altered the fundamental nature of the processes of medicalization). Sociologists need to examine the impact of advances in biotechnology, the influence of pharmaceutical industry marketing and promotion, the role of consumer demand, the enabling and constraining aspects of managed care and health insurance, the impact of the Internet, the changing role of the medical profession, and the pockets of medical and popular resistance to medicalization. Because so many of these social phenomena involve collective action, contestation, and organized protest, the expansion and evolution of theories of medicalization will necessarily need to incorporate more systematically HSM activity.

The Institutional Political Economy of Health

A political economic critique considers a broader frame of power relations than the personal and group empowerment approaches we discussed in the prior section. Once individuals become mobilized into a collectivity, HSMs may launch different kinds of challenges depending on their form and substantive focus. In our own work, for example, we have described how EHMs challenge the medical, scientific, governmental, and media institutions that delineate a biomedicalized definition of disease, a limited set of etiologic explanations for its origins, and a medically circumscribed set of treatment options. We term this the DEP (see Fig. 7.1). Key here is that from the perspective of HSMs, many institutions matter to human health and well-being, including political-economic systems. Thus, to understand HSMs claims, interests, and actions, medical sociologists must adopt an institutional and political economic perspective. The DEP model provides just such a framework.

By drawing upon key concepts from medical sociology such as popular epidemiology (Brown and Mikkelsen 1990), the literature on the social construction and articulation of social problems and theories from science and technology studies, the DEP presents a model for understanding the complexities of disease discovery; how certain scientific, governmental, and media actors work to support a dominant view of the disease; and how a range of actors may mount challenges to that vision (Brown et al. 2001). Participants in HSMs must contend with various institutions, such as science, government, policymakers, and the media, in an effort to shift the DEP, reshape public understanding of a disease's etiology, and redirect the resources for prevention or treatment.

We have focused much of our research on how EHMs, as a class of HSM, organize their movement goals and strategic plans to counter specific components of this DEP. Scholars who have examined other kinds of HSMs have constructed similar models and frameworks for exploring how the movement groups they study organize and mount challenges to medical authority as it articulates and acts through a variety of institutions. A recent study of Health Access Movements, for example, examined how stakeholder mobilization has been used at various times over the twentieth century to block efforts to provide universal access to healthcare (Quadagno 2004). By identifying the stakeholders and analyzing their structural positions, however, it becomes possible to understand partial victories in the effort to provide some expanded access. Quadagno points out, however, that the parallel federated structures of the labor movement and the American Medical Association made it possible for these two advocacy groups to cooperate and lobby for passage of the Medicare Act in the middle of the twentieth century. Donald Light has contributed the notion of *countervailing powers* to delineate various axes of change that have transformed the medical marketplace from one that was provider driven to one that is more buyer driven in an age of managed care (Light 2004). These axes of change include not only clinical and technological innovations but also political, economic, and organizational changes that have transformed medical practice and weakened medical professional authority.

In general, HSMs offer a strong critique of contemporary science, medicine, and policy by calling out how ideological and political-economic factors shape medical research and treatment to systematically overlook the contribution of environmental factors in disease. In doing so, movement groups often leverage scientific data and medical information and marshal strategic resources to produce their own scientific knowledge, through what we term "citizen-science alliances" (Brown et al. 2001). An institutional political economy of health perspective combined with an understanding of empowerment through the mobilization of politicized collective illness identities provide the necessary tools to develop a multilayered analysis of HSMs. It is to such an analysis that we turn next.

Through the Lens of the EBCM

The EBCM exemplifies EHMs as a type of HSM in that it presses the medical and scientific establishments as well as the broader breast cancer movement to focus on environmental causes. This has fundamentally changed how breast cancer is researched and publicly perceived. For example, EBCM organizations like Breast Cancer Action have consistently challenged the corporate control of Breast Cancer Awareness Month. As part of its "think before you pink" campaign, Breast Cancer Action advocates sought to shift revenues raised from the US Postal Service's official breast cancer stamp from the National Institutes of Health and Department of Defense medical research program (which conducts mostly treatment research) to the National Institute of Environmental Health Sciences Breast Cancer and the Environment Research Centers (which funds research on breast cancer etiology). EBCM activists work with many other types of groups including EHMs such as minority women's cancer groups and HSMs such as toxics-use-reduction groups (McCormick et al. 2003). Examining alliances and collaborations among different types of HSMs opens up a range of questions about coalition formation that would be useful not only to medical sociologists but also to social movements researchers.

Changing the Illness Experience

Illness from the Patient's Perspective. Ever since Parsons (1951) introduced the notion of the "sick role," a concept describing the duties and obligations of a patient during a time of illness, more critical medical sociologists (e.g., Conrad 1987; Charmaz and Olesen 1997) have offered a patient-oriented perspective to transcend the image of the passive, obedient patient. In such a view, the individual moves through diverse social and institutional spheres to form a unique illness experience, often by challenging the boundary between physician and patient through such practices as self-diagnosis and acquisition of expert medical knowledge. By following the patient through the boundary-crossing process, we can construct more representative accounts of health and illness.

The complex, multifaceted process of making sense of illness often results in an illness identity, or the individual sense of oneself shaped by the physical constraints of illness and by others' reactions to that illness (Charmaz 1991). This identity, along with the illness experience, is expressed by sufferers in the form of narratives, a strategy on the part of the sufferer to create a sense of order in the midst of what Bury (1982) refers to as the "biographically disruptive" event of illness onset. Williams (1984) characterizes this adaptive response as "narrative reconstruction." Since a person's illness experience is influenced by a broad array of social as well as medical factors, narrative reconstruction empowers the patients to become actively involved in their own health and make sense of their illness in the context of their entire life experience. Unlike professional accounts of illness, which tend to be narrow in scope, illness narratives have the capacity to provide a more comprehensive depiction of illness, because they originate directly from the voice of the lived patient – the common denominator in the multifaceted story of illness (Bell 2000) – without being filtered through the lens of medical authority.

We amplify this by noting that narratives are not only individual based but can also be movement based. HSM narratives explain disease causation and illness experience through a larger lens. These narratives exist at the microlevel but are more inclusive than the individual narratives. Individual sufferers, then, can have two forms of narratives: their own personal narrative and a movement narrative that encompasses that movement's history of discovery and transformation of disease understanding, causation, treatment impacts, and policy implications. Both narrative forms are empowering tools that patients utilize to understand their experience and its connection to the broader social sphere. Klawiter (2005) offers a vivid example of how one woman's experience of breast cancer was radically different at two different points in her life, in part because no social movement had existed when she was initially diagnosed, in the 1970s. When her cancer recurred, in the 1990s, she found that the intervening rise in social movement activism significantly transformed her experience of the illness, including support from breast cancer movement activists, and how she interacted with her physician as a more educated and engaged patient. The breast cancer movement transformed the "regime of breast cancer" so that "collective identities, emotional vocabularies, popular images, public policies, institutionalized practices, social scripts, and authoritative discourses" give women with breast cancer today a fundamentally changed experience from 20 to 30 years ago (Klawiter 2005).

Politicized Collective Illness Identity in the EBCM. During much of its history, breast cancer was a disease that women dealt with privately. In some instances, women hid the disease so well that not even immediate family members would know exactly what type of cancer was killing their sister, mother, or daughter. Eventually support groups, initiated by the American Cancer Society to help women support one another following a radical mastectomy, transformed into incubators of collective illness identity that helped form the contemporary breast cancer movement (Casamayou 2001). In its early days, this movement embraced individual responsibility as the primary weapon in breast cancer prevention by encouraging women to get mammograms and change their diets and lifestyles. The politicized collective illness identity challenged the mainstream movement when many activists, prompted by the women's health movement, railed against the unquestioned use of radical mastectomies long after they were proven unnecessary (Lerner 2001) and against the demand that women focus their attention on their appearance. This does not diminish the importance of traditional support groups since they provided a venue wherein sufferers could share their frustration with the medical system and perhaps move toward the politicized collective illness experience.

But the mainstream movement that emerged from these support groups remains firmly ensconced in a DEP that emphasizes treatment over research into causes, and that focuses on personal responsibility in reducing women's risk of breast cancer. The EBCM challenges this paradigm by generating public policies and scientific knowledge that address environmental causes of breast cancer, and it claims that an individualized approach is one that lays blame on women, rather than the political and social structures that allow them to be exposed to carcinogens. EBCM activists benefited early on from having been politicized through their work in other movements such as the women's movement. Meyer and Whittier (1994) refer to this sort of effect as "social movement spillover." Organizations within the EBCM (e.g., Breast Cancer Action, Breast Cancer Fund, and Massachusetts Breast Cancer Coalition) employed their politicized collective illness identities in a number of ways – they took critical stances about funding sources they would accept, and campaigned against the mainstream movement's licensing of the pink ribbon in order to raise money through the sale of some of the very products linked to the causes of breast cancer. In these and other examples, the EBCM illustrates how a politicized collective illness identity focuses attention on the role of power and politics in shaping the forces that lead to a disease in the first place. Similarly, it also demonstrates how politicized collective illness identities become mobilized to engage in a critique of the institutional political economy of health.

Lay-Professional Conflict and Cooperation

For decades, work by Elliot Freidson (1970) sparked our awareness of lay-professional conflict. The experience of illness differs according to race, class, gender, religion, ethnicity, and locality, and the typical provider, no matter how sympathetic to patient involvement and/or local culture, could not grasp all those contexts. While some lay challenges concerning etiology and treatment are the product of individual interaction (Freidson 1970), our work indicates that the strongest effects come from social movement activity.

HSMs examine the social and scientific discovery of diseases and their causes, ask why particular conditions are identified at particular times, what action was taken or not, who benefits or loses by identification and action, and how divergent perspectives on disease merge or clash. As these questions point to barriers to professional awareness and action, understanding the strategies that activists employ in asking them is a central concern of scholarship on HSMs. Such questions are important since we now know that ulterior motives occasionally shape medical and professional responses to disease. For example, some corporate physicians deny job-related diseases or environmental causation, such as Johns-Manville Corporation physicians who hid evidence and lied to patients about asbestos-caused mesothelioma (Brodeur 1985). Professionals may also be resistant to challenging larger social norms, as with health professionals' failure to act on child abuse and spouse abuse (Pfohl 1977). Pharmaceutical and other firms exert huge control over the research process itself, hiding harmful effects from publication (Markowitz and Rosner 2002; Krimsky 2003). Particular approaches to disease may also simply be the result of physicians and researchers following the status quo. In many ways, this was the challenge faced by the EBCM as it attempted to urge physicians to see breast cancer as a potential outcome of women's positions in a toxic environment, and as it worked to get researchers to expand their understanding of potential causes beyond the narrow genetic and lifestyle factors that dominated most research. EBCM activists found that these efforts were often more successful when they built relationships with the professionals on whom they were depending. But health professionals are often wary of accepting lay perspectives on environmentally induced diseases, fearing that novel hypotheses will discredit them or isolate them from their colleagues.

Another example of how HSMs challenge the diagnosis and treatment status quo can be found in the previously mentioned challenges the women's movement made to radical mastectomy and postcancer adjustment (Casamayou 2001; Lerner 2001). Breast cancer activists demanded cancer diagnosis and full consent before radical mastectomies, opposing the standard regimen of proceeding directly from biopsy to mastectomy without allowing the woman to waken from anesthesia so that she could be actively involved in a decision about her care. This set the stage, along with the emergence of evidence in demonstrating the efficacy of alternatives, for later critiques of medical approaches to breast cancer, including the choice in the postradical mastectomy era for breast-conserving surgery and adjuvant treatment as an alternative to mastectomy. These are clearly forms of empowerment by women, in which they reject medical authority concerning proper treatment and disease prevention strategies. For example, the EBCM vehemently challenged the FDA and pharmaceutical manufacturers regarding the long-term hazards of prescribing the hormonal drug Tamoxifen to "prevent" breast cancer in healthy women who may be at high risk for breast cancer, but who have not yet had the disease (Klawiter 2006). EBCM activists also opposed widespread prescription of hormone replacement therapy (HRT) to prevent osteoporosis and to reduce the risk of cardiovascular events among postmenopausal women, due to early scientific evidence suggesting that cardioprotective effects did not outweigh the increased risk of breast cancer associated with HRT. Ultimately, the EBCM position on HRT was proven to be correct, as the Women's Health Initiative trial, a prospective cohort study of HRT for the prevention of coronary heart disease, was brought to an early end in 2002 when it was found that the hormone regimen increased women's risk of breast cancer, stroke, heart attack, and blood clots, and was not effective in preventing heart disease. Now, HRT use among postmenopausal women is strongly discouraged (Writing Group for the WHI Investigators 2002).

Despite challenges and conflicts, we also find potential for lay-professional cooperation. One reason is the emergence of professional activism within medicine and allied health fields. Much of this activism concerns access to health care, which has been curtailed by third party payment control over health professionals, such as McKinlay and Arches' (1985) notion of proletarianization, Light's (1991) concept of countervailing power, and other work on professional loss of power. When this is combined with a broader professional campaign for democratic access and a challenge to health inequalities, there is much potential for professional activism. For example, Physicians for a National Health Program represented a significant organizing effort that exposed fundamental flaws in the health care system, and critiqued third party payers and their assault on professional authority (Physicians Working Group 2003). This has the potential to radicalize physicians into other efforts, such as occupational and environmental health concerns through Health Care Without Harm, a large coalition that seeks safer hospital products and waste disposal (see www.noharm.org). Growing legitimation of environmental causation of disease has made it more possible for health professionals and researchers to accept invitations from EBCM and other similar environmental health activists to conduct innovative research. Further, some of that research is done in the form of community-based participatory research, leading to further capacity-building for movement organizations (Minkler and Wallerstein 2003).

For medical sociology, looking at HSMs extends our analytic focus beyond doctor–patient relationships to relationships between patient–activists and researchers/scientists around questions of disease causation, diagnosis, and treatment. It also extends our focus to relationships between patient–activists and funders/policy-makers around funding for research on what constitutes disease prevention versus what treatment and funding streams prioritize genetic and lifestyle factors.

Challenges to Medical Institutions and the Production of Scientific Knowledge

Science and Medicine as Targets of Challenge. Although science and medicine have increasingly come under scrutiny by social movements, they differ from other institutions, especially the state, that are commonly targeted by social movements. These differences make science and medicine open to a range of strategies that may not be available in other cases of contestation. They present four types of opportunities to social movement actors. First, rapid changes in scientific innovation, investment in new areas of research, and the lack of a strongly held consensus on a scientific issue may create *windows of opportunity* for protest and action. Second, the heterogeneous field of actors involved in creating and maintaining the DEP presents *multiple points of leverage* for social movement activists. Third, science policy is enacted at *multiple levels*, and activists can target local, statewide, or federal agencies. Finally, science policy presents *multiple targets* in the formulation of science policy and the translation of scientific findings in regulations, presenting activists with multiple arenas for action.

First, medicine and science are in a nearly constant state of flux as the growth and advancement of scientific knowledge progresses. In addition to creating new stores of knowledge that may be contested by social movement actors, this process may also serve to destabilize rules and relationships that govern institutions. When an organization receives a large influx of research dollars, experiences rapid growth in membership or staffing, or when the expansion of the knowledge base triggers a paradigm shift, this destabilizes the organization and may open up opportunities for social movement actors to challenge the institutions. In such circumstances, the institution often lacks a unified center of gravity, or a single center of power to vet the validity of scientific knowledge. As Moore (1999) notes, a scientific field undergoing rapid change presents "multiple locations of challenge and access for protesters and dissenting scientists (113)." Moore argues that social movement actors (including sympathetic scientists or the general lay public) can alter institutional practices when they capitalize on these windows of opportunity. For example, as breast cancer research funding expanded rapidly, it opened opportunities for different kinds of challenges, such as that related to improvement for detection devices and for better treatment (Casamayou 2001), and to very different types of demands about causes (McCormick et al. 2003).

Second, medical and scientific institutions are rarely as unified around a single set of institutional structures. The DEP is developed and maintained by a diverse group of actors, including academic and government scientists, the media, and patient advocacy groups. With respect to breast cancer, while the DEP is dominated by an outlook that emphasizes individual and behavioral risk factors for disease, rather than environmental or social factors, some elements of the DEP may be more accepting of environmental hypotheses (Zavestoski et al. 2005). For example, some scientific institutions have embraced the endocrine disruption hypothesis (Krimsky 2000), some journals have devoted attention to the precautionary principle (Davis et al. 1998), and some institutes within the National Institutes of Health (e.g., NIEHS) have funded extensive research on environmental causation of disease (McCormick et al. 2004). While this is still a controversial idea, and some segments of the DEP still de-emphasize the investigation of environmental causation in favor of individualized factors such as genes, diet, and health behaviors such as drinking or smoking, the existence of sympathetic elites in parts of the science policy arena creates opportunities for social movement actors to press their agenda. A lack of consensus among the scientific actors involved in creating or maintaining the DEP may make it possible for social movement actors to gain entry into an institution of authority. This example shows that the DEP may not necessarily be monolithic, and the presence of controversy and dissent among the actors create multiple possible points of entry for activists who are trying to influence the scientific agenda (Zavestoski et al. 2005).

Third, activists may encounter medical and scientific institutions at multiple levels: locally, regionally, or nationally. Each scale adds a space for contestation. There may be locally based research institutions that are responsive to local advocate interests. Silent Spring Institute is one such organization, founded by the Massachusetts Breast Cancer Coalition to conduct research on women's health and the environment with a strong component of citizen involvement (McCormick et al. 2003). In addition, national-level research initiatives like those within NIEHS can respond to national organizations with sufficient credibility and membership. Medical institutions that attempt to resolve illnesses similarly operate on a multiplicity of scales. While local practitioners may see disease phenomena on a microlevel that relate to community concerns, more macrolevel health care foundations and philanthropic institutions get involved with movement leadership and elites that have transcended the concerns of one community. This has taken place with the panoply of breast cancer foundations like Komen for the Cure and the Breast Cancer Research Foundation that drive public attention (McCormick and Baralt 2006).

Finally, many scientific and medical institutions are connected to the state through regulatory channels, which creates another potential target for social movement action. Scientific research is dependent on funding, and activists can mount challenges by questioning funding decisions or demanding additional funding for certain projects. For example, forcing the passage of the Long Island Breast Cancer Study Project in 1993 was a part of breast cancer activists' establishment of a new agenda focused on prevention, rather than treatment and cure (McCormick forthcoming). After this took place, activism began to burgeon around environmental links to breast cancer both in Long

Island and across the country. This gave activists the credibility to ask for state and local level regulation of the chemicals that were being studied. As an institution, medical practice is regulated by the state, which provides another avenue for activism and contentious politics. Thus, by challenging these connections, movements and public groups, in essence, challenge both the state and institutions simultaneously.

EHMs and Challenges to Science

As a subtype of HSM, EHMs enact particular kinds of challenges to both the scientific basis of medical authority and the application of that authority in practice. In doing so, EHMs critique the medicalization of social problems and the scientization of society more generally. In our prior work on EHMs and breast cancer, we have identified three realms of scientific knowledge production: doing science, interpreting science, and acting on science. The three realms are interrelated and simultaneous, and paradigm contestations may occur in all three (Brown et al. 2006).

Doing scientific research involves a critique by HSMs of the actual design and conduct of scientific studies. Activists may question how scientists select particular topics and hypotheses, why they ignore or discard other questions or hypotheses, how they proceed with their investigations, and how they view their relations with funding, research, and support organizations. Scientific research is often limited by disciplinary boundaries, or is circumscribed by prior theoretical and methodological approaches, or so-called bandwagons (Fujimura 1995). The EBCM has challenged a scientific agenda that has focused heavily on lifestyle or genetic factors (Davis 2002) and instead pressed for more attention to social or environmental factors (McCormick et al. 2003). A critique of doing research also addresses how organizations shape the conduct and funding of science. Silent Spring Institute, for example, has brought women affected by breast cancer into the research process, inviting them to collaborate on the design of the research, collection of the data, and interpretation of the findings (McCormick et al. 2004).

Interpreting science involves a critique by HSM actors of the ways in which scientists make sense of data. Normal science relies heavily on two standards: the weight of evidence approach and standards of proof. Standards of proof are determined by and reinforce the position that science is neutral and value free, that scientific work is a universal reflection of reality, and that the scientific community can separate its work from personal interests (Harding 1998). Standards of proof include metrics such as strength of association, a statistical level of significance, temporality, biological plausibility, etc. Activists and scholars alike have pointed out that these standards of proof exemplify the built-in conflict between professional standards (which prefers to err on the side of a false negative) and clinical or lay preferences (which would argue for erring on the side of uncertainty and avoid a false positive) (Ozonoff and Boden 1987). Activists who critique the standards of proof often argue for shifting this pattern of thinking to instead err on the side of precaution and protecting public health (Brown et al. 2006).

The weight of evidence approach to risk assessment reviews data from many different disciplines (e.g., human and animal studies, in vitro studies) to arrive at an overall assessment of a chemical's safety. For example, Colborn et al. (1997) synthesized many different bodies of research to argue that endocrine-disrupting compounds have multiple adverse impacts on many different species in many different contexts. Collins' (1983) notion of "interpretive flexibility," however, informs us that different conclusions can be drawn from the same data. Multiple scientific "truths" can coexist or lead to disputes over what constitutes "sound" methodology and proof of causation. Activists from the EBCM have challenged the weight of evidence approach by advocating for the incorporation of information on endocrine disrupting effects on wildlife and on human developmental, sexual, and neurological effects, including gray literature. Generally speaking, a critique of the interpretation of science may challenge the processes by which studies are selected for inclusion in an evaluation, setting standards of proof, and assessing the weight of evidence.

Acting on science involves a critique of how scientific evidence is enacted in policy or public health interventions. A crucial part of acting on science is the recognition of knowledge gaps, what Hess (2002, p. 79) terms "undone science." This relates to the EBCM in terms of "toxic ignorance" (Roe et al. 1997), a situation in which over 85,000 chemicals are registered for commercial use in the United States, but only a small portion of them have been tested for carcinogenicity, and even fewer have been fully and comprehensively tested for non-cancer outcomes. Activists and scientists have called for increased human and environmental monitoring to generate crucial information about the origins and potential long-term effects of chemicals. In essence, acting on science involves choosing whether to act and how to act.

An Ecosocial View of Epidemiology and the Social Production of Disease

The EBCM is also reshaping theoretical and methodological approaches in medical and public health science for understanding causes of breast cancer and disparities in disease incidence and mortality among diverse populations. It has pushed for a paradigm shift in how the regulatory community, policy-makers, health care providers, and research scientists address the disease. This shift has led to what Klawiter (2003) characterizes as two models for addressing the disease: (1) a *biomedical model* that seeks to elucidate disease biology in order to develop more effective treatments (surgery, chemotherapy, or radiation) and earlier detection technologies to increase survival; versus (2) the *environmental model* that focuses on understanding the role of suspected carcinogens in disease causation and promotion, and the development and dissemination of regulatory strategies to reduce individual and population exposures to environmental hazards. An excellent example of how the EBCM has sought to redirect science and policy on the latter model is manifested in the struggle over the meaning and implications of the term "breast cancer prevention." Historically, prevention had been framed largely in biomedical terms by breast cancer activists and scientists alike and generally refers to strategies such as chemotherapy (to prevent disease mortality or extend survival time), chemoprevention (to decrease breast cancer recurrence or incidence in potentially high-risk individuals), and breast self-examination combined with screening mammography (to detect tumors earlier).

EBCM activists have resisted this biomedical framing of prevention on several levels. First, they have argued persuasively that screening does not actually prevent disease, but merely detects it. Indeed, by the time most breast cancer tumors appear in mammograms, they have been present in the body for 6–8 years (Love 1990); therefore, just how much mammography has contributed to reducing mortality, particularly in younger women remains contested within the scientific community (Gøtzsche and Nielsen 2007). Second, EBCM activists contend that better treatment will not effectively reduce the rising incidence of breast cancer; therefore, true disease prevention requires a radical shift in research and intervention toward understanding fundamental causes of the disease, which are more likely to be structural in nature. This necessitates a better understanding of environmental and social factors (Morello-Frosch et al. 2006).

This upstream perspective on breast cancer prevention raises formidable methodological challenges that are inherent to the fields of environmental and social epidemiology, including adequately measuring the timing, levels, and impacts of chronic and intermittent exposures to environmental hazards, and operationalizing individual and area-level measures of social drivers of inequities in breast cancer incidence and mortality among diverse populations. Indeed, although mortality rates from breast cancer appear to be declining overall, studies indicate persistent social inequities in mortality and incidence rates among racial/ethnic groups. For example, studies demonstrate that African–American women present with breast cancer at an earlier age with later stage disease and with more aggressive tumors than their white counterparts. Moreover, the survival rates of African–American women are worse than for Whites (Polite and Olufunmilayo 2005).

This trend has encouraged the EBCM to link its advocacy to an environmental justice framework, which highlights how various forms of discrimination shape current spatial distributions of environmental hazards among different communities and explicitly connects the political economy of social inequality with discrimination, environmental degradation, health and disease. EBCM advocates have also connected race and class inequities in exposures to environmental hazards and to the inadequacy of US chemicals policy. The EBCM argues that public agencies continue to rely on conventional end-of-pipe controls, and that they have insufficient authority to compel hazard data development, extended producer responsibility, and fail to protect health and ecosystems on the basis of early warnings of harm. Lack of effective environmental health regulation is made even more challenging by globalized forms of production in which industry has also sought enhanced mobility and production flexibility to cut back labor costs and evade regulatory requirements in the workplace and communities (Morello-Frosch 2002).

Linking breast cancer and environmental justice activism has encouraged both the EBCM and scientists to theorize more deeply about how social drivers of environmental health disparities might explain current patterns of breast cancer and highlight more upstream opportunities for intervention and disease prevention. In order to elucidate the origins and persistence of breast cancer distribution patterns and trends, research must integrate two lines of inquiry that examine disease causation (e.g., due to environmental hazards) as well as social and regulatory drivers of the distribution of disease burden and health disparities (e.g., due to class- and race-based discrimination in the health care and regulatory systems).

Ecosocial theory has been integral to new scientific thinking on this question by emphasizing the cumulative interplay of exposure and susceptibility over the life course and how individuals and populations incorporate biologically social experiences where they live, work, and play in ways that impact health, disease, and well-being (Krieger 1994, 2005). Indeed, such a model can suggest how the complex interplay of societal, environmental, and individual events over the life cycle can have long-term biological repercussions, manifesting in specifically adverse cellular outcomes that lead to breast cancer. In this way, adverse health outcomes such as breast cancer can result from social drivers of environmental health disparities and socially mediated reproductive patterns due to race- and class-based discrimination (Masi and Olopade 2005; Krieger 1989). Thus, to the extent that societal and individual events vary systematically with race, ethnicity or class, biological outcomes such as breast cancer may ultimately result from social inequalities. Figure 7.2 below demonstrates this ecosocial view, advocated by the EBCM, that connects social inequality to community-level conditions that disproportionately expose communities of color to environmental hazards and stressors. These community- and individual-level stressors potentially amplify vulnerability to the toxic effects of pollution that lead to breast cancer. EBCM advocates along with their environmental justice allies have argued that this dynamic may partially explain persistent racial and class-based health disparities in breast cancer incidence and mortality among young women that may be environmentally mediated.

Conclusion: Further Steps to Develop the Study of HSMs

Health has emerged as a singularly powerful frame for many grievances. Although HSMs are by no means a new phenomenon, there remains a vast and largely unexplored terrain in terms of understanding their impact on health policy, environmental regulation, and how they shape the production of scientific knowledge and the delivery of health care in diverse medical and nonmedical settings. First, much work remains to be done in the field of medical sociology in terms of developing adequate criteria and measures for evaluating the effects of HSMs in diverse realms. This evaluation must emphasize both process and outcomes. For example, how have HSMs strengthened the capacity of social movements more broadly to advance policy-making goals in the realms of environmental and public health policy, health care policy, and the regulation of industrial production? Have they

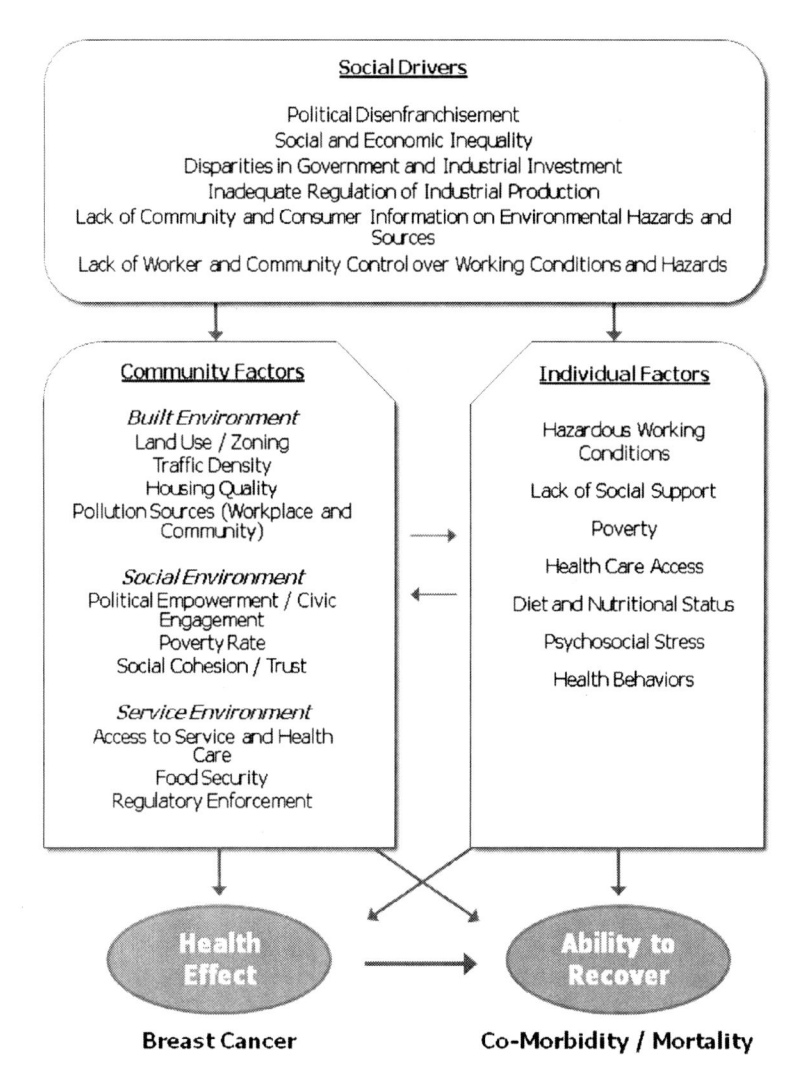

Fig. 7.2 Links between environmental health disparities and breast cancer: an ecosocial view

managed to reframe and reshape the scientific enterprise in any significant ways, and if so, has this occurred through their direct engagement with science, or their strict opposition to it?

Second, why do HSMs address certain diseases and not others? For example, the EBCM emerged from the women's health movement. This is a result of social movement spillover and its role in framing the illness experience in politicized terms. Similarly, Gulf War veterans drew from the experiences of Vietnam veterans who were denied compensation for Agent Orange exposure in order to frame their own symptoms as a form of injustice. However, we have not seen similar movement spillover emerging from the Grey Panthers, to address chronic conditions that particularly impact the elderly. Instead, these groups have tended to emphasize awareness campaigns and resource advocacy within the mainstream medical system, rather than challenging dominant perspectives of disease causation or seeking democratic participation in the research enterprise. Similarly, when a condition has no specific diagnosis or name to give it medical legitimacy, the formation of illness identities, and thus a politicized identity, may be more constrained, as in the case of Gulf War Syndrome.

Third, what is the role of more traditional identity politics and subaltern movement formation based on class, race, and gender in HSMs? Specifically, this points to the need to more deeply examine those factors that enable or compel the formation of movement coalitions, especially among constituencies that may initially seem to be unlikely partners, such as labor–environment, breast cancer–AIDS, and breast cancer–environmental justice coalitions. How do these coalitions frame issues related to empowerment, medicalization, collective illness experience, and the political economy of disease in order to challenge the scientific and medical enterprises and move policy and regulation toward strategies for disease prevention? Have any of these coalitions resulted in more broad-based transnational linkages aimed at addressing global public health and environmental challenges (such as HIV or climate change) that require targeting international scientific institutions, trade organizations, or multinational firms and industries? How do these movements remain beholden to their constituency demands, while building sustainable and effective coalitions?

Future research answering these and other related questions will enhance medical sociology's understanding of the institution of medicine. Particularly, study of HSMs will continue to illuminate how the institution of medicine is shaped by the situation of individuals and social movement organizations within a given society's political economy. This chapter demonstrates how theoretical and analytic concepts – such as a typology of HSMs, the notions of medicalization and empowerment, and an understanding of the political economy of disease as a function of the DEP – can advance our understanding of the intersection of social movements and medicine.

Acknowledgements We thank Alison Cohen, Alissa Cordner, Mercedes Lyson, and Ruth Simpson for their comments on the manuscript.

References

Bell S (2000) Experiencing illness in/and narrative. In: Chloe Bird, Peter Conrad, Allen Fremont, Sol Levine, eds., Handbook of Medical Sociology, fifth edition, Prentice-Hall
Brodeur P (1985) Outrageous misconduct: the asbestos industry on trial. Pantheon, New York, NY
Brown P (1984) The right to refuse treatment and the movement for mental health reform. J Health Polit Policy Law 9:291–313
Brown P (2007) Toxic exposures: contested illnesses and the environmental health movement. Columbia University Press, New York
Brown P, Mikkelsen EJ (1990) No safe place: toxic waste, leukemia, and community action. University of California Press, Berkeley, CA
Brown P, Zavestoski S, McCormick S, Mandelbaum J, Luebke T, Linder M (2001) A gulf of difference: disputes over gulf war-related illnesses. J Health Soc Behav 42:235–257
Brown P, Zavestoski S, McCormick S, Mayer B, Morello-Frosch R, Gasior R (2004) Embodied health movements: uncharted territory in social movement research. Sociol Health Illn 26:1–31
Brown P, McCormick S, Mayer B, Zavestoski S, Morello-Frosch R, Altman RG, Senier L (2006) "A lab of our own:" environmental causation of breast cancer and challenges to the dominant epidemiological paradigm. Sci Technol Human Values 31(5):499–536
Bullard R (ed) (1994) Confronting environmental racism: voices from the grassroots. South End Press, Boston, MA
Bury M (1982) Chronic illness as biographical disruption. Sociology of Health and Illness 4(2):167–82
Casamayou MH (2001) The politics of breast cancer. Georgetown University Press, Washington, DC
Charmaz K (1991) Good days, bad days: the self in chronic illness and time. Rutgers University Press, New Brunswick, NJ
Charmaz K, Olesen V (1997) Ethnographic research in medical sociology. Sociological Methods and Research 25:452–494
Clarke A, Shim J, Mamo L, Fosket J, Fishman J (2003) Biomedicalization: theorizing technoscientific transformation of health, illness, and U.S. biomedicine. Am Sociol Rev 68:161–194
Colborn T, Dumanoski D, Myers JP (1997) Our Stolen Future: Are we threatening our fertility, intelligence and survival? A scientific detective story. Penguin Books, New York

Collins H (1983) An empirical relativist program in the sociology of scientific knowledge. In: Knorr-Cetina K, Mulkay M (eds) Science observed. Sage, Beverly Hills, CA

Conrad P (1987) Wellness in the workplace: Potentials and Pitfalls of Work-Site Health Promotion. Milbank Quarterly 65(2):255–275

Conrad P, Bird C, Fremont A (2000) Handbook of Medical Sociology (5th edition) Prentice Hall, Upper Saddle River, NJ

Conrad P, Leiter V (2004) Medicalization, Markets and Consumers. Journal of Health and Social Behavior 45:158–176.

Conrad P, ed. (2005) Sociology of Health and Illness: Critical Perspectives (7th edition). Worth Publishing, New York

Corburn J (2005) Street science: community knowledge and environmental health justice. MIT, Cambridge, MA

Davis D (2002) When smoke ran like water: tales of environmental deception and the battle against pollution. Basic Books, New York

Davis D, Axelrod D, Bailey L, Gaynor M, Sasco AJ (1998) Rethinking breast cancer risk and the environment: the case for the precautionary principle. Environ Health Perspect 106(9):523–29

Della Porta D, Diani M (1999) Social movements: an introduction. Blackwell, Malden, MA

Epstein S (1996) Impure science: AIDS, activism, and the politics of knowledge. University of California Press, Berkeley, CA

Epstein S (2007) Patient groups and health movements. In: Hackett EJ, Amsterdamska O, Lynch M, Wajcman J (eds) The handbook of science and technology studies. MIT, Cambridge, MA, pp 499–539

Figert AE (1996) Women and the ownership of PMS: the structuring of a psychiatric disorder. Aldine de Gruyter, Hawthorne, NY

Freidson E (1970) Profession of medicine: a study of the sociology of applied knowledge. University of Chicago Press, Chicago, IL

Fujimura J (1995) Ecologies of action: recombining genes, molecularizing cancer, and transforming biology. In: Star SL (ed) Ecologies of knowledge: work and politics in science and technology. SUNY Press, Albany, NY

Gøtzsche P, Nielsen M (2007) Review: adequately randomized trials showed that mammography screening did not significantly reduce breast cancer, cancer, or all cause mortality but increased breast surgeries. Evid Based Nurs 10:80

Goldstein M (1999) Alternative health care: medicine, miracle, or mirage? Temple University Press, Philadelphia, PA

Harding S (1998) Is science multicultural? Indiana University Press, Bloomington, IN

Hess DJ (2002) Technology-oriented social movements and the problem of globalization. Unpublished paper

Klawiter M (2003) Chemicals, cancer, and prevention: the synergy of synthetic social movements. In: Casper M (ed) Synthetic planet: chemical politics and the hazards of modern life. New York, Routledge, pp 155–176

Klawiter M (2005) Breast cancer in two regimes. In: Brown P, Zavestoski S (eds) Social movements in health. Blackwell, London, pp 161–189

Klawiter M (2006) Regulatory shifts, pharmaceutical scripts, and the new consumption junction: configuring high-risk women in an era of chemoprevention. In: Frickel S, Moore K (eds) The new political sociology of science: institutions, networks, and power. University of Wisconsin Press, Madison, WI

Krieger N (1989) Exposure, susceptibility and breast cancer risk: a hypothesis regarding exogenous carcinogens, breast tissue development, and social gradients, including black/white differences, in breast cancer risk. Breast Cancer Res Treat 13:205–223

Krieger N (1994) Epidemiology and the web of causation: has anyone seen the spider? Soc Sci Med 39:887–903

Krieger N (2005) Defining and investigating social disparities in cancer: critical issues. Cancer Causes Control 16:5–14

Krimsky S (2000) Hormonal chaos: the scientific and social origins of the environmental endocrine hypothesis. Johns Hopkins University Press, Baltimore, MA

Krimsky S (2003) Science in the private interest: has the lure of profits corrupted biomedical research? Rowman and Littlefield, Lanham, MD

Lerner B (2001) *The* breast cancer wars: hope, fear, and the pursuit of a cure in twentieth-century America. Oxford University Press, New York

Light D (1991) Professionalism as a countervailing power. J Health Polit Policy Law 16:499–506

Light DW (2004) Ironies of success: a new history of the American health care system. J Health Soc Behav 45(extra issue):1–24

Loh P, Sugerman-Brozan J (2002) Environmental justice organizing for environmental health: case study on asthma and diesel exhaust in Roxbury, Massachusetts. Ann Am Acad Pol Soc Sci 584:110–124

Love SM, Lindsey K (1990) Dr. Susan Love's Breast Book. Addison-Wesley, New York

McAdam D (1982) Political process and the development of black insurgency, 1930–1970. University of Chicago Press, Chicago, IL

McCally M, Haines A, Fein O, Addington W, Lawrence RS, Cassel CK, Blankenship E (2007) Poverty and ill health: physicians can, and should, make a difference. In: Brown P (ed) Perspectives in medical sociology, 4th edn. Waveland Press, Prospect heights, IL

McCormick S (Forthcoming) No family history: finding the environmental links to breast cancer. Rowman and Littlefield, New York

McCormick S, Baralt L (2006) Social movement success?: the breast cancer movement. Paper presented at Annual Meeting of Society for the Study of Social Problems. Montreal, Canada.

McCormick S, Brown P, Zavestoski S (2003) The personal is scientific, the scientific is political: the public paradigm of the environmental-breast cancer movement. Sociol Forum 18(4):545–76

McCormick S, Polk R, Brown P, Brody J (2004) Public involvement in breast cancer research: an analysis and prototype. Int J Health Serv 34(4):625–646

McKinlay JB, Arches J (1985) Towards the proletarianization of physicians. Int J Health Serv 15:161–195

Markowitz G, Rosner D (2002) Deceit and Denial: The Deadly Politics of Industrial Pollution. University of California Press, Berkeley

Masi C, Olopade O (2005) Racial and ethnic disparities in breast cancer: a multilevel perspective. Med Clin North Ama 89:753–770

Meyer DS, Whittier N (1994) Social movement spillover. Soc Probl 41:277–298

Minkler M, Wallerstein N (eds) (2003) Community-based participatory research for health. Jossey-Bass, San Francisco, CA

Moore Kelly (1999) Political protest and institutional change: the anti-Vietnam War movement and American science. In: Giugni M, McAdam D, Tilly C (eds) How social movements matter, vol 10. University of Minnesota Press, Minneapolis, MN

Moore K (2006) Powered by the people: varieties of participatory science as challenges to scientific authority. In: Frickel S, Moore K (eds) The new political sociology of science: institutions, networks, and power. University of Wisconsin Press, Madison, WI

Morgen S (2002) Into our own hands: the women's health movement in the United States, 1969–1990. Rutgers University Press, New Brunswick, NJ

Morello-Frosch R (2002) The political economy of environmental discrimination. Environ Plann C 20:477–496

Morello-Frosch R, Zavestoski S, Brown P, McCormick S, Mayer B, Gasior R (2006) Social movements in health: responses to and shapers of a changed medical world. In: Moore K, Frickel S (eds) The new political sociology of science: institutions, networks, and power. University of Wisconsin Press, Madison, WI

Ozonoff D, Boden L (1987) Truth and consequences: health agency responses to environmental health problems. Sci Technol Human Values 12(3–4):70–77

Parsons T (1951) The Social System. Free Press, Glencoe, IL

Physicians Working Group for Single-Payer National Health Insurance (2003) Proposal of the physicians working group for single-payer national health insurance. JAMA 290(6):798–805

Pfohl SJ (1977) The 'discovery' of child abuse. Soc Probl 24:310–323

Poletta F, Jasper JM (2001) Collective identity and social movements. Annu Rev Sociol 27:283–305

Polite BN, Olufunmilayo IO (2005) Breast cancer and race: a rising tide does not lift all boats equally. Perspect Biol Med 48:166–175

Quadagno J (2004) Why the United States has no national health insurance: stakeholder mobilization against the welfare state, 1945–1996. J Health Soc Behav 45(extra issue):25-44

Roe D, Pease W, Florini K, Silbergeld E (1997) Toxic ignorance: the continuing absence of basic health testing for top-selling chemicals in the United States. Environmental Defense Fund, New York

Rosner D, Markowitz G (1987) Dying for work: workers' safety and health in twentieth-century America. Indiana University Press, Indianapolis, IN

Ruzek SB (1978) The women's health movement: feminist alternatives to medical control. Praeger, New York

Ruzek SB, Olesen VL, Clarke AE (eds) (1997) Women's health: complexities and differences. Ohio State University Press, Columbus, OH

Scheper-Hughes N, Lock MM (1987) The mindful body: a prolegomenon to future work in medical anthropology. Med Anthropol Q 1(1):6–41

Shapiro J (1993) No pity: people with disabilities forging a new civil rights movement. Random, New York

Sharp LA (2000) The commodification of the body and its parts. Annu Rev Anthropol 29:287–328

Shepard PM, Northridge ME, Prakash S, Stover G (2002) Preface: advancing environmental justice through community-based participatory research. Environ Health Perspect 110(Suppl 2):139–140

Szasz A (1994) Ecopopulism: toxic waste and the movement for environmental justice. University of Minnesota Press, Minneapolis, MN

Sze J (2007) Noxious New York: the racial politics of urban health and environmental justice. MIT, Cambridge, MA

Waitzkin H (2000) The second sickness: contradictions of capitalist health care. Rowman and Littlefield, Lanham, MD

Waitzkin H (2001) At the front lines of medicine: how the health care system alienates doctors and mistreats patients. Rowman and Littlefield, Lanham, MD

Williams G (1984) The genesis of chronic illness: narrative re-construction Sociology of Health and Illness 6:175–200

Writing Group for the Women's Health Initiative Investigators (2002) Risks and benefits of estrogen plus progestin in healthy postmenopausal women: principal results from the Women's Health Initiative randomized controlled trial. JAMA 288(3):321–332

Zavestoski S, McCormick S, Brown P (2005) Gender, embodiment and disease: environmental breast cancer activists' challenge to science, the biomedical model, and policy. Sci Cult 13(4):563–586

Zola IK (1972) Medicine as an institution of social control. Sociol Rev 20:487–504

Chapter 8
Layering Control: Medicalization, Psychopathy, and the Increasing Multi-institutional Management of Social Problems

Tait R. Medina and Ann McCranie

Introduction

Scholars interested in the medicalization of deviance tend to draw a clear line between major institutions of social control – namely law, religion, and medicine – and describe a process whereby medicine becomes more dominant than other institutions in terms of defining and controlling problematic behavior (Friedson [1970]1988). This is not surprising, as the study of the medicalization of deviance has been primarily about a shift in both the definition and the locus of control of a problem from one institutional domain into another (Conrad 1975; Conrad and Schneider [1980]1992). However, some forms of deviant behavior cross-cut institutional arenas and the medicalization of these problems happen concurrently with other institutional controls, such as increased criminalization of mental illness, or the reverse, increased medicalization of criminal behavior (Hiday 1999). Instead of nudging aside law and religion in favor of medicine, these cases demonstrate the *layering* of institutional control and the increasing multi-institutional management of social problems.

Because of their substantive focus on medicine, medical sociologists have too often neglected the interplay of medicine and other dominant institutions when considering the management of social problems. Dingwall (2008) refers to this as a failure to look outside the medical "silo" and notes that, at least in the U.S., there has been a simultaneous expansion of the medical and legal systems that heretofore has largely been considered separately. Our aim in this chapter is to present a new approach to understanding medicine's role in the institutional management of social problems, one that considers overlapping institutional environments. It is our contention that what has been referred to as partial or "degrees of medicalization" (Conrad and Schneider [1980]1992) can often be better understood as a *layering* of institutional control over social problems. Multiple institutions – namely medicine, the law, and religion – can be involved simultaneously and with "profound complicity" (Foucault 2006, p. 85) in controlling a social problem. Instead of an either/or approach that views medicalization as a process that reduces the primacy of a religio-moral or legal understanding and control of a problem, we argue that medicalization is but one interesting institutional layer of an increasingly formalized process of social control over problems in modern life.

Here we focus on current debates and research on psychopathy as our illustrative case. Psychopathy is an increasingly recognized "personality disorder" that has as its hallmark the lack of moral conscience and empathy for the suffering of others. We argue that psychopathy stands at the intersection of law, medicine, and morality and highlights the institutional layering of deviance.

T.R. Medina (✉)
Department of Sociology, Indiana University, Ballantine 744, Bloomington, IN 47405, USA
e-mail: tmedina@indiana.edu

While medical language and imagery is used to understand the problem of psychopathy, there are virtually no treatment regimens available for individuals diagnosed with this medical condition. Thus, while psychopathy is increasingly named and framed as a medical or biological problem, it is largely contained within a legal arena or through other social exclusion mechanisms. In fact, this illness designation often leads to harsher punishments in the legal system, as opposed to the reduction in responsibility often afforded to people diagnosed with other mental health conditions. The concept of psychopathy has also been exported into both lay and professional communities as a risk management tool designed to exclude "psychopaths" from social interactions and protect individual and business interests. Further, the concept of psychopathy continues to be laden with discourse about morality and, in particular, evil.

As such, the case of psychopathy raises key issues regarding the relationship among institutions of social control, namely medicine and the law, in the management of social problems. While the medicalization thesis often focuses on a linear progression from non-medical to medical (and perhaps back to non-medical) understandings of a social problem, this case highlights the need to look *across* institutions and consider *linked interactions* between these fields of knowledge.

We begin this chapter with a brief description of medicalization and medical social control and introduce the "twin process" of criminalization. Next, we define and explain the institutional layering approach to the study of deviant behavior. We then provide an introduction to the case of psychopathy as well as the related concepts of sociopathy and anti-social personality disorder. We use the case of psychopathy to illustrate institutional layering and the increasing multi-institutional management of deviance. Finally, we conclude with a discussion of future lines of research.

Medicalization, Criminalization, and the Institutional Management of Deviance

The medicalization of deviant behavior has been a prominent area of inquiry in medical sociology since at least Irving Zola's (1972) work on medicine and social control. Conrad and Schneider's publication, *Deviance and Medicalization: From Badness to Sickness*, has become a standard in this field of study and describes medicalization as "the definition and labeling of deviant behavior as a medical problem, usually an illness, and mandating the medical profession to provide some type of treatment for it" (Conrad and Schneider [1980]1992, p. 29). The medicalization concept has been applied to a broad array of behaviors including hyperactivity (Conrad 1975), excessive drinking (Schneider 1978), gambling (Rossol 2001), compulsive shopping (Lee and Mysyk 2004), and becoming "dependent" on welfare assistance (Schram 2000). However, this concept has also been used to discuss the medicalization of "difference," rather than behavior – such as the medicalization of family relations through new genetic information (Finkler et al. 2003) and aging (Estes and Binney 1989).

While the focus of medicalization scholars varies – with some focusing on the medical profession (e.g., medical imperialism and professional dominance) and others on the changing definition and conceptualization of deviant behavior (see Clarke and Shim 2010) – most classical theorists agree that medicalization has resulted in a weakening of the jurisdiction of more traditional institutions of social control, such as law and religion (Conrad and Schneider [1980]1992; Friedson 1970). Through its ability to officially label deviance as illness, medicine has expanded into areas that were previously understood and managed in a non-medical way (Conrad and Schneider [1980]1992; Conrad 2005). Increased medicalization is not just a product of medical professionals, to be sure (Conrad and Potter 2000), and it may be enacted outside a traditional allopathic medical context (Appleton 1995), but it continues to gain ground in the control of social problems at the expense of more traditional institutions of social control.

Some of the earliest sociological work in the area of criminalization was by Edwin Sutherland, who wrote about the creation and diffusion of sexual psychopath laws through the United States (Jenness 2004; Sutherland 1950). A key aspect to this diffusion was the roles of media and expert opinion. While criminalization lacks the same definitional core that Conrad provided for medicalization, the usage of the term appears to parallel Michalowski (1985), who describes it as a process whereby previously legal acts are transformed into crimes and individuals into criminals. Jenness (2004, p. 150) argues that "changes in structural conditions provide the impetus for the development of law that targets a set of activities perceived to be attached to a social group deemed 'in need of control' by those in a position to stimulate, define, and institutionalize criminal law." She maps a broad literature on criminalization and the many approaches used to study it, including social entrepreneurs, triggering events, interest groups and social movements, political opportunism, and structural factors. While criminalization work appears focused more on the structural position of the deviant person vis-à-vis the controlling agent than medicalization theory does, the emphasis on definitional issues is similar. Thus, while medicalization scholars are interested in how behavior comes to be defined and treated as medical, criminalization scholars examine the processes by which behavior becomes defined and punished as criminal. For this reason, medicalization and criminalization are often juxtaposed as twin processes with one ebbing as the other increases in its dominance (Jenness 2004).

For their part, sociologists have a long history of studying institutions of social control. Parsons (1951) explicitly defined medicine as an institution of social control and set medicine alongside law in this regard. In *The Social System*, Parsons discussed the practices and processes that contribute to stability in societies and argued that the criminal role and sick role exemplify two different mechanisms of social control. The criminal role functions primarily through defining criminal acts as illegitimate, holding the criminal responsible for his behavior, and punishing the criminal by excluding him from the social group. The sick role functions primarily through placing deviants under the care of a "technically competent expert" (Parsons 1951, p. 314), releasing them from responsibility for the onset of their conditions, and creating a therapeutic relationship that will assist in the return to the social group. While the criminal role is illegitimate, the sick role is conditionally legitimate. That is, the deviant act (illness) is legitimate as long as the sick person expresses a desire to get well and cooperates in this process. In this way, therapeutic support is given in exchange for taking on the obligation to get well. Because the therapeutic relationship is more effective than punishment in reintegrating the deviant back into society, Parsons believed that, given a choice, diverting deviants into the sick role was a more effective social control mechanism.

The pioneers of medicalization theory, namely Freidson, Zola, and Conrad, were influenced, sometimes to the contrary, by Parson's conceptualization of medicine as an institution of social control. These early scholars continued to make the treatment versus punishment distinction between medicine and law and to associate these discrete approaches to the imputation of responsibility. Freidson called this the "institutional division of labor for deviance" (Freidson [1970]1988, p. 247). In this division of labor, law punishes individuals who are held responsible for their deviance and medicine treats individuals who are labeled as ill it is this institutional division of labor for deviance that we address in the next sections. Specifically, we challenge the treatment/punishment distinction and its relationship to the label of illness as well as the claim that the extension of medicine into new realms necessarily weakens the jurisdiction of law (and the influence of a religio-moral discourse). While we do view medicalization and criminalization as twin processes, each highlighting a different form of social control, we shift our focus to the simultaneous development of a criminal and medical model of understanding, the co-occurrence of which highlights the increasing multi-institutional management of social problems.

However, before moving into our discussion of institutional layering, we address two concepts that motivate our approach: levels of medicalization and degrees of medicalization.

Institutional Layering and the Increasing Formalized Social Control of Problems

Classic theories of medicalization are flexible enough to accommodate the idea of layering and multi-institutional management of social problems, even if the explicit focus has not been applied before. Concepts of levels and degrees of medicalization provide a starting point. Conrad and Schneider (1980) suggested that medicalization can occur on at least three levels: *conceptual*, *institutional*, and at the *doctor–patient relationship*. In later formulations (Conrad 1992; Conrad and Schneider [1980]1992), the institutional is also referred to as *organizational* and the doctor–patient interaction is described more broadly as the *interactional* level. Medicalization at the conceptual level consists of using medical language or a medical frame to define and treat a problem (see also Brown 1995). Medicalization occurs at the organizational/institutional level if an organization adopts a medical definition of a problem in which it specializes. Conrad's and Schneider's use of "institution" appears to be focused on identifiable, specific organizations rather than the "more enduring features of social life" (Giddens 1986) that we prefer to use. At the level of the interaction/doctor–patient relationship, medicalization occurs when a problem in an individual is diagnosed and treated medically, most often by a doctor.

In addition to levels of medicalization, Conrad and Schneider argue that "medicalization is not an either/or phenomenon; it is better seen in terms of degrees" ([1980]1992, p. 278) and that older non-medical definitions of a problem can continue to exist alongside medical definitions. For instance, they claim that while madness has been fully medicalized, opiate addiction has been partially medicalized and sex addiction has been only minimally medicalized. Factors likely to affect the degree of medicalization include the availability of medical treatments and the existence of competing, non-medical definitions. State and popular support of the medical profession, availability of treatments, and financial incentives (such as insurance coverage) could also contribute to the degree of medicalization achieved. Further, the authors suggest that "medical social control does not preclude the simultaneous and even coordinated operation of legal controls" ([1980]1992, p. 283). While we are in fundamental agreement with this statement, we argue that this phenomenon has not been fully explicated, nor has a theoretical foundation for understanding this simultaneous and coordinated operation been presented. This is what we propose to do.

It is our contention that the social control of deviance is not a zero-sum equation, where one institution can gain only at the expense of another institution's control. In many of the classic studies of institutional social control of deviance, there appears to be an inversely proportionate amount of control that one institution (e.g., medicine) can have over the other, such as the criminal justice system. For instance, early efforts to have homosexuality viewed as a medical condition were focused on relieving the persecution of homosexuals through the protection of medicine, though that medical social control itself later became a source of contestation (Conrad and Schneider [1980]1992; Conrad and Angell 2004).

And yet, there are some instances in which the easy equation of decriminalization and increased medicalization do not hold. Armstrong's (2003) study of the case of fetal alcohol syndrome (FAS) shows that the increasing medicalization of FAS leads to an inherent maternal–fetal conflict and more restrictive and punitive approaches toward pregnant women. The outcome of the creation of the diagnosis of FAS is increased social control over all pregnant women and their alcohol-drinking habits. Armstrong is focusing on a conflict between the traditional Parsonian understanding of the sick role, which diminished personal responsibility in the face of illness and has a "restituitive" and "restorative" approach toward those who fall into its purview. But in the case of FAS, medicine is "neither restituitive nor restorative" (Armstrong 2003, p. 210). This paradox, we argue, is similar to that of psychopathy.

To account for conflicts in the theoretical underpinning of medicalization, we propose the idea of *institutional layering*. By this we mean that the social control of a problem can become the focus of multiple institutions – such as medicine, law, and religion – simultaneously. While one institution may, over time, come to dominate control over a problem, we propose that multiple definitions and loci of control can exist simultaneously. Further, these institutions can either be cooperative, in conflict, or be agnostic toward one another in the construction and containment of the problem. In the particular case of psychopathy, they are so intertwined as to be inseparable.

The Psychopath, the Sociopath, and Others

"Psychopaths" have been described as "intraspecies predators" (Hare 1998, p. 196), people who lack in conscience and who use superficial charm, manipulation, and sometimes violence to satisfy their own needs. Popular press and media accounts tend to use the terms *sociopath* and *psychopath* interchangeably, to discuss people who hurt others without remorse or empathy. However, in the scientific literature, there is a distinction drawn between the terms. Both the *sociopath* and the *psychopath* are "characterized by a lack of the restraining influence of conscience and of empathic concern for other people" (Lykken 2006, p. 11). What distinguishes the *psychopath* in this formulation is that the individual "has failed to develop conscience and empathic feelings, not because of a lack of socializing experience, but, rather, because of some inherent psychological peculiarity which makes him especially difficult to socialize" (Lykken 2006, p. 11). The etiology of this "inherent psychological peculiarity" is at the root of much heated debate, but the understanding that sociopaths are made through some sort of social conditions while psychopaths are born with a predisposition of some sort not uncommon among researchers. In fact, Hare suggests that the terms *psychopath* and *sociopath* may well reflect the different understandings of the "origins and determinants of the problem" (Hare 1999b, p. 23). For instance, Hare states that social scientists tend to prefer the term sociopathy to emphasize environmental and social antecedents to the problem, whereas those who hold more closely to the "psychological, biological and genetic factors" prefer the term psychopathy (Hare 1999b, pp. 23–24).

Those who study anti-social behaviors sometimes claim that *sociopaths* are the real practical concern because they are "metastasizing" quickly (Lykken 2006, p. 4), are much more numerous, and as a group are responsible for a high percentage of violent crime. However the rare, curious, and potentially dangerous *psychopath* attracts more scientific attention. In 2005, a group of researchers founded an organization called "The Society for the Scientific Study of Psychopathy." This international society with biannual conferences numbers more than 160 members, according to the published accounts on the society's website in late 2009. The majority of members are from the United States, but Canada, Europe, and Asia are also well represented.

As scientific consensus has developed about what a *psychopath* is, Robert Hare's Psychopathy Checklist-Revised (PCL-R; Hare 1991, 2003) became the dominant diagnostic tool. Analyses of the coherence of the items (Hare and Neumann 2006; Neumann et al. 2007) yielded four major dimensions of psychopathy. The interpersonal dimension is associated with glibness and superficial charm, grandiose behavior, and conning or manipulative behavior. The affective dimension targets callousness, and lack of remorse, guilt, or empathy. The lifestyle dimension includes impulsivity, parasitic orientation, and stimulation-seeking behavior. Finally, the anti-social dimension highlights behavioral issues such as criminality or a history of delinquent behavior.

From that, they conclude: "…psychopathy is essentially a personality disorder involving a failure to: (a) adopt the common interpersonal conventions of honesty, modesty, and trustworthiness, (b) experience full-fledged emotions concerning one's relation to others (e.g., love, empathy, guilt), (c) adopt widely shared sociocultural norms pertaining to financial responsibility and safe conduct, and (d) obey the laws of society." (Neumann et al. 2007, p. 104)

Further related and potentially confusing categories are those included in *The Diagnostic and Statistical Manual of Mental Disorders* (DSM IV-TR; American Psychiatric Association 2000).

The DSM IV-TR sees both sociopathy and psychopathy as synonymous with the diagnosis of *antisocial personality disorder* (APD), an Axis II disorder. This simple linking between APD and psychopathy, not surprisingly, is rejected by those who study psychopathy, specifically (Hare 1999b; Lykken 2006; Widiger 2006). APD is defined by a pattern (manifesting in some form from at least age 15) of acting with callous disregard for the rights of others that might be characterized by recklessness, breaking the law, or acting with little remorse upon mistreating, stealing from, or harming others.[1] While the description of the behaviors, namely breaches of social norms, is similar to the clinical definition of psychopathy, missing are the personality dimensions of psychopathy, such as callousness, egocentricity, and lack of remorse.[2] Hare has suggested that this is not a fundamental disagreement, but rather a "concept drift" (Hare et al. 1991, p. 393) by drafters of the DSM IV due to the concern that clinicians would be unable to reliably assess personality traits connected with this condition (see also, Hare 1999b).

It is also important to keep the research field's distinction between *psychopathy* and *psychosis* distinct, though it is clear that in popular media the terms *psychopath* and *psychotic* are used interchangeably to define individuals who are mentally ill, who behave in reckless and dangerous ways. While the term *psychosis*, introduced into the English language in the mid-19th century, originally referred to all manner of mental illness (OED 2007), its meaning has, at least in the psychiatric field, become a signifier for a constellation of symptoms (not all of which must be present for the label to be applied) such as delusions, hallucinations, disorganized speech, or disorganized or catatonic behavior. In DSM-IV, these symptoms usually would lead to an Axis I (clinical) disorder. While this constellation of symptoms is an important feature for several disorders (i.e., schizophrenia and schizophreniform, schizoaffective, and delusional disorders), psychosis is the defining characteristic of other disorders that are recognized to have distinct etiologies: psychotic disorder due to a general medical condition and substance-induced psychotic disorder. In addition, psychosis is recognized as an important potential feature in other disorders, such as those categorized primarily on their mood effects such as major depressive disorder and bipolar disorder. Finally, three disorders: brief psychotic disorder, shared psychotic disorder, and psychotic disorder not otherwise specified, cement this constellation of problems as a recognizable disorder when other conditions have been ruled out or the etiology is unclear. The DSM IV-TR notes this confusing mélange of terms (American Psychiatric Association 2000, pp. 297–298) and provides some distinction, though it offers nothing definitive.

To further muddy the waters, *psychosis* and the related term *psychotic* are often used outside of medical contexts (for instance, in films and books) to connote breaks with reality, particularly those that lead to frenzied, unpredictable, or possibly violent or murderous behavior. Occasionally, the terms *psychopath* and *psychotic* are used interchangeably to connote violent mentally ill individuals, though this conflation will often bring condemnation from those who wish to separate the "mad" with psychosis from the stigma of the "bad" with psychopathy.[3] However, within a psychiatric framework, psychosis is viewed as clearly distinct from psychopathy, which is characterized by more realistic thinking and knowledge of social norms. Some studies (for example, Nestor et al. 2002) have found the two disorders to occur largely exclusive of one another, though there can be some co-morbidity. In fact, there are numerous studies that isolate psychopathic tendencies or APD markers as one of the best predictors for violent or recidivistic behavior among people with schizophrenia (Mueser et al. 2007; Nolan et al. 1999; Rice and Harris 1992; Tengström et al. 2000).

---

[1] Conduct Disorder is a diagnostic category similar to APD, but applied to children under the age of 18.

[2] The tension that this issue has caused may well lead to changes in the criteria that will be adopted in the DSM V, currently scheduled for 2013. At least two workgroups, the ADHD and Disruptive Behavior Disorders Work Group and the Personality and Personality Disorders Work Group, are considering related issues.

[3] Two illustrative letters to the editor in the New York Times illustrate this perceived misuse and correction: one written by Jack Olsen, Feb 26, 1986, "Psychotic or Psychopathic" and another written by Janet Hebb, March 17, 1991, "Psychopaths on film; What's in a Name?"

Finally, the general term *psychopathology* refers to the field of study of mental illness or abnormal behavior (such as depression, psychosis, or anxiety) or maladaptive behaviors or personality characteristics. *Psychopathy* is but one pattern of behavior or set of personality characteristics that could be considered *psychopathological*.

Psychopathy and Institutional Layering: Who Takes Precedence?

Key to our proposed *institutional layering* approach is the claim that the increasing institutional control of a social problem in one domain (such as medicine) should not – and sometimes cannot – be considered in isolation from other domains. In what follows, we demonstrate that it is impossible to sort the institutional control of psychopathy into either a purely legal or a medical field, nor is it possible to consider medical, criminal, and religio-moral understandings of the problem in isolation. Instead it is necessary to focus on the increasingly complex relations between medicine and the criminal/legal system in simultaneously managing the problem of psychopathy, as well as the multiple frameworks used to order and conceptualize the problem (the person is sick, bad, evil, etc.). Once the state of "being a psychopath" becomes named and framed, efforts to contain (or quarantine or exclude) individuals so named become more pronounced in multiple arenas.

Medical Understandings of Psychopathy

Over time, a clear diagnostic history, codification of the clinical entity in diagnostic tools, and several well-developed etiological theories have developed, indicating that psychopathy has been medicalized to some degree. However, the attempt to contain this problem through medical means (i.e., treatment) has thus far largely failed. This does not represent degrees of medicalization; rather, we argue that medicalization is just one layer of the social control of psychopathy.

History of the Diagnosis

The definition of psychopathy has a long and varied history. In the 1800s, French psychiatrist Philippe Pinel developed the clinical construct *manie sans delire* (or madness without delirium) to describe a class of individuals who engaged in impulsive and socially unacceptable behavior while being fully aware of the irrational and potentially self-destructive nature of these actions (Herve 2007). What set this condition apart from other disruptive psychological conditions was the lack of any identifiable psychosis (Hare and Neumann 2006). At around the same time as Pinel, the American physician Benjamin Rush noted a similar condition that he called *moral derangement* or *anomia* (Herve 2007). Marked by the presence of manipulative, deceitful, and socially disruptive behaviors performed without remorse or guilt, Rush linked this condition to an impairment of the moral faculty, which he believed had a biological basis (Verplaetse 2009).

The British physician J.C. Pritchard later labeled this disorder *moral insanity*. Like Pinel and Rush, he noted that individuals with this condition had no impairment in understanding and intellect, but lacked a sense of decency, fairness, and responsibility. Pritchard argued that individuals with this condition were highly prone to criminal activity and because they lacked the ability to learn from their mistakes and could not be rehabilitated through punishment (Herve 2007). The term *psychopathic* was introduced to the psychiatric literature by the German psychiatrist J.L. Koch, who labeled the condition *psychopathic inferiority*. Koch argued that this disorder was chronic in nature and had an underlying biological or organic cause (Herve 2007). Koch's contemporary, Kraepelin, refined this definition and described a set of p*sychopathic personalities* or *psychopathies*, each of which was marked by a deficiency in both emotions and will (Herve 2007).

Throughout the course of the 20th century there were many attempts to refine the construct; however, it was American psychiatrist Hervey Cleckley who exerted the most influence on future definitions (Herve 2007). In his seminal volume, *The Mask of Sanity*, Cleckley presents extensive case studies of psychopathic individuals conducted while in residence at a large neuropsychiatric hospital. He describes the psychopathic personality as one marked by an outward appearance of good mental health that masks a severe behavioral maladjustment. Importantly, Cleckley presents 16 specific criteria which stand as the defining characteristics of the disorder, including superficial charm, lack of remorse or shame, and a general poverty in major affective reactions (see Cleckley [1941]1964, pp. 362–400 for a full description). While prior psychiatrists defined the condition solely in terms of anti-social behavior, Cleckley argued that psychopathy was both behavioral and social–emotional in nature. He believed that a deficit in emotional reactivity was central to this disorder and argued that while the psychopathic personality had no deficit in emotions such as rage and frustration, a severe deficit in emotions such as love and empathy existed. This lack of complex social emotions makes the psychopathic personality immune to normal forms of social control, which either compels a person to act according to social norms out of love or out of fear of experiencing feelings of shame, remorse, and guilt (Cleckley [1941]1964; Herve 2007).

These "Clecklian" traits were operationalized in the Hare (1991) Psychopathy Checklist (PCL-R), which stands today as the dominant diagnostic tool (Conoley and Impara 1995; Hill et al. 2004). Developed in the 1980s and refined in the 1990s, the PCL-R is a clinical construct rating scale initially designed to identify incarcerated males who matched Cleckley's description of the psychopathic personality. The PCL-R consists of 20 items and is scored on the basis of an extensive file review and a semi-structured interview. Early analyses found two broad dimensions: Factor 1 characterized by a callous and unemotional interpersonal style and Factor 2 by impulsive and anti-social behavior. More recently a four-factor model – comprised of interpersonal, affective, lifestyle, and anti-social behavior dimensions – has been proposed and validated (Hare and Neumann 2008).

While the PCL-R was primarily constructed and validated using a forensic population, it has been adapted for use in the general population and among juvenile offenders. The PCL-Screening Version (Hart et al. 1995), which was developed for the MacArthur Violence Risk Assessment Study, is a 12-item scale based on a subset of PCL-R items that can be used in "psychiatric evaluations, personnel selection, and community studies" (Hare n.d.). The PCL–Youth Version is a 20-item rating scale for the assessment of psychopathic traits in juvenile offenders (Forth et al. 2003). A number of self-report measures have also been developed for use in the general population (Campbell et al. 2009). These include the Psychopathic Personality Inventory–Revised (Lilienfeld and Widows 2005), Levenson's Self-Report Psychopathy Scale (Levenson et al. 1995), and the Self-Report Psychopathy Scale–II (Hare et al. 1989).

The identification of psychopathy in children and adolescents has taken on greater interest in recent years. Because psychopathy is seen as a relatively stable disorder that is linked to aggressive behavior in adulthood, it is argued that the early identification of psychopathy in children could allow for early intervention measures that can protect the public from the "fledgling psychopath" (Seagrave and Grisso 2002).[4]

---

[4] Researchers also hope that studying psychopathy in children can contribute to the understanding of the developmental pathways that lead to adult psychopathy (Lynam et al. 2009). The most commonly used assessment tools for identifying psychopathic traits in children and adolescents (Campbell et al. 2009) include the Antisocial Process Screening Device (Frick and Hare 2001), the Childhood Psychopathy Scale (Lynam 1997), and the Youth Psychopathic Traits Inventory (Andershed et al. 2002).

Medical and Biological Theories of Psychopathy

If psychopathy is a brain disorder, what is its basis? The most dominant theories are described below.[5]

Fear-Conditioning Deficit. The low-fear hypothesis of psychopathy was proposed by Lykken in 1957 and continues today to spark great interest and debate (Fowles and Dindo 2006). Lykken (1957) suggested that psychopathic individuals suffered from defective emotional reactivity. He hypothesized that psychopathic individuals are comparatively less able to develop fear/anxiety in response to warning signals. Because of this defect, such individuals are incapable of learning to avoid circumstances that produce fear/anxiety or result in punishment. Using a series of experiments based on the classical conditioning paradigm, he found support for these hypotheses. For example, compared to controls, psychopathic individuals showed less electrodermal activity (a measure of sweat gland activity) to a conditioned stimulus associated with a shock, as well as poor avoidance of shocked responses on a mental maze game (Lykken 1957). Subsequent studies have provided further support for the low-fear hypothesis (Fowles and Dindo 2006).

Psychoanalytic Models. Those working within the psychoanalytic tradition argue that disturbed early relations are central to psychopathy (Blackburn 2006). The internalization of group standards is believed to be underdeveloped in psychopathic individuals due to poor parenting, specifically parental rejection, neglect, abuse, and abandonment. While the focus of these models is on disturbed relations that lead to attachment deficits, some researchers posit an underlying biological or genetic disorder that predisposes the psychopathic individual to react aggressively in response to traumatic early experiences (Kernberg 1992). Studies have found that psychopathic individuals display signs of an attachment deficit; however, there has been only moderate support for the connection between childhood abuse and neglect and psychopathy. For example, childhood abuse appears to be high among all young male offenders, both psychopathic and non-psychopathic (see Blackburn 2006 for more).

Cognitive Theories. Dysfunctions in cognition tend to be associated with either a deficit in cognitive processing (decoding, encoding, retrieval, and attention) or a distortion in cognitive structures (beliefs, schemas, and tacit assumptions) (Blackburn 2006). Those working within the deficit approach (e.g., Newman 1998) suggest that psychopathic individuals have poor response modulation that inhibits their ability to shift attention away from goal-directed behavior in order to accommodate environmental feedback. Several studies have found that in the face of cues that suggest the modification of behavior (e.g., loss of money or punishment), psychopathic individuals persist in their behavior (Blackburn 2006). Those working within the distortion approach (e.g., Beck 1976) suggest that psychopathic individuals experience cognitive distortions that cause them to employ dysfunctional strategies when interacting with the social world. Psychopathic individuals have dysfunctional schemas about the self, the world, and the future (e.g., "If I don't exploit/manipulate/attack others, I will never get what I deserve/need/want") which lead to distorted interpretations of events. Few studies have examined the relationship between distorted schemas and deviant behavior (Blackburn 2006).

Neurocognitive Theories. The burgeoning area of structural and functional brain imaging spawned numerous neurocognitive theories of psychopathy which try to link the theories above to abnormalities or impairments in the brain. For example, the hippocampus has been shown to play a critical role in fear conditioning (LeDoux 1996), with impairments linked to psychopathic behavior (Raine et al. 2004; Laakso et al. 2001). Blair and colleagues have proposed that the psychopath is ill

---

[5] The large majority of the studies mentioned rely on the PCL-R to identify their "test" (e.g., psychopathic individuals) and control populations and most, but not all (i.e., Raine et al. 2004; Blair et al. 2001) recruit their "test" subjects from forensic settings.

equipped to engage in emotional learning due to genetic abnormalities that disrupt the functioning of the amygdala (Blair et al. 2005), the center of fear and empathic processing (Blair et al. 2001). Studies have found decreased activation in the amygdala among psychopathic individuals when viewing negative affective images (Kiehl et al. 2004), and children with psychopathic tendencies have been found to have difficulty recognizing sad and fearful expressions, mistaking them for other types of expressions (Blair et al. 2001).

Psychopathy has also been linked to structural abnormalities in what is called the "moral brain" (de Oliveira-Souza et al. 2008). Using functional magnetic resonance imaging, researchers have identified a series of brain networks (e.g., the orbital and medial sectors of the prefrontal cortex and the superior temporal sulcus region) that are thought to specialize in the development of moral emotions, emotions that have to do with the welfare of others (Moll et al. 2002). Studies have found that psychopathic individuals display more structural abnormalities in the "moral brain" then do non-psychopathic individuals (de Oliveira-Souza et al. 2008).

The Treatment of Psychopathic Individuals

One critical part to medicalization is the understanding and adoption of a treatment regimen for the affected. However, in the case of psychopathy, the prevailing clinical view is that it is incurable (Minzenberg and Siever 2006). No single set of established protocols or approaches exists, and there is a general sense of pessimism about the prospects of effectively treating or curing psychopathy.

Even Hare, who, along with Wong (Wong and Hare 2005) published a set of widely cited guidelines for the treatment of psychopaths, has signaled caution: "There is little evidence that psychopaths can be, or even believe that they should be, rehabilitated..." Unfortunately, psychopaths already are aware of their own motivations, see little wrong with them, and do not believe they need to change" (Carozza 2008).

Not only have effective treatments for psychopathy been largely elusive, but the message that treatment might actually be *counterproductive* has also found its way into the treatment literature and public understanding about psychopathy. One effort to reform psychopaths through a therapeutic community was not only ineffective, but actually had the opposite effect – the psychopathic subjects were more likely to violently reoffend, while non-psychopathic subjects who went through the same program were less likely to do so (Rice et al. 1992). Other published studies found alarming increases in violent recidivism after treatment (Seto and Barbaree 1999; D'Silva et al. 2004; Harris and Rice 2006; Lee 1999).

The case of the medical understanding of psychopathy indicates that the problem has not been fully medicalized. The lack of a psychopharmaceutical "silver bullet" and the muddled picture for the behavioral treatment, coupled with an increasing adoption of the medical and biological framework for understanding the etiology of the problem, have led to some frustration. Yet there is no retreat by psychopathy researchers who have formed a professional society dedicated to psychopathy studies and to research into nosological and etiological issues, and with pilot programs for treatment options.

Medico-Criminal Understandings of Psychopathy

While the case of psychopathy has been partially medicalized, the fact that its dominant diagnostic tool, the PCL-R, is situated within the field of forensic psychiatry and psychology clearly indicates an overlapping of the medical and the crimino-legal arenas. By examining the use of the PCL-R within the field of forensic psychiatry/psychology (a field that stands at the interface of medicine and the law[6]), we argue that psychopathy as a diagnostic entity illustrates the "profound complicity" of these twin mechanisms of social control.

The PCL-R, developed and validated using a forensic population, has been shown to predict both recidivism (Hart et al. 1988; Serin et al. 1990) and future violence (Rice et al. 1990). For offender populations, the PCL-R has been hailed as being "unparalleled as a measure for making risk assessments" (Salekin et al. 1996, p. 211). For example, while 25% of non-psychopathic individuals reoffended within 3 years, 80% of individuals classified as psychopathic reoffended (Hart et al. 1988). The PCL-R has become the gold standard in psychopathy research in large part because of its ability to predict recidivism and violence (Salekin et al. 1996).

Courts of law have become increasingly reliant on expert opinions regarding the possible risk of violence among individuals standing trial or receiving sentencing (Salekin et al. 1996), and clinical assessment instruments are highly regarded among forensic psychologists/ psychiatrists for evaluating the mental state at the time of the offense, risk for violence, and competency to stand trial (Archer et al. 2006). Among members of the American Psychology-Law Society Division of the American Psychological Association and the American Board of Forensic Psychology, the PCL-R is the most commonly used assessment tool for evaluating violence risk assessment and psychopathy (Archer et al. 2006).

While a diagnosis of schizophrenia, mania, or depression can serve as a defensive claim, reducing one's responsibility for the crime, a diagnosis of psychopathy is used, most often, as an aggravating factor (Morse 2008). A case law survey of published U.S. court cases involving the PCL–R from 1991 through 2004 found that the PCL–R was used in 87 reported cases (76 state cases and 11 federal cases), with the frequency of use increasing precipitously over time. Fewer than two cases were reported per year in the years 1991–1999, but from 2000 to 2004, 10–30 cases per year were reported (DeMatteo and Edens 2006). In most of the state cases and in all of the federal cases, the PCL-R was introduced by the prosecution to argue that the defendant is dangerous and should be (or continue to be) removed from society, particularly the sexually violent predator (SVP) subject to involuntary and indefinite civil commitment. The second most frequent use of the PCL-R was to determine future risk of danger in parole and probation hearings. In fact, a diagnosis of psychopathy is quite compelling in this area. A 2007 study found that a diagnosis of psychopathy was the strongest predictor of whether or not a patient would be recommended for release from a maximum security forensic hospital (Manguno-Mire et al. 2007). Finally, in capital cases, the PCL-R has been used during sentencing to determine the presence of aggravating factors required to impose a death sentence (DeMatteo and Edens 2006). A diagnosis of psychopathy is actually suspected to have a negative impact on sentencing decisions for an accused criminal. A recent study (Edens et al. 2005) found that jurors in a mock trial were far more likely to recommend the death sentence for a murderer who was labeled with the diagnosis of psychopathy (60%) than someone with no diagnosis (38%). A diagnosis of psychosis, in stark contrast, offered a protective effect (30%).

Importantly, a diagnosis of psychopathy is not considered a sufficient basis for raising an insanity defense (Morse 2008). The Model Penal Code, which includes an insanity test later adopted by many states, indicates that "the terms mental disease or defect do not include an abnormality manifested only by repeated criminal or otherwise anti-social conduct" (American Law Institute 1962). While psychopathy has been argued to have a strong biological and affective component, the association of this diagnosis with anti-social behavior often precludes it from being considered in an insanity defense (Campbell 1990). As Hare himself argues, this "would be appalling" (Hare 1996, p. 47).

---

[6] The Ethics Guidelines for the Practice of Forensic Psychiatry states that: "Forensic psychiatrists practice at the interface of law and psychiatry, each of which has developed its own institutions, policies, procedures, values, and vocabulary. As a consequence, the practice of forensic psychiatry entails inherent potentials for complications, conflicts, misunderstandings and abuses" (*Source*: http://www.aapl.org/pdf/ethicsgdlns.pdf, accessed January 27, 2010).

Beyond its widespread use in legal trials, the PCL-R is used frequently in decisions about treatment suitability in forensic settings (Gacono et al. 2001; Archer 2006). Because psychopathy is generally understood as an immutable personality disorder that increases one's propensity for violence, the diagnosis often disqualifies a person from participation in treatment programs (Skeem et al. 2002). As Megargee (2003, p. 374) explains: "In correctional facilities where treatment resources are scarce and access must be limited to those most likely to profit from interventions, such findings suggest that psychopaths should have lower priority than other offenders." Since the prognosis for effectively treating psychopathy "is practically zero," Kernberg (1998, p. 377) goes further to argue that "the main therapeutic task is to protect the family, the therapist, and the society from such a patient." In this setting, psychopathy is a clinical diagnosis that signals institutional management via containment and social exclusion rather than through medical means such as treatment. This reaction challenges in a fundamental way the claim that increased medicalization allows an individual to gain access to the privileges of the sick role (Gacono et al. 2001).

The medicalization thesis indicates that medicine has jurisdiction over anything that is labeled illness and that once deviance is recast as illness the problem moves into the jurisdiction of medicine. This claim was complicated, however, by the case of psychopathy. Instead of a weakening of legal jurisdiction over a problem in favor of a medical solution, the case of psychopathy highlights Foucault's notion of "profound complicity" (Foucault 2006, p. 85) between these twin mechanisms of social control. The problem is ordered using medical language, but medicine remains largely impotent with regard to containing the problem. Indeed, the diagnosis sometimes precludes individuals in forensic settings from receiving medical treatment. In this way, psychopathy is an illness designation that is controlled, not through treatment, but through punishment. The criminal justice system can be successful in containing psychopathic offenders for a time, but has no reach over the problem (to be discussed below) of those "successful psychopaths" who do not break laws in their abusive behavior.

A key component of the medicalization thesis is that labeling deviance as illness comes with certain humanitarian benefits, namely management via treatment rather than punishment. Conrad and Schneider [1980]1992) cite the insanity defense as a key example of this phenomena. However, a diagnosis of psychopathy is rarely, if ever used, as an insanity defense (Morse 2008) and some within the medical profession argue that it *should not* be used (Hare 1996). The label itself appears to be more effective in the prosecution rather than defense of a criminal.

While psychopathy is a medical diagnosis, the psychopath is hardly accepted as sick in the Parsonian sense (1951) and instead represents a complicated bad-sick hybrid role. The psychopath is understood to have a brain dysfunction that increases his propensity to commit criminal acts and he is held legally accountable for his actions. Once in a forensic setting, the label "illness" does not alter the imputation of responsibility and as such the management of the psychopath remains within the jurisdiction of the criminal justice system. Psychopathy, it seems, is a medical diagnosis that not only excludes individuals from treatment but leads to harsher punishment.

The Appropriation of Evil: Moral Discourse and the Medico-Criminal Understanding of Psychopathy

Scientists working within the field of psychopathy describe the psychopath as the personification of evil (Blair et al. 2005). This conceptualization, which combines disparate systems of knowledge, namely medical and religio-moral, is held by lay and professionals alike. *Evil Genes*, a popular press book, for example, expresses this hybrid understanding of psychopathy, one that attempts to explain evil through an appeal to biology. Some forensic psychiatrists argue for the incorporation of the concept of evil into the field of forensic psychiatry, arguing that the only way to understand some predatory killers is to incorporate evil alongside biological, psychological, and social understandings of the problem (Stone 2009). This has led to a move by psychiatrists and psychologists to standardize the definition of evil, especially as it is used in courts of law to identify crimes that are "depraved" and "heinous" (Welner 2009). Psychiatrist Michael Stone argues that the discussion of the concept of evil has, in recent years, undergone a "sea-change." Once the exclusive province of religion, "evil has become an acceptable subject for study by the mental health professions, including general psychiatry, forensic psychiatry, and neuroscience. Rather than relying on the Bible (of whatever religion) for explanations about the nature and roots of evil, we now look where we should have been looking all along: the human brain" (Stone 2010, p. 15).

The attempt to localize evil, or more broadly morality, to the brain, is a bourgeoning area of study in the brain sciences. For example, Moll et al. (2002) claim to have identified, using functional magnetic resonance imaging, a series of brain networks that specialize in the development of moral emotions. de Oliveira-Souza and colleagues (2008) have applied this concept of the "moral brain" to psychopathy, arguing that individuals with psychopathic tendencies display more structural abnormalities in the "moral brain" then those who lack such tendencies.

While some scientists argue that the concept of evil deserves attention, others are less convinced. For example, Dr Saul Faerstein, a forensic psychiatrist, explains: "I don't know that we want psychiatrists as gatekeepers, making life-and-death judgments in some cases, based on a concept that is not medical" (Carey 2005). But regardless of whether or not the concept should be used in formal medical discourse, it is being used, at least on the ground. In a study of mental health professionals working in a high-security psychiatric hospital in the U.K., Mason, Richman, and Mercer discovered a complicated relationship between medical ideological discourse and lay notions of evil. Nurses not only use the term evil in their day-to-day interactions and considered patients with a diagnosis of psychopathy as "representing the epitome of evil" (Mason et al. 2002, p. 85), but nursing care plans were impacted by these lay notions of evil (Mercer et al. 2001). Nurses viewed patients with psychotic disorders as sick and developed nursing care plans based on a medical, symptom-centered, approach. Patients with a diagnosis of psychopathy, however, were viewed as evil, and nursing plans were constructed, as one nurse puts it, "for the commissioner. No one takes them seriously. Everyone knows they are meaningless, a front, that's all" (Mason et al. 2002, p. 87).

While religion is an institution of social control, it cannot be considered, at least in the United States, an official or state-sanctioned social control institution. The Constitutional separation of church and state precludes it from being so (Freidson [1970]1988). However, religion is thought to "leave its mark" on official institutions of social control through its influence on public opinion (Freidson [1970]1988, p. 248). Alternately, the medicalization thesis argues that a supernatural understanding of deviant behavior that invokes the concept of evil has been largely excluded from our lay and professional discourse and replaced by the more modern concept of illness. Conrad and Schneider ([1980]1992, p. 251) explain: "Medicalization contributes to the exclusion of concepts of evil in our society." Like the label crime, the label sin, and with it the power of religion to manage society, has been pushed aside in favor of the label illness and the medical management of society.

While the medicalization thesis argues that the concept of evil has become less important in both the lay and professional understanding of deviance, it does not argue that illness designations are morally neutral. For example, Freidson (1970) contends that while the label illness *appears* as morally-neutral, the person is nonetheless held morally responsible to rid himself of the disease. Zola (1972, p. 514) echoes this, writing: "Though his immoral character is not demonstrated in his having a disease, it becomes evident in what he does about it."

While the medicalization thesis suggests that the concept of evil has become less central to the discourse surrounding deviance, the case of psychopathy illustrates a complicated medical-religio-moral framing of the problem. Psychopathy is a medical diagnosis that continues to be linked, even by medical professionals, to the concept of evil. Further, there appear to be some attempts to use medical technologies to explain evil via an appeal to biology. This case highlights the liminal space that lies at the intersection of medical, religious, and moral understandings of deviance. Even at the conceptual level, although the problem has been officially named and framed by medicine, at the edges, psychopathy is comprised of disparate dimensions. It seems likely that a certain class of phenomena is more vulnerable to this type of fragmentation. Problems that are highly socially and morally abhorrent and are not amenable to medical treatment, such as child abuse and pedophilia, are likely to be ordered using medical language yet infused with strong moral overtones. These behaviors pose a troublesome moral conundrum to societies that value humanitarianism and assume that people are rational and voluntary actors. Medicalization scholars would do well to examine more closely this class of deviant behavior. Advances in the brain sciences, especially around psychopathy, have complicated our notions of badness and sickness. While medical sociologists have been interested in the process through which badness gets remade as sickness, the claim that morality is localized in the prefrontal cortex and that murder, torture, and rape could be due to a brain disorder, forces us to move beyond a description of the medicalization process and into a much more complicated arena. While the question of how a set of behaviors once considered bad come to be considered sick is a necessary question, medical conceptualizations that incorporate religio-moral dimensions force us to look across dominant institutions and to examine the socio-political consequences of this institutional ideological interface where social and moral issues are reframed within a medical ideology.

The concept of evil appears to have both a moral and religious dimension. While some associate evil quite explicitly with Satan or evil spirits, others use the term to connote a moral transgression that is particularly socially abhorrent. Future research should examine what type of evil is being invoked with regards to deviance such as psychopathy. When lay and professionals use the term "evil," are they connecting this with the devil, or does this term connote an extreme transgression of the social contract?

The Irony of Psychopathy in Modern Society

An increasingly popular concept of the "successful psychopath" suggests that not all individuals identified as psychopaths are located in forensic settings. Both Cleckley and Hare argue that many individuals who could be classified as psychopaths never become involved with the criminal justice system; some are able to use the primary characteristics of the disorder, namely, superficial charm and lack of remorse or guilt to lead successful non-criminal careers. In fact, Hare writes: "I always said that if I wasn't studying psychopaths in prison, I'd do it at the stock exchange" (Deutschman 2007). Hare and others estimated that between 1% and 5% of the general population meets the clinical criteria for psychopathy (Hare 1999a; Hart et al. 1995; Salekin et al. 2001).

More recently, Hare collaborated with an organizational psychologist, Paul Babiak, to adapt the PCL-R into a screening device for use in the workplace. The Business Scan (B-Scan) is an instrument designed to "identify developmental needs in management and supervisory staff" and can be used to spot employees with psychopathic traits (Babiak and Hare (2006); http://www.b-scan.com). Hare and Babiak discuss the "corporate psychopath" as well as the B-Scan in numerous trade publications including Harvard Business Review, FastCompany, and Fraud Magazine as well as their popular press book *Snakes in Suits: When Psychopaths go to Work*.

So, in this way, psychopathy has leaked into multiple institutional contexts. Not only is psychopathy a medical condition that requires non-medical control and intervention, it is a medical diagnosis that has escaped the bounds of medicine, and the clinical rating scale has been adapted for use by the lay public. The public likely holds multiple and seemingly disparate knowledge about psychopathy simultaneously. Understanding the patterned and multi-dimensional ways the public makes sense of "deviant" behavior will help us to understand the layering of institutional control.

Discussion: The agenda for Sociology

While medicalization theory has provided very fertile ground for research, it has found itself in the crosshairs recently as a conceptual muddle. Davis (2006), for instance, argues that medicalization has "lost its way" by encompassing talk of medicalization without medicine. Dingwall (2006) notes that the sociological language of medicalization has slipped into everyday language and taken on new contexts. Hafferty (2006) wonders if medicalization has become less about medicine and more about science.

Clearly the concept of medicalization has encouraged scholars to apply it to phenomenon that do not stop at the interaction between the physician and the patient or on the policing of the sick role. Clarke and colleagues (2003) call this transformation biomedicalization, and consider it a radical shift in the way our society is organized. Conrad (2005) prefers to think of it as shifting engines, and has noted that physicians are not necessarily the primary drivers of medicalization.

We have attempted to step back from all of the instances of medicalization or partial medicalization and to reassess how it functions as a mechanism of social control in concert with other mechanisms. That is, medicine is but one set of potential *layerings* of institutional control over deviance that can be employed by different sets of actors with different goals. While this solution will likely not please those who wish to relegate medicalization to something that can only properly occur in the institution of medicine (Davis 2006, for instance), we think it can offer some conceptual clarity to those who find themselves dealing with cases of "incomplete" or "partial" medicalization and to those that see the parallels to processes in other fields that look quite similar. We would like for medicalization studies to step out of the "silo" (Dingwall 2006) that they are often a part of and consider how the layering of institutional control over deviance plays a part in the labeling and treatment of problems, whether they medical, scientific, technical, etc.

It is useful to think for a moment about the other "-izations" that are sometimes mentioned alongside medicalization. Criminalization is often used as a conceptual foil to medicalization, but it is far from the only other understanding of the nature of a problem. *Geneticization* (Freese and Shostak 2009) offers another window into the reach and march of science into understanding individual difference and similarity. *Biologization* is a less often used term, but Williams has used it to refer to the move within psychology to account for behaviors, emotions, intentions, etc. in biological terms (Williams et al. 2001). Habermas and Shapiro (1971) used the term *scientization* as part of a critique of the transformation of questions previously encompassed in a moral or political sphere into a techno-scientific sphere. The term has also been used to refer to the increasing levels of surveillance and prescriptiveness of recommendations about issues previously considered less "technical," such as infant nutrition or motherhood (Kimura 2008).

Medicalization is a very well-developed theory of the individualization of a social problem, both in definition and treatment. It provides a nice parallel to criminalization, which individualizes deviance as a personal fault and contains it accordingly. While geneticization, biologization, and scientization as concepts do not rely on the individualization of a problem (though often they do exactly this) they do provide a shift in institutional control. All five of these "-izations" can overlap, and sometimes do. They can all share some conceptually similar processes. As a case study, psychopathy has something for everyone: medicine, crime, genetics, biology, and scientization.

The relationship between medicine, science, law, and morality is becoming increasingly complex as we make our way into the 21st century. As such, the "siloed" approach to studying social problems can only take us so far. Instead we would be well served to draw on the most unique feature of sociology, the ability to look across institutions. Sociology as a discipline is not predominantly tied to any one institution but instead allows for a broad view across institutional arenas. The increasingly overlapping and cross-cutting nature of the organizations and institutions of the 21st century requires a broader perspective. The institutional layering approach is one such perspective.

How societies conceptualize and react to individuals who breach social norms, break the rules, and violate the social contract is a central area of inquiry for sociology. However, studies that start with the premise that a problem has been medicalized and attempt to document this process are limited, as they do not examine multiple mechanisms and processes of social control. The different -izations discussed above suggest a ramping up of a more formalized or institutionalized management of social problems. An approach to social problems that considers only one system of social control necessarily misses this phenomenon. A careful consideration of the layered conceptualizations of and reactions to the problem, the institutions and players involved, as well as the mechanisms, features, processes, and characteristics of each can shed a broader light on the fundamental organizing principles of a society.

Future Questions

Our work in the area of institutional layering is not complete and many questions remain. For example: Is institutional layering more likely when deviance is understood as being particularly abhorrent or threatening? Is there something about the problem itself – in this case, the inability to form a moral conscience and to empathize with others, which many might define as key components of "humanness" – that sets these types of problems apart? What are the causal processes and structures that underlie institutional layering of the increased institutional management of social problems? Can the institutional layering perspective shed light on the processes through which new scientific findings are interpreted, framed, and used by medical professionals, law makers, judges, juries and the lay public and how in turn these findings are remade within the scientific and medical realms? Can the institutional layering perspective shed light on how science is employed in different ways and in different institutional arenas to in the tension between private rights and public safety? The answers to these questions may lie outside traditional subjects of medicalization work, but we are confident that the strong base of medicalization theory – coupled with an increased attention to the other institutions of social control that surround a problem – will help yield the answers.

References

American Law Institute (1962) Model penal code (proposed official draft). The Executive Office, The American Law Institute, Philadelphia, PA
American Psychiatric Association (2000) Diagnostic and statistical manual of mental disorders (4th edn, text revision). American Psychiatric Association, Washington, DC
Andershed H, Kerr M, Stattin H, Levander S (2002) Psychopathic traits in non-referred youths: a new assessment tool. In: Blaauw E, Sheridan L (eds) Psychopaths: current international perspectives. Elsevier, The Hague, pp 131–158
Appleton LT (1995) Rethinking medicalization: alcoholism and anomalies. In: Best J (ed) Images of issues: typifying contemporary social problems. Aldine de Gruyter, Hawthorne, NY, pp 59–80
Archer RP (2006) Forensic uses of clinical assessment instruments. Lawrence Erlbaum, Mahwah, NJ
Archer RP, Buffington-Vollum JK, Stredny RV, Handel RW (2006) A survey of psychological test use patterns among forensic psychologists. J Pers Assess 87:84–94
Armstrong EM (2003) Conceiving risk, bearing responsibility: fetal alcohol syndrome and the diagnosis of moral disorder. Johns Hopkins University Press, Baltimore, MD
Babiak P, Hare RD (2006) Snakes in suits: when psychopaths go to work. Regan Books, New York, NY
Beck AT (1976) Cognitive therapy and the emotional disorders. International Universities Press, New York
Blackburn R (2006) Other theoretical models of psychopathy. In: Patrick CJ (ed) Handbook of psychopathy. Guilford Press, New York, pp 35–57

Blair J, Mitchell D, Blair K (2005) The psychopath: emotions and the brain. Blackwell, Malden, MA

Blair RJR, Colledge E, Murray L, Mitchell DGV (2001) A selective impairment in the processing of sad and fearful expressions in children with psychopathic tendencies. J Abnorm Child Psychol 29:491–498

Brown P (1995) Naming and framing: the social construction of diagnosis and treatment. J Health Soc Behav Extra Issue 34–52

Campbell E (1990) The psychopath and the definition of "mental disease of defect" under the model penal code test of insanity: a question of psychology or a question of law? Neb Law Rev 69:190–229

Campbell MA, Doucette NL, French S (2009) Validity and stability of the youth psychopathic traits inventory in a nonforensic sample of young adults. J Pers Assess 91:584–592

Carey B (2005) For the worst of us, the diagnosis may be 'evil'. New York Times, pp F-1

Carozza D (2008). These men know 'snakes in suits': identifying psychopathic fraudsters: Interview with Dr. Robert D. Hare and Dr. Paul Babiak. Fraud Magazine

Clarke AE, Shim JK (2010) Medicalization and biomedicalization revisited: technoscience and transformations of health, illness, and American medicine. In: Pescosolido BA, McLeod JD, Martin JK, Rogers A (eds) The handbook of the sociology of health, illness, and healing: blueprint for the 21st century. Springer, New York

Clarke AE, Shim JK, Mamo L, Fosket JR, Fishman JR (2003) Biomedicalization: technoscientific transformations of health, illness, and US biomedicine. Am Sociol Rev 68:161–194

Cleckley H ([1941]1964) The mask of sanity: an attempt to clarify some issues about the so-called psychopathic personality. Mosby, St. Louis, MO

Conoley JC, Impara JC (1995) 12th mental measurement yearbook. Buros Institute, Lincoln, NE

Conrad P (1975) The discovery of hyperkinesis: notes on the medicalization of deviant behavior. Soc Probl 23:12–21

Conrad P (1992) Medicalization and social control. Annu Rev Sociol 18:209–232

Conrad P (2005) The shifting engines of medicalization. J Health Soc Behav 46:3–14

Conrad P, Angell A (2004) Homosexuality and remedicalization. Society 41:32–39

Conrad P, Potter D (2000) From hyperactive children to ADHD adults: observations on the expansion of medical categories. Soc Probl 47:559–582

Conrad P, Schneider JW (1980) Looking at levels of medicalization: a comment on strong's critique of the thesis of medical imperialism. Soc Sci Med A 14:75–79

Conrad P, Schneider JW ([1980]1992) Deviance and medicalization: from badness to sickness. Temple University Press, Philadelphia, PA

Davis JE (2006) How medicalization lost its way. Society 43:51–56

de Oliveira-Souza R, Hare RD, Bramati I, Garrido G, Ignacio F, Tovar-Moll F, Moll J (2008) Psychopathy as a disorder of the moral brain: fronto-temporo-limbic grey matter reductions demonstrated by voxel-based morphometry. Neuroimage 40:1202–1213

DeMatteo D, Edens JF (2006) The role and relevance of the psychopathy checklist-revised in court – A case law survey of US Courts (1991–2004). Psychol Public Policy Law 12:214–241

Deutschman A (2005) Is your boss a psychopath? Fast Company Issue 96

Dingwall R (2006) Imperialism or encirclement? Society 43:30–36

Dingwall R (2008) Peter Conrad, the medicalization of society: on the transformation of human conditions into treatable disorders. Society 45:382–384

D'Silva K, Duggan C, McCarthy L (2004) Does treatment really make psychopaths worse? A review of the evidence. J Pers Disord 18:163–177

Edens JF, Colwell LH, Desforges DM, Fernandez K (2005) The impact of mental health evidence on support for capital punishment: are defendants labeled psychopathic considered more deserving of death? Behav Sci Law 23:603–625

Estes CL, Binney EA (1989) The biomedicalization of aging: dangers and dilemmas. Gerontologist 29:587–96

Finkler K, Skrzynia C, Evans JP (2003) The new genetics and its consequences for family, kinship, medicine, and medical genetics. Soc Sci Med 57:403–412

Forth AE, Kosson DS, Hare RD (2003) The psychopathy checklist: youth version. Multi-Health Systems, Toronto, ON

Foucault M (2006) Madness and civilization. Routledge, New York

Fowles DC, Dindo L (2006) A dual-deficit model of psychopathy. In: Patrick CJ (ed) Handbook of psychopathy. Guilford Press, New York, pp 14–34

Freidson E [1970] 1988 The profession of medicine: a study of the sociology of applied knowledge. The University of Chicago Press, Chicago, IL

Freese J, Shostak S (2009) Genetics and social inquiry. Annu Rev Sociol 35:107–128

Frick PJ, Hare RD (2001) The antisocial process screening device. Multi-Health Systems, Toronto, ON

Gacono CB, Nieberding RJ, Owen A, Rubel J, Bodholdt R (2001) Treating conduct disorder, antisocial, and psychopathic personalities. In: Ashford JB, Reid WH, Sales BD (eds) Treating adult and juvenile offenders with special needs. American Psychological Association, Washington, DC, pp 99–129

Giddens A (1986) The constitution of society: outline of a theory of structuration. University of California Press, Berkeley, CA
Habermas J, Shapiro JJ (1971) The scientization of politics and public opinion. In: Scott W, Butler J (eds) Toward a rational society: student protest, science, and politics. Beacon Press, Boston, MA, pp 62–80
Hafferty FW (2006) Medicalization reconsidered. Society 43:41–46
Hare RD (1991) The hare psychopathy checklist – revised. Multi-Health Systems, Toronto, ON
Hare RD (1996) Psychopathy: a clinical construct whose time has come. Crim Justice Behav 23:25–54
Hare RD (1998) Psychopaths and their nature: implications for the mental health and criminal justice systems. In: Millon T, Simonson E, Burket-Smith M, Davis R (eds) Psychopathy: antisocial, criminal, and violence behavior. Guilford Press, New York, pp 188–212
Hare RD (1999a) Psychopathy as a risk factor for violence. Psychiatr Q 70:181–197
Hare RD (1999b) Without conscience: the disturbing world of the psychopaths among us. Guilford Press, New York
Hare RD (2003) The hare psychopathy checklist – Revised, 2nd edn. Multi-Health Systems, Toronto, ON
Hare RD (n.d.) Without conscience: Robert Hare's web site devoted to the study of psychopathy. Retrieved Nov 12, 2009, from: http://www.hare.org/scales/pclsv.html
Hare RD, Neumann CS (2006) The PCL-R assessment of psychopathy: development, structural properties, and new direction. In: Patrick CJ (ed) Handbook of Psychopathy. Guilford Press, New York, pp 58–88
Hare RD, Neumann CS (2008) Psychopathy as a clinical and empirical construct. Annu Rev Clin Psychol 4:217–246
Hare RD, Harpur YJ, Hemphill JF (1989) Scoring pamphlet for the self-report psychopathy scale: SRP-II. Unpublished manuscript. Simon Fraser University, Vancouver, B C
Hare RD, Hart SD, Harpur TJ (1991) Psychopathy and the DSM-IV criteria for antisocial personality disorder. J Abnorm Psychol 100:391–398, Special issue: diagnoses, dimensions, and DSM IV: The science of classification
Harris GT, Rice MF (2006) Treatment of psychopathy: a review of empirical findings. In: Patrick CJ (ed) Handbook of psychopathy. Guilford Press, New York, pp 555–572
Hart SD, Kropp PR, Hare RD (1988) Performance of male psychopaths following conditional release from prison. J Consult Clin Psychol 56:227–232
Hart SD, Cox DN, Hare RD (1995) The Hare psychopathy checklist: screening version, 1st edn. Multi-Health Systems, Toronto, ON
Herve H (2007) Psychopathy across the ages: a history of the hare psychopath. In: Herve H, Yuille JC (eds) The psychopath: theory, research, and practice. Lawrence Erlbaum, Mahwah, NJ, pp 31–56
Hiday VA (1999) Mental illness and the criminal justice system. In: Horwitz AV, Scheid TL (eds) A handbook for the study of mental health. Cambridge University Press, New York, pp 508–525
Hill CD, Neumann CS, Rogers R (2004) Confirmatory factor analysis of the psychopathy checklist: screening version in offenders with axis I disorders. Psychol Assess 16:90–95
Jenness V (2004) Explaining criminalization: from demography and status politics to globalization and modernization. Annu Rev Sociol 30:147–171
Kernberg O (1998) The psychotherapeutic management of psychopathic, narcissistic, and paranoid transferences. In: Millon T, Simonson E, Burket-Smith M, Davis R (eds) Psychopathy: antisocial, criminal, and violent behavior psychopathy: antisocial, criminal, and violence behavior. Guilford Press, New York, pp 372–382
Kernberg O (1992) Aggression and personality disorders and perversions. Yale University Press, New Haven, CT
Kiehl KA, Smith AM, Mendrek A, Forster BB, Hare RD, Liddle PF (2004) Temporal lobe abnormalities in semantic processing by criminal psychopaths as revealed by functional magnetic resonance imaging. Psychiatry Res Neuroimaging 130:27–42
Kimura AH (2008) Who defines babies' "needs"?: the scientization of baby food in Indonesia. Soc Polit Int Stud Gend State Soc 15:232–260
Laakso MP, Vaurio O, Koivisto E, Savolainen L, Eronen M, Aronen HJ (2001) Psychopathy and the posterior hippocampus. Behav Brain Res 118:187–193
LeDoux J (1996) The emotional brain: the mysterious underpinnings of emotional life. Simon and Schuster, New York
Lee JH (1999) The treatment of psychopathic and antisocial personality disorders: A review. Clinical Decision Making Support Unit, Broadmoor Hospital, Berkshire
Lee S, Mysyk A (2004) The medicalization of compulsive buying. Soc Sci Med 58:1709–1718
Levenson MR, Kiehl K, Fitzpatrick CM (1995) Assessing psychopathic attributes in a noninstitutionalized population. J Pers Soc Psychol 68:151–158
Lilienfeld SO, Widows MR (2005) Psychopathic personality inventory-revised. Psychological Assessment Resources, Lutz, FL
Lykken DT (1957) A study of anxiety in the sociopathic personality. J Abnorm Soc Psychol 55:6–10

Lykken DT (2006) Psychopathic personality: the scope of the problem. In: Patrick CJ (ed) Handbook of psychopathy. Guilford Press, New York, pp 3–13

Lynam DR (1997) Pursuing the psychopath: capturing the fledgling psychopath in a nomological net. J Abnorm Psychol 106:425–438

Lynam D, Charnigo R, Moffitt TE, Raine A, Loeber R, Stouthamer-Loeber M (2009) The stability of psychopathy across adolescence. Dev Psychopathol 21:1133–1153

Manguno-Mire GM, Thompson JW Jr, Bertman-Pate LJ, Burnett DR, Thompson HW (2007) Are release recommendations for NGRI acquittees informed by relevant data? Behav Sci Law 25:43–55

Mason T, Richman J, Mercer D (2002) The influence of evil on forensic clinical practice. Int J Ment Health Nurs 11:80–93

Megargee EI (2003) Psychological assessment in correctional settings. In: Weiner IB, Freedheim DK, Graham JR, Naglieri JA (eds) Handbook of psychology: assessment psychology. Wiley, Hoboken, NJ, pp 365–388

Mercer D, Mason T, Richman J (2001) Professional convergence in forensic practice. Aust NZ J Ment Health Nurs 10:105–115

Michalowski RJ (1985) Order, law and crime. Random House, New York

Minzenberg M, Siever LJ (2006) Neurochemistry and pharmacology of psychopathy. In: Patrick CJ (ed) Handbook of psychopathy. Guilford Press, New York, pp 251–278

Moll J, de Oliveira-Souza R, Eslinger PJ, Bramati IE, Mourao-Miranda J, Andreiuolo PA, Pessoa L (2002) The neural correlates of moral sensitivity: a functional magnetic resonance imaging investigation of basic and moral emotions. J Neurosci 22:2730–2736

Morse S (2008) Psychopathy and criminal responsibility. Neuroethics 1:205–212

Mueser KT, Drake RE, Ackerson TH, Alterman AI, Miles KM, Noordsy DL (2007) Antisocial personality disorder, conduct disorder, and substance abuse in schizophrenia. J Abnorm Psychol 106:473–477

Nestor PG, Kimble M, Berman I, Haycock J (2002) Psychosis, psychopathy, and homicide: a preliminary neuropsychological inquiry. Am J Psychiatry 159:138–140

Neumann CS, Hare RD, Newman JP (2007) The super-ordinate nature of the psychopathy checklist-revised. J Pers Disord 21:102–107

Newman JP (1998) Psychopathic behavior: an information processing perspective. In: Cooke DJ, Forth AE, Hare RD (eds) Psychopathy: theory, research and implications for society. Kluwer, Dordrecht, pp 81–104

Nolan KA, Volavka J, Mohr P, Czobor P (1999) Psychopathy and violent behavior among patients with schizophrenia or schizoaffective disorder. Psychiatr Serv 50:787–792

Parsons T (1951) The social system. The Free Press of Glencoe, Glencoe

Psychosis n (2007) The Oxford English dictionary. 2007. Oxford: Oxford University Press. June 11, 2009 <http://dictionary.oed.com/cgi/entry/50191674>

Raine A, Ishikawa SS, Arce E, Lencz T, Knuth KH, Bihrle S, LaCasse L, Colletti P (2004) Hippocampal structural asymmetry in unsuccessful psychopaths. Biol Psychiatry 55:185–191

Rice ME, Harris GT (1992) A comparison of criminal recidivism among schizophrenic and nonschizophrenic offenders. Int J Law Psychiatry 15:397–408

Rice ME, Harris GT, Quinsey VT (1990) A followup of rapists assessed in a maximum security psychiatric facility. J Interpers Violence 5:435–448

Rice ME, Harris GT, Cormier CA (1992) Evaluation of a maximum security therapeutic community for psychopaths and other mentally disordered offenders. Law Human Behav 16:399–412

Rossol J (2001) The medicalization of deviance as an interactive achievement: the construction of compulsive gambling. Symbolic Interact 24(3):315–341

Salekin RT, Rogers R, Sewell KW (1996) A review and meta-analysis of the psychopathy checklist and psychopathy checklist-revised: predictive validity of dangerousness. Clin Psychol Sci Pract 3:203–215

Salekin RT, Trobst KK, Krioukova M (2001) Construct validity of psychopathy in a community sample: a nomological net approach. J Pers Disord 15:425–441

Schneider JW (1978) Deviant drinking as disease: alcoholism as a social accomplishment. Soc Probl 25:361–372

Schram SF (2000) In the clinic: the medicalization of welfare. Social Text 18(1):82–107

Serin RC, Peters RD, Barbaree HE (1990) Predictors of psychopathy and release outcome in a criminal population. Psychol Assess J Consult Clin Psychol 2:419–422

Seagrave D, Grisso T (2002) Adolescent development and the measurement of juvenile psychopathy. Law Human Behav 26:219–239

Seto MC, Barbaree HE (1999) Psychopathy, treatment behavior, and sex offender recidivism. J Interpers Violence 14:1235–1248

Skeem JL, Monahan J, Mulvey EP (2002) Psychopathy, treatment involvement, and subsequent violence among civil psychiatric patients. Law Human Behav 26:577–603

Stone MH (2009) The anatomy of evil. Prometheus Books, Amherst, NY

Stone MH (2010) Evil in historical perspective: at the intersection of religion and psychiatry. In: Verhagen PJ, van Praag HM, Lopez-Ibor JJ Jr, Cox JL, Moussaoui D (eds) Religion and psychiatry: beyond boundaries. Wiley-Blackwell, Hoboken, NJ, pp 13–38

Sutherland EH (1950) The diffusion of sexual psychopath laws. Am J Sociol 56:142–148

Tengström A, Grann M, Långström N, Kullgren G (2000) Psychopathy (PCL-R) as a predictor of violent recidivism among criminal offenders with schizophrenia. Law Human Behav 24:45–58

Verplaetse J (2009) Localizing the moral sense: neuroscience and the search for the cerebral seat of morality, 1800–1930. Springer, New York

Welner M (2009) The justice and therapeutic promise of science-based research on criminal evil. J Am Acad Psychiatry Law 37:442–449

Widiger TA (2006) Psychopathy and DSM-IV psychopathology. In: Patrick CJ (ed) Handbook of psychopathy. Guilford Press, New York, pp 156–171

Williams RN, Slife BD, Barlow SH (2001) The biologization of psychotherapy: understanding the nature of influence. In: Slife BD, Williams RN, Barlow SH Critical issues in psychotherapy: Translating new ideas into practice. Sage, Thousand Oaks, CA, pp 51–68

Wong S, Hare RD (2005) Guidelines for a psychopathy treatment program. Multi-Health Systems, Toronto, ON

Zola IK (1972) Medicine as an institution of social control. Sociol Rev 20:487–504

Chapter 9
Community Systems Collide and Cooperate: Control of Deviance by the Legal and Mental Health Systems

Virginia Aldigé Hiday

Introduction

For most of history, society controlled mentally disordered behavior informally; but with modernization it developed formal organizational controls for the behavior it recognized as mentally disordered. This chapter examines relatively recent formal attempts by two systems, the legal and mental health systems, to define and execute control over persons with mental illness whose behavior violates societal norms. It begins with a brief history of the posture of the legal and mental health systems toward mentally disordered persons prior to the mid-twentieth century. It then describes the collision which occurred following civil rights reforms which made the legal system the arbiter of the mental health system's decisions in treatment and hospitalization, especially involuntary treatment and hospitalization. It describes societal forces beyond the two systems which brought about conditions leading to their cooperation. It then examines the new cooperation that is beginning to occur, giving some detail to one promising program of cooperation. Finally, it discusses directions for future inquiry by researchers who study the two systems' efforts in controlling deviance of persons with mental illness.

Background: The Social History of Two Systems

Both the legal system and the mental health system control deviant behavior; but they developed separately with different social control mechanisms. The former assumes willfulness and dispenses punishment, and the latter assumes sickness and delivers treatment; but both attempt to control persons whose deviance becomes public, often by removing them from the community. The much older legal system, with its roots in early civilizations, was the formal organization which controlled most public deviance, often in conjunction with the religious system. Even as society adopted the moral stance that a person's madness should preclude punishment for his crime, the legal system held responsibility for control of publicly disturbing deviance of mentally ill persons. Less disturbing deviance was controlled informally, mostly by the family (Grob 1994; Rochefort 1997; Rothman 1980).

There was no mental health system until the first half of the nineteenth century when society created asylums for the humane care of persons with mental illness. As states built and expanded state mental hospitals during that century, the legal system stopped incarcerating persons with mental

V.A. Hiday (✉)
Department of Sociology, North Carolina State University, Rm. 355, 1911 Building, Raleigh, NC 27695-8107, USA
e-mail: ginny-aldige@ncsu.edu

illness in jails and almshouses, and basically turned over mentally ill persons to these new institutions for care and control. In the face of etiologies that viewed the city as a breeding ground of mental disease and that promised cure in rural asylums, society came to believe that mental hospitals were the best place for all mentally ill persons requiring care; thus, it left admission, although involuntary and sanctioned by law, in the hands of family and physicians. With the exception of a few periods of reform following revelations of abuse, the legal system acted paternalistically for over a century, allowing the mental health system to coerce hospitalization on anyone hospital administrators or psychiatrists judged to be mentally ill and in need of treatment (Grob 1994).

With such practice and with escalating public deviance as industrialization, urbanization, and the large third wave of immigration transformed society, state mental hospitals became recipients of great numbers of deviants deemed mentally ill by the latter part of the nineteenth century. Their patient rolls grew to such an extent that treatment became rare while custody seemed to be their only function (Grob 1994). As the progressive belief in rehabilitation in penology evolved in the early twentieth century, the legal system added to state mental hospital patient rolls by turning over mentally ill offenders to psychiatrists to be rehabilitated. These once humane institutions, which began with a hope of cure, became overcrowded; often filthy and foul warehouses for persons with mental disorders and, not uncommonly, for various other deviants who had no mental disorder (Grob 1994; Kittrie 1971).

Mid-twentieth century saw new developments which created pressures that dramatically changed the operation of state mental hospitals and the practices of psychiatrists. Journalistic exposés of shameful state hospital conditions; sociological studies of the bias of labeling and the harm of institutionalization and stigma; newly developed psychoactive drugs; and the community mental health philosophy with its promise of freedom, treatment, and inclusion combined to set the stage for an increasingly successful civil rights movement to spread from other disadvantaged groups to mental patients (Appelbaum 1994; Goffman 1961; Hiday 1983; La Fond and Durham 1992). Led by a nascent mental health bar, it focused on abuses which had occurred under the paternalistic neglect of the prior era and on the essential punitive nature of all involuntary hospitalization and the harm it entails, aiming to check those abuses and minimize coerced mental hospitalization (Hiday 1983; Wexler 2008).

Before describing the ensuing collision between the two systems, it should be noted that both systems have more functions than that of control agents for the deviance of persons with mental illness. In addition, the mental health system may function to provide or assist in obtaining meals, housing, skills training, activities, employment, education, and disability income from other agencies as well as its more basic functions of diagnosing and treating disorders with medication and psychotherapy. Besides confining mentally ill persons, who are dangerous and/or violate laws, the legal system functions to protect persons with mental illness. At least as far back as the feudal ages, the legal system was concerned with protecting estates of wealthy insane persons from unscrupulous family members who would take advantage of their mental vulnerabilities (Dershowitz 1974). From that function grew its responsibility to assure care and custody not only of insane persons with property but also of insane family members of poor parishioners (Dershowitz 1974). The legal system still functions in a social welfare role in adjudicating competence, assigning guardianship, and assuming ultimate responsibility for severely disabled persons as wards of the state. With the American with Disabilities Act (ADA) of 1990 and the Fair Housing Act Amendment of 1988, the legal system has functioned to bar discrimination in employment, public access, transportation, telecommunications, and housing because of a mental disability (Bonnie and Monahan 1996; Petrila and Ayers 1994; Scheid 2005).

Collision: The Two Systems Collide Over Rights

Beginning in the 1960s, court rulings and legislation changed the relationship between the legal system and the mental health system (La Fond and Durham 1992). The legal system began to affirm individual rights of persons with mental illness and continued expanding the scope of these rights throughout the mental health system into the early 1980s. In so doing, it limited how and why psychiatrists dealt with patients, and limited who and under what conditions psychiatrists could treat individuals against their wills. The legal system constrained psychiatrists' decisions with substantive boundaries and procedural rules to protect individuals from abuses which had occurred from paternalistic neglect of the prior era. To be civilly committed to a mental hospital, an individual now had to be legally dangerous as well as mentally ill; and the decision to hospitalize was reviewed, if not ultimately made, by a legal authority. Alleged mentally ill individuals now had basic due process rights long held by criminal defendants, such as counsel, notice, hearings, confrontation of witnesses, and regular review. In the criminal law, mentally ill offenders also gained due process rights such as greater use of habeas corpus release petitions, hearings on transfers between prison and mental hospitals, and review at expiration of their sentences. Both civil and criminal mental patients gained rights to treatment, to refuse treatment, and to be treated in the least restrictive alternative (Hiday 1983; La Fond and Durham 1992; Wexler 1981).

Initially, many psychiatrists were in favor of these new procedural measures in hospital commitment, and new limits to involuntary treatment and to the role of state mental hospitals. Indeed, the earlier Community Mental Health Movement aimed to reduce or even close state mental hospitals; and some mental health practitioners had called for patient treatment rights (Appelbaum 1994; Grob 2008). Some practitioners viewed the new commitment procedures as therapeutic; and a few collaborated in legal suits brought to obtain patient rights (Appelbaum 1994). But the scope and intensity of these newly mandated civil rights were so great that most psychiatrists came to perceive them as a "legal onslaught against the psychiatric profession and the mental health system" (Halleck 1979) and met them with "great resistance" (Dietz 1977; McGarry 1976; Sadoff 1979). Indeed, one legal scholar described these new mental health laws affirming patient rights as "part of the antipsychiatry movement" (Wexler 2008).

A vocal group of psychiatrists wrote of negative experiences under the new laws. They claimed that the laws prevented them from caring for mentally ill persons in need of treatment which would lead to patients "dying with their rights on," (Treffert 1973) or "rotting with their rights on" (Appelbaum and Gutheil 1980). Some psychiatrists feared that the new dangerousness standard would produce such an accumulation of violent patients in mental hospitals, many of whom would be untreatable, that it would be impossible for hospitals to be therapeutic (Stone 1975). Other psychiatrists argued that the new laws which made it more difficult for psychiatrists to hospitalize mentally ill persons would lead to the arrest and criminal incarceration of mentally ill patients who could no longer be hospitalized (Abramson 1972; Rachlin et al. 1975).

Despite attorneys' leading the mental patients' civil rights reform movement and psychiatrists' feeling attacked by the legal system (Kahle et al. 1978), most practicing lawyers and judges in courts dealing with mentally disordered persons were not antagonistic towards psychiatrists and mental hospitals. To the contrary, they tended to view mental hospitals, including large state mental hospitals, as legitimate medical institutions to aid and benefit persons with mental illness; but they recognized weaknesses in them and saw them only as a last resort after other ways of helping had failed (Hiday 1982). They also respected psychiatrists as professionals with expertise in mental illness. Such favorable opinions were operative in civil commitment proceedings where most attorneys followed a "best interests" model, that is, they were non-adversarial and did what they thought best for their clients as recommended by psychiatrists, even if it were involuntary hospitalization. Only a small minority of attorneys assumed an adversarial role, challenging psychiatric recommendations for hospitalization when their clients did not want it (Hiday 1982; Warren 1984). Nonetheless, courts upheld the new dangerousness criterion, and in so doing reduced the number of potential involuntary hospitalizations (Hiday and Markell 1981; Hiday and Smith 1987).

Psychiatrists' extreme fears of the deleterious effects of the new civil rights laws, however, were not realized. Criminalization did not occur; persons with mental illness who were dangerous only to self or gravely disabled could still be hospitalized when they did not voluntarily seek treatment; hospitals did not fill up with untreatable violent persons; most patients did not refuse medication or persist in refusal after consultation on type and dose; medication could be forced in emergencies; and patients whose physical and mental problems required long-term nursing and psychiatric care were able to obtain them in state mental hospitals (Engel and Silver 2001; Fisher et al. 2001; Hiday 1988, 1991, 1992a, b 1999; Hoge et al. 1988; La Fond and Durham 1992; Monahan et al. 1979; Teplin 1984; Teplin and Pruett 1992). The legal system did restrict psychiatric discretion; but eventually psychiatrists learned to cope with legal regulation of their medical practices in the new environment (Halleck 1979).

Beyond the Two Systems: Economic Forces Create New Problems

By the late 1980s, changes mandated by the legal system slowed and even retreated; there was a move to return to less stringent commitment criteria with the legal system supporting psychiatrists in hospitalization decisions (Appelbaum 1994; La Fond and Durham 1992). On the other hand, economic forces continued to diminish the role of large mental hospitals in the care of persons with mental illness, first with Medicaid as states moved patients out of state mental hospitals to shift costs to the federal government and later with managed care as it severely restricted admissions and stays (Grob 2008; Manderscheid et al. 1999; Mechanic 1999). Even when courts approved psychiatric recommendations in ordering civil commitment, psychiatrists under financial constraints often released patients well before their legal orders expired. Commonly after discharge, patients received little or no treatment in the community which led to a revolving door whereby patients cycled in and out of the hospital (Hiday and Scheid-Cook 1987). With this changed environment, attention of both legal and mental health reformers shifted to assuring that mental patients in the community obtained treatment (Petrila 2001).

Because numerous discharged patients were unwilling or unable to comply voluntarily with treatment, some psychiatrists called for outpatient commitment, that is, they called for legislation authorizing community treatment orders for patients unwilling or unable to comply voluntarily with treatment. In most states, civil rights lawyers had already obtained legislation permitting outpatient commitment as a less restrictive alternative to involuntary hospitalization (Hiday and Goodman 1981; Keilitz and Hall 1985; McCafferty and Dooley 1990). Now, some legal and mental health reformers called for extending outpatient commitment to allow intervention before a person deteriorated to the point that involuntary hospitalization became necessary, an intervention which required broadening the legal criteria to allow preventive action (Hiday 2003). Other attorneys and psychiatrists successfully fought these efforts as unnecessarily and unconstitutionally abridging individual freedom (see Wales and Hiday 2006 for explication of these arguments). Despite the controversy surrounding these community treatment orders, especially preventive action, psychiatrists have used outpatient commitment only infrequently because of ignorance of the law, liability concerns, funding conflicts, and inertia (Appelbaum 1986; Hiday and Scheid-Cook 1991; Petrila and Christy 2008; Wales and Hiday 2006).

The large number of discharged mental patients without treatment in the community was then and is now not mainly a matter of needing to force treatment on persons who do not want it (Wales and Hiday 2006). More important then and now is inadequate funding to provide both mental health treatment and other needed services for severely disordered persons who want such help. Lack of funds to provide these essential resources has led to a growing population of untreated or only intermittently treated persons with severe mental illness, many of whom often self-medicate with alcohol and illegal drugs. By the mid-1980s, society became aware that sizeable numbers of them were ending up on the streets, adding to the emerging larger societal problem of homelessness (Jencks 1994; Lamb 1984).

Inadequate treatment of persons with severe mental illness was made worse by managed care which came to dominate mental health care coverage in both private insurance and public programs in the 1990s (Scheid and Greenberg 2007). The shifting of control of mental health care from providers to payers and their representatives in our multi-tiered system promoted "dumping" from the private to the public sectors and "dumping" from the public programs to the streets (Manderscheid et al. 1999; Mechanic 2007).

Although the legal system's regulation of the mental health system did not directly lead to criminalization, spreading drug culture and growing homelessness introduced conditions which inevitably brought and continue to bring mentally disordered persons into the criminal justice system. Most studies have found the offenses of persons with mental illness to be primarily minor ones involving nuisance behavior (disturbing the peace as they argue with their voices in the mall), survival acts ("dine and dash," breaking into empty buildings as they seek shelter), drug use and procurement (stealing to support an addiction), and assaults (fighting with other intoxicated persons and resisting law officers); but they lead to arrest (Desai et al. 2000; Engel and Silver 2001; Fisher et al. 2007; Hartwell 2004a; Hiday 1991; Hiday and Wales 2003; Junginger et al. 2006; Swaminath et al. 2002; Swartz and Lurigio 2007). Two recent 10-year retrospective studies of severely mentally ill and disadvantaged public mental health clients reported arrest patterns with more serious offending patterns, most being charged with felonies in one (Fisher et al. 2007) and over one-third being charged with violent offenses in the other (Cuellor et al. 2007). Few of these offenses, however, are driven by psychosis; rather they are caused by the same factors that cause offending among the general population (Bonta et al. 1998; Fisher et al. 2005; Hiday 1999; Hiday and Wales 2003; Junginger et al. 2006). Furthermore, cases of unreasoned violence, sensationalized by the media and feared by the public, are rare.

Police try to settle disputes and disturbances involving mentally disordered persons without arrest just as they try to settle disputes and disturbances involving others (Engel and Silver 2001; Teplin and Pruett 1992; Watson and Angell 2007). Nonetheless, numerous persons with mental illness have come to be arrested and detained in jails, in part because mental health practitioners have been disinclined, if not loathe, to treat criminal offenders and substance abusers (Borum et al. 1998; Lamb et al. 1999; Lamb and Weinberger 2005; Teplin 1984; Watson and Angell 2007).

For some time, disproportionate numbers of persons with mental illness have been criminally incarcerated. Estimates of mentally disordered jail and prison populations range from 6 to 22% of all inmates with variation depending on demographic group, methodology, and definition (Ditton 1999; Teplin 1990a; Teplin et al. 1996).[1] Indeed, it has reached the point that more persons with severe mental illness are detained in jails than are admitted to mental hospitals (Morrissey et al. 2007).

While in jail, there is little likelihood that treatment will be provided and high likelihood that mental deterioration will occur; on exit, linkage to community services is unlikely (Hartwell 2004b; Lamb and Weinberger 2005; Teplin 1990b). Such neglect of these offenders has produced a second revolving door syndrome of arrest, jail, and release back into the community where the same conditions which led to the earlier offenses lead to re-offending and re-arrest. Repeat mentally ill offenders became noticeable in overcrowded jails and on overburdened court dockets (Lamb and Weinberger 2005; Moore and Hiday 2006).

---

[1] A 2006 report, using an unreasonably expansive definition, raised the estimate to over half of those incarcerated in jails and prisons (James and Glaze 2006).

Cooperation: Recognizing the Need

In some jurisdictions, the legal system realized that traditional criminal justice processing and punishment were inadequate to slow this revolving door. It reached out to the mental health system seeking ways to divert mentally ill defendants from the criminal justice system into mental health treatment on the assumption that untreated mental illness was the root cause of their offending. The two systems in these jurisdictions cooperated to establish various types of diversion programs. Reports of their success in popular media and professional journals caused other jurisdictions facing the same seemingly intractable problems to follow their lead. The federal government through on-going funding from both its law and health agencies (the Institute of Justice, Bureau of Justice Assistance, National Institutes of Health, and Substance Abuse and Mental Health Administration), and special allocations from Congress has encouraged their proliferation by giving financial and organizational support to local efforts. Some national organizations, such as the Council of State Governments, the Gains Center, and TAPA Center with federal government support, have joined these efforts to promote effective diversion programs (see Consensus Project 2008).

There had been diversion out of the legal system into the mental health system earlier, even before large-scale deinstitutionalization; but it was not formally organized. Then, as now, defense counsel, through plea-bargains, would gain from courts' dismissal of charges against their mentally ill clients on the condition that their clients would be hospitalized or enter outpatient mental health treatment (Hiday 1999). Police officers, even before arrest, diverted mentally ill persons from the legal system as they carried out their long-assumed role of street-corner psychiatrists by cooling altercations, giving helpful suggestions, making referrals to agencies, and taking mentally disordered persons to emergency rooms for psychiatric intervention (Teplin 1984; Teplin and Pruett 1992). But such earlier diversion required little or no cooperation between the two systems. Essentially, the legal system had disowned responsibility for mentally disordered persons in turning them over as the mental health system's problem to fix.[2] In contrast, the two systems in jurisdictions dispersed across the country are now both accepting responsibility and cooperating in development and operation of the new diversion programs.

Diversion Programs: Attempts to Solve Criminalization

Local jurisdictions are attempting assorted approaches to divert persons with mental illness at different points along the path from police encounter to arrest, detention, prosecution, and incarceration. Prebooking interventions aimed at avoiding arrest have included training police in handling mentally disordered subjects, providing in-house mental health consultation to police in the field, and establishing specialized police units for mental health crises (Draine et al. 2005). The most successful ones of these include a no-refusal mental health center where police can take mentally ill offenders at any time of any day (Borum et al. 1998; Steadman et al. 1995). Post-booking interventions aimed at getting treatment and possibly an alternative to incarceration at the earliest point have included screening and needs assessment programs for jail detainees, in-jail treatment and case

---

[2] The legal system had established forensic mental health units to deal with competency evaluations, competency treatment, not-guilty-by-reason-of-insanity (NGRI) treatment, and treatment for prisoners whose mental illness was recognized after incarceration (Steadman and Monahan 1982); but these units did not constitute diversion programs. Additionally, courts sometimes ordered treatment as a condition of probation and parole; but formal programs in the community were few (see Bloom et al. 1986 for an exception) and, as stated earlier, mental health practitioners avoided treating mentally ill offenders.

management, treatment as a condition of probation, pretrial court services, mental health courts, and re-entry treatment and services with linkage to community agencies. The most successful ones of these have early identification, integrated substance-abuse and mental health treatment, and cooperative mechanisms of regular key agency meetings and designated boundary spanners in both systems (Borum et al. 1998; Steadman et al. 1995).

Studies of early diversion programs show that they can reduce days in jail, increase time in the community, and increase services without increasing arrests, psychotic behavior, or substance abuse (Broner et al. 2004; Moore and Hiday 2006). Unfortunately, the reported increase in many programs' services for those diverted compared to non-diverted controls, while significant, has been quite small (Broner et al. 2004; Boothroyd et al. 2003). In such cases, even though arrests showed no increase, there was no hoped-for reduction in the number of offences and arrests (Broner et al. 2004; Christy et al. 2005; Cosden et al. 2003, 2005). Commonly, diversion in these programs was only *out of* the legal system but *not into* the mental health system, despite cooperation agreements (Broner et al. 2004), or was to mental health services-as-usual rather than to specialized services which address the criminal behavior of defendants (Fisher et al. 2005; Morrissey et al. 2007). To the extent that prebooking programs avoid arrest and post-booking programs remove mentally disordered offenders from jail at an early point, jail days will be reduced and community time will increase; but that does not mean that the root problem is being addressed as these programs intend. Many mentally ill persons diverted out of the legal system but left without needed treatment and services return to their earlier ways, to former associates and to previous neighborhoods which predictably lead to their re-offending and being re-arrested.

One of the diversion models garnering much attention is the mental health court. Perceiving it to hold great promise not only for reducing offending, but also for reducing jail and prison crowding, court workload and criminal justice costs, jurisdictions across the country have created more than 200 such courts in the past decade; and federal and state governments have created formal programs to promote their adoption and best practices, and to understand what works (see Consensus Project 2008).

Mental health courts attempt to address offenders' mental illness and its disadvantages with mental health treatment and support services coupled with court monitoring to give structure, supervision, support, and encouragement for a sustained period. These courts are different from traditional criminal courts in that defendants voluntarily participate and agree to comply with both treatment and behavioral mandates which include appearing at regularly scheduled court sessions. Mental health courts also differ in that each court has: (1) a separate docket, (2) one or two dedicated judges who preside at all hearings, (3) dedicated prosecution and defense attorneys; and (4) a nonadversarial team approach involving consensus decisions by law and mental health professionals. The team, including judge, prosecutor, defense counsel, probation officers, mental health liaison, and care providers such as mental health clinicians and case managers, social workers, and substance abuse counselors, reviews each defendant prior to court sessions in terms of progress in behavioral change, cooperation with treatment, and need for modification of treatment and services. It then decides what message the judge should deliver to the defendant in open court (encouragement, praise, reprimand, or warning) and what rewards or sanctions to apply. Team members, anticipating defendants' likely slippage and reversals, offer assistance in compliance and multiple second chances both through the judge in open court and individually when working with them. After successful completion of an individualized mandated treatment plan, the court dismisses a defendant's criminal charges or jail/prison term depending on whether court entry was pre- or post-adjudication of the charges.

Mental health courts vary in limiting eligibility. Some allow only misdemeanants, fearing public outcry over more serious offenders being handled too softly; while some allow only felons, believing that more time [longer sentences] and a stronger sanction [return to prison] are necessary to effect treatment compliance and behavioral change. Others limit cases to nonviolent offenders, fearing serious harm from violent defendants. They all, however, have reported positive results.

Empirical studies show that mentally ill defendants obtain more treatment while participating in mental health courts than they did before entry and more treatment than mentally ill defendants in matched traditional criminal courts (Boothroyd et al. 2003; Cosden et al. 2003, 2005; Herinckx et al. 2005; McNiel and Binder 2007; Ridgely et al. 2007). Additionally, regardless of offense, mental health court defendants are less likely to offend than they did before entering mental health court, and no more likely to re-offend than comparable defendants in traditional criminal court, even though they spend more time in the community (Hendrixx et al. 2005; Moore and Hiday 2006; McNiel and Binder 2007; Ridgely et al. 2007). Early results on whether they are *less likely* to offend than comparable traditional criminal court defendants were mixed; but the most recent studies show that mental health courts reduce recidivism beneath the level of traditional criminal courts (McNiel and Binder 2007; Moore and Hiday 2006; Ridgely et al. 2007).

Directions for Future Inquiry

Although the legal and mental health systems of some jurisdictions now cooperate in controlling the public deviance of persons with mental illness, questions arise as to whether this cooperation will continue beyond the tenure of current innovative leaders. Will cooperation become embedded with roles and rules in the bureaucracies of both systems so as to survive the innovators' departures? Will it continue to spread to other jurisdictions so that it becomes the modus operandi of the two systems throughout the country in controlling publicly deviant persons with mental illness? The answer to these questions depends in part on how successful the federal government and the Council of State Governments are in their efforts to synthesize and spread the best practices of current mental health courts such that the charisma of innovators becomes routinized. It also depends on whether evidence continues to accumulate demonstrating reduced offending and subsequent benefits to the legal system for longer periods than the average 1-year follow-up of most extant studies.

Therapeutic jurisprudence, a new theory of how courts should operate (Wexler and Winick 1996), may advance continued cooperation. In promoting therapeutic goals which aim to make the law have a positive impact on psychological well-being while at the same time upholding traditional due process, and in providing an articulated framework, logic, and vocabulary to attorneys, judges, and law professors, therapeutic jurisprudence is likely to assist multiplication of cooperative policies and structures such as mental health courts. Its influence on the course of the two systems' cooperation should be studied.

Another set of questions calling for study addresses the reasons some diversion programs work and others do not. What are the components of each diversion type necessary to have it work? Are there essential components to the operation of all successful diversion programs regardless of diversion type? Are there similar structures and rules for the two systems' interactions in successful programs? What are the roles of legal and mental health professionals in these programs? What are the stressors and strains in these roles that might undermine the goals of diversion?

Because coerced treatment is involved when the legal system joins with the mental health system to control persons with mental illness, both practical and normative questions arise about its use in criminal as well as in civil law. Empirical research has shown that coercion in mental health and substance abuse treatment can work in producing positive clinical and behavioral outcomes (Hiday 2003; Gottfredson et al. 2007; Marlowe et al. 2005). But is it necessary in all diversion programs and with all types of defendants? If so, what is the minimal coercion which works? How much and what kind of integration in the coercive measures is required of the legal system once an initial diversion to the mental health system is made?

Attention needs to be paid to how changes in one system affect the other. We have earlier pointed to the contributing role played by the mental health system to increased arrests by its limitation of hospital admissions and stays. What happens to voluntary, non-offending clients of the mental health system when the legal system orders involuntary treatment for mentally ill persons who would otherwise not be treated? If cooperative diversion programs and outpatient commitment programs are fully funded with new allocations, there should be no detrimental effect on other clients. More commonly, there is inadequate or no additional money for such programs. The possible consequence that legally mandated treatment without adequate additional resources would push voluntary clients out of treatment or reduce the services available to them calls for investigation.

Finally, researchers need to investigate how the two systems attend not only to needed treatment of mentally ill offenders but also to those components of the lives of persons with mental illness which are causal in their offending: unemployment, broken families, poverty, victimization, substance abuse, homelessness, and disorganized, crime-ridden neighborhoods. These are problems of the larger society which the legal and mental health systems cannot solve; but if they are to be successful in their joint effort of reducing recidivism, they will insure that mentally ill persons who come into their programs receive needed social services such as disability income, employment, and housing assistance as well as clinical treatment.

References

Abramson MF (1972) The criminalization of mentally disordered behavior: possible side-effects of a new mental health law. Hosp Community Psychiatry 23:101–105
Appelbaum PS (1986) Outpatient commitment: the problems and the promise. Am J Psychiatry 143:1270–1272
Appelbaum PS (1994) Almost a revolution: mental health law and the limits of change. Oxford University Press, New York
Appelbaum PS, Gutheil TG (1980) The Boston state hospital case: 'involuntary mind control', the constitution and the 'right to rot'. Am J Psychiatry 137:720–723
Bloom JD, Rogers JL, Manson SM, Williams MH (1986) Lifetime police contacts of discharged psychiatric security review board clients. Int J Law Psychiatry 8:189–202
Bonnie RJ, Monahan J (1996) Mental disorder, work disability, and the law. University of Chicago Press, Chicago, IL
Bonta J, Law M, Hanson K (1998) The prediction of criminal and violent recidivism among mentally disordered offenders: a meta-analysis. Psychol Bull 123:123–142
Boothroyd RA, Poythress NG, McGaha A, Petrila J (2003) The Broward mental health court: process, outcomes, and service utilization. Int J Law Psychiatry 26:55–71
Borum R, Deane MW, Steadman HJ, Morrissey J (1998) Police perspectives on responding to mentally ill people in crisis: perceptions of program effectiveness. Behav Sci Law 16:393–405
Broner N, Lattimore PK, Cowell AJ, Schlenger WE (2004) Effects of diversion on adults with co-occurring mental illness and substance use: outcomes from a national multi-site study. Behav Sci Law 22:519–541
Christy A, Poythress NG, Boothroyd RA, Petrila J, Mehra S (2005) Evaluating the efficiency and community safety goals of the Broward County mental health court. Behav Sci Law 23:227–243
Consensus Project (2008) https://consensusproject.org
Cosden M, Ellens J, Schnell J, Yamini-Diouf Y, Wolfe M (2003) Evaluation of a mental health treatment court with assertive community treatment. Behav Sci Law 21:415–427
Cosden M, Ellens J, Schnell J, Yamini-Diouf Y (2005) Efficacy of a mental health treatment court with assertive community treatment. Behav Sci Law 23:199–214
Cuellor AE, Snowden LM, Ewing T (2007) Criminal records of persons served in the public mental health system. Psychiatr Serv 58:114–120
Dershowitz A (1974) The origins of preventive confinement in Anglo-American law – Part I: the English experience. Univ Cincinnati Law Rev 43:1–60
Desai RA, Lam J, Rosenheck RA (2000) Childhood risk factors for criminal justice involvement in a sample of homeless people with serious mental illness. J Nerv Ment Dis 188:324–332
Dietz PE (1977) Social discrediting of psychiatry: the protasis of legal disenfranchisement. Am J Psychiatry 134:1356–1370
Ditton PM (1999) Mental health and treatment of inmates and probationers. Bureau of Justice Statistics, Washington, DC, NCJ 174463

Draine J, Blank A, Kottsieper P, Solomon P (2005) Contrasting jail diversion and in-jail services for mental illness and substance abuse: do they serve the same clients? Behav Sci Law 23:171–181

Engel RS, Silver E (2001) Policing of disordered suspects: a reexamination of the criminalizatrion hypothesis. Criminology 39:225–252

Fisher W, Barreira PJ, Geller JL, White AW, Lincoln AK, Sudders M (2001) Long State patients in state psychiatric hospitals at the end of the 20th century. Psychiatr Serv 52:1051–1056

Fisher W, Silver E, Wolff N (2005) Beyond criminalization: toward a criminologically informed mental health policy and services research. Adm Policy Ment Health 33:544–547

Fisher W, Roy-Bujnowski K, Grudzinskas AJ, Clayfield JC, Banks SM, Wolff N (2007) Arrest in a mental health service use cohort. Psychiatr Serv 57:1623–1628

Goffman E (1961) Asylums. Anchor Books, New York

Gottfredson DC, Kearley BW, Najaka SS, Rocha CM (2007) How drug treatment courts work: an analysis of mediators. J Res Crime Delinq 44:3–35

Grob GN (1994) The mad among us: a history of the care of America's mentally ill. Harvard University Press, Cambridge, MA

Grob GN (2008) Mental health policy in the liberal state: the example of the United States. Int J Law Psychiatry 31:89–100

Halleck SL (ed) (1979) Coping with the legal onslaught. Jossey-Bass, San Francisco, CA

Hartwell SW (2004a) Comparison of offenders with mental illness only and offenders with dual diagnosis. Psychiatr Serv 55:145–149

Hartwell SW (2004b) Triple stigma: persons with mental illness and substance abuse problems in the criminal justice system. Crim Justice Policy Rev 15:89–99

Herinckx HA, Swart SC, Ama SM, Dolezal CD, King S (2005) Rearrest and linkage to mental health services among clients of the Clark County mental health court program. Psychiatr Serv 56:853–857

Hiday VA (1982) The attorney's role in involuntary civil commitment. North Carol Law Rev 60:1021–1056

Hiday VA (1983) Sociology of mental health law. Sociol Soc Res 67:111–128

Hiday VA (1988) Civil commitment: a review of empirical research. Behav Sci Law 6:15–43

Hiday VA (1991) Hospitals to jails: arrests and incarceration of civil commitment candidates. Hosp Community Psychiatry 42:729–734

Hiday VA (1992a) Civil commitment and arrests: an investigation of the criminalization thesis. J Nerv Ment Dis 180:184–191

Hiday VA (1992b) Coercion in civil commitment: process, preferences, and outcome. Int J Law Psychiatry 15:359–377

Hiday VA (1999) Mental illness and the criminal justice system. In: Horwitz A, Scheid TL (eds) The handbook of the sociology of mental health. Cambridge University Press, New York, pp 508–525

Hiday VA (2003) Outpatient commitment: the state of empirical research on its outcomes. Psychol Public Policy Law 9:8–32

Hiday VA, Goodman RR (1981) The least restrictive alternative to involuntary hospitalization, outpatient commitment: its use and effectiveness. J Psychiatry Law 10:81–96

Hiday VA, Markell SJ (1981) Components of dangerousness: legal standards in civil commitment. Int J Law Psychiatry 3:405–419

Hiday VA, Scheid-Cook T (1987) The North Carolina experience with outpatient commitment: a critical appraisal. Int J Law Psychiatry 10:215–232

Hiday VA, Scheid-Cook T (1991) Outpatient commitment for "revolving door" patients: compliance and treatment. J Nerv Ment Dis 179:85–90

Hiday VA, Smith LN (1987) Effects of the dangerousness standard in civil commitment. J Psychiatry Law 15:433–454

Hiday VA, Wales HW (2003) Civil commitment and arrests. Curr Opin Psychiatry 16:575–580

Hoge SK, Sachs G, Appelbaum PS, Greer A, Gordon C (1988) Limitations on psychiatrists' discretionary civil commitment authority by the Stone and dangerousness criteria. Arch Gen Psychiatry 45:764–769

James DJ, Glaze LE (2006) "Mental health problems of prison and jail inmates. Bureau of Justice Statistics, Washington, DC, NCJ 213600

Jencks C (1994) The homeless. Harvard University Press, Cambridge, MA

Junginger J, Claypoole K, Laygo R, Crisanti A (2006) Effects of serious mental illness and substance abuse on criminal offenses. Psychiatr Serv 57:879–882

Kahle LR, Sales BD, Nagel S (1978) On unicorns blocking commitment law reform. J Psychiatry Law 6:89–105

Keilitz I, Hall T (1985) State statutes governing involuntary civil commitment. Ment Phys Disabil Law Rep 9:378–397

Kittrie NN (1971) The right to be different. The Johns Hopkins University Press, Baltimore, MD

La Fond JQ, Durham ML (1992) Back to the asylum: the future of mental health law and policy in the United States. Oxford University Press, New York

Lamb HR (ed) (1984) The homeless mentally ill: a task force report of the American Psychiatric Association. American Psychiatric Association, Washington, DC

Lamb HR, Weinberger LE (2005) The shift of psychiatric inpatient care from hospitals to jails and prisons. J Am Acad Psychiatry Law 33:529–534

Lamb HR, Weinberger LE, Gross BH (1999) Community treatment of severely mentally ill offenders under the jurisdiction of the criminal justice system: a review. Psychiatr Serv 50:907–913

Manderscheid RW, Henderson MJ, Witkin MJ, Atay JE (1999) Contemporary mental health systems and managed care. In: Horwitz AV, Scheid TL (eds) A handbook for the study of mental health. Cambridge University Press, New York, pp 412–426

Marlowe DB, Festinger DS, Foltz C, Lee PA, Patapis NS (2005) Perceived deterrence and outcomes in drug court. Behav Sci Law 23:183–198

McCafferty G, Dooley J (1990) Involuntary outpatient commitment: an update. Ment Phys Disabil Law Rep 14:276–287

McGarry AL (1976) The holy legal war against state hospital psychiatry. N Engl J Med 294:318–320

McNiel D, Binder RL (2007) Effectiveness of a mental health court in reducing criminal recidivism and violence. Am J Psychiatry 164:1395–1403

Mechanic D (1999) Mental health and social policy: the emergence of managed care. Allyn and Bacon, Boston, MA

Mechanic D (2007) Truth about health care: why reform is not working in America. Rutgers University Press, New Brunswick, NJ

Monahan J, Calderia C, Friedlander HD (1979) Police and the mentally ill: a comparison of committed and arrested persons. Int J Law Psychiatry 2:509–518

Moore ME, Hiday VA (2006) Mental health court outcomes: a comparison of re-arrest and re-arrest deverity between mental health court and traditional court participants. Law Human Behav 30:659–674

Morrissey J, Meyer P, Cuddeback G (2007) Extending assertive community treatment to criminal justice settings: origins, current evidence and future directions. Community Ment Health J 43:527–544

Petrila J (2001) From constitution to contracts: mental disability law at the turn of the century. In: Frost LA, Bonnie RJ (eds) The evolution of mental health law. American Psychological Association, Washington, DC, pp 75–100

Petrila J, Ayers K (1994) Enforcing the fair housing amendments act to benefit people with mental disability. Psychiatr Serv 45:156–160

Petrila J, Christy A (2008) Florida's outpatient commitment law: a lesson in failed reform? Psychiatr Serv 59:21–23

Rachlin S, Pam AK, Milton J (1975) Civil liberties versus involuntary hospitalization. Am J Psychiatry 132:189–191

Ridgely MS, Engberg J, Greenberg MD, Turner S, DeMartini C, Dembosky JW (2007) Justice, treatment, and cost: an evaluation of the fiscal impact of Allegheny county mental health court. RAND No. TR-439-CSG. RAND Corporation, Santa Monica, CA

Rochefort DA (1997) From poorhouses to homelessness: policy analysis and mental health care, 2nd edn. Auburn House, Westport, CN

Rothman DJ (1980) Conscience and convenience: the asylum and its alternatives in progressive America. Little Brown, Boston, MA

Sadoff RL (1979) Changes in the mental health law: progress for patients – problems for psychiatrists. In: Halleck SL (ed) Coping with the legal onslaught. Jossey-Bass, San Francisco, CA, pp 1–12

Scheid TL (2005) Stigma as a barrier to employment: psychiatric disability and the impact of the American with disabilities act. Int Acad Psychiatry Law 28:670–690

Scheid TL, Greenberg G (2007) An organizational analysis of mental health care. In: Avison WR, McLeod JD, Pescosolido BA (eds) Mental health, social mirror. Springer, New York, pp 379–406

Steadman HJ, Monahan J (eds) (1982) Mentally disordered offenders: perspectives from law and social science. Plenum, New York

Steadman HJ, Morris S, Dennis D (1995) The diversion of mentally ill persons from jails to community based services: a profile of programs. Am J Public Health 85:1630–1635

Stone AA (1975) Mental health and the law: a system in transition. NIMH, Center for Studies of Crime and Delinquency, Rockville, MD

Swaminath RS, Mendonca JD, Vidal C, Chapman P (2002) Experiments in change: pretrial diversion of offenders with mental illness. Can J Psychiatry 47:450–458

Swartz JP, Lurigio AJ (2007) Severe mental illness and arrest: the generalized mediating effect of substance use. Crime Delinq 53:581–609

Teplin LA (1984) Criminalizing mental disorder: the comparative arrest rate of the mentally ill. Am Psychol 39:794–803

Teplin LA (1990a) The prevalence of severe mental disorder among male urban jail detainees: comparison with the Epidemiological Catchment Area Program. Am J Public Health 80:663–669

Teplin LA (1990b) Detecting disorder: the treatment of mental illness among jail detainees. J Consult Clin Psychol 58:233–36

Teplin LA, Pruett NS (1992) Police as street corner psychiatrists: managing the mentally ill. Int J Law Psychiatry 15:157–170

Teplin LA, Abram KM, McClelland GM (1996) The prevalence of psychiatric disorder among incarcerated women. Ann Gen Psychiatry 53:505–512

Treffert DA (1973) Dying with their rights on. Am J Psychiatry 130:1041

Wales HW, Hiday VA (2006) PLC or TLC: is outpatient commitment the/an answer? Int J Law Psychiatry 29:451–468

Warren CAB (1984) Court of last resort. University of Chicago Press, Chicago, IL

Watson AC, Angell B (2007) Applying procedural justice theory to law enforcement's response to persons with mental illness. Psychiatr Serv 58:787–793

Wexler D (1981) Mental health law: major issues. Plenum, New York

Wexler D (2008) Two decades of therapeutic jurisprudence. Touro Law Rev 24(1):17–29

Wexler D, Winick BJ (eds) (1996) Law in a therapeutic key: developments in therapeutic jurisprudence. Carolina Academic Press, Durham, NC

Part III
Connecting To Medicine:
The Profession and Its Organizations

Chapter 10
Medicalization and Biomedicalization Revisited: Technoscience and Transformations of Health, Illness and American Medicine

Adele E. Clarke and Janet Shim

Introduction

Medicalization theory has been at the heart of medical sociology or the sociology of health and illness for nearly 40 years (Zola 1972; Freidson 1970) and is also vital to medical anthropology (Hogle 2002; Lock 2001, 2004), the history of medicine (Nye 2003; Sinding 2004), medicine itself (Chervenak and McCullough 2005), bioethics (Bergeron 2007), and beyond. The still robust medicalization thesis is that the legitimate jurisdiction of Western or scientific medicine began expanding by including new domains of human life (such as alcoholism, drug addiction, and obesity) by redefining or reconstructing them as falling properly within *medical* (rather than legal, religious, etc.) domains (e.g., Ballard and Elston 2005; Conrad 1992, 2005, 2007; Conrad and Schneider 1980a, b).

In the late 1990s, a group of medical sociologists, including ourselves, began to find classic medicalization theory inadequate to the intellectual tasks of explaining what we were seeing in our varied research projects as new and different "conditions of possibility" vis-à-vis health, illness, and biomedicine. We conceptualized *biomedicalization* as an extension of medicalization theory to capture these shifts. While conventional medicalization practices typically emphasize exercising *control over* medical phenomena – diseases, illnesses, injuries, bodily malfunctions – biomedicalization practices, in contrast, emphasize *transformations of* them by technoscientific means. These are accomplished largely through quick high-tech interventions not only for treatment but increasingly also for enhancement or optimization. The fundamental processes of medicalization as the extension of medical jurisdiction into new arenas through new medical definitions continue today, likely unabated (cf. Ballard and Elston 2005). At the same time, we argue, across the full array of biomedical and health-related practices, emphasis is shifting to the elaboration of technoscientific modes of intervention, (re)organization, transformation, and the remaking of identities and socialities characteristic of biomedicalization (Clarke et al. 2000, 2003, 2004, 2010a).

Theoretically, biomedicalization is situated as part of the broader shift from what Foucault (1975) termed "the clinical gaze" dominant since the eighteenth century to what Nikolas Rose (2007a) recently called "the molecular gaze" now reformulating "vital politics" and "life itself" in the twenty-first century (Clarke et al. 2010b). If the twentieth century was the "century of physics" (thanks, for example, to the atomic bomb, silicon chip and the Internet), then the twenty-first century is not merely the "century of the gene" (Keller 2000), but more broadly the "century of biology"

A.E. Clarke (✉)
Department of Social and Behavioral Sciences, University of California – San Francisco,
3333 California St., #LHts-455, San Francisco, CA 94143-0612, USA
e-mail: adele.clarke@ucsf.edu

(Brenner 2000) and nanotechnology. Biomedicalization theory directly engages these new and elaborating technoscientific developments.

Biomedicalization theory too is becoming central to medical sociology (e.g., Clarke et al. 2009), medical anthropology (e.g., Burri and Dumit 2007), and so on. It is also very lively in the transdisciplinary field of science and technology studies (STS) where its originators also dwell.[1] Others have also sought to push the boundaries of medical sociology, anthropology and history to include relations of medicine with sciences and technologies more broadly within their purview (e.g., Casper and Berg 1995; Star 1995; Casper and Koenig 1996; Shim 2002; Hogle 2002). We attempt to sustain those efforts here. Specifically, we seek to introduce contemporary science and technology studies perspectives that should be useful as technoscientific innovations increasingly transform biomedicine in the USA and transnationally. We hope this chapter performs some of the necessary work to build productive bridges and exciting sites of intersection for future work on medicalization and biomedicalization in but not limited to medical sociology.

We next discuss some of the history of medicalization theory and recent areas of research emphasis. We then define and historicize biomedicalization more thoroughly. Following that, we situate it in relation to the broader theoretical backdrop emerging from medical sociologists, anthropologists, and historians centered around "the politics of life itself" and how these are engaged individually, collectively, and at the level of population. This includes issues of bioeconomy and biocapital. There are, of course, critiques of biomedicalization theory and we lay these out and respond to them. Although its "life" is still short, biomedicalization theory has been taken up fairly widely and we next offer an overview of biomedicalization theory in action, detailing key ways it has been utilized and the kinds of work it is doing. In conclusion, we discuss the relations among medicalization, biomedicalization, and medical sociology and offer an agenda for future research.

Medicalization Theory Today

Medicalization theory per se has been recently debated and updated. Historically, one strand of scholarship has tended to emphasize the professional dominance thesis, with a relative focus on doctors as (the) main agents of medicalization, and a critique of professional aggrandizement and medical imperialism. This is characteristic of some early work in medicalization theory and Marxist perspectives (e.g., Illich 1975; Jasso-Aquilar, Waitzkin and Landwehr 2004; Navarro 1986, 2007; Waitzkin 1989, 2000). British sociologists' conceptualizations of medicalization have also often (but not always) been characterized by an emphasis on professional dominance (e.g., Strong 1979, 1984; Murcott 2006; Williams 2004; Dingwall 2006). There has also, in fact, been some recent and especially British lament over the concept of medicalization becoming "a complete muddle" (Davis 2006), with many scholars ruing the inclusion in medicalization theory of patients as consumers (e.g., Henderson and Petersen 2002), and pharmaceutical companies' promotional efforts which they call "selling sickness" and "disease mongering" (e.g., Moynihan and Cassels 2005) as promoting medicalization (Furedi 2006).

A second direction, on the other hand, has long emphasized the definitional, jurisdictional and institutional aspects of medicalization with a focus on examining the processes, complexities, and consequences of how things are actually made "medical" (rather than legal, religious, personal, etc.). American sociologists have more commonly shared such inflections (Zola 1972). In fact, it

---

[1] Fully nine chapters of a total of 38 in *The Handbook of Science and Technology Studies* focus on medical topics (Hackett et al. 2007). While presentations on medical topics at the Society for Social Studies of Science meetings have gone from 11% in 1988 to 29% in 2001 (Amsterdamska and Hiddinga 2004), both broader and deeper knowledge *across* these disciplines remains rare.

was in response to the critique of medical imperialism that Conrad and Schneider (1980b) elaborated three levels of medicalization: the conceptual (the use of medical language or a medical model to redefine a problem); the institutional (where organizations use the medical approach to address particular problems, legitimating and institutionalizing medical management); and the level of the physician–patient interaction. Since then, the relative focus in studies of medicalization has been on how a phenomenon is discursively defined – socially constructed – as falling within medical jurisdiction and how that is elaborated (Conrad and Schneider 1980a, esp. pp. 17–38, Conrad 1992, pp. 277–279; Conrad 2005, 2007).[2]

Analyses of agents, actions, and processes involved in wide-ranging domains of health and medicine have progressively become more nuanced and complicated, and theorizing medicalization has followed suit. These analyses have emerged, according to Nye (2003), especially from social and political histories of medicine and public health and from enhanced appreciation of the work of Foucault. Issues of medical professional dominance are also taken up in this strand of scholarship, but within such contexts as the professions per se (Freidson 1970, 2001), the role and effects of third party payers (e.g., McKinlay and Marceau 2002; Quadagno 2005; Scott et al. 2000), and the issue of professional discretion vs. clinical practice guidelines (e.g., Timmermans and E. Kolker 2004). Such scholars, rather than assuming medical imperialism is necessarily linked to medicalization, have worked to decouple professional dominance from medicalization (e.g., Furedi 2006) and to treat medicalization as an open empirical and theoretical question rather than a foregone conclusion.

In addition to emphasizing definitional and institutional aspects, these medical sociologists have explicitly pointed beyond the profession of medicine to entities such as "big pharma," suppliers of hospital equipment and technologies, and patients increasingly acting as consumers of biomedical goods and services, for example, in their discussions of the increasing medicalization of society. Their arguments focus on how the power of medicalization and persistence of specific forms and contents of medical care rest on economic interests and motivations of multiple and varied actors situated in different institutions of society (e.g., Conrad and Schneider 1980a; Conrad 1992, 2005, 2006, 2007). Recent American work has further emphasized nonphysician actors such as insurance companies (e.g., Quadagno 2005), managed care organizations (Scott et al. 2000), and last and far from least philanthropic organizations from the great (e.g., Rockefeller, Carnegie and now Gates Foundations) to the persistent, smaller, local private giving that over the past century has deeply entrenched medical schools and hospitals institutionally in every major city in the USA in ways largely taken-for-granted historically (Pescosolido and Martin 2004; Pescosolido 2006).

The major sustained American contributor here is Peter Conrad who has recently (2006, 2007; Conrad and Leiter 2004) emphasized the increasing salience of the market. In 2006, he asserted that "the shifting engines of medicalization" today are biotechnology (in which he includes the pharmaceutical industry as well as genomic research and medicine), consumers and managed care. His book, *The Medicalization of Society* (2007), takes up both the extension of medicalization (to men via medicalization of andropause, baldness and sexual dysfunction), and its expansion (across age categories such as children's hyperactivity morphing into adult ADHD). Conrad also sees new forms of bodily improvement (e.g., use of human growth hormone) as falling within the traditional framework of medicalization, and frames the appeal of such interventions as "temptations" of biomedical enhancement.

Demedicalization – the ending of medical jurisdiction over some activities or attributes – has also been an issue in medicalization theory for some time (e.g., Fox 2001). The classic case was the demedicalization of homosexuality by its exclusion as an illness from the psychiatric Diagnostic and Statistical Manual; but Conrad (2007) now points to the potential of its remedicalization through the

---

[2] How much these national differences might be attributable to living under radically different health systems remains unclear, but this debate is ongoing. See special section in *Society* 43(6):14–56, (2006).

emergence of gender identity disorder, and the geneticization of sexual orientation. More broadly, Ballard and Elston (2005) point to several ongoing trends that may either increase the potential for medicalization or lead to demedicalization. Heightened concerns over risk, for example, could work in both directions, as they might both undermine faith in the efficacy and safety of medical interventions, as well as motivating individuals to pursue them in order to reduce disease risks. Thus, Williams and Calnan (1996) have argued that people can be simultaneously more skeptical of and more dependent upon medicine, and resisting as well as embracing medicalization (see also Fox and Ward 2006). Similarly, several scholars (e.g., Ballard and Elston 2005; Tomes 2007) have observed that the confluence of new medical technologies, continued efforts to maximize cost control and cost effectiveness, and new emphases on self-care and preventive medicine also contributes to the oscillation between the medicalization and demedicalization of everyday life. Moreover, many others (e.g., Pescosolido 2006; Bury 2006) have observed that although the professional autonomy of physicians has certainly been eroded, the dominance of medical technosciences and interventions, and of the sociocultural and economic sector of medicine, remain powerful.

In terms of research, one area of growing interest is the medicalization of risk itself (Crawford 2004; Halpern 2004), called "risk trafficking" by Dumit (2005). This also involves the possibility of the treatment of risk – such as mastectomy for breast cancer risk (Gibbon 2007) and consumption of hormones during pregnancy to prevent fetal intersexuality (Casper and Muse 2006). Additionally, recent research on medicalization has taken up mental health (e.g., Horwitz 2002; Martin et al. 2007; Wheaton and Clarke 2003), "unruly" children (e.g., Rafalovich 2005), shyness (Scott 2006), autism (e.g., Nadesan 2005), and compulsive buying (Lee and Mysyk 2004). A significant proportion of recent research on medicalization is concerned with gender (e.g., Gibbon 2007; Lorber and Moore 2002; Mamo 2007a, b; Mamo and Fosket 2009; Riska 2004, 2009; Rosenfeld and Faircloth 2006; Schulz and Mullings 2006; and Shim 2002, 2009).[3]

One of the enduring challenges of medicalization theory has been the increasing need to parse the meanings and distinctions among medicalization, medicine, the medical profession, and the social and cultural landscapes and economic sectors with deep and complicated ties to the provision of health care. It is now fairly widely accepted that these do not march in lockstep; deprofessionalization, for example, does not necessarily indicate demedicalization. Our synthetic attempts to assess this complicated picture thus led to the articulation of *bio*medicalization, in order to better account for how medicine is now so much more than the profession, or the clinical provision of treatments, or even the health care system. Instead, expanding domains of everyday life, technoscientific and economic activities and strategies, and socio-cultural shifts are implicated today in new ways in the biomedical transformation of life itself.

Defining and Historicizing Biomedicalization Theory

The intellectual origins of biomedicalization theory lie in large part in attempts to come to terms with the implications of science and technology studies as a transdisciplinary field for medical sociology. Key epistemological and ontological assumptions of the sociology of knowledge that are featured in STS, such as the intrinsically social nature of sciences, technologies, and knowledges more broadly (Fleck 1935, 1979), are also central to medicine generally and to biomedicalization theory.[4]

---

[3] Little has been written directly on race and (bio)medicalization, but see Clarke et al. (2009b), Kahn (2009), and Shim (2002, 2009).

[4] See Armstrong (1983, 2002), Jordanova (2004), Hess (1997), Wright and Treacher (1982), Restivo and Croissant (2007), and Hackett et al. (2007). On medical technologies, see Mechanic (2002), Lock (2008), and Hogle (2008).

Defining

The crux of biomedicalization theory is that *bio*medicine broadly conceived is being transformed from the inside out by densely elaborating technoscientific interventions and the coproduced social arrangements that allow their implementation (Clarke et al. 2000, 2003, 2010b).[5] These include computer and information sciences as well as all the *bio*sciences and technologies such as molecular biology, genetics, genomics, biotechnology, pharmacogenomics, nanotechnologies, and medical technologies including those of visualization. Along with our growing and largely individualized responsibilities for our biological /somatic citizenship (e.g., Ginsberg and Rapp 1995; Nguyen 2005; Novas and Rose 2000; Petryna 2002), these technosciences both allow and provoke new kinds of interventions in health, illness, healing, the organization of medical care, and ultimately how we think about and live "life itself."

In terms of the in-practice dynamics of biomedicalization, Clarke and colleagues (2003, pp. 166) argued that it "is coconstituted and manifest through five central (and overlapping) processes (1) major political economic shifts; (2) a new focusing on health and risk and surveillance biomedicines; (3) the technoscientization of biomedicine; (4) transformations of the production, distribution, and consumption of biomedical knowledges; and (5) transformations of bodies and identities." We next discuss each briefly.[6]

First, the political economic reorganization of biomedicine is part of the emergent if not already coalescent "biopolitical economy" of health, illness, life, and death (discussed further below). This concept emphasizes the *corporatized* and *privatized* (rather than state-funded) research, products, and services made possible by technoscientific innovations that further biomedicalization. The USA spends more on health care per person than any other nation in the world, now approximately 15.2% of the GDP, and expected to reach 19.5% by 2017 (Centers for Medicare and Medicaid Services 2008a). Projections estimate that the USA will spend in 2007 $2.26 trillion on health care or $7,439 per person (Centers for Medicare and Medicaid Services 2008b). The most notable socioeconomic changes in health care indicative of and facilitating biomedicalization are corporatization and commodification; centralization, rationalization, and devolution of services; and stratification. Significantly, the very *legitimacy* of medicalization and increasingly of biomedicalization is foundational to the generation of biocapital – nationally and transnationally.[7]

The second key process of biomedicalization is an intensifying focus on health itself and the elaboration of risk and surveillance biomedicines. In commodity cultures such as the USA, health becomes another commodity and the biomedically (re)engineered body becomes a prized possession. Health matters have taken on a "life of their own" (Radley et al. 1997, pp. 8), and health is increasingly viewed as a moral obligation (Crawford 2004) of "biological citizens" (Petryna 2002; Rose and Novas 2004). Risk and surveillance concerns shape both the technologies and discourses of biomedicalization as well as the spaces within which biomedicalization processes occur.

Third, the increasingly technoscientific nature of the practices and innovations of biomedicine are, of course, key features of biomedicalization. While sciences and technologies became increasingly constitutive of medicine across the twentieth century, in its final decades, technoscientific transformations both altered in their fundamental natures and gained momentum. The three main areas in which the technoscientization of biomedicine manifest are computerization and data banking; molecularization and geneticization of biomedicine and drug design; and medical technology design, development, and distribution.

---

[5] On coproduction see especially Jasanoff (2005).

[6] See Clarke et al. (2003) for thorough elaboration of these processes.

[7] One recent transnational development of note is the elaboration of medical tourism. See, e.g., Ramirez de Arellano (2007) and Turner (2007).

Fourth, biomedicalization concerns transformations of biomedical knowledge production, information management, distribution, and consumption. Today, information on health and illness is proliferating through all kinds of media, especially newspapers, on the Internet, in magazines, and through direct-to-consumer prescription. More than being a subculture, biomedicine is today so much a fundamental element of mass culture that Bauer (1998) suggested that its constant presence points to the medicalization of not only of science news but of society generally, which Conrad (2007) emphasized. Thus the production and transmission of health and medical knowledges are key sites of biomedicalization in terms of both the transformation of their sources and distribution channels and the reformulation of who is responsible for grasping and applying such knowledges.

In the fifth and last key process of biomedicalization, the shift from control to transformation is central, enabling "transformations of" bodies to include desired new properties and technoscientific identities (Clarke 1995). Regulation through biomedicalization works "from the inside out" as a type of biomedical governance, achieved through alterations of subjectivities and desires for transformed bodies and selves. The body becomes "a project" (Brumberg 1997). Such opportunities and imperatives, however, are stratified in their availability – imposed, made accessible, and/or promoted differentially to different populations and groups. New technoscientific identities – identities knowable only through the application of technoscience (e.g., DNA, BRCA risk) – may be taken up individually, often ramifying through families. They may also engender biosocialities (Rabinow 1992a, 2008) – collective identities – through "patient groups" (e.g., Atkinson et al. 2007; Gibbon and Novas 2008).

In terms of researching the biomedicalization of a particular phenomenon, analyzing any and all of these processes offers useful entrée. Within different phenomena, different processes are often fore-grounded (e.g., Clarke et al. 2010a case studies). At this historical moment, we think it important to place greater emphasis on engagements with enhancements, or what Rose (2007a, pp. 7) more broadly calls *optimization* in terms of the increasing legitimacy of securing "the best possible futures." Specifically, we are asserting the need for empirical social science research to better understand how users/consumer/patients and providers/scientists/producers are engaging new technologies so that policies and procedures for their use might be improved to better meet people's needs and desires – as individuals, as participants in patient groups, and as biological citizens (e.g., Boero 2010; Fishman 2010; Mamo 2007a, 2010).[8] To date, pharmaceuticals have been a major focus here.[9]

We also wish to point out that biomedicalization is not intended inherently or only as a critique (of medicine), but instead as an analytic term used to identify and describe a new set of phenomena. Thus, we also want to emphasize here that there exist varied counter-trends against medicalization and biomedicalization. Foremost, there has been in the USA as well as transnationally a too-often ignored history of medical pluralism – the simultaneous availability of multiple kinds of medicines (e.g., Unschuld 1987; Kelner et al. 2000; Sharma 2000; Lock 2002b). Alternatives to conventional medicalization and biomedicalization alike have been available and increasingly well utilized (Eisenberg et al. 1998). However, medical pluralism is complicated by what Clarke (2010b) calls "medical partialisms" – the only partial and often contingent availabilities of various kinds of medicines in many sites. Stratified medicalization (unequal development, distribution, and access to scientific medicine) and stratified biomedicalization (unequal distribution and access to high-tech biomedicine) are ongoing, partializing those processes (Clarke et al. 2003, 2010b).

---

[8] Recent work has focused, e.g., on the pursuit of perfection (Rothman and Rothman 2003), human growth hormone (Conrad and Potter 2004), antiaging (Binstock and Fishman 2010), "replaceable you" (Serlin 2004), hormone treatments (Mamo and Fosket 2009; Watkins 2007), treatment of male and female sexual dysfunction (Fishman 2004; Loe 2004), depression (e.g., Healy 2002), and pharmacogenetics (Hedgecoe 2004).

[9] Martin (2006) describes "the pharmaceutical person" and Davis-Berman and Pestello (2005) "the medicated self." Tomes (2005) and Tone and Watkins (2007) analyze the evolving relationship between doctors, patients, and prescription drugs; Daemmrich (2004) takes up drug regulation as pharmacopolitics. See also Critser (2005) and Lakoff (2008).

Today we are also seeing increased questioning of the value and appropriateness of (bio)-medicalization such as Brownlee's (2007) *Overtreated: Why Too Much Medicine is Making Us Sicker and Poorer,* and Horton's (2000) "How Sick is Modern Medicine?" Intervening in "nature" has long been controversial (e.g., Clarke 1990, 1998; Nelkin 1995; Nelkin and Lindee 2004) and controversies are elaborating along with new technological capacities (Gottweis 2005; Jasanoff 2005). Murray (2009) views biomedicalization as part of the biofascism of Western health care, sorely in need of critical bioethical reforms.

Moreover, patients/users/consumers of new technoscientific alternatives are themselves often ambivalent and "reluctant" users (e.g., Kerr and Franklin 2006; Landzelius 2006a; Malacrida 2004). Even Viagra prescriptions are not always renewed (Berenson 2005). The ethically charged situations when one person such as a parent is deciding for another such as a child, or vice versa, are particularly fraught, such as surgical modifications (e.g., Parens 2006), cochlear implants (e.g., Hahn and Belt 2004), vaccination (Landzelius 2006b), and (male) circumcision (Darby 2005). Clinical providers and producers of technoscientific interventions themselves also express ambivalence and anxiety, including around end of life care (e.g., Kaufman 2005) and in terms of tinkering with both human (Franklin and Roberts 2006), and plant and animal reproduction (Haraway 2007; Friese 2007; Thompson 2010). It will be interesting to see whether these trends expand and in what directions.

Historicizing

Biomedicalization theory is historical, predicated on an understanding of three eras in the history of American medicine (Clarke et al. 2003, pp. 164–6; Clarke 2010a). The first was the rise of "scientific" medicine[10] as densely webbed networks of organizations and institutions devoted to the production, sales and delivery of an array of commodities, and services linked to diagnostics and treatments of what are deemed illnesses, conditions, and diseases. In the USA, the *rise of medicine era* occurred c1890–1945. It has been described as the first "social transformation of American medicine" (Starr 1982) and fully established the medical sector of the US political economy by the end of World War II (Brandt and Gardner 2000). Even during the Great Depression, Americans spent over $3.5 billion annually on medical services and commodities, and the health care sector already ranked sixth among American industries, above automobile, iron and steel, oil and coal sectors, with 4–5% of the GDP (Tomes 2001, pp. 524–6).

During the *medicalization era,* c1940–1985, the *jurisdiction* of medicine expanded dramatically if not exponentially. Initially, medicalization was seen to occur as particular social problems deemed morally problematic and often affecting the body (e.g., alcoholism, homosexuality, abortion, and drug abuse) were moved from the professional jurisdiction of the law to that of medicine (Zola 1972). Drawing upon symbolic interactionist labeling theory, Conrad and Schneider (1980a) termed this a transformation from "badness to sickness" as socially designated deviant behaviors were increasingly labeled and treated as medical problems. By conceptually redefining particular phenomena in medical terms, and thereby effacing them as *social* problems, medicine as an institution became understood as an important new agent of social control. This occurs at multiple levels – conceptually, institutionally, in popular culture and other discourses, and in provider–patient relationships (Conrad and Schneider 1980b; Conrad 1992; Lock 2004). Gradually in the USA, the concept

---

[10] While there are many kinds of medicines and healing systems on our planet, we focus on what seems best termed "scientific medicine," with major roots in the West, also known as Western medicine. Today, however, it both dwells in many places in its "local" forms and is continuously (re)constituted through developments generated in many sites beyond the West.

of medicalization was extended to any and all instances when new phenomena were deemed medical problems under medical jurisdiction – from infertility to hyperactivity and so on (Conrad 2007).[11]

Since 1985, dramatic, largely technoscientific changes in the constitution, organization and practices of contemporary biomedicine have coalesced into the *biomedicalization era*, the second major transformation of American medicine (Clarke et al. 2000, 2003, 2010a). Biomedicalization practices emphasize transformations largely through immediate high-tech interventions not only for treatment but increasingly also for health maintenance, enhancement and "optimization" – the growing sense of individual obligation or responsibility to literally "make the best" of oneself (Rose 2007a). The pervasiveness of biomedicalization practices – their ubiquity in the USA today – has recently been described as "the biomedicalization of society" (Burri and Dumit 2007, pp. 5).

To generate this analysis of three eras, we generated a dense historical chart (Clarke et al. 2010c). Here we offer a synopsis version; please see Fig. 10.1: From the Rise of Medicine to Biomedicalization (Clarke 2010a).

	c1890 – 1945 Rise of Medicine	c1940 – 1985 Medicalization	c1980 – present Biomedicalization
Infrastructure	Organizational	Physical	Digital
Basic Social Processes	Specification Legitimation	Control Elaboration	Transformation Molecularization/ Geneticization
Focus of Clinical Gaze	Acute Illnesses/ Communicable Diseases	Chronic Illnesses/ Diseases	Risk factors/ Medicalization of health
Main Mode of Clinical Action	Surgical Success & Clinical Skills	Routinization of Medical Care	Drugs /Devices /Technologies
Main Focus of Biomedical Sciences	Germ Theory / Disease Classification	Biochemistry / Pharmaceutical Sciences	Molecular Biology Genetics / Genomics
Main Focus of Biomedical Technology	Amplifying Bodily Indicators & Imaging	Imaging, Procedures & Treatments	Biotechnologies & Nanotechnologies
Medical Construction of Patients / Identities	Fortunate to be Patients Illness/ Disease Identities in Known Biographies	Passive Patients Diagnostic Identities	Responsible Consumers, Technoscientific Identities & Biosocialities

Fig. 10.1 From the rise of medicine to biomedicalization

---

[11] See also Armstrong (2002), Conrad (1992, 2006a, b), Conrad and Schneider (1980a), and Freidson (1970). For historical overviews, see Ballard and Elston (2005), Nye (2003), and Pfohl (1985). On organizational dimensions, see esp. Light (2004) and Scott et al. (2000); on pharmaceuticals see Tone and Watkins (2007).

Of course, the eras are fuzzily bounded and bleed into one another, and processes or phenomena in different eras are matters of emphasis not exclusion.[12] Innovations of all kinds are *cumulative over time* such that older practices approaches are usually available simultaneously somewhere.

Situating Biomedicalization Theory: Twenty-First Century Questions of Life Itself

How does biomedicalization theory fit in with other contemporary theorizing, especially but not only in sociology and anthropology? In this section, we situate biomedicalization theory first in terms of its roots in Foucault and then vis-à-vis currently coalescing retheorizing of questions of changes in the nature of "life itself." Our basic argument is that the fundamentals of the situation of medicine itself have changed, requiring biomedicalization theory that goes beyond medicalization theory. Here we elaborate upon how the situation has shifted in societal, governmental (in both conventional and Foucauldian senses), collective, and individual strategies to address health, disease, and the body.

The "bio" in the concept of *bio*medicalization does several kinds of work. First and foremost, it signals the increasing importance of biology – the life sciences broadly speaking as institutions, sets of practices, knowledges, and so on – to biomedicine today. Second, the "bio" signals that Foucauldian questions of biopower and biopolitics are each and all integral to our project.[13] Foucault (1975, 1984) argued that biopower emerged out of the modernization and industrialization of western societies during the eighteenth and nineteenth centuries. In contemporary society, biopower represents a new kind of "microphysics of power" and takes the form of knowledges coupled with technologies to exert diffuse yet constant forces of surveillance and control over human bodies and their behaviors, sensations, physiological processes, and pleasures – both individually and in terms of populations.

For Foucault, power is automatically "built in" and mobile, embodied in social practices and norms rather than "invested" in particular individuals or institutions – including the state. Nor are technologies of power comprised simply of specific punitive measures, repression, and other "negative" mechanisms enacted by institutions. Instead, they are embedded within infinitesimal machineries and productive micropractices aimed at knowing and exploring the human body, breaking it down, and rearranging it – "positively" and "pleasurably" as well as otherwise. Power-knowledges create a *normalizing imperative* that effects the self-judgment and self-regulation of individuals (through "technologies of the self") as well as the regulation through social policies of groups and populations. Modern disciplines of power-knowledge thereby "produce subjected and practised bodies, 'docile' bodies" (Foucault 1979, pp. 138). And all of this is naturalized – becomes taken for granted (Lock 2004; Sinding 2004).

In the decade since we began writing on biomedicalization, a related body of scholarship has coalesced that articulates what has been changing so dramatically which biomedicalization theory addresses. This work builds upon and extends Foucauldian analysis around the premise that, as Rose (2007a, b, c, pp. 7) eloquently argues, today "we are inhabiting an emergent form of life." One of the key questions Foucault (1970) raised, following Canguilhem (1966), was "What is life?"

---

[12] On the question of historical periodization, see Clarke (2010a).

[13] Over the past 30 plus years, the Foucauldian turn has permeated the sociology, anthropology and history of medicine, perhaps more deeply in Europe and the UK but increasingly in the USA as well. See e.g., Armstrong (1983, 2002), Jones and Porter (1994), Peterson and Bunton (1997), Lupton (2003), Rabinow and Rose (2006), Sinding (2004), and Turner (1997).

Canguilhem had asserted that what "life" is changes over time and circumstance, and constitutes what Williams (1976) called a "keyword" – a site indicator of social change that should be routinely reassessed. Today the question "What is life?" is increasingly taken up again as the study of life processes has shifted from cellular to molecular levels over the last half of the twentieth century. Important seeds were sown in the pioneering work of some social scientists and historians seeking to theorize biotechnologies – for example, the works of Yoxen (1981, 1982) on life as a productive force and the capitalizing of molecular biology, Pauly (1987) on "controlling life" through biological engineering, and Kay (1993) on "life as technology" and "molecularizing."

Since the original development of biomedicalization theory (Clarke et al. 2000, 2003), these theoretical concerns have increasingly intersected with projects of biomedicine. There are three main overlapping areas of recent theorizing that are critical: changing notions of "vital politics" and "life itself;" new theories of biocapital and bioeconomies; and research about how people are engaging innovative technoscientific interventions as users/consumers, as scientists, as activists, and as citizens – individually, collectively, and as populations.

"Life Itself": From the Clinical Gaze to the Molecular Gaze

A number of scholars have been discussing (with growing intensity since 2000) changing conceptions of life, death, birth, and nature. For example, Lock (1993, pp. 48) argued that "Nature will be 'operationalized' for the good of society" – remade in the service of "man." Haraway (2004, pp. 202) has argued that the better term is "nature-culture" as the two are inextricable – coconstitutive (see also Latour 1987). Clarke (1998, pp. 273 and 275) argued that "the biomedicalization of life itself (human, plant and animal) was the key *social* process." Fischer (1999) asserted that we should attend to "emergent forms of life." Lash (2001) discussed "technological forms of life."

Franklin and Lock (2003) have argued that we are in the midst of "remaking life and death" through increasing technoscientific capacities to intervene at its beginnings and ends. At its beginnings lie new reproductive technologies: to prevent life through contraception (e.g., Clarke 2000); to make life through infertility treatments (Franklin and Roberts 2006; Thompson 2005; Mamo 2007a, b); to transform agricultural production (Clarke 2007; Schrepfer and Scranton 2004); and to prevent death through extraordinary means (e.g., Kaufman 2005; Shim et al. 2006, 2007; Kaufman and Morgan 2005). In a path-breaking essay, Franklin (2000, pp. 188) captured the broader thrust of recent changes:

> We are currently witnessing the emergence of a new genomic governmentality – the regulation and surveillance of technologically-assisted genealogy. This is necessitated by the removal of the genomes of plants, animals and humans from the template of natural history that once secured their borders, and their reanimation as forms of corporate capital, in the context of a legal vacuum ... Nature ... has been de-traditionalized. It has been antiquated, displaced and superseded ... nature is in a spin.

Another path-breaking contributor theorizing current "conditions of possibility" is Rose (Rose 2007a, pp. 3 and 262; Rose 2007c) who takes up the politics of "life itself":

> The vital politics of our own [21st] century...is neither delimited by the poles of illness and health, nor focused on eliminating pathology to protect the destiny of the nation. Rather it is concerned with our growing capacities to control, manage, engineer, reshape, and modulate the very vital capacities of human beings as living creatures.[14]

---

[14]With multiple parallels to biomedicalization, Rose (2007a), pp. 5–6) argues more broadly that "contemporary biopolitics has not been formed by any single event," but by changes along five key dimensions which he calls "mutations": *Molecularization* as a "style of thought"; *optimization* as securing "the best possible futures"; *subjectification* in terms of recoding the "duties, rights, and expectations of human beings" in terms of health and illness; *somatic expertise* as the growing numbers and kinds of subprofessions dedicated to managing aspects of somatic existence; and last, *economies of vitality* such that "biopolitics has become inextricably intertwined with bioeconomics."

Rose's assertion that we are in the midst of an epistemic shift from the clinical gaze initiated in the eighteenth century to the molecular gaze of today seems fundamental precisely because it signals a change in what Foucault called "the conditions of possibility" of how life can be/should be lived.

Biocapital and Bioeconomics

The terms "bioeconomy" and "biocapital" (e.g., Franklin 2006a; Rajan 2006; Harrington et al. 2006) capture the new ways in which capital itself is being (re)conceptualized and (re)organized by virtue of imbrications with the biological sciences and technologies, including biomedicine, the megacorporate pharmaceutical industry, and so on. In short, a very significant and growing proportion of capital globally (whether private, state, hybrid, etc.) is linked with things biological, biotechnological, and/or biomedical, including plant and animal agribusiness and "academic capitalism" (Slaughter and Rhoades 2004). The term bioeconomy is used to refer to this vast set of activities. In contrast, biocapital is used both as part of bioeconomy but also, as we shall see, in reference to the capacity of certain things – such as organs and tissues – to produce surplus value (e.g., Waldby and Mitchell 2006).

Rajan (2005, pp. 21, emphasis added) defines biocapital as "not only the systems of exchange and circulation involved in the contemporary workings of the life sciences but also a *regime of knowledge* pertaining to the life sciences as they become increasingly foundational epistemologies for our times." Based on comparative ethnographic research on biotech worlds in both the USA and India, he argues that biocapital as the fusion of capital and biotech is becoming transnationally dominant. He provocatively calls this technoscientific capital "lively capital" as part of "speculative capitalism."

Thompson (2005, pp. 248–9) captures a particularly important sense of potential and hype in her concept of "promissory capital" – capital raised for speculative ventures on the promise of future returns. She argues that there is a shift of importance from production to reproduction. "The biomedical mode of reproduction …has its own characteristic systems of exchange and value, notions of the lifecourse, epistemic norms, hegemonic political forms, security, and hierarchies and definitions of commodities and personhood." She asserts that generating biocapital by these means is a form of extraction that involves isolating and mobilizing the "primary reproductive agency" of specific body parts, particularly cells. In these exchanges, cells operate as soil does in agriculture – playing the "principal" role, as Marx described it. Cellular reproduction has certainly riveted the world of late, especially although far from only, vis-à-vis cloning and stem cells.[15]

Franklin (2003) discusses what she terms "ethical biocapital" as a new form of cultural capital produced in the UK through sustained governmental attention to the bioethical issues raised by genetics, cloning, stem cells, etc., and the British establishment of detailed regulations of such activities generated through citizen/expert collaborative processes. The "ethical biocapital" generated over time has allowed the UK to proceed rapidly with its government-supported research agendas and production of "biocapital" – in sharp contrast to a number of other industrialized nations such as the US and Germany (Gottweis 1998, 2005; Jasanoff 2005).

A significant part of biocapital is the growing transnational traffic in human tissues (blood, organs, and cell lines) that Hogle (2003, 2008) frames as the potential for "life/time warranties" in terms of rechargeable cells and extendable lives. Waldby and Mitchell (2006) have analyzed biocapital in terms of this traffic as "the global tissue economy" wherein "biogifts" are transformed into "biocommodities" as tissue "freely" given is transformed into products bought and sold. They refer to a major legal case

---

[15] See, e.g., Franklin (2003, 2005, 2007), Friese (2007), Ganchoff (2004, 2007), Thompson (2008), and the Special Issue on the Hwang affair of *East Asian Science, Technology and Society: An International Journal* 2(1).

in the USA (Moore v. The Regents of the University of California, et al.) of tremendous advantage to biocapital, which decided that individuals do not "own" or even hold fiscal rights in our body parts once they are separated from "us" (Rabinow 1992b). Cells and tissue may be taken for "free" regardless of our preferences and regardless of their "biovalue" in the world. Cohen (2005) terms this "bioavailability" using the example of poor people in India selling a kidney for transplantation.

Another domain of activity of biocapital that links to biomedicalization is what is being called "bioprospecting" (searching for new and available bioresources) and "biopiracy" (extracting and removing those resources from their sites of origin without adequate if any compensation). Hayden (2003) has been especially interested in the corporate pursuit of patentable biodiversity largely in less-developed and less-regulated nation states. More direct biopiracy is being pursued through the appropriation of "indigenous" medicines – much more usable and also patentable in the USA and elsewhere (e.g., Adams 2002).

Clearly politicoeconomic trends originally identified as part of biomedicalization in 2003 including corporatization and commodification – have been elaborating such that the very boundaries of bioeconomy are expanding.

Engaging "Life Itself": Individuals, Collectives, Populations

A third area of important theoretical work on changing conditions of possibility concerns how people are animated by and actively engaging these new biomedical potentialities individually (as embodied selves, vis-à-vis enhancements, and as users/consumers), collectively (especially in terms of health social movements), and as populations (especially in terms of "biological citizenship"). For example, Collier and Lakoff (2005, pp. 22–23) argue that "living" is becoming increasingly ethically problematic in terms of issues of biopolitics and technologies. Key sites of such ethical stakes often involve issues of *individual* enhancement, "unlike previous efforts in modernity to achieve progress through social and political institutions" (Hogle 2005, pp. 695). Knorr Cetina (2005, pp. S76–77) asserts that these constitute the rise of a "culture of life" within which developments in the biological sciences are encouraging the move away from concerns with humans in society and social salvation and toward ideals of individual perfectibility and enhancement. For example, Singh and Rose (2006, pp. 97) ask: "Can individuals resist/access the pharmaceutically powered drive toward perfection; is their personal agency sufficient to resist/access enhancing drugs, especially if they are very young, or poor, an ethnic minority, a convicted felon – or, for that matter, if they are students at elite competitive universities?" As we finalized this chapter, a local newspaper headline read "Experts Call for Wider Use of Brain Enhancing Drugs" (Tansey 2008, pp. A1).

Collectively, engaging "life itself" is largely the purview of "health social movements" or "patients' organizations," which also may engage ethical issues.[16] A major trend has been seeking further biomedicalization. For example, the AIDs movement challenged national biomedical research agendas (Epstein 1996), and civil rights and feminist movements contested the organizational principles of clinical trials in terms of gender and race vis-à-vis access and inclusion (Epstein 2007, 2008). Most distinctive is the trend toward direct sponsorship of research by patient groups themselves (Callon 2003), shaping new social identities based in both science and activism (Callon and Rabeharisoa 2003). These hybridities are remaking lay–expert relations and can be seen to both scientize social movements and mobilize scientists in new ways (Epstein 1996; Hess 1997; Ganchoff 2007). The salience of affect in such relations is also being explored (e.g., Silverman 2010).

---

[16]"Health social movements" or "patients' organizations" differ from other social movements in several key ways too complex to detail here. See Brown (2007), Brown and Zavetoski (2005), Allsop et al. (2004), Novas (2006), Landzelius (2006a), and Epstein (2008).

In terms of "life itself," new and reconstituted movements are now working for stem cell research (Ganchoff 2004, 2007), provoking research on environmental illnesses (Frickel 2004; Washburn 2009) and focusing on a wide array of diseases and conditions that may be treatable and perhaps even preventable using molecular technologies (e.g., Shostak 2003, 2004, 2005). Sites where life itself is engaged at the level of populations are also framed as "biocitizenship," often nation-state related.[17] Perhaps the broadest framing includes citizens' rights to both the protection and promotion of their health and well-being. For example, affirming claims of Chernobyl victims, Petryna (2002) has argued that citizens have rights to health services and social support – both care and protection as "biological citizens." For Americans, the profound inadequacies of governmental response to Hurricane Katrina were assessed through often tacit assumptions of biological citizenship.

In sum, these various incarnations of "bios," "life itself," and "vital politics" can be understood as forming an emergent and already dense theoretical web within which biomedicalization theory per se makes deeper sense. With Rabinow and Rose (2006), we do not see these changes as having a totalizing coherence but rather that fragmentation and contingency are rife as life itself is constantly negotiated afresh.

Critiques of Biomedicalization Theory

Conrad (2005, 2007) has offered the major critiques of biomedicalization theory to date. He (2005, pp. 5) has argued that the concept of biomedicalization paints with too broad a brush, and "attempts to be so comprehensive and inclusive" that it "loses focus on the definitional issues, which have always been a key to medicalization studies." While he (2007) agrees with much of what we identified as the rising complexities of biomedicine, he believes these changes are more a matter of expansion and degree, rather than representing "qualitatively different phenomena" (Conrad 2005, pp. 5). For him, these changes are better captured as shifts in the engines driving medicalization processes.

Conrad's points do echo issues that audiences have raised when we have presented biomedicalization theory in the USA and abroad. The main critiques have been (1) How much of this is actually new? (2) Is the concept too all-encompassing? (3) Is the concept overly determinative, attending too little to contingencies, counter-efforts, unintended consequences and the like? We address each in turn.

First, is biomedicalization qualitatively different? Is there something that is happening that can be characterized in ways distinct from medicalization? In the section above on "Situating Biomedicalization," we have elaborated how the contemporary situation has shifted in fundamental ways in societal, governmental (in both conventional and Foucauldian senses), and individual strategies to address health, disease, and the body. To recap, qualitatively different conditions of possibility for making jurisdictional claims about phenomena as "medical" derive today from all of the following: the now crucial importance of the biosciences and the biopolitical economy to the medical enterprise (indeed their imbrication), the rise and spread of biopower and biopolitics, and a progressive shifting in focus toward *transformation of* in addition to *control over* life itself.

In the concept of biomedicalization, we have kept intact the definitional processes that lie at the heart of medicalization theory. However, we do believe that these changing conditions, especially

---

[17] There is a growing literature on such forms of citizenship (e.g., Ginsberg and Rapp 1995; Nguyen 2005; Novas and Rose 2000; Petryna 2002; Rose 2001; Rose and Novas 2004).

vis-à-vis technoscience, indelibly affect both the range and kinds of processes, strategies, dynamics, and consequences of medicalization in important ways. Few American medical sociologists attend to the centrality of the life sciences or the computer and information sciences that are currently reorganizing them for biomedicine, or the changes happening in how we are conceptualizing "life itself." However, Hafferty (2006, pp. 42) recently argued that there are two "missing witnesses" in terms of understanding medicalization today: the capital market and science. This is indeed our argument. More broadly, the nature of biomedical interventions (as increasingly "inside out" and aimed at transformation), the interpenetration of sciences and technologies, and the increasing simultaneity of research–development–application (now institutionalized in the form of US governmental support for "clinical translational science") indicate more far-ranging pathways and qualitatively different approaches through which biomedical redefinition could happen. In our estimation, all this clearly called for a revised concept – biomedicalization – that directly gestures to the escalating complexity, multisitedness, and multidirectionality that are enabled by these twenty-first century conditions.

Second, is there not a sense in which biomedicalization is everything and everywhere? In response, we would emphasize that, as with medicalization, the five key processes of biomedicalization may or may not be present in any given empirical situation – which must be empirically examined. That said, however, we do believe that many more institutions (e.g., biotech start-ups and pharmaceutical companies), sociocultural ideas (e.g., about risk), technologies (both medical and informatic), and so on contribute to making medical jurisdictional claims, and participate in interventions on health, the body, life and death, than before. Through an examination of the literature and in the course of doing our own research, we identified the key processes as implicated in redefining all kinds of phenomena as "medical." That our listing includes so much is an indication of the enduring – and, many would argue (e.g., Franklin 2006a; Rose 2007a, c), growing – power of medical science and interventions.

But no one process is necessary or sufficient in and of itself and, conversely, all or most of them need not be present in order for some measure of biomedicalization to occur. Biomedicalization and its five key processes are, like any other theory, tools to think with. We and others have used biomedicalization as an overarching framework and its key processes as sensitizing concepts to systematically identify and trace what in an empirical site might potentially lead to the expansion of biomedical jurisdiction, and conversely, what might not (Clarke et al. 2010a).

Specifically, one could examine a particular topic of interest in terms of (1) the dynamics of its biopolitical economy; (2) precisely how it intensifies the focus on health (in addition to illness, disease, injury), on enhancement by technoscientific means, and on the elaboration of risk and surveillance at individual, group, and population levels; (3) how it elaborates the technoscientization of concrete biomedical practices; (4) how it engenders transformations of biomedical knowledge production, information management, distribution, and consumption; and/or (5) the kinds of transformations of bodies, selves, and new individual and collective technoscientific identities that are promoted. We believe that these analytics offer sociologists and others a "blueprint for the twenty-first century" – the project of this *Handbook* – for investigating the boundary-making activities of biomedicine. By following the lines of inquiry along the five processes of biomedicalization that we have identified, we hope that medical sociological research will better and more specifically illuminate how biomedicalization might vary across sites – and as importantly, how it is a fluid and ongoing process, as we discuss next.

Finally, a third critical perception of biomedicalization theory is that it feels overly deterministic. This observation could be an artifact of the second critique: the perception that biomedicalization is everything and everywhere contributes to the sense that it is also inescapable and inevitable. Thus, in addition to our response to the omnipresence critique above, we would add here that biomedicalization (and even its converse of de-biomedicalization) in many sites is a contingent, ongoing, provisional process, and not an achieved outcome that remains forever stable.

Moreover, an array of counter-trends against both medicalization and biomedicalization has gained momentum since World War II. These varied "pushbacks" include ongoing critiques of medicine, medicalization, and biomedicalization; people seeking help from beyond the boundaries of biomedicine, thereby expanding American medical pluralism; understanding patienthood as an increasingly fraught state; the elaboration of health social movements resistant to medicalization and biomedicalization; patient and related movements against specific forms of biomedicalization; a (re)emergent public discourse that "*more* (bio)medicine is not necessarily *better*"; and a growing discourse attempting to articulate "appropriate" levels and forms of biomedical intervention from the beginnings to the end of life (somewhat akin to the "appropriate technology movement") (see Clarke et al. 2010b).

Let us offer an example of the complexities. Certainly in many domains of health and illness in the West, the legitimacy of biomedicine as the first line of attack is largely unquestioned: for instance, in the treatment of AIDS, advanced heart disease, or diabetes. But even in such cases, one can find sites where biomedicalization is being contested and potentially contingent. For example, debates over the relative importance of genetic vs. behavioral vs. social causes of heart disease will have impacts on the kinds of interventions and disciplinary jurisdictions selected as policy. Possibilities here include pharmacogenomic therapies, public health lifestyle modification programs, and/or societal policies aimed at reducing social inequalities. The approach deemed most efficacious will inform whether biomedicalization occurs or not in that arena, and how, to what degree, and under what conditions (Shim 2002, 2010).

In sum, although we have characterized biomedicalization as a basic social process today, this does not presume that it is a fait accompli. It must be implemented – or not – again and again. Perhaps most of all, we see the possibilities and practices of biomedicalization and debiomedicalization as sites for exciting and innovative empirical work. Biomedicalization and medicalization are best understood as "keywords" in the social sciences that carry significant cultural weight (Williams 1976). Their deployment, definitions, and contours will therefore require ongoing interrogation and analysis.

Biomedicalization Theory in Action

The concept of biomedicalization has traveled widely and been used in multiple ways since its 2003 publication. We briefly summarize these here. Williams (2004), for example, views the "bio" in biomedicalization to imply that medical sociologists and others should be more deeply engaged with developments in biology per se in order to more fully comprehend "the biological body." We agree but would extend this to more fully comprehending relations between biomedical sciences and clinical practices.

A number of works use the concept of biomedicalization as an overarching process (like globalization). At times it was used seemingly instead of using medicalization, especially in aging research (e.g., Estes and Binney 1989; Estes et al. 2003). At times it was quite negatively inflected. For example, Midanik (2004, 2006; Midanik and Room 2005) critique biomedicalization as a social trend in the health field as legitimating biological reductionism – "seeing" alcohol(ism) solely in biological terms, excluding the social. Critical bioethicist Murray (2009) views the conjuncture of contemporary biomedicalization, neoliberalism, and biosocial/biocultural discourses as ultimately biofascist in relentlessly promoting biomedical approaches that seek not only to exclude but also to delegitimate alternative approaches and broader ethical considerations. While we might agree about such tendencies, for us, medicalization and biomedicalization need to be complicated. They can refer to "medical miracles" that wondrously alleviate pain and suffering *as well as* overpromoting their value. They refer to so many different things happening in such wildly divergent situations that we tend to agree with Bury (2006, pp. 38) that "drawing inferences about the impact of [bio] medicalization…is hazardous." Instead, using the five processes of biomedicalization as analytics to tease out the dynamics of particular cases (as detailed above) seems more useful than using the concept as a terminal critique.

Another group of scholars has interestingly used the concept of biomedicalization as framing emergent forms of "technogovernance." Here May et al. (2006; May 2007) argue that in clinical encounters, information technologies representing evidence-based data (e.g., population data), the guidelines, protocols, and decision-making tools themselves become nonhuman actors in clinical settings, mediating experiences of *both* patients and physicians (see also Timmermans and Kolker 2004; Vailly 2006; Novaes 2006). Such structural changes "reframe the clinical encounter in *corporate* rather than *private* time and space, and move key elements of interactional work within it between the *moral* and *managerial* practices of the clinical encounter" (May 2007, pp. 1022).

An array of risk studies has utilized biomedicalization theory. One emphasis has been biomedicalization as *treatment* for risk, such as Fosket's (2004) research on chemoprevention as treatment for breast cancer risk via an assessment tool available on the Internet. Fosket (2010) asserts that breast cancer risk is now biomedicalized as a disease per se. Preda (2005) argues that lifestyle as risk has been biomedicalized, especially vis-à-vis HIV/AIDS, portraying how quantification is very much a part of biomedicalization. In the domain of mental health, Orr (2006) examined the biomedicalization of panic disorder over half a century. Her current work (2010) takes up biopsychiatry and the ways in which risk diagnostics are produced in informatics and also made available on the Internet.

Studies of aging have found biomedicalization theory a helpful lens. Joyce and Mamo (2006) assert that research should "gray the cyborg" – attend to the intersectionality of age, technology, science, and gender. Using the five key processes of biomedicalization as analytics, they argue that how each is taken up in aging could be interrogated for its specifically ageist tropes. Processes of biomedicalization are also transforming late life. Technoscientific innovations are pushing when old age is believed to occur further into a receding future – one that is increasingly mutable and reversible, in stark contrast to previous expectations of age-associated decline (Kaufman et al. 2004; Shim et al. 2006). The broadening scope of medicine over the management of old age per se (rather than pathologies) (Kaufman et al. 2004), and the redefinition of old age as site for risk prevention (Shim et al. 2006) exemplify biomedicalization's intensified focus on health and the elaboration of risk. The case of kidney transplants to seniors from living donors, often their children, demonstrates how late-life extensions are reconfiguring familial obligations in new ways (Kaufman et al. 2006a). The French film "A Christmas Tale" vividly portrays the complexities of child-to-parent donation of bone marrow. And aging patients are taking up a new kind of "clinical life" (Shim et al. 2007), one that often includes an unprecedented willingness to allow intervention (Kaufman et al. 2006a), within a framework of emergent ethical obligations to promote ever-longer life (Kaufman et al. 2004).

Pursuing the molecular gaze with the analytics of biomedicalization, Prainsack (2006) frames the regulation of human cloning and stem cell research in Israel as "negotiating life."[18] She argues that it is not only religious commitments that have resulted in Israeli openness to cloning, but also population issues – viz. "the demographic threat" of Israelis being outnumbered by Palestinians. Patient organizations and movements around stem cell research are also pursued with the lenses of biomedicalization by Ganchoff (2004, 2007 see also Landzelius 2006a).

Other new work sustains our argument that health itself is being biomedicalized. For example, Nichter and Thompson's (2006) study of dietary supplements found they were "for my wellness,

---

[18] A conference on "Biomedicalization, New Social Conflicts, and the Politics of Bioethics" was held at the University of Vienna, Fall 2002, sponsored by Professor Herbert Gottweis. See also Prainsack and Siegal (2006).

not just my illness." Wheatley's (2005) ethnography of heart disease takes up rehabilitation and the biomedicalization of fitness. Cockerham (2005) argues that within this era of biomedicalization, there is a need for a healthy lifestyle theory that attends to structural dimensions. Yet others have utilized biomedicalization theory in terms of changes at the beginning and end of life (Kaufman and Morgan 2005; Timmermans and Mauck 2005), the Western and largely corporate appropriation of indigenous medicines (Waldram 2004; Barnes and Sered 2005), disability (Tremain 2005), Viagra and the biomedicalization of sexual dysfunction (Loe 2004; Potts et al. 2006; Fishman 2010), gender and headache (Kempner 2006), infertility (Friese et al. 2006), pharmaceutical interventions to prevent posttraumatic stress disorder (Henry et al. 2007), and disease representation and diagnosis (Clarke and Everest 2006; Joyce 2005, Joyce 2009; Rosenberg 2007).

Finally, we and our other colleagues have provided a set of nine case studies through which one can view "biomedicalization in action" (Clarke et al. 2010a). The case studies largely cluster around two main groupings: difference and enhancement. Studies of the biomedicalization of difference include the use of imaging technologies (Joyce 2010), lesbian conceptive practices (Mamo 2010; see also Mamo 2007a, b), the molecularization of environmental health (Shostak 2010), and race-based pharmaceuticals (Kahn 2010) and epidemiology (Shim 2010). Studies of biomedicalization via enhancement include bariatric surgery (Boero 2010), drugs for sexual dysfunction (Fishman 2010), drugs for preventing cancer (Fosket 2010), and biopsychiatry (Orr 2010).

As we predicted, the range of sites of biomedicalization keeps expanding. Burri and Dumit (2007, pp. 2–5) have recently asserted that there is a biomedicalization of society per se.

Medicalization, Biomedicalization, and Medical Sociology: An Agenda for the Future

One of the most enduring, if erroneous, critiques of medical sociology has been that it is atheoretical and merely applied.[19] Obviously medicalization and biomedicalization theories continue to provide serious challenges to this critique. Medicalization theory today is alive, well and highly productive in terms of generating and theoretically informing research. And from its inception, biomedicalization theory explicitly countered such assertions on several fronts: linkages to Foucault, to science, technology and medicine studies, and to the sociology of knowledge (Clarke et al. 2000, 2003). Today, biomedicalization theory is further situated theoretically vis-à-vis the exciting new generation of work centered around the biopolitical economy of health, illness, life, and death (above; see also Clarke et al. 2010b). The life sciences "matter" today both *within* medicine in terms of its technoscientific capacities, and *for* medicine in terms of setting the "conditions of possibility" vis-à-vis the legitimacy of intervening in "life itself" and optimizing its potential futures.

Biomedicalization theory dwells within the increasingly dense webs and assemblages being woven among biopolitical economy, the life sciences, technological interventions, human/animal/plant tissues and parts, and biological forms of citizenship transforming life itself. It provides enhanced traction through using the five key processes as analytics to empirically trace not only how biopolitical economy matters, but also how the precise sites of action and transformation of life itself do so as well. Biomedicalization theory has been recognized as pioneering in terms of extending medicalization theory to more broadly grasp and engage market/biocapital elements and the tremendous salience of

---

[19] In the American Sociological Association, the Medical Sociology Section is among the largest, reflecting the varied sites of employment of sociologists in teaching and research (e.g., NIH), as well as our domain of scholarly commitment. There is also a large Mental Health Section. However, medical sociology has not been prestigious in terms of curricular inclusion in leading American departments of sociology, although this situation seems to be changing.

the life sciences in the new millennium (e.g., Prainsack 2006; Hafferty 2006; Gottweis 2005; Cockerham 2005), especially in terms of "mapping the new genomic era" (Clarke et al. 2010d). Moreover, through theorizing biopolitical economy as integral to biomedicalization, we further link medical sociology to both economic sociology and political sociology/political science.[20] And through taking science and technology seriously, we link to science and technology studies and medical anthropology (e.g., Good and Good 2007; Inhorn 2007). All these disciplinary and specialty boundaries do seem to be highly porous if not melting in the face of vital politics and biomedicalization.

Future directions for research might include using the now nicely honed lenses of consumption studies to examine the modes and consequences of patients becoming consumers and biomedicine using the language and sales strategies of other consumer products and services (e.g., advertising).[21] Studying optimization would include what Frank (2004, pp. 21) has called technoluxe: "'Technoluxe' depends, first, on a view of the body as something to shape and of life as a project of shaping. It depends equally on the idea that projects are realized through acts of consumption."

An emergent topic in the literature is what we term the biomedicalization of defense – the growth of biomedical approaches to the development of weaponry (Vogel 2008) and warfare including the biological alteration of warriors by technoscientific means (Hogle 2003, 2005, 2008) and biosecurity (King 2005; Lentzos 2006; Braun 2007; Lakoff and Collier 2008), sadly a "growth industry." Another possible point of engagement for biomedicalization theory is to explore the potential consequences of evidence-based medicine for, for example, the growing tendency to move directly to highly sophisticated interventions rather than proceeding more "conservatively" medically, one rung up the ladder of care and intervention at a time (e.g., May et al. 2006; Mykhalovskiy and Weir 2004). The notion of biomedicalization offers possibilities for gaining better purchase on how new biomedical techniques, knowledges, and interventions impact prevailing definitions of difference and hierarchical relations. In turn, we need a better grasp on how ideas about race, gender, class, sexuality and so on propel selective and uneven biomedical efforts to transform, regulate, and optimize bodies and futures.

Also sorely needed are more explicit investigations of how biomedicalization is stratified in its objects, practices, and effects. That is, the unevenness of both medicalization and biomedicalization have been insufficiently theorized and researched. While this is of obvious importance in the USA and the West more broadly, the theory itself needs to be further elaborated to "take" analyses of biomedicalization global (e.g., Clarke 2009, 2010b). Studies of medical tourism will elaborate these concerns (e.g., Ramirez de Arellano 2007; Turner 2007).

Within biomedicalization theory, the legitimacy and practices of what Rose (2007a) calls "optimization" – efforts to enhance and secure "the best possible futures" for oneself – are becoming increasingly central. Beyond engaging with biocommodities and other biomedical enhancements in order to actualize optimal futures, optimization also involves new forms of engagement with regimes of risk and surveillance, of heightened responsibilities for knowledge accumulation and consumption. Optimization also involves the taking up of new kinds of biologically inflected individual and collective (including familial) identities, originally described as technoscientific identities (Clarke et al. 2003, pp. 182). Together, these new forms of subjectification point to the duties and burdens of authorizing and making one's own – and others' – futures.

This constant orientation towards the future – which socioculturally parallels the bioeconomic and biopolitical focus on promissory capital – gives a greater temporal dimension to biomedicalization theory. In these senses, then, biomedicalization theory is anticipatory – offering a conceptual frame for analyzing the emergent, the about-to-be, the evanescent (Adams et al. 2009). This is a useful part of a "blueprint for medical sociology in the twenty-first century" indeed!

---

[20] Other recent work has also linked science and technology studies to these fields as well (e.g., Callon 2003; Gottweis 1998, 2005; Mirowski 2004).

[21] Henderson and Petersen (2002) have pursued this viz. medicalization. On consumption studies, see e.g., Applbaum (2004), Hearn and Roseneil (1999), and Lury (2004).

Acknowledgements The authors are deeply indebted to Laura Mamo, Jennifer Fosket and Jennifer Fishman with whom we developed much of the work on biomedicalization upon which we draw here, and for comments on an earlier version of this chapter.

References

Adams V (2002) Randomized controlled crime: postcolonial sciences in alternative medicine research. Soc Stud Sci 32:659–690.
Adams V, Murphy M, Clarke AE (2009) Anticipation: technoscience, life, affect, temporality. Subjectivity 28:246–265
Allsop J, Jones K, Baggott R (2004) Health consumer groups in the UK: a new social movement? Sociol Health Illn 26(6):737–756
Amsterdamska O, Hiddinga A (2004) Trading zones or citadels? Professionalization and intellectual change in the history of medicine. In: Huisman F, Warner JH (eds) Locating medical history: the stories and their meanings. The Johns Hopkins University Press, Baltimore, MD, pp 237–261
Applbaum K (2004) The marketing era: from professional practice to global provisioning. Routledge, New York
Armstrong D (1983) Political anatomy of the body: medical knowledge in Britain in the twentieth century. Cambridge University Press, Cambridge, UK
Armstrong D (2002) A new history of identity: a sociology of medical knowledge. Palgrave, London
Atkinson P, Glasner P, Greenslade H (eds) (2007) New genetics, new identities. Routledge, London
Ballard K, Elston ME (2005) Medicalization: a multi-dimensional concept. Soc Theory Health 3:228–241
Barnes LL, Sered SS (eds) (2005) Religion and healing in America. Oxford University Press, New York
Bauer M (1998) The medicalization of science news: from the 'rocket-scalpel' to the 'gene-meteorite' complex. Social Science Information/Information sur les Sciences Sociales 37:731–751
Berenson A (2005) Sales of drugs for impotence are declining. The New York Times. 4 Dec 2005, p 34
Bergeron V (2007) The ethics of cesarean section on maternal request: a feminist critique of the American College of Obstetricians and Gynecologists' position on patient-choice surgery. Bioethics 21(9):478–487
Binstock RH, Fishman JR (2010) Social dimensions of anti-aging science and medicine. In: Dannefer D, Phillipson C (eds) SAGE handbook of social gerontology. University of Chicago Press, Chicago
Boero N (2010) Bypassing blame: bariatric surgery and the case of biomedical failure. In: Clarke A, Fosket J, Mamo L, Shim J, Fishman J (eds) Biomedicalization: technoscience and transformations of health and illness in the US. Duke University Press, Durham, NC, pp 307–330
Brandt AM, Gardner M (2000) The golden age of medicine? In: Cooter R, Pickstone J (eds) Medicine in the twentieth century. Harwood, Amsterdam, pp 21–38
Braun B (2007) Biopolitics and the molecularization of life. Cult Geogr 14:6–28
Brenner S (2000) Genomics: the end of the beginning. Science 287(5461):2173–2174
Brown P (2007) Toxic exposures: contested illnesses and the environmental health movement. Columbia University Press, New York
Brown P, Zavetoski S (eds) (2005) Social movements in health. Blackwell, Malden, MA
Brownlee S (2007) Overtreated: why too much medicine is making us sicker and poorer. Bloomsbury, London
Brumberg JJ (1997) The body project: an intimate history of American girls. Random House, New York
Burri RV, Dumit J (eds) (2007) Biomedicine as culture: instrumental practices, technoscientific knowledge, and new modes of life. Routledge, New York
Bury M (2006) Dominance from above and below. Society 43(6):37–40
Callon M (2003) The increasing involvement of concerned groups in R&D policies: what lessons for public powers? In: Geuna A, Salter AJ, Steinmueller WE (eds) Science and innovation: rethinking the rationales for funding and governance. Edward Elgar, Cheltenham, UK, pp 30–68
Callon M, Rabeharisoa V (2003) Research "in the wild" and the shaping of new social identities. Technol Soc 25(2):193–204
Canguilhem G (1966/1994) The concept of life. In: Delaporte F (ed) A vital rationalist: writings from Georges Canguilhem (trans. Arthur Goldhammer). Zone Books, New York, pp 302–320
Casper MJ, Berg M (1995) Introduction to special issue on constructivist perspectives on medical work: medical practices in science and technology studies. Sci Technol Hum Values 20(4):395–407
Casper MJ, Koenig B (1996) Introduction: reconfiguring nature and culture: intersections of medical anthropology and technoscience studies. Med Anthropol Q 10(4):523–536
Casper MJ, Muse C (2006) Genital fixations: what's wrong with treating intersex in the womb? American Sexuality Magazine (NSRC). www.nsrc.sfsu.edu/MagArticle.cfm?Article=595&ReturnURL=1

Centers for Medicare and Medicaid Services (2008a) National health expenditure data: NHE fact sheet. http://www.cms.hhs.gov/NationalHealthExpendData/25_NHE_Fact_Sheet.asp. Accessed 26 Feb 2008

Centers for Medicare and Medicaid Services (2008b) NHE Projections 2007–2017, Forecast summary and selected tables. http://www.cms.hhs.gov/NationalHealthExpendData/Downloads/proj2007.pdf. Accessed 20 Mar 2008

Cetina KK (2005) The rise of a culture of life. EMBO Rep 6:S76–S80

Chervenak FA, McCullough LB (2005) An ethical critique of boutique fetal imaging: a case for the medicalization of fetal imaging. Am J Obstet Gynecol 192(1):31–33

Clarke AE (1995) Modernity, postmodernity and reproductive processes ca. 1890–1990 or, 'mommy, where do cyborgs come from anyway?' In Gray, CR Figueroa-Sarriera, H Mentor S (eds) The cyborg handbook. Routledge, New York, pp 139–156

Clarke AE (1990) Controversy and the development of reproductive sciences. Soc Probl 37(1):18–37

Clarke AE (1998) Disciplining reproduction: modernity, American life sciences, and 'the problems of sex. University of California Press, Berkeley

Clarke AE (2000) Maverick reproductive scientists and the production of contraceptives c1915–2000. In: Saetnan A, Oudshoorn N, Kirejczyk M (eds) Bodies of technology: women's involvement with reproductive medicine. Ohio State University Press, Columbus, pp 37–89

Clarke AE (2007) Reflections on the reproductive sciences in agriculture in the UK and US, c1900-2000. Hist Philos Biol Biomed Sci 38(2):316–339

Clarke AE (2010a) From the rise of medicine to biomedicalization: U.S. healthscapes and iconography c1890-present. In: Clarke A, Fosket J, Mamo L, Shim J, Fishman J (eds) Biomedicalization: technoscience and transformations of health and illness in the US. Duke University Press, Durham, NC, pp 104–146

Clarke AE (2010b) Biomedicalization in its transnational travels. In: Clarke A, Fosket J, Mamo L, Shim J, Fishman J (eds) Biomedicalization: technoscience and transformations of health and illness in the US. Duke University Press, Durham, NC, pp 380–406

Clarke AE (2009) Introduction: gender and reproductive technologies in East Asia. East Asian Sci Technol Stud 2(3):303–326

Clarke AE, Mamo L, Fosket JR, Fishman JR, Shim JK (2000) Technoscience and the new biomedicalization: Western roots, global rhizomes. [In French]. Sciences Sociales et Sante 18(2):11–42

Clarke AE, Shim JK, Mamo L, Fosket JR, Fishman JR (2003) Biomedicalization: technoscientific transformations of health, illness, and U.S. biomedicine. Am Sociol Rev 68:161–194

Clarke AE, Fishman JR, Fosket JR, Mamo L, Shim JK (2004) Biomedicalization: technoscientific transformation of health, illness and US biomedicine. In Conrad P (ed) The sociology of health and illness, 7th edn. St. Martin's, New York, pp 442–455

Clarke AE, Fosket JR, Mamo L, Shim JK, Fishman JR (eds) (2010a) Biomedicalization: technoscience and transformations of health and illness in the U.S. Duke University Press, Durham, NC

Clarke AE, Shim J, Mamo L, Fosket J, Fishman J (2010b) Biomedicalization: a theoretical and substantive introduction. In: Clarke A, Fosket J, Mamo L, Shim J, Fishman J (eds) Biomedicalization: technoscience and transformations of health and illness in the US. Duke University Press, Durham, NC, 1–46

Clarke AE, Shim JK, Mamo L, Fosket JR, Fishman JR (2010c) Charting (bio)medicine and (bio)medicalization in the United States, 1890-present. In: Clarke A, Fosket J, Mamo L, Shim J, Fishman J (eds) Biomedicalization: technoscience and transformations of health and illness in the US. Duke University Press, Durham, NC, pp 88–103

Clarke AE, Shim JK, Shostak S, Nelson A (2009) Biomedicalisation of Health and Identity. In: Atkinson P, Glasner P, Lock M (eds) Handbook of genetics and society: mapping the new genomic era. Routledge, London

Clarke JN, Everest MM (2006) Cancer in the mass print media: fear, uncertainty and the medical model. Soc Sci Med 62(10):2591–2600

Cockerham WC (2005) Health lifestyle theory and the convergence of agency and structure. J Health Soc Behav 46(1):51–67

Cohen L (2005) Operability, bioavailability and exception. In: Ong A, Collier SJ (eds) Global assemblages: technology, politics, and ethics as anthropological problems. Blackwell, Malden, MA, pp 79–90

Conrad P (1992) Medicalization and social control. Annu Rev Sociol 18:209–232

Conrad P (2005) The shifting engines of medicalization. J Health Soc Behav 46(1):3–14

Conrad P (2006) Up, down, and sideways. Society 43(6):19–20

Conrad P (2007) The medicalization of society: on the transformation of human conditions into treatable disorders. Johns Hopkins University Press, Baltimore

Conrad P, Leiter V (2004) Medicalization, markets and consumers. J Health Soc Behav 45:158–176

Conrad P, Potter D (2004) Human growth hormone and the temptations of biomedical enhancement. Sociol Health Illn 26(2):184–215

Conrad P, Schneider J (1980a/1992) Deviance and medicalization: from badness to sickness. Mosby, St. Louis/ Temple University Press, Philadelphia, exp. ed

Conrad P, Schneider J (1980b) Looking at levels of medicalization: a comment on strong's critique of the thesis of medical imperialism. Soc Sci Med 14A:75–79
Crawford R (2004) Risk ritual and the management of control and anxiety in medical culture. Health 8(4):505–528
Critser G (2005) Generation RX: how prescription drugs are altering American lives, minds, and bodies. Houghton Mifflin, New York
Daemmrich A (2004) Pharmacopolitics: drug regulation in the United States and Germany. University of North Carolina Press, Chapel Hill
Darby R (2005) The sorcerer's apprentice: why can't we stop circumcising boys? Contexts 4(2):34–39
Davis JE (2006) How medicalization lost its way. Society 43(6):51–56
Davis-Berman J, Pestello FG (2005) The medicated self. Stud Symbol Interact 28:283–308
Dingwall R (2006) Imperialism or encirclement? Society 43(6):30–36
Dumit J (2005) Virtually unlimited health imperatives: risk trafficking and prescription maximization. Presentation at the Stanford Seminar on Science, Technology, and Society, Spring
Eisenberg DM, Davis RB, Ettner SL, Appel S, Wilkey S, Van Rompay M, Kessler RC (1998) Trends in alternative medicine use in the U.S., 1990–1997: results of a follow-up national survey. J Am Med Assoc 280:1569–1575
Epstein S (1996) Impure science: AIDS, activism, and the politics of knowledge. University of California Press, Berkeley
Epstein S (2007) Inclusion: the politics of difference in medical research. University of Chicago Press, Chicago
Epstein S (2008) Patient groups and health movements. In: Hackett EJ, Amsterdamska O, Lynch M, Wajcman J (eds) Handbook of science and technology studies. MIT Press, Cambridge, MA, pp 499–540
Estes CL, Binney E (1989) The biomedicalization of aging: dangers and dilemmas. Gerontologist 29:587–595
Estes CL, Biggs S, Phillipson C (2003) Biomedicalization, ethics and aging. In: Estes CL, Biggs S, Phillipson C (eds) Social theory, social policy and aging. Open University Press, Maidenhead, pp 79–101
Fischer M (1999) Emergent forms of life: anthropologies of late or postmodernities. Annu Rev Anthropol 28:455–478
Fishman JR (2004) Maufacturing desire: the commodification of female sexual dysfunction. Soc Stud Sci 34(2)187–218
Fishman JR (2010) Viagra and the biomedicalization of sexual dysfunction. Clarke A, Fosket J, Mamo L, Shim J, Fishman J (eds) Biomedicalization: technoscience and transformations of health and illness in the US. Duke University Press, Durham, NC, pp 289–306
Fleck L (1935/1979) Genesis and development of a scientific fact. University of Chicago Press, Chicago IL
Fosket J (2004) Constructing 'high risk' women: the development and standardization of a breast cancer risk assessment tool. Sci Technol Hum Values 29(3):291–323
Fosket JR (2010) Breast cancer risk as disease: biomedicalizing risk. In: Clarke A, Fosket J, Mamo L, Shim J, Fishman J (eds) Biomedicalization: technoscience and transformations of health and illness in the US. Duke University Press, Durham, NC, pp 331–352
Foucault M (1970) The order of things: an archeology of the human sciences. Vintage, New York
Foucault M (1975) Birth of the clinic: an archaeology of medical perception. Vintage, New York
Foucault M (1979) Discipline and punish. Vintage, New York
Foucault M (1984) Biopower. In: Rabinow P (ed) The Foucault reader. Pantheon Books, New York, pp 258–289
Fox RC (2001) Medical uncertainty revisited. In: Bendelow G, Carpenter M, Vautier C, Williams S (eds) Gender, health and healing: the public/private divide. Routledge, London, pp 236–253
Fox N, Ward K (2006) Health identities: from expert patient to resisting consumer. Health 10(4):461–479
Frank AW (2004) Emily's scars: surgical shapings, technoluxe, and bioethics. Hastings Cent Rep 34(2):18–29
Franklin S (2000) Life itself: global nature and the genetic imaginary. In: Franklin S, Lurie C, Stacey J (eds) Global nature, global culture. Sage, London, pp 188–227
Franklin S (2003) Ethical biocapital: new strategies of cell culture. In: Franklin S, Lock M (eds) Remaking life and death: toward an anthropology of the biosciences, School of American research advanced seminar series. Santa Fe, New Mexico, pp 97–128
Franklin S (2006a) Mapping biocapital: new frontiers of bioprospecting. Cult Geogr 13(2):301–304
Franklin S (2006b) Embryonic economies: the double reproductive value of stem cells. BioSocieties 1(1):71–90
Franklin S (2007) Dolly mixtures: the remaking of genealogy. Duke University Press, Durham, NC
Franklin S, Lock M (2003) Animation and cessation: the remaking of life and death. In: Franklin S, Lock M (eds) Remaking life and death: toward an anthropology of the biosciences, School of American research advanced seminar series. Santa Fe, New Mexico, pp 3–22
Franklin S, Roberts C (2006) Born and made: an ethnography of preimplantation genetic diagnosis. Princeton University Press, Princeton NJ
Freidson E (1970) Profession of medicine: a study in the sociology of applied knowledge. University of Chicago Press, Chicago
Freidson E (2001) Professionalism: the third logic. University of Chicago Press, Chicago IL

Frickel S (2004) Chemical consequences: environmental mutagens, scientist activism, and the rise of genetic toxicology. Rutgers University Press, New Brunswick, NJ

Friese, C Becker, G Nachtigal, R (2006) Rethinking the Biological Clock: Eleventh-hour Moms, Miracle Moms, and Meanings of Age-Related Infertility. Social Science and Medicine 63(6): 1550–1560

Friese C (2007) Enacting conservation and biomedicine: cloning animals of endangered species in the cultures of late modernity. Ph.D. dissertation, Department of Social and Behavioral Sciences, University of California, San Francisco

Furedi F (2006) The end of professional dominance. Society 43(6):14–18

Ganchoff C (2004) Regenerating movements: embryonic stem cells and the politics of potentiality. Sociol Health Illn 26:757–774

Ganchoff C (2007) Regenerating movements: stem cells and the politics of potentiality, Ph.D. dissertation. Department of Social and Behavioral Sciences, University of California, San Francisco

Gibbon S (2007) Breast cancer genes and the gendering of knowledge: science and citizenship in the cultural context of the 'new' genetics. Palgrave, London

Gibbon S, Novas C (2008) Introduction. In: Gibbon S, Novas C (eds) Biosocialities, genetics and the social sciences: making biologies and identities. Routledge, London, pp 1–18

Ginsberg F, Rapp R (eds) (1995) Conceiving the new world order: the global politics of reproduction. University of California Press, Berkeley

Good M-JD, Good B (2000) Parallel sisters': medical anthropology and medical sociology. In: Bird CE, Conrad P, Fremont AM (eds) Handbook of medical sociology, 5th edn. Prentice Hall, Upper Saddle River, NJ

Gottweis H (1998) Governing molecules: the discursive politics of genetic engineering in Europe and the United States. MIT Press, Cambridge, MA

Gottweis H (2005) Governing genomics in the 21st century: between risk and uncertainty. New Genetics and Society 24(2):175–193

Hackett EJ, Amsterdamska O, Lynch M, Wajcman J (eds) (2008) Handbook of science and technology studies. MIT Press, 3rd ed. Cambridge, MA

Hafferty FW (2006) Medicalization reconsidered. Society 43(6):41–46

Hahn H, Belt TL (2004) Disability identity and attitudes toward cure in a sample of disabled activists. J Health Soc Behav 45(4):453–464

Halpern SA. (2004) Lesser harms: the morality of risk in medical research. University of Chicago Press, Chicago, IL

Haraway D (2004) The Haraway reader. Routledge, New York

Haraway D (2007) When species meet (posthumanities). University of Minnesota Press, Miimeapolis, MN

Harrington A, Rose N, Singh I (2006) Editors' introduction. BioSocieties 1(1):1–5

Hayden C (2003) When nature goes public: the making and unmaking of bioprospecting in Mexico. Princeton University Press, Princeton

Healy D (2002) Let them eat Prozac. New York University Press, New York

Hearn J, Roseneil S (eds) (1999) Consuming cultures: power and resistance. Macmillan, London

Hedgecoe A (2004) The politics of personalised medicine: pharmacogenetics in the clinic. Cambridge University Press, Cambridge

Henderson S, Petersen A (eds) (2002) Consuming health: the commodification of health care. Routledge, London and New York

Henry M, Fishman JR, Youngner SJ (2007) Propranolol and the prevention of post-traumatic stress disorder: is it wrong to erase the 'sting' of bad memories? Am J Bioeth 7(9):12–20

Hess DJ (1997) Science studies: an advanced introduction. NYU Press, New York

Hogle L (2002) Introduction: jurisdictions of authority and expertise in science and medicine. Med Anthropol 21:231–246

Hogle L (2003) Life/time warranty: rechargeable cells and extendable lives. In: Franklin S, Lock M (eds) Remaking life and death: toward an anthropology of the biosciences, School of American research advanced seminar series. Santa Fe, New Mexico, pp 61–96

Hogle LF (2005) Enhancement technologies and the body. Annu Rev Anthropol 34:695–716

Hogle L (2008) Emerging medical technologies. In: Hackett EJ, Amsterdamska O, Lynch M, Wajcman J (eds) The new handbook of science and technology studies. MIT Press, Cambridge, MA, pp 841–874

Horton R (2000) How sick is modern medicine? The New York Review. 2 Nov 2000, pp 46–50

Horwitz AV (2002) Creating mental illness. University of Chicago Press, Chicago IL

Illich I (1975) Medical nemesis. Pantheon, New York

Inhorn M (2007) Medical anthropology at the intersections. Medical Anthropology Quarterly 21(3): 249–55

Jasanoff S (2005) Designs on nature: science and democracy in Europe and the United States. Princeton University Press, Princeton

Jasso-Aquilar R, H Waitzkin, Landwehr A (2004) Multinational corporations and health care in the United States and Latin America. J Health Soc Behav 45(Extra Issue):136–157

Jones C, Porter R (eds) (1994) Reassessing Foucault: power, medicine and the body. Routledge, London

Jordanova L (2004) The social construction of medical knowledge. In: Huisman F, Warner JH (eds) Locating medical history: the stories and their meanings. The Johns Hopkins University Press, Baltimore, pp 338–363

Joyce K (2010) The body as image-commodity: an examination of the economic and political dynamics of magnetic resonance imaging and the shift towards visualization. In: Clarke A, Fosket J, Mamo L, Shim J, Fishman J (eds) Biomedicalization: technoscience and transformations of health and illness in the US. Duke University Press, Durham, NC, pp 197–217

Joyce, K (2005) Appealing Images: Magnetic Resonance Imaging and the Production of Authoritative Knowledge. Soc Stud Sci 35(3):437–462

Joyce K, Mamo L (2006) Graying the cyborg: new directions in feminist analyses of aging, science, and technology. In: Calasanti T, Slevin KF (eds) Age matters: realigning feminist thinking. Routledge, New York, pp 99–122

Kahn J (2010) Surrogate markers and surrogate marketing in biomedicine: the regulatory etiology and commercial progression of "ethnic" drug development. In: Clarke A, Fosket J, Mamo L, Shim J, Fishman J (eds) Biomedicalization: technoscience and transformations of health and illness in the US. Duke University Press, Durham NC, pp 263–288

Kaufman SR (2005) …And a Time to Die: how American Hospitals Shape the End of Life. Scribner, New York

Kaufman SR, Morgan L (2005) The anthropology of the beginnings and ends of life. Annu Rev Anthropol 34:317–341

Kaufman SR, Shim JK, Russ AJ (2004) Revisiting the biomedicalization of aging: clinical trends and ethical challenges. Gerontologist 44(6):731–738

Kaufman SR, Russ AJ, Shim JK (2006a) Aged bodies and kinship matters: the ethical field of kidney transplant. Am Ethnol 33(1):81–99

Kaufman SR, Shim JK, Russ AJ (2006b) Old age, life extension, and the character of medical choice. J Gerontol Soc Sci 61B(4):S175–S184

Kay LE (1993) Life as technology: representing, intervening and molecularizing. Rivista di Storia Scienza [NS] 1(2):85–103

Keller EF (2000) The century of the gene. Harvard University Press, Cambridge, MA

Kelner MJ, Wellman B, Pescosolido B, Saks M (2000) Complementary and alternative medicine: challenge and change. Gordon and Breach, Amsterdam

Kempner J (2006) Gendering the migraine market: do representations of illness matter? Soc Sci Med 63(8):1986–1997

Kerr A, Franklin S (2006) Genetic ambivalence: expertise, uncertainty and communication in the context of new genetic technologies. In: Webster A (ed) New technologies in healthcare: challenge, change and innovation. Palgrave, London, pp 40–56

King NB (2005) The ethics of biodefense. Bioethics 19(4):432–446

Lakoff A (2005) Pharmaceutical reason: knowledge and value in global psychiatry. Cambridge University Press, West Nyack, NY

Lakoff A (2008) The right patients for the drug: pharmaceutical circuits and the codification of illness. In: Hackett EJ, Amsterdamska O, Lynch M, Wajcman J (eds) The new handbook of science and technology studies. MIT Press, Cambridge, MA, pp 741–760

Lakoff A, Collier SJ (eds) (2008) Biosecurity interventions: global health and security in question. Columbia University Press, New York

Landzelius K (2006a) Introduction: patient organization movements and new metamorphoses in patienthood. Soc Sci Med 62(3):529–537

Landzelius K (2006b) The incubation of a social movement? Preterm babies, parent activists, and neonatal productions in the U.S. context. Soc Sci Med 62(3):668–682

Lash S (2001) Technological forms of life. Theory Cult Soc 18(1):105–120

Latour B (1987) Science in action: how to follow scientists and engineers through society. Harvard University Press, Cambridge, MA

Lee S, Mysyk A (2004) The medicalization of compulsive buying. Soc Stud Med 58:1709–1718

Lentzos F (2006) Rationality, risk and response: a research agenda for biosecurity. BioSocieties 1(4):453–464

Light DW (2004) Introduction: ironies of success – a new history of the American health care 'system'. J Health Soc Behav 45(Extra Issue):1–24

Lock M (1993) Encounters with aging: mythologies of menopause in Japan and North America. University of California Press, Berkeley

Lock M (2001) Medicalization: an expansive concept. In: Smelser NJ, Baltes PB (eds) International encyclopedia of the social and behavioral sciences. Elsevier, Oxford, UK

Lock M (2002a) Biomedical technologies: anthropological approaches. In: Ember CR, Ember M (eds) Encyclopedia of medical anthropology: health and illness in the world's cultures. Springer, New York, pp 86–95

Lock M (2002b) Introduction: from documenting medical pluralism to critical interpretations of globalized health knowledge, policies, and practices. In: Nichter M, Lock M (eds) New horizons in medical anthropology: essays in honour of Charles Leslie. Routledge, London, pp 1–34

Lock M (2004) Medicalization and the naturalization of social control. In: Ember CR, Ember M (eds) Encyclopedia of medical anthropology: health and illness in the world's cultures. Springer, New York, pp 116–125

Lock M (2008) Biomedical technologies, cultural horizons, and contested boundaries. In: Hackett EJ, Amsterdamska O, Lynch M, Wajcman J (eds) The new handbook of science and technology studies. MIT, Cambridge, MA, pp 875–900

Loe M (2004) The rise of Viagra: how the little blue pill changed sex in America. New York University Press, New York

Lorber J, Moore LJ (2002) Gender and the social construction of illness, 2nd edn. Walnut Creek, Rowman & Littlefield, California

Lupton D (2003) Medicine as culture: illness, disease and the body in Western society, 2nd edn. Sage, London

Lury C (2004) Brands: the logos of the global economy. Routledge, London

Malacrida C (2004) Medicalization, ambivalence and social control: mothers' descriptions of educators and ADD/ADHD. Health 8(1):61–80

Mamo L (2007a) Queering reproduction: achieving pregnancy in the age of technoscience. Duke University Press, Durham, NC

Mamo L (2007b) Negotiating conception: lesbians' hybrid-technological practices. Sci Technol Hum Values 32(3):369–393

Mamo L (2010) Fertility Inc.: consumption and subjectification in lesbian reproductive practices. In: Clarke A, Fosket J, Mamo L, Shim J, Fishman J (eds) Biomedicalization: technoscience and transformations of health and illness in the U.S. Duke University Press, Durham, NC, pp 173–196

Mamo L, Fosket JR (2009) Scripting the body: pharmaceuticals and the (re)making of menstruation. Signs 34(4):925–949

Martin E (2006) The pharmaceutical person. BioSocieties 1(3):273–288

Martin JK, Pescosolido BA, Olafsdottir S, McLeod JD (2007) The construction of fear: Americans' preferences for social distance from children and adolescents with mental health problems. J Health Soc Behav 48(1):50–67

May C (2007) The clinical encounter and the problem of context. Sociology 41(1):29–45

May C, Rapley T, Moreira T, Finch T, Heaven B (2006) Technogovernance: evidence, subjectivity, and the clinical encounter in primary care medicine. Soc Sci Med 62(4):1022–1030

McKinlay JB, Marceau LD (2002) The end of the golden age of doctoring. Int J Health Serv 32(2):379–416

Mechanic D (2002) Socio-cultural implications of changing organizational technologies in the provision of care. Soc Sci Med 54:459–467

Midanik LT (2004). Biomedicalization and alcohol studies: implications for policy. J Public Health Policy 25(2):211–228

Midanik LT (2006) Biomedicalization of alcohol studies. Transaction, Piscataway, NJ

Midanik L, Room R (2005) Contributions of social science to the alcohol field in an era of biomedicalization. Soc Sci Med 60:1107–1116

Mirowski P (2004) The effortless economy of science? Duke University Press, Durham, NC

Moynihan R, Cassels A (2005) Selling sickness: how the world's biggest pharmaceutical companies are turning us all into patients. Nation Books, New York

Murcott A (ed) (2006) Sociology and medicine: selected papers by P.M. Strong. Ashgate, Burlington VT

Murray SJ (2009) The perils of scientific obedience: bioethics under the spectre of biofascism. In: Murray SJ, Holmes D (eds) Critical interventions in the ethics of healthcare: challenging the principle of autonomy in bioethics. Ashgate, Surrey, UK

Mykhalovskiy E, Weir L (2004) The problem of evidence-based medicine: directions for social science. Soc Sci Med 59:1059–1069

Nadesan M (2005) Constructing autism. Routledge, New York

Navarro V (1986) Crisis, health and medicine. Tavistock, New York

Navarro V (ed) (2007) Neoliberalism, globalization and inequalities: consequences for health and quality of life. Baywood, Amityville, NY

Nelkin D (1995) Scientific controversies. In: Jasanoff S, Markle GE, Petersen JC, Pinch T (eds) Handbook of science and technology studies. Sage, Thousand Oaks, CA, pp 444–456

Nelkin D, Lindee MS (2004) The DNA mystique: the gene as a cultural icon. University of Michigan Press, Ann Arbor, MI

Nguyen V-K (2005) Antiretroviral globalism, biopolitics and therapeutic citizenship. In: Ong A, Collier SJ (eds) Global assemblages: technology, politics, and ethics as anthropological problems. Blackwell, Malden, MA, pp 124–144

Nichter M, Thompson JJ (2006) For my wellness, not just my illness: North Americans' use of dietary supplements. Cult Med Psychiatry 30(2):175–222

Novaes HMD (2006) From production to evaluation of health systems technologies: challenges for the 21st century. Revista de Saude Publ 40(spl issue):133–140

Novas C (2006) The political economy of hope: patients' organizations, science and biovalue. BioSocieties 1(3):289–306

Novas C, Rose N (2000) Genetic risk and the birth of the somatic individual. Econ Soc 29(4):485–513

Nye RA (2003) The evolution of the concept of medicalization in the late twentieth century. J Hist Behav Sci 39(2):115–129

Orr J (2006) Panic diaries: a genealogy of panic disorder. Duke University Press, Durham, NC

Orr J (2010) Biopsychiatry and the informatics of diagnosis: governing mentalities. In: Clarke A, Fosket J, Mamo L, Shim J, Fishman J (eds) Biomedicalization: technoscience and transformations of health and illness in the U.S. Duke University Press, Durham, NC, pp 353–379

Parens E (2006) Surgically shaping children: technology, ethics and the pursuit of normality. Johns Hopkins University Press, Baltimore, MD

Pauly PJ (1987) Controlling life: Jacques Loeb and the engineering ideal in biology. Oxford University Press, New York

Pescosolido BA (2006) Professional dominance and the limits of erosion. Society 43(6):21–29

Pescosolido BA, Martin JK (2004) Cultural authority and the sovereignty of American medicine: the role of networks, class and community. J Health Health Policy Law 29(4–5):735–755

Petryna A (2002) Life exposed: biological citizens after Chernobyl. Princeton University Press, Princeton, NJ

Pfohl SJ (1985) Images of deviance and social control: a sociological history. McGraw Hill, New York

Potts A, Grace VM, Vares T, Gavey N (2006) 'Sex for life'? Men's counter-stories on 'erectile dysfunction', male sexuality and aging. Sociol Health Illn 28(3):306–329

Prainsack B (2006) 'Negotiating life': the regulation of human cloning and embryonic stem cell research in Israel. Soc Stud Sci 36(2):173–205

Preda A (2005) AIDS, rhetoric, and medical knowledge. Cambridge University Press, New York

Quadagno J (2005) One nation, uninsured: why the U.S. has no national health insurance. Oxford University Press, New York, NY

Rabinow P (1992a) Artificiality and enlightenment: from sociobiology to biosociality. In: Crary J, Kwinter S (eds) Incorporations. Zone, New York, pp 234–252

Rabinow P (1992b) Severing the ties: fragmentation and dignity in late modernity. Knowl Soc Anthropol Sci Technol 9:169–187

Rabinow P (2008) Afterword: concept work. In: Gibbon S, Novas C (eds) Biosocialities, genetics and the social sciences: making biologies and identities. Routledge, London, pp 188–192

Rabinow P, Rose N (2006) Biopower today. BioSocieties 1:195–217

Radley A, Lupton D, Ritter C (1997) Health: an invitation and an introduction. Health 1:5–21

Rafalovich A (2005) Relational troubles and semiofficial suspicion: educators and the medicalization of 'unruly' children. Symbol Interact 28(1):25–46

Rajan KS (2006) Biocapital: the constitution of postgenomic Life. Duke University Press, Durham NC

Ramirez de Arellano A (2007) Patients without borders: the emergence of medical tourism. Int J Health Serv 37:193–198

Restivo, 5, Croissant J (2007) Social constructionism in science and technology studies. In Holstein JA, Gubrium, JF (eds) Handbook of constructionist research, Guilford Press, New York, NY, pp 2 13–230

Riska E (2004) Masculinity and men's health: coronary heart disease in medical and public discourse. Rowman & Littlefield, Lanham, MD

Riska E (2010) Gendering the medicalization and biomedicalization theses. In: Clarke A, Fosket J, Mamo L, Shim J, Fishman J (eds) Biomedicalization: technoscience and transformations of health and illness in the US. Duke University Press, Durham, NC, pp 147–172

Rose N (2007a) The politics of life itself: biomedicine, power and subjectivity in the twenty-first century. Princeton University Press, Princeton, NJ

Rose N (2007b) Beyond medicalisation. Lancet 369:700–702

Rose N (2007c) Molecular politics, somatic ethics and the spirit of biocapital. Soc Theory Health 5:3–29

Rose N, Novas C (2004) Biological citizenship. In: Ong A, Collier SJ (eds) Global assemblages: technology, politics, and ethics as anthropological problems. Blackwell, Malden MA, pp 439–463

Rosenberg CE (2007) Our present complaint: American medicine, then and now. The Johns Hopkins University Press, Baltimore

Rosenfeld D, Faircloth CA (eds) (2006) Medicalized masculinities. Temple University Press, Philadelphia

Rothman SM, Rothman DJ (2003) The pursuit of perfection: the promise and perils of medical enhancement. Pantheon, New York

Schrepfer SR, Scranton P (eds) (2004) Industrializing organisms: introducing evolutionary history. In: Hagley Perspectives on business and culture, vol. 5. Routledge, New York

Schulz AJ, Mullings L (eds) (2006) Gender, race, class, and health: intersectional approaches. Jossey-Bass, San Francisco, CA

Scott S (2006) The medicalization of shyness: from social misfits to social fitness. Sociol Health Illn 28(2):133–153

Scott WR, Ruef M, Mendel PJ, Caronna CA (2000) Institutional change and healthcare organizations: from professional dominance to managed care. University of Chicago Press, Chicago

Serlin D (2004) Replaceable you: engineering the body in postwar America. University of Chicago Press, Chicago

Sharma U (2000) Medical pluralism and the future of CAM. In: Kelner MJ, Wellman B, Pescosolido B, Saks M (eds) Complementary and alternative medicine: challenge and change. Gordon and Breach, Amsterdam, pp 211–222

Shim JK (2002) Understanding the routinised inclusion of race, socioeconomic status and sex in epidemiology: the utility of concepts from technoscience studies. Sociol Health Illn 24(2):129–150

Shim JK (2010) Stratified epidemiology and the imperative of health: the biomedicalization of race, gender, and class in heart disease. In: Clarke A, Fosket J, Mamo L, Shim J, Fishman J (eds) Biomedicalization: technoscience and transformations of health and illness in the US. Duke University Press, Durham, NC, pp 218–241

Shim JK, Russ AJ, Kaufman SR (2006) Risk, life extension, and the pursuit of medical possibility. Sociol Health Illn 28(4):479–502

Shim JK, Russ AJ, Kaufman SR (2007) Clinical life: expectation and the double edge of medical promise. Health 11(2):245–264

Shostak S (2003) Locating gene-environment interaction: at the intersections of genetics and public health. Soc Sci Med 56:2327–2342

Shostak S (2004) Environmental justice and genomics: acting on the futures of environmental health. Sci Cult 13(4):539–562

Shostak S (2005) The emergence of toxicogenomics: a case study of molecularization. Soc Stud Sci 35(3):367–404

Shostak S (2010) Marking populations and persons at risk: molecular epidemiology and environmental health. In: Clarke A, Fosket J, Mamo L, Shim J, Fishman J (eds) Biomedicalization: technoscience and transformations of health and illness in the US. Duke University Press, Durham, NC, pp 242–262

Silverman C (2010) Desperate and rational: of love, biomedicine, and experimental community. In: Rajan KS (ed) Lively capital: biotechnology, ethics and governance in global markets. Duke University Press, Durham, NC (forthcoming)

Sinding C (2004) The power of norms: Georges Canguilhem, Michel Foucault, and the history of medicine. In: Huisman F, Warner JH (eds) Locating medical history: the stories and their meanings. The Johns Hopkins University Press, Baltimore, MD, pp 262–284

Singh I, Rose N (2006) Neuro-forum: an introduction. BioSocieties 1(1):97–102

Slaughter S, Rhoades G (2004) Academic capitalism: politics, policies and the entrepreneurial university. Johns Hopkins University Press, Baltimore, MD

Star SL (1995) Epilogue: work and practice in social studies of science, medicine and technology. Sci Technol Hum Values 20(4):501–507

Starr P (1982) The social transformation of American medicine: the rise of a sovereign profession and the making of a vast industry. Basic Books, New York

Strong P (1979) Sociological imperialism and the profession of medicine: a critical examination of the thesis of medical imperialism. Soc Sci Med 13A:199–215

Strong P (1984) The academic encirclement of medicine. Sociol Health Illn 6:339–358

Tansey B (2008) Experts call for wider use of brain enhancing drugs. San Francisco Chronicle 8 Dec 2008:A1,7

Thompson C (2005) Making parents: the ontological choreography of reproductive technologies. MIT, Cambridge, MA

Thompson C (2008) Stem cells, women, and the new gender and science. In: Schiebinger L (ed) Gendered innovations in science and engineering. Stanford University Press, Stanford, CA, pp 109–130

Thompson C (2010) Charismatic megafauna and miracle babies: essays in selective pronatalism. (in prep)

Timmermans S, Kolker E (2004) Clinical practice guidelines and the implications of shifts in knowledge for sociological accounts of professional power. J Health Soc Behav 45(Extra Issue):177–193

Timmermans S, Mauck A (2005) The promises and pitfalls of evidence-based medicine. Health Aff 24(1):18–28

Tomes N (2001) Merchants of Health: Medicine and Consumer Culture in the United States, 1900–1940. Journal of American History 88(2):519–547

Tomes N (2005) The great American medicine show revisited. Bull Hist Med 79:627–663

Tomes N (2007) Patient empowerment and the dilemmas of late-modern medicalisation. Lancet 369:698–700

Tone A, Watkins ES (eds) (2007) Medicating modern America: prescription drugs in history. New York University Press, New York

Tremain SL (ed.) (2005) Foucault and the government of disability. University of Michigan Press, Ann Arbor, MI

Turner B (1997) From governmentality to risk: some reflections on Foucault's contribution to medical sociology. In: Petersen A, Bunton R (eds) Foucault, health and medicine. Routledge, London and New York, pp ix–xxii

Turner L (2007) 'First world health care at third world prices': globalization, bioethics and medical tourism. BioSocieties 2:303–325

Unschuld PU (1987) Traditional Chinese medicine: some historical and epistemological reflections. Soc Sci Med 24(12):1023–1029

Vailly J (2006) Genetic screening as a technique of government: the case of neonatal screening for cystic fibrosis in France. Soc Sci Med 63(12):3092–3101

Vogel KM (2008) Framing Biosecurity: An Alternative to the Biotech Revolution Model? Science and Public Policy 35(1):45–54

Waitzkin H (1989) Social structures of medical oppression: a Marxist view. In: Brown P (ed) Perspectives in medical sociology, 1st edn. Waveland, Belmont, CA, pp 166–178

Waitzkin H (2000) The second sickness: contradictions of capitalist health care. Rowman & Littlefield, Lanham, MD

Waldby C, Mitchell R (2006) Tissue economies: blood, organs, and cell line in late capitalism. Duke University Press, Durham

Waldram JB (2004) Revenge of the Windigo: the construction of the mind and mental health of North American aboriginal peoples. University of Toronto Press, Toronto

Washburn R (2009) Measuring the 'pollution in people': biomonitoring and constructions of health and environment. Ph.D. dissertation, Department of Social and Behavioral Sciences, University of California, San Francisco

Wheatley EE (2005) Disciplining bodies at risk: cardiac rehabilitation and the medicalization of fitness. Journal of Sport and Social Issues 29(2):198–221

Wheaton B, Clarke P (2003) Space meets time: integrating temporal and contextual influences on mental health in early adulthood. Am Sociol Rev 68(5):680–706

Williams R (1976/1985) Keywords: a vocabulary of culture and society. Oxford University Press, New York

Williams SJ (2004) Beyond medicalization-healthicization? A rejoinder to Hislop and Arber. Sociol Health Illn 26(4):453–459

Williams SJ, Calnan M (1996) The 'limits' of medicalisation? Modern medicine and the lay populace in 'late' modernity. Soc Sci Med 42:1609–1620

Wright P, Treacher A (eds) (1982) The problem of medical knowledge: examining the social construction of medicine. Edinburgh University Press, Edinburgh, UK

Yoxen E (1981) Life as a productive force: capitalizing the science and technology of molecular biology. In: Levidow L, Young R (eds) Science, technology and the labour process. Free Association Books, London, pp 66–122

Yoxen E (1982) Giving life a new meaning: the rise of the molecular biology establishment. In: Elias N, Martins H, Whitley R (eds) Scientific establishment and hierarchies. D. Reidel, Boston, MA

Zola IK (1972) Medicine as an institution of social control. Sociological Review 20:487–504

Chapter 11
Two Cultures: Two Ships: The Rise of a Professionalism Movement Within Modern Medicine and Medical Sociology's Disappearance from the Professionalism Debate

Frederic W. Hafferty and Brian Castellani

Two Cultures

In 1959, the novelist and physicist C. P. Snow, delivered his famous lecture on *'Two Cultures'* at the University of Cambridge. Snow argued that while the humanities and the sciences (in particular, the natural sciences) form the two great cultural traditions humans use to make sense of their lives, these domains of knowing remain strangers to one another. Like ships passing in the night, science and art reflect a cultural divide for which no easy rapprochement exists.

In 1957, the sociologist Robert Straus, made a similar, albeit less dramatic, distinction between medicine and medical sociology (Straus 1957). Strauss's prescient realization was that medicine and sociology represent two very different – and "incompatible" (for Straus – page 203) cultural traditions, each with a distinctive language, associated concepts, methods, intellectual traditions, and authoritative literature. Even when discussing a similar topic such as medical professionalism – the focus of this chapter – one finds sociology and medicine going about their work in very different ways.

To highlight this cultural divide, Robert Straus differentiated between a *sociology of* and a *sociology in* medicine – a distinction August Hollingshead later would label a "watershed in the subsequent development of the field" (Hollingshead 1973). On the one side were those sociologists whose ideas worked in the service of medicine, the *sociology in medicine* community; on the other side were sociologists who remained within the culture of sociology and studied medicine as anthropologically strange – the *sociology of medicine* community.

Straus gave form to this dichotomy at a time of considerable disciplinary ferment (Anderson and Seacat 1957; Freeman and Reeder 1957; Hawkins 1958). Medical sociology was in its infancy and there was considerable ambiguity and tension within its ranks. Disciplinary anchors such as the *Journal of Health and Human Behavior* (its first journal) and section status in the *American Sociological Society* (the association's name at that time) were still 3 years (1960) into the future. Concerns about where medical sociologists might occupationally migrate – along with the concomitant integrity of their sociological gaze – were rife (Anderson and Seacat 1962; Bloom 2002; New and May 1965; Rosengren 1967). Straus was particularly concerned that sociologists operating within an occupationally powerful sector such as medicine might come to identify more with the educational, research or clinical agendas of their employer or setting, thus subverting their sociological gaze. For Straus, the core tension was between an ever-broadening disciplinary acceptance (e.g., including employment in nontraditional settings) and the field's ongoing disciplinary integrity.

F.W. Hafferty (✉)
Department of Behavioral Sciences, University of MN Medical School,
1035 University Drive, Duluth, MN 55812-2487, USA
e-mail: phaffert@charter.net

Although now 50 years old, Straus' basic distinction – and underlying concerns – remain a useful lens from which to examine the highly textured (and evolving) interface between sociology and medicine. Organized medicine (debates as to its diminished status as a profession notwithstanding) continues to wield substantial powers in framing the problems it addresses and the relative legitimacy of solutions it endorses. Over the years, only a handful of sociologists (e.g., David Mechanic and John McKinlay are two examples) have maintained a presence (with cross and conjoint credibility) on both sides of the sociology-medicine fence. In short, while the worlds of medical sociology and medicine have continued to evolve, they have largely done so as separate domains rather than in anything that might be described as a substantive partnership.

In the following pages we will explore a modern day cultural divide, a divide between sociology's study of professions during the 1970s and 1980s and the subsequent rise of a professionalism movement within organized medicine – a movement that began just as sociology's interest in the topic of medicine's professionalism prospects began to wane. However, just as medicine remained largely indifferent to sociology's analytical preoccupations during the 1960s and 1970s, sociology, in turn, has focused its own indifferent eye to medicine's current (and ongoing) efforts to reestablish its professionalism prospects. It is as if we have had two ships passing in the night – now on two occasions, and counting. To better explore these two waves of indifference, we briefly review the rise of a sociology *of* professions, culminating with the emergence of a "great debate" in the 1970s and 1980s between Eliot Freidson and his critics. Next, we explore the subsequent rise of a professionalism movement *within* organized medicine – spending more time on this iteration largely because of sociology's relative silence about this movement. In this latter story, we take particular interest in the relative (and longstanding) absence of a sociological perspective within medicine's emerging discourse on professionalism, and how the rise of a new literature on professions (a "new professionalism" literature) may well signal a shift within medicine from an almost exclusive focus on motives (e.g., the call to physicians to rediscover their professional roots) to one recognizing the structural conditions facing professions (e.g., how structural factors may hinder or facilitate agency) may offer sociology a strategic seat at the head of the analytic table. The degree to which sociology will accept this opportunity, however, is an empirical question and one that has not yet been answered.

The Case of Professionalism

The topic of profession, its study as an organizational form of work and as an object of occupational status, represents an opportunity to examine the disjunctures that currently exist between sociology and medicine. The basic story is quite simple – if nuanced. In the 1970s and 1980s, medical sociology was a hotbed of discussion about the nature of medicine as a profession. Concepts flew (e.g., professional dominance, deprofessionalization, proletarianization, corporatization, countervailing powers), notables (e.g., Eliot Freidson, Marie Haug, Donald Light, John McKinlay) wrangled, while points and counterpoints accumulated. Organized medicine, however, remained essentially oblivious to sociology's particulars, even though the debate detailed substantive challenges to medicine's ongoing control over the content, structure and process of its work. At best, there might be a fleeting reference in the medical literature to Paul Starr's *Social Transformation of American Medicine* (Starr 1982). By the early 1990s, even this had passed. Sociological interest in this debate began to wane. Various camps proclaimed conceptual victory, yet without apparent closure on key issues.

About this time, and as if linked in some unfathomable fashion to sociology's dwindling enthusiasm, organized medicine began to lumber and unfurl its own professionalism banner. Buffeted by what it would increasingly identify as the "scourge of commercialism," and reeling before the onset of "industry," medicine began to launch a self-proclaimed "professionalism project" with formal statements of organizational purpose, broad participation across a number of medical organizations, international codes and charters, and substantial investments of time, money, and other resources (Hafferty 2006b; Hafferty and Castellani 2008). Twenty years later, this movement continues unabated, yet sociology has remained substantively quiet (with few exceptions, see below) to what has become a veritable social movement within a dominant occupational sector.

We have, then, a tale of two ships. Each has chosen to navigate a similar sea (medical professionalism), but at different times and with each operating in seeming indifference to the presence and efforts of the other. How this has come to pass is the focus of this chapter. In turn, we examine the implications of these "passings" for each discipline, along with the possibility for future joint excursions and mutual cooperation.

The Emerging Sociology of Professions

Profession has been a topic of sociological interest since sociology's emergence as an academic discipline. While important figures in the history of sociology such as Herbert Spencer (2002 [1896]) and Emile Durkheim (1933), helped to frame initial arguments, they were not alone. At the turn of the twentieth century, sociologists were engaged in examining a number of occupational groups for their "professional characteristics," including accounting (Sterrett 1906), city managers (Ridley and Nolting 1934), social work (Rubinow 1925), nursing (Brown 1936), life insurance (Fouse 1906), "handling men" (Bloomfield 1915), engineering (Cooke 1915; Newell 1922), law (Jessup 1922), and even sociology (Chapin 1934). Medicine was one among many and would not emerge from within this chorus line of players until the 1940s. By the late 1920s, enough work had accumulated for Carr-Saunders and Wilson to edit a highly influential volume on the topic (Carr-Saunders and Wilson 1928). As was true for much of what was taking place within sociology in the 1930s, 1940s, and 1950s, the driving force for medicine's ascending identity as "the prototype profession" was Talcott Parsons.

Talcott Parsons and Medicine as a Profession

The tipping point in sociology's fascination with medicine came in 1939 when Talcott Parsons published an article on professions ("The professions and social structure") in *Social Forces* (Parsons 1939). In this article, Parsons employed a comparative framework to challenge what he saw as a well-entrenched public perception (something actively cultivated by organized medicine) that medicine and business were radically different domains of work reflecting fundamentally different value systems (Light 2000) – a difference Parsons characterized as; "the most radical cleavage conceivable in the field of human behavior" (Parsons 1939, p. 458). Parsons' analysis of this schism is of interest here for several reasons. First, it is an important window into how one might frame issues of professions from a sociological (albeit functionalist) perspective. For example, and as we will explore later, Parsons argued that one should focus on institutional and structural factors – and not personal motivations – while tackling the "problem of self-interest." Parsons viewed the popular distinction between egoistic and altruistic motives as a "false dichotomy," and one that "obscure(s) the importance of...other elements, notably rationality, specificity of function, and universalism" (Parsons 1939, p. 467).

A second window of relevance is Parsons' views on what he saw as current threats to medicine's occupational hegemony. Key here is the fact that Parsons was casting his analytical gaze during a time (the 1930s) we now consider as a period of *ascendancy* in medicine's professional powers (Starr 1982). Although the evolving conflict between the medical profession (characterized by Parsons as retaining "organizational independence") and the forces of industrialism was not a central theme in his 1939 work, Parsons remained keenly interested (see Parsons 1963) in the topic.

Between 1939 *and* 1963, Parsons would publish several treatises on medicine as a profession – the most famous being "Chapter Ten," (*Social Structure and Dynamic Process: The Case of Modern Medical Practice*) in his classic *The Social System* (Parsons 1951). Across this 14 year span, Parsons traced medicine's structural shifts, including the increasing complexity and internal differentiation of medical work, new patterns of financing medical care, and how these shifts were threatening the "organizational independence" of physicians and the highly personal nature of the physician–patient relationship – the latter of which Parsons saw (at the time) as "not subject to intervention on bureaucratic' grounds" (Parsons 1963, p. 26). Parsons also felt that "the *relative* (ital. in original) role of the physician in the total complex of health care has been steadily diminishing" because of an increasingly complex division of labor (Parsons 1963, p. 30). Finally, Parsons contrasted organized medicine's "great historic tradition of concern for the welfare of any and all patients" with more recent shifts (since the 1920s) toward organizational self-protectionism and a more conservative political realignment – in a theme that would anticipate the proletarianization and deprofessionalization debates of the 1970s and 1980s (see below).

In sum, while Parsons' characterizations of medicine and physicians may appear functionally fawning to contemporary eyes, it is clear that he was concerned with how corporate and bureaucratic forces were threatening the organization of physician work, weakening the gemeinschaft-like physician–patient relationship, and how all of this would alter the normative structure of medical education – all themes that would preoccupy the *sociology of* professions during the 1960, 1970s and 1980s.

Professions Post Parsons: The Debate Ensues

The fact that Parsons would see sociological significance in studying professions (with a particular focus on the differences/similarities between medicine as a profession and medicine as a business) functioned as a powerful legitimating influence within sociology. Beginning in the 1950s, but particularly by the 1960s (paralleling the emergence of medical sociology as an academic sub-discipline), sociologists began to study the profession in its own right. Examples (a very partial list) include works by Everett C. Hughes (Hughes 1960), Bernard Barber (Barber 1963), Fred Davis and Virginia Olesen (Davis and Olesen 1963), William J. Goode (Goode 1957, 1960, Goode 19691969), Wilbert Ellis Moore (Moore 1970), Harold Wilensky (Wilensky 1964), and the 1966 edited volume *Professionalization* by Howard Vollmer and Donald Mills (Vollmer and Mills 1966).

This surge notwithstanding, use of the terms "profession" and "professional" within sociology during the 1960s remained more descriptive than analytical – and when directed towards medicine, tended to affirm medicine's elite status. In other instances, the concept of profession was not used as a theoretical construct. Murray Wax's analysis of "public dissatisfaction with the medical profession" (Wax 1962) is an excellent example in this latter respect. In his study, Wax documents; (1) a growing tension between the public and medicine over issues of cost, (2) the distancing of the physician from the "familiar and emotional life of the patient," (3) the growing preoccupation of physicians with the laboratory and a move by physicians to esoteric treatments and diagnoses, (4) the fact that the general population was forced to purchase "medical services as if they were commodities" while having a "decreasing ability to judge their potential value and efficiency" – all leading to medicine becoming less "intelligible" to the public (Wax 1962). Nonetheless, Wax never invokes profession and/or professionalism as an analytic lens – and this in spite of the fact that virtually all of his data speak of the issues of professionalism.

The work of Parsons and others notwithstanding, the true rise of a theory of professions would have to wait until 1970 and the conjoint publication of Eliot Freidson's *Professional Dominance*

(Freidson 1970b) and *Profession of Medicine* (Freidson 1970a). In a nutshell, Freidson used the concept of profession to organize his understanding of how certain occupational groups, medicine in particular, gain social closure over their work through the implementation of a complex set of occupational strategies, including the establishment of a professional ethic and corresponding professionalism. In its extreme form, this social closure emerges as almost total occupational control, which Freidson referred to as professional dominance.

Although the 1970s and 1980s would come to house a broad range of sociological insights into the nature of professions (Abbott 1988; Johnson 1972; Larson 1977; Ritzer and Walczak 1988; Starr 1982), and while a moderate flurry of work would extend into the 1990s and 2000s (e.g., Brint 1994; Freidson 2001; Krause 1996; Pescosolido 2006; Pescosolido et al. 2001), *the* signature event during the 1970s and 1980s was the emergence of a "great debate" within sociology between Eliot Freidson and his critics.

The Great Debate

The ink was hardly dry on Freidson's two tomes before alternative characterizations of medicine's professional status began to surface. While challenges came from multiple sources (see above), a notable core in this wave of criticisms included the deprofessionalization arguments of Marie Haug (Haug 1973, 1975, 1976, 1977; Haug and Lavin 1981, 1983) and the proletarianization thesis of John McKinlay (McKinlay 1973, 1977, 1982; McKinlay and Arches 1985, 1986; McKinlay and Stoeckle 1988). Over time, Donald Light (Light and Levine 1988) and McKinlay (McKinlay and Marceau 2002) would advance a "corporatization" thesis, with Light then moving to frame professionalism issues from a "countervailing powers" perspective (Light 1991, 1993, 1995, 2000; see also Mechanic 1991).

Freidson, meanwhile, responded to his critics, argument-by-argument and in some cases concept-by-concept (Freidson 1983, 1984, 1986, 1993, 1994, 2001, 2003). In some instances the arguments were cumulative, with a critique of Freidson, countered by a Freidson, with Freidson's criticisms fodder for the next round of criticism. Edited compilations highlighting the various arguments included a 1988 special issue of *Milbank Memorial Fund Quarterly* (McKinlay 1988) and a related book by Hafferty and McKinlay (1993). Additional overviews were provided by Hafferty and Wolinsky (1991), Hafferty and Light (1995), Timmermans and Kolker (2004), and Pescosolido (2006). Although not a literal part of this debate, later work by Mechanic on trust and changes in medical organization (Mechanic 1996, 1998, 2004; Mechanic and Meyer 2000, Mechanic and Schlesinger 1996), and Pescosolido's work on the role of capital, and her social network and institutional resources model (Pescosolido 2006) have built upon this foundation.

In addition to its flurry of claims and counter-claims, this debate also was notable for its major noncombatants. Although clearly players in sociology's professionalism discussions, two of sociology's most notable theorists on professions – Paul Starr and Andrew Abbott – had little presence in these sociologically-public arguments. Neither had much to say in their own work about the various players (e.g., Freidson, Haug, McKinlay, Larson, Light, etc), and neither drew much ire from Freidson's curmudgeonous pen during this time period. For example, Starr, mentions Freidson only twice (page 20 and a footnote on page 495) in his 1982 Pulitzer Prize winning *The Social Transformation of American Medicine* (Starr 1982), while Freidson had little to say about Starr in either of his two post-debate books on professionalism (e.g., *Professionalism Reborn* (Freidson 1994) and *Professionalism: The Third Logic* (Freidson 2003). Evidence of additional disconnects would come in 2004 when Starr's *Social Transformation* was the object of a 22 year reassessment – in a journal that was neither mainstream medical nor sociological (Wailoo et al. 2004). This special issue of the *Journal of Health Policy, Politics and Law* included commentaries by a bevy of notable social scientists, with an extended rejoinder by Starr (Starr 2004). Nonetheless, neither Freidson nor Abbott participated in the special issue, nor did Starr reference the tumultuous conceptual sparring that took place in the 1970s and 1980s.

By the mid to late 1980s the fireworks were all but over. Haug had retreated somewhat from her earlier claims (Haug 1988), while McKinlay turned his energies to health services research and to establishing a large international research institute – with only intermittent excursions into his proletarianization roots (McKinlay and Marceau 2002, 2008). Stripped of these authoritative voices, the debate sputtered, surfacing occasionally in the study of topics such as cross-professional boundaries (Halpern 1992), malpractice (Majoribanks et al. 1996), computerization of the workplace (Burris 1998), physician satisfaction (Warren et al. 1998), legal professionalism (Kritzer 1999), and political legitimacy (Schlesinger 2002).

While the deaths of Haug in 2001 and Freidson in 2005 clearly had an impact on the ongoing nature of this debate, the relative quiet that has existed within sociology since the mid 1980s about issues of medicine's professional status did provide Freidson with a seeming "last word" on the subject. In 2001, Freidson published his last book on professions (*Professionalism: The Third Wave* (Freidson 2001). Here, Freidson employed an ideal-type methodology to contrast profession with the two other forms of organizing work (free market and bureaucratic), a trilogy he saw operating in an overall dynamic of countervailing pressures. In his closing two chapters (*Assault on Professionalism* and *The Soul of Professionalism*), Freidson continued to rebut theoretical alternatives to his theory of professional dominance. Two years later, a review symposium of Freidson's book was published – once again in *JHPPL* – this time it was composed of three commentaries (Hafferty, Havighurst, and Relman) and what would be Freidson's truly final word on the topic (*Comments on JHPPL Review Symposium*; Freidson 2003). Parenthetically, Freidson would use both *The Third Wave* and his review symposium comments to advance some rather Parsonian-sounding observations on the institutional "soul of professionalism" (e.g., the necessary presence of transcendent values that add "moral substance to the technical content of disciplines"; Freidson 2001, p. 222).

The extinguishing of this once-vibrant debate did have its consequences. For one, and as we will explore in just a moment, this waning of interest in medicine's professionalism prospects left sociology ill inclined to respond to a major – if belated – set of movements within organized medicine during the mid 1980s to reconnect with its roots as a scientific and service oriented profession. These movements included medicine's own professionalism project, buttressed by an evidence-based medicine (EBM) and a patient safety movement. As literatures in all three areas began to accumulate during the last decade of the twentieth century in the case of professionalism and EBM, and in the opening years of the twenty-first in the case of patient safety, there would be nary a sociological voice in sight – Timmermans and Kolker's examination of four models of medical professionalism (functionalism, professional dominance, deprofessionali-zation, and countervailing powers) and how they account for the rise of EBM and practice guidelines, and their impact on physician autonomy, being a rather lonely exception (Timmermans and Kolker 2004).

Finally, and before formally moving into medicine's own discovery – and embrace – of professionalism, it is important to reemphasize that sociology's debate during the 1970s and 1980s received virtually no recognition within the medical literature during this time period. While there would be the occasional reference to issues of professionalism and commercialism in an isolated *American Medical Association* (AMA) presidential address (e.g., Coury 1986; Ring 1991) – these were more rhetoric and exhortation than analysis. Rome may have been burning (according to the sociologists), but the Romans were otherwise engaged. Those few analytic pieces that did appear (e.g, Arnold Relman's *The New Medical-Industrial Complex*; Relman 1980; David Mechanic's *Public Perceptions of Medicine*; Mechanic 1985; and Reed and Evan's *The Deprofessionalization of Medicine: Causes, Effects, and Responses*; Reed and Evans 1987) generated few citations within the medical literature at this time.

The one sociological presence that did surface in the medical literature during the 1970s and 1980s was Starr's aforementioned *The Social Transformation of American Medicine* (Starr 1982). Unlike Freidson's earlier and Abbott's later tomes, Starr's book was reviewed in major medical journals (e.g., *NEJM* and *JAMA*) and by important figures within those publications (former editors Arnold Relman for the *NEJM* and Lester King for *JAMA*) (King 1983; Relman 1983). Although it is unclear how many physicians actually consumed Starr's five hundred and eight page tome (see Howell 2004), the book stands virtually alone as a presence for the *sociology of medicine* within the medical literature during the 1970s–1990s.

The Rise of Professionalism (With) in Organized Medicine

Over the course of its hundred-plus year emergence as a profession, and with some exceptions (see above) organized medicine has treated its professional status as proper, deserved, and aphoristic. While there were – and will continue to be – battles at the organizational level, particularly over the desire of other occupations to secure powers and privileges such as clinical independence and access to direct reimbursement, medicine has long considered the attainment of professional status at the trainee level to be axiomatically tied to the completion of one's formal training (Sigerist 1960). No additional attainments were necessary. The degree (M.D.) defined and established everything. In turn, carrying out one's clinical work in a "conscientious manner" established that one was practicing medicine in a professional manner. Freidson's warning in 1970 that professionalism might engender organizational insularity leading to a "self-deceiving view of the objectivity and reliability of knowledge and the virtues of its members" (Freidson 1970b) quickly appeared prophetic – as physicians began to treat professionalism as something they were owed by a "grateful" public.

By the early 1980s, medicine's self-congratulatory hubris was beginning to shatter. One bellwether date was August 13, 1982 when the U.S. stock market shifted from what had been a decade-long bear market into what would become this nation's second longest bull market (stretching almost to the year 2000). Investors (e.g., think pension funds rather than individuals) poured billions of dollars into a cornucopia of nascent industries. "Dot.com era" may have been the prevailing marquee, but investors also directed a substantial portion of their fortunes into health care. What had been a rather sleepy and staid industry of pharmaceuticals and medical equipment manufacturers quickly ballooned into a dynamic and internally differentiated "health care marketplace." Analysts responded and ever more refined tools were developed. MSN.com's *Money Central* (moneycentral.msn.com) for example, now groups "health" stocks into nine different sectors: (1) Medical Instruments and Supplies, (2) Medical Appliances and Equipment, (3) Health Care Plans, (4) Long-Term Care Facilities, (5) Hospitals, (6) Medical Laboratories and Research, (7) Home Health Care, (8) Medical Practitioners, and (9) Specialized Health Services. And this is in addition to "Drugs," with its own seven subcategories (from "Drug Manufacturers-Major" to "Diagnostic Substances").

Such stratospheric change took place at the individual-company level as well. For example, in 1987, a tiny company opened its corporate doors with two hospitals in El Paso, Texas. A mere 10 years later, this company (Columbia/HCA–HCA today) had become the nation's largest hospital chain and its 49th most valuable company (stock price times number of shares). Although Columbia/HCA's rise was meteoric, it was not unique. Any number of companies (within health care and without) shared a similar trajectory.

Organized medicine struck back. Beginning in the mid 1980s (and more fully by the early 1990s), medical leaders began to unleash a torrent of articles, editorials, and commentaries denouncing the arrival of "corporate medicine" (Angell 1993, 2000; Barondess 2003; Burnham 1982; Davis 1988; Kassirer 1995, 1997; Lundberg 1985, 1988, 1990, 1997; McLeod 1982, Relman 1987, 1991, 1993, 1997; Relman and Angell 2002; Ring 1991). This body of work identified a common enemy – "commercialism" – something also labeled as "corrosive" and "antithetical" to professionalism. In turn, medicine called upon its members to "rediscover" and to "recommit" themselves to "an ethic of professionalism" (Hafferty 2006b). Medical journals, such as *Academic Medicine* (the flagship journal of the *Association of American Medical Colleges*) became a virtual caldron of work on professionalism – informing the medical education community that professionalism was to be medicine's new magic bullet (see Fox 1990). By the mid 1990s, courses on professionalism were being deployed at virtually every medical school in the country. Unfortunately, most of these initiatives were shoehorned into an already overburdened course schedule – something which spoke volumes (via medicine's hidden curriculum) about medical education's true priorities and general organizational inertia (Bloom 1988; Hafferty and Franks 1994).

Medicine's call to rally the troops, however, reflected the same type of parochialism and insularity that had concerned Freidson. In spite of the fact that medicine's outcry would highlight many of the same social forces identified by sociology across the preceding 80 years (but particularly during the previous 2 decades), there were virtually no references to sociological work and references within the medical literature. In short order, medicine's outpouring of concerns, fears, and denouncements began to create a different professionalism than the debate within sociology. In a nutshell, where sociology had emphasized social structures, jurisdictional issues of influence, and themes such as power and privilege, medicine's own professionalism was more about the motives and behaviors of individual practitioners and students. Furthermore, the backbone of medicine's professionalism discourse was a particular version of professionalism – something sociologists would come to label "nostalgic professionalism" (Castellani and Hafferty 2006). This particular framing, with its emphasis on altruism and personal sacrifice, would not sit well with students and would form the basis of a subcultural backlash against something (professionalism) students felt was being "crammed down our throats" (see below; Hafferty 2002, 2006a, 2008; Humphrey et al. 2007).

Medicine may have been ignorant of sociology's long-standing scholarship, but medicine's call for a resurgence of its own professionalism was broadly based, impressively sustained (the initiative has been evolving for over 20 years) and fascinating in its details (Hafferty and Castellani 2008). In very short order, a number of national medical organizations (e.g., *AMA*, *AAMC*), specialty groups (e.g., *American Board of Internal Medicine – ABIM*), accrediting bodies (e.g., *Accreditation Council of Graduate Medical Education – ACGME*), and even private companies (e.g. *National Board of Internal Medicine – NBME*) began work on what internally was termed as medicine's "professionalism project." Led by the *ABIM Foundation*, early writers first sought to "outline the problem," followed by formal efforts to define and then measure medical professionalism (Arnold 2002; Hafferty and Levinson 2008; Stern 2005). Various professional societies (e.g., oncology, orthopedics, pathology, etc.) began to publish articles on the "problem of professionalism" and the need for physicians and organized medicine to "rediscover their professional roots" (see Talbott 2006 as one example).

Efforts to formalize these calls, definitions, and measurement tools began almost immediately. Various medical schools and residency programs began to develop curriculum that would "teach" professionalism, while specialty organizations began to develop new codes of conduct. Among the many other projects was an internationally endorsed *Physicians' Charter* – a joint product of the *ABIM Foundation, the ACP–ASIM Foundation, and the European Federation of Internal Medicine* (ABIM Foundation, ACP-ASIM Foundation, and European Federation of Internal Medicine 2002). The *Charter* is structured around three "fundamental principles" (primacy of patient welfare, patient autonomy, social justice) and ten "professional responsibilities" (e.g., commitment to professional competence, honesty with patients, patient confidentiality, etc.). Its primary focus is on professionalism at the individual practitioner level. Over a hundred physician groups worldwide have endorsed the *Charter*.

A second major organizational initiative is tied to the residency program accreditation. In the late 1990s, the *ACGME*, which accredits the nation's 9,000-odd residency programs, decided to shift its accreditation practices from a rather exclusive focus on structure and process (e.g., courses completed, type, length and ordering of that coursework, hospital beds, patient volume, and diagnostic procedure counts) to a focus on outcome (What can students perform/accomplish – clinically – at different stages of their training?). Specifically, the *ACGME* identified six "core competencies" in the training of residents – one of the six being professionalism (ACGME 1999). The *ACGME* devised definitions, instructional materials, and an assessment "toolbox." While programs were free to develop their own materials, the *ACGME* did require them to teach and assess all six competencies at the individual resident level, with programs firmly on notice that their accreditation status (which determined their ability to receive federal funding) would be directly tied to their willingness and ability to meet these standards. The implementation and impact of these new standards are being closely followed within medicine (Arnold 2002; Bataldan et al. 2002; Blank et al. 2003; Cohen 2006).

A Brief Look at Medicine's Discourse of Professionalism

Two facts already noted bracket organized medicine's professionalism project (at least within the context of this chapter). First, medicine's discourse of professionalism is a different discourse than framed by sociology during the 1970s and 1980s. Where sociologist had focused on conditions of work, organized medicine targeted the motives and behaviors of students and practitioners. Where sociology had been interested in analyzing (and understanding) a particular social force (profession) and its impact on broader social issues, medicine (in the face of perceived external threats) was interested in rediscovering "lost" principles, and then applying these principles to counter the "threats of commercialism" (*the* key "enemy" in medicine's discourse). Organized medicine wanted to rally and incite its troops. Sociology wanted to understand the war.

Medicine's penchant for framing professionalism as an issue of motives is readily discernible within the vast number of documents (e.g., articles, editorials, books, reports, policy proposals, etc.) produced during the late 1980s and across the 1990s. Two notable examples are the aforementioned *Physician Charter* and the *ACGME's* professionalism competency. Both define professionalism at the individual practitioner/student level and both call upon individuals (in a variety of rather specific ways) to rediscover their roots. For example, the *ACGME* expects residents to; "demonstrate respect, compassion, and integrity; a responsiveness to the needs of patients and society that supersedes self-interest; accountability to patients, society, and the profession; and a commitment to excellence and on-going professional development." Conversely, there would be little recognition with medicine that social structures, including how medical training and practice were organized, might well limit – or even circumvent – even the most dedicated of trainees from manifesting these principles (Cohen et al. 2007).

The second bracket turns medicine's prior distance from sociology on its head with the fact that now it was sociology that appeared unfamiliar with and unenthusiastic about exploring organized medicine's contemporary embrace of professionalism. Although there had been an occasional interest in particular issues of profession since the 1990s (see discussion above), there has been no real effort to study what has become a massive organizational undertaking by organized medicine to "rediscover" and "reestablish" (according to medicine) its core identity. Ironically, what little effort there has been to bridge this gap has come from within medicine (See Cruess and Cruess 1997; Wynia et al. 1999a; Relman 2007 as notable examples). Arnold Relman's recent denouncement of commercialism and professionalism as antithetical (Relman 2007) is notable for several reasons. In addition to being an icon within academic medicine, Relman's warnings about the medical-industrial complex and the corrosive effects of commercialism on medical professionalism are long-standing and legion (see above). Second, this most recent article appears in *JAMA*, which along with *NEJM*, form the two most legitimate "voices" within academic medicine. Finally, and in a giant nod to sociology, Relman opens his essay – and thus his depiction of professionalism – with a two-paragraph synopsis of Eliot Freidson's *Professionalism: The Third Logic* (Freidson 2001). In these paragraphs, Relman reminds medical readers that, at root, profession is one of three foundational strategies for the organization of work. Sociology could not have done it any better.

Some Contemporary Events that Continue to Shape Medicine's Discourse of Professionalism

Relman's sociological leanings notwithstanding, the bulk of medical efforts to conceptualize, define, and measure professionalism have focused on the individual. They also have advanced a rather "nostalgic" or "old school" version of professionalism (Castellani and Hafferty 2006). Nostalgic professionalism calls upon physicians (both explicitly and tacitly) to embrace core values of altruism ("selfless service"), and to value (as a rallying cry) autonomy, discretionary control over clinical decision-making, and occupational dominance in the health care system. In comparison, there has been relatively little interest in wrestling with issues of how organizations might be framed in terms of professionalism or even how to assess organizations in terms of their ability (or lack thereof) to promote professionalism among trainees or practitioners.

If there is one "professionalism topic" that has focused more on context than motives, and more on structure than personality, it is conflict of interest (COI). While COI is only one type of professionalism issue, concerns about the impact of pharmaceutical and medical equipment companies on medical education have escalated during the past few years (Alpert 2005; Bekelman et al. 2003; Brett et al. 2003; Campbell et al. 2006; Campbell et al. 2007a, b; Chimonas et al. 2007; Ross et al. 2007; Steinman et al. 2001). One particularly influential article in this body of work is a 2006 "policy proposal" published in *JAMA* and authored by a bevy ($N=10$) of medical leaders in addition to one sociologist – Neil Smelser (Brennan et al. 2006). This proposal, among many things, called for academic medical centers (AHCs) to develop formal COI policies and to ban most forms of industry gift-giving. It also denounced two self-labeled COI "myths," the myth of small gifts (e.g., small gifts generate less COI than larger gifts), and the myth of full disclosure (e.g., disclosing a conflict mitigates the conflict). While COI represents a major topic in its own right, the major issue here is a reframing of the traditional COI approaches, which called upon individuals to "just say no," to a new focus on restructuring the relationships and interactions (interpersonal and otherwise) between academic medicine and industry (particularly the pharmaceutical and medical device industries), and to ridding medical student (and resident) learning environments of a hidden curriculum of COI practices. To date, several medical schools, led by Stanford University, and more recently the Cleveland Clinic have implemented versions of this proposal.

A second problem with the nostalgic model of professionalism is that it clashes with a more contemporary, nuanced, and student-based set of expectations about what it means (and should mean) to be professional. Although this is a complicated topic in its own right, medical students and residents are not as inclined as previous generations of student–physicians to frame commercialism as the antithesis of professionalism. Moreover, these trainees are unabashedly lukewarm – and even moderately suspicious – about traditional definitions (e.g., Swick 2000) of professionalism that place altruism at its core (Castellani and Hafferty 2006; Hafferty 2002). The image of a physician's work as underscored by an ethic of "selfless service" runs counter to a series of contemporary ethics stressing "lifestyle," "self-care," and the value of "family." Contemporary medical students argue that there should be a "balance" between work and what they see as their "private time" (Croasdale 2003; Dorsey et al. 2003; Tholhurst and Stewart 2004). Within this general context, students can be quite suspicious of faculty calls to altruism, viewing such expectations "as just another way to get us to do more work" or "a surefire path to burnout" (Hafferty 2002). Faculty, in turn (and particularly older faculty), have been prone to label such students as "lazy" and unwilling to make the kinds of commitments faculty feel are "necessary" in order to place the "needs of the patient above all else." To date, organized medicine in the U.S. has not sought to reconcile its more traditional definitions of professionalism with these more contemporary constructions of what it means to be a physician.

Another document indicating a possible shift in organized medicine's discourse of professionalism, published in *JAMA*, and lead authored by the former president of the *AAMC*, argues that "institutional and organizational settings of contemporary medical practice pose significant impediments to achieving several of the responsibilities to be assumed by physicians" and therefore that many of the core principles stated in the *Physician Charter* (detailed above) cannot be addressed at the individual practitioner level. The authors call for "system wide change" and the emergence of a "functional alliance" (shades of Parsons) between medicine and society (Cohen et al. 2007). Again, whether organized medicine's current discourse of professionalism, with its almost singular focus on the motives and behaviors of individuals, can make the shift to a structurally-based paradigm remains to be seen.

The Rise of a "New Professionalism" Literature

The broad range of forces shaping the organization and delivery of health care, including what some believe to be the unyielding presence of commercialism within medicine, has generated calls for a "new professionalism." Some of these calls emanate from within organized medicine (e.g., Sir Donald Irvine, Irvine 2006; Ronald Epstein, Epstein 1999), some from sociology (e.g., David Mechanic, Mechanic 2000), while others come from elsewhere within the social sciences (e.g., David Frankford, Frankford and Konrad 1998, and William Sullivan (Sullivan 2005). What is of interest here (besides the differences in the content and conceptual structuring of these respective calls) is that they represent a distinctive break with the more traditional (e.g., nostalgic) views of professionalism that continue to dominate organized medicine's professionalism movement. These different framings also have clear sociological underpinnings. For one, the different calls clearly reflect their country of origin (Hafferty and Castellani 2006). For example, Sir Donald Irvine's (Britain) call for a "patient centered professionalism" with its focus on formal participation of the public in all levels of medical decision-making and oversight is a fundamentally different professionalism than Epstein's (USA) focus on self reflection as the "sine qua non of the successful professional and essential to the expression of core values in medicine such as empathy, compassion, and altruism" (Epstein 1999). The fact that Britain has a national health care system while the U.S. reflects a more individualistic and market-driven approach is not coincidental.

There also is a distinctly sociological flavor to this new professionalism literature, particularly when they explicitly call for medicine to socially reconnect with the public/communities (be they social and/or geographic), and/or when this literature links professionalism to other social movements such as quality of care. For example, Michael Whitcomb (the former editor of *Academic Medicine*) has called for a new ethic of "civic professionalism" and on medical education to facilitate this move by focusing more on health policy and on helping medical students understand the U.S. health care system (Whitcomb 2005). Similarly, the influential medical voice of Troyen Brennan secured a place in *JAMA* to argue for a patient-safety focused professional responsibility grounded in what he conjointly labels "civic professionalism" and "activist professionalism" (Brennan 2002). A third example, once again appearing in *JAMA*, highlights the concept of "physician–citizens, in meeting public roles and professional obligations" (Gruen et al. 2004). In this latter example, the authors stress both quality of care initiatives and "political or grassroots advocacy to bring about changes in the structure of the health care financing system."

In short, and whether it be the "new professionalism" of Mechanic (Mechanic 2000, 2005), the "civic professionalism" of Sullivan (Sullivan 1999, 2004, 2005), the "reflective/responsive professionalism" of Frankford (Frankford and Konrad 1998; Frankford et al. 2000), or the "democratic" or "activist" professionalism of other writers, these calls usually contain some explicit call for medicine to reengage the public and to do so within a context (e.g., social contract, quality, evidence, safety) that stresses a link between medicine's traditional values of technical expertise and public service with the changing conditions of medical work – particularly the involvement of large health systems and the presence of a capital marketplace. Although these new professionalists do not use the term, "nostalgic professionalism" they clearly do not view medicine's traditional discourse as an appropriate (dare we say "functional?") orientation toward medical work.

Finally, we need once again to note that while these calls for a new professionalism have a presence (albeit marginal) within the medical literature, they have virtually no presence in the sociology literature. Thus, when sociologist Mechanic calls for a new professional ethic, he does so in a health policy (*Health Affairs*) or a law (*Houston Journal of Law & Policy*) journal (Mechanic 2000, 2005). Likewise, Sullivan's work on civic professionalism and Frankford's on responsive medical professionalism reflect a similar – and non sociological – choice in venue.

Conclusions

This is a tale of two ships. Each has chosen to navigate a similar sea, but at different times and on a different course. Were a novice to dive into the medical professionalism literature today, he or she would encounter a distinctive *professionalism in medicine*, with physicians writing on professionalism citing other physicians writing on professionalism, all for a physician-readership. There would be, however, little evidence that a *professionalism of medicine* literature had ever existed.

Meanwhile, operating from their own port of call, sociologists continue to conduct their own (largely internal) discussions about the nature of the profession, although with nowhere near the same intensity as what took place in the 1970s and 1980s, and with little attempt to address the significant changes that took place within medicine. One consequence of medicine's distance and sociology's disinterest is the lack of a sociological framework for understanding medicine's current and substantive move to embrace professionalism – along with the prospect that sociology might create a far different understanding of the profession as a social institution than the one currently being constructed by medicine.

It does not have to be this way. There is much sociology *can* say to medicine and the public about all that is unfolding within medicine's professionalism project – and there is much sociology *should be* saying about these changes. Nonetheless, what is being said comes mainly from the non-sociological pens of physicians. Thus, we are left with "mini references," such as Arnold Relman's two-paragraph summary of Freidson's *The Third Wave* or to the occasional reference to the concepts of trust or the social contract. This marginalization of sociology is compounded by the fact that there are few individuals within medicine who have either the expertise or interest to reach into sociology to expand medicine's understanding of professions. Examples of sociologically savvy physician writers, such as the physician team of Richard and Sylvia Cruess (Cruess and Cruess 1997, 2006; Cruess et al. 2008) or physician Matthew Wynia (Wynia et al. 1999b) can be counted on one hand. There are physicians with formal (Ph.D.) training in sociology (e.g., Howard Waitzkin; Nicholas Christakis) but they are interested in issues other than professionalism (Christakis 1999; Waitzkin 2001). Christakis, for example, has used social network theory (and social networks as an independent variable) to explore the rise in adult obesity (Christakis and Fowler 2007), smoking (Christakis and Fowler 2008), and the spread of happiness (all using data from the Framingham Heart Study; Fowler and Christakis 2008). It is not without irony that we note that work on social networks and health/medicine is more likely to be found in the medical (e.g., *JAMA*) than in the sociology (e.g., *JHSB*) journals (ISI Web of Science 2008 #71452). As a matter of record, and in this specific context (social networks), the major social science journal linking medicine and sociology is *Social Science and Medicine*.

We can also revisit the debate.....

What else could medicine learn (if it was so willing) from sociology – focusing now on medicine's current professionalism initiative? The nature of this initiative as a social movement is one example. To date, organized medicine continues to call upon its "troops" to rally behind a distinctly "old school" view of professionalism – with little acknowledgement that there are serious schisms within medicine's ranks (particularly among trainees) about what it means to be a professional in an age of "big business" and corporately controlled health care systems. Furthermore, medicine's entire professionalism movement is predicated on the need – as identified by medicine – to reestablish public trust, but with that goal grounded in the belief that the public will uncritically and unreservedly respond to medicine's overtures (the field of dreams scenario). The new professionalism literature does call for a more dynamic interface between the public and medicine, but this literature has no presence within sociology and has yet to penetrate the major journals (e.g., *JAMA, NEJM, Annals of Internal Medicine, Journal of General Internal Medicine*). Even recognizing that its preferred version of professionalism represents a form of privileged discourse (Wear and Kuczewski 2004) would be in the right (sociological) direction for medicine.

Organized medicine also could benefit from embracing Parsons' distinction between motives and social institutions. Even if medicine were somehow to infuse individual physicians with a renewed sense of nostalgic professionalism (something the younger generation of physicians is resisting), there still remains the unaddressed issue of how medicine's increasing complex non-system of health care will nurture and reflect this ethic of selfless service. Finally, and as just noted, it is not altogether clear whether the public (as the ultimate source of medicine's professional standing) will respond positively to medicine's belated acknowledgement that it has indeed abused and violated that trust. To date, organized medicine has no real plan to link its physician and medical student-directed efforts to any related programs of public awareness and eventual (hopeful) acceptance. To date, there is only the faintest of glimmers within the medical literature recognizing that motivating physicians to "be more professional" is not a sustainable action plan (Cohen et al. 2007).

A third entry point for sociology is the clash between medicine's "nostalgic" view of professionalism, its institutionalization of that view via new mandates to teach professionalism in the formal curriculum, and the emergence of a more lifestyle-centered view of professionalism among trainees and recent graduates. The issue is multifactorial and is reflected in (among other things) the increasing popularity of "lifestyle specialties," a new label within medicine and one attached to specialties (radiology, anesthesiology, emergency medicine, and dermatology) seen as having more "reasonable" work hours and demands (Dorsey et al. 2003, 2005; Newton et al. 2005). How these trends reflect yet other workforce realignments such as the flight of recent graduates from primary care, the rising distaste of new practitioners for night and weekend call, or ER and OB coverage, the move into shared, part-time, or temporary (e.g., locum tenens) practice arrangements, the increasing tendency of practitioners to retire at an earlier age, and the fact that a majority of today's physicians would not recommend the practice of medicine to newcomers, all have important ramifications for medicine's status as profession.

A fourth and related example of a sociologically "hot" topic touches upon medicine's continuing internal differentiation and how more recent permutations of this differentiation will impact on medicine's status as a profession. Many new types of medical workers (e.g., intensivist, hospitalist, nocturnalist, proceduralist) are not reflected (organizationally speaking) within traditional specialty groups (or specialty training) and thus with the control of work settings and the specification of the terms and conditions of work increasingly defined and specified by employers. This shift has definite implications for the medicine's professional prospects. There are numerous other examples.

Finally, there is an ongoing need for sociology to sharpen its sociological gaze, particularly with respect to Freidson's warnings about insularity and self-deception within medicine's professionalism rhetoric and practices. Organized medicine may claim that commercialism and professionalism are antitheticals, but there are innumerable examples of industry influence within the realms of clinical practice and medical research (e.g., physician ownership of freestanding surgi-centers or storefront MRI diagnostic facilities; or selling Amway products as a revenue-enhancer being one set of examples; industry funding of research another) and, to date, organized medicine has shown little inclination to officially label the entrepreneurial and commercial activities of physicians as "unprofessional" (Hafferty 2006b). Adopting a *sociology of* professionalism and calling medicine to task for actions in the light of rhetoric remains an important sociological responsibility.

The issue here is not whether sociology has anything to say to medicine about matters of health and health care (it does), or even whether sociology has anything to say about profession in general (it does), but rather whether sociology (and in particular medical sociology) is willing to tackle medicine's current professionalism project – and to do so by exploring the multitude of social factors and forces that continue to buffer medicine today.

We believe that medicine's embrace of professionalism as a de facto social movement offers sociology a myriad of possibilities to develop its sociological gaze – and that this gaze, in turn, can provide new insights into medicine's evolving status as a social institution.

References

Abbott A (1988) The system of professions: an essay on the division of expert labor. University of Chicago Press, Chicago, IL

ABIM Foundation, ACP-ASIM Foundation, and European Federation of Internal Medicine (2002) Medical professionalism in the new millennium: a physician charter. Ann Intern Med 136:243–246

ACGME (1999) Accreditation Council for Graduate Medical Education – Outcome Project

Alpert J (2005) Doctors and the drug industry: how can we handle potential conflicts of interest? Am J Med 118:99–100

Anderson OW, Seacat MS (1957) The nature and status of medical sociology. In: Anderson OW, Seacat MS (eds) The behavioral scientists and research in the health field. Health Information Foundation, Chicago, IL, pp 1–3

Anderson OW, Seacat M (1962) An analysis of personnel in medical sociology. Health Information Foundation, Chicago, IL

Angell M (1993) The doctor as double agent. Kennedy Inst Ethics J 3:279–286

Angell M (2000) Is academic medicine for sale? N Engl J Med 342:1516–1518

Arnold L (2002) Assessing professional behavior: yesterday, today, and tomorrow. Acad Med 77:502–515

Barber B (1963) Some problems in the sociology of the professions. Daedalus 92:669–679

Barondess JA (2003) Medicine and professionalism. Arch Intern Med 163:145–149

Batalden P, Leach D, Swing S, Dreyfus H, Dreyfus S (2002) General competencies and accreditation in graduate medical education: an antidote to overspecification in the education of medical specialists. Health Aff 21:103–111

Bekelman JE, Li Y, Gross CP (2003) Scope and impact of financial conflicts of interest in biomedical research: a systematic review. J Am Med Assoc 289:454–465

Blank L, Kimbal H, McDonald W, Merino J, for the ABIM Foundation, and European Federation of Internal Medicine (EFIM) (2003) Medical professionalism in the new millennium: a physician charter 15 months later. Ann Intern Med 138:839–841

Bloom SW (1988) Structure and ideology in medical education: an analysis of resistance to change. J Health Soc Behav 29:294–306

Bloom SW (2002) The word as a scalpel: a history of medical sociology. Oxford University Press, New York

Bloomfield M (1915) The new profession of handling men. Ann Am Acad Pol Soc Sci 61:121–126

Brennan TA (2002) Physicians' professional responsibility to improve the quality of care. Acad Med 77:973–980

Brennan TA, Rothman DJ, Blank LL, Blumenthal D, Chimonas SC, Cohen JJ, Goldman J, Kassirer JP, Kimball HR, Naughton J, Smelser N (2006) Health industry practices that create conflicts of interest: a policy proposal for academic medical centers. J Am Med Assoc 292:1044–1050

Brett AS, Burr W, Moloo J (2003) Are gifts from pharmaceutical companies ethically problematic? Ann Intern Med 163:2213–2218
Brint S (1994) In an age of experts: the changing role of professionals in politics and public life. Princeton University Press, Princeton, NJ
Brown EL (1936) Nursing as a profession, 2nd edn. Russell Sage, New York
Burnham J (1982) American medicine's golden age: what happened to it? Science 215:474–479
Burris BH (1998) Computerization of the workplace. Annu Rev Sociol 24:141–157
Campbell EG, Weissman JS, Vogeli C, Clarridge BR, Abraham M, Marder JE, Koski G (2006) Financial relationships between institutional review board members and industry. N Engl J Med 355:2321–2329
Campbell EG, Gruen RL, Mountford J, Miller LG, Cleary PD, Blumenthal D (2007a) A national survey of physician-industry relationships. N Engl J Med 356:1742–1750
Campbell EG, Weissman JS, Ehringhaus S, Rao SR, Moy B, Sandra Feibelmann S, Goold SD (2007b) Institutional academic-industry relationships. J Am Med Assoc 298:1779–1786
Carr-Saunders AM, Wilson PA (1928) The professions. Clarendon Press, Oxford
Castellani B, Hafferty FW (2006) Professionalism and complexity science: a preliminary investigation. In: Wear D, Aultman JM (eds) Medical professionalism: a critical review. Springer, New York, pp 3–23
Chapin FS (1934) The present state of the profession. Am J Sociol 39:506–508
Chimonas S, Brennan TA, Rothman DJ (2007) Physicians and drug representatives: exploring the dynamics of the relationship. J Gen Intern Med 22:184–190
Christakis N (1999) Death foretold: prophecy and prognosis in medical care. University of Chicago Press, Chicago, IL
Christakis NA, Fowler JH (2007) The spread of obesity in a large social network over 32 years. N Engl J Med 357:370–379
Christakis NA, Fowler GA (2008) The collective dynamics of smoking in a large social network. N Engl J Med 358:2249–2258
Cohen JJ (2006) Professionalism in medical education, an american perspective: from evidence to accountability. Med Educ 40:607–617
Cohen JJ, Cruess S, Davidson C (2007) Alliance between society and medicine: the public's stake in medical professionalism. J Am Med Assoc 298:670–673
Cooke ML (1915) Ethics and the engineering profession. Ann Am Acad Pol Soc Sci 101:68–72
Coury JJ Jr (1986) Physicians' fundamental responsibility. J Am Med Assoc 256:1005
Croasdale M (2003) Professional issues: balance becomes key to specialty pick: family practice and general surgery are taking the biggest hit, but fewer students are choosing medicine overall. AMNews.com
Cruess RL, Cruess SR (1997) Teaching medicine as a profession in the service of healing. Acad Med 72:941–952
Cruess SR, Cruess RL (2006) The role of professionalism in the social contract. In: Parsi K, Sheehan M (eds) Educating for professionalism. Rowan and Littlefield, Lanham, MD, pp 9–23
Cruess RL, Cruess S, Steinert Y (2008) Teaching medical professionalism. Cambridge University Press, New York
Davis JE (1988) Let's work together! A call to America's physicians and the public we serve. J Am Med Assoc 260:834
Davis F, Olesen VL (1963) Initiation into a women's profession: identity problems in the status transition of coed to student nurse. Sociometry 26:89–101
Dorsey ER, Jarjoura D, Rutecki GW (2003) Influence of controllable lifestyle on recent trends in specialty choice by U.S. medical students. J Am Med Assoc 290:1173–1178
Dorsey ER, Jarjoura D, Rutecki GW (2005) The influence of controllable lifestyle and sex on the specialty choices of graduating U.S. medical students, 1996–2003. Acad Med 80:791–796
Durkheim E (1933) The division of labor in society. Macmillan, New York
Epstein RM (1999) Mindful practice. J Am Med Assoc 282:833–839
Fouse LG (1906) The life insurance profession. Ann Am Acad Pol Soc Sci 28:70–81
Fowler JH, Christakis NA (2008) Dynamic spread of happiness in a large social network: longitudinal analysis over 20 years in the Framingham heart study. BMJ 337:370–379
Fox RC (1990) Training in caring competence: the perennial problem in North American medical education. In: Hendrie HC, Lloyd C (eds) Educating competent and humane physicians. Indiana University Press, Bloomington, IN, pp 199–216
Frankford DM, Konrad TR (1998) Responsive medical professionalism: integrating education, practice, and community in a market-driven era. Acad Med 73:138–145
Frankford DM, Patterson M, Konrad TR (2000) Transforming practice organizations to foster lifelong learning and commitment to medical professionalism. Acad Med 75:708–717
Freeman HE, Reeder LG (1957) Medical sociology: a review of the literature. Am Sociol Rev 22:73–81
Freidson E (1970a) Profession of medicine: a study of the sociology of applied knowledge. Harper and Row, New York
Freidson E (1970b) Professional dominance: the social structure of medical care. Atherton Press, New York

Freidson E (1983) The reorganization of the professions by regulation. Law Hum Behav 7:279–290
Freidson E (1984) The changing nature of professional control. Annu Rev Sociol 10:1–20
Freidson E (1986) Professional powers: a study of the institutionalization of formal knowledge. University of Chicago Press, Chicago, IL
Freidson E (1993) How dominant are the professions? In: Hafferty FW, McKinlay JB (eds) The changing medical profession: an international perspective. Oxford University Press, New York, pp 54–66
Freidson E (1994) Professionalism reborn: theory, prophecy, and policy. University of Chicago Press, Chicago, IL
Freidson E (2001) Professionalism: the third logic. University of Chicago Press, Chicago, IL
Freidson E (2003) Review symposium on Eliot Freidson's professionalism: the third logic: comments on JHPPL Review Symposium. J Health Polit Policy Law 28:168–172
Goode WJ (1957) Community within a community: the professions – psychology, sociology and medicine. Am Sociol Rev 25:902–914
Goode WJ (1960) Encroachment charlatanism, and the emerging profession: psychology, sociology, and medicine. Am Soc Rev 25:902–914
Goode WJ (1969) The theoretical limits of professionalization. In: Etzioni A (ed) The semi-professions and their organization. Free Press, New York
Gruen R, Pearson SD, Brennan TA (2004) Physician–citizens public roles and professional obligations. J Am Med Assoc 291:94–98
Hafferty FW (2002) What medical students know about professionalism. Mt Sinai J Med 69:385–397
Hafferty FW (2006a) The elephant in medical professionalism's kitchen. Acad Med 81:906–914
Hafferty FW (2008) Professionalism and the socialization of medical students. In: Cruess RL, Cruess SR, Steinert Y (eds) Teaching medical professionalism. Cambridge University Press, New York, pp 53–70
Hafferty FW, Castellan B (2010) The two cultures of professionalism: sociology and medicine. In: Pescosolido BA, Martin J, McLeod J, Rogers A (eds) The handbook of health, illness & healing: blueprint for the 21st century. Springer, New York
Hafferty FW, Castellani B (2006) Medical Sociology. In: Bryant CD, Peck DL (eds) Handbook of twenty-first century sociology. Sage, Thousand Oaks, CA, pp 331–338
Hafferty FW, Franks R (1994) The hidden curriculum, ethics teaching, and the structure of medical education. Acad Med 69:861–871
Hafferty FW, Levinson D (2008) Professionalism perspective: moving beyond nostalgia and motives towards complexity science view of medical professionalism. Persp Biol Med 51:599–614
Hafferty FW, Light DW Jr (1995) Professional dynamics and the changing nature of medical work. J Health Soc Behav (Extraissue):132–153
Hafferty FW, McKinlay JB (1993) The changing medical profession: an international perspective. Oxford University Press, New York
Hafferty FW, Wolinsky FD (1991) Conflicting characterizations of professional dominance. In: Levy J (ed) Current research on occupations and professions. JAI Press, Greenwich, CT, pp 225–249
Hafferty FW (2006b) Professionalism and commercialism as antitheticals: a search for 'unprofessional commercialism' within the writings and work of American medicine. In: Parsi K, Sheehan M (eds) Healing as vocation: a medical professionalism primer. Rowen and Littlefield, New York, NY, pp 35–59
Halpern S (1992) Dynamics of professional control: internal coalitions and cross-professional boundaries. Am J Sociol 97:994–1021
Haug MR (1973) Deprofessionalization: an alternate hypothesis for the future. Sociol Rev Monogr 20:195–211
Haug MR (1975) The deprofessionalization of everyone? Sociol Focus 3:197–214
Haug MR (1976) The erosion of professional authority: a cross-cultural inquiry in the case of the physician. Milbank Mem Fund Q Health Soc 54:83–106
Haug MR (1977) Computer technology and the obsolescence of the concept of profession. In: Haug M, Dofny J (eds) Work and technology. Sage, Beverly Hills, CA, pp 215–228
Haug MR (1988) A re-examination of the hypothesis of physician deprofessionalization. Milbank Q 66:48–56
Haug MR, Lavin B (1981) Practitioner or patient: who's in charge? J Health Soc Behav 22:212–229
Haug MR, Lavin B (1983) Consumerism in medicine: challenging physician authority. Sage, Beverly Hills, CA
Hawkins NG (1958) Medical sociology: theory, scope and method. Charles C. Thomas, Springfield, IL
Hollingshead AB (1973) Medical sociology: a brief review. Milbank Mem Fund Q Health Soc 51:531–542
Howell JD (2004) What the doctors read. J Health Polit Policy Law 29:781–798
Hughes EC (1960) The professions in society. Can J Econ Polit Sci 26:54–61
Humphrey HJ, Smith K, Reddy S, Scott D, Madara JL, Arora VM (2007) Promoting an environment of professionalism: the university of Chicago "roadmap". Acad Med 82:1098–1107
Irvine D (2006) New ideas about medical professionalism. Med J Aust 184:204–205
Jessup HW (1922) The ethics of the legal profession. Ann Am Acad Pol Soc Sci 101:16–29
Johnson T (1972) Professional and power. Macmillan, London
Kassirer JP (1995) Managed care and the morality of the marketplace. N Engl J Med 333:50–52

Kassirer J (1997) Our endangered integrity – it can only get worse. N Engl J Med 336:1666–1667
King L (1983) Review: the social transformation of American medicine. J Am Med Assoc 249:2237
Krause E (1996) Death of the guilds: professions, states, and the advance of capitalism-1930 to the present. Yale University Press, New Haven, CT
Kritzer HM (1999) The professions are dead, long live the professions: legal practice in a postprofessional World. Law Soc Rev 33:713–759
Larson MS (1977) The rise of professionalism: a sociological analysis. University of California Press, Berkeley, CA
Light DW Jr (1991) Professionalism as a countervailing power. J Health Polit Policy Law 16:499–506
Light DW Jr (1993) Countervailing power: the changing character of the medical profession in the United States. In: Hafferty FW, McKinlay JB (eds) The changing medical profession: an international perspective. Oxford University Press, New York, pp 69–79
Light DW Jr (1995) Countervailing powers: a framework for professions in transition. In: Johnson T, Larkin G, Saks M (eds) Health professions and the state in Europe. Routledge, London
Light DW Jr (2000) The medical profession and organizational change: from professional dominance to countervailing power. In: Bird CE, Conrad P, Fremont AM (eds) Handbook of medical sociology, 5th edn. Prentice Hall, Upper Saddle River, NJ, pp 201–216
Light DW Jr, Levine S (1988) The changing character of the medical profession: a theoretical overview. Milbank Q 66:10–32
Lundberg GD (1985) Medicine – a profession in trouble? J Am Med Assoc 253:2879–2880
Lundberg GD (1988) Editorial: American medicine's problems, opportunities, and enemies. J Am Med Assoc 259:3174
Lundberg GD (1990) Countdown to millennium: balancing the professionalism and business of medicine: medicine's rocking horse. J Am Med Assoc 263:86–87
Lundberg GD (1997) A pendulum swings and a rocking horse rocks. J Am Med Assoc 278:1704
Majoribanks T, Good Mary-Jo Delvecchio, Lawthers AG, Peterson LM (1996) Physicians' discourses on malpractice and the meaning of medical practice. J Health Soc Behav 37:163–178
McKinlay JB (1973) On the professional regulation of change. In: Paul Halmos (ed) Professionalisation and social change, sociological review monographs 20. University of Keele, Staffordshire, pp 61–84
McKinlay JB (1977) The business of good doctoring or doctoring as good business: reflections on Freidson's view of the medical game. Int J Health Serv 7:459–487
McKinlay JB (1982) Toward the proletarianization of physicians. In: Derber C (ed) Professionals as workers: mental labor in advanced capitalism. G.K. Hall, Boston, MA, pp 37–62
McKinlay JB (1988) The changing character of the medical profession: introduction. Milbank Q 66:1–9
McKinlay JB, Arches J (1985) Towards the proletarianization of physicians. Int J Health Serv 15:161–195
McKinlay JB, Arches J (1986) Historical changes in doctoring: a reply to Milton Roemer. Int J Health Serv 16:473–477
McKinlay JB, Marceau LD (2002) The end of the golden age of doctoring. Int J Health Serv 32:379–416
McKinlay JB, Marceau LD (2008) When there is no doctor: reasons for the disappearance of primary care physicians in the U.S. during the early 21st century. Soc Sci Med 67:1481–1491
McKinlay JB, Stoeckle JD (1988) Corporatization and the social transformation of doctoring. Int J Health Serv 18:191–205
McLeod AJ (1982) Maintaining professionalism in a material age. Can Med Assoc J 126:847–848
Mechanic D (1985) Public perceptions of medicine. N Engl J Med 312:181–183
Mechanic D (1991) Sources of countervailing power in medicine. J Health Polit Policy Law 16:485–498
Mechanic D (1996) Changing medical organization and the erosion of trust. Milbank Q 74:171–189
Mechanic D (1998) Public trust and initiatives for new health care partnerships. Milbank Q 76:281–302
Mechanic D (2000) Managed care and the imperative for a new professional ethic: a plan to address the growing misfit between traditional medical professionalism and emerging health care structures. Health Aff 19:100–111
Mechanic D (2004) In my chosen doctor I trust. BMJ 329:11418–11419
Mechanic D (2005) The media, public perceptions and health, and health policy. Hust J Law Policy 5:187–211
Mechanic D, Meyer S (2000) Concepts of trust among patients with serious illness. Soc Sci Med 51:657–668
Mechanic D, Schlesinger MJ (1996) The impact of managed care on patients' trust in medical care and their physicians. J Am Med Assoc 275:1693–1697
Moore WE (1970) Professions: roles and rules. Russell Sage, New York
New PK-M, May JT (1965) Teaching activities of social scientists in medical schools and public health schools. Soc Sci Med 2:447–460
Newell FH (1922) Ethics of the engineering profession. Ann Am Acad Pol Soc Sci 101:76–85
Newton DA, Grayson MS, Thompson LF (2005) The variable influence of lifestyle and income on medical students' career specialty choices: data from two U.S. medical schools, 1998–2004. Acad Med 80:809–814
Parsons T (1939) The professions and social structure. Soc Forces 17:457–467

Parsons T (1951) The social system. Free Press, New York
Parsons T (1963) Social change and medical organization in the United States: a sociological perspective. Ann Am Acad Pol Soc Sci 346:21–33
Pescosolido BA (2006) Professional dominance and the limits of erosion. Society 43:30–36
Pescosolido BA, Tuch SA, Martin JK (2001) The profession of medicine and the public: examining Americans' changing confidence in physician authority from the beginning of the 'health care crisis' to the era of health care reform. J Health Soc Behav 42:1–16
Reed RR, Evans D (1987) The deprofessionalization of medicine: causes, effects, and responses. J Am Med Assoc 258:3279–3282
Relman AS (1980) The new medical-industrial complex. N Engl J Med 303:963–970
Relman AS (1983) Review: the social transformation of American medicine. N Engl J Med 308:466
Relman AS (1987) Practicing medicine in the new business climate. N Engl J Med 316:1150–1151
Relman AS (1991) Shattuck lecture: the health care industry: where is it taking us? N Engl J Med 325:854–859
Relman AS (1993) What market values are doing to medicine. Natl Forum 73:17–21
Relman AS (1997) Dr. Business. Am Prospect 8:91–95
Relman AS (2007) Medical professionalism in a commercialized health care market. J Am Med Assoc 298:2668–2670
Relman AS, Angell M (2002) America's other drug problem: how the drug industry distorts medicine and politics. New Repub 227:27–41
Ridley CE, Nolting OF (1934) The city-manager profession. University of Chicago Press, Chicago, IL
Ring JJ (1991) President's address: the right road for medicine: professionalism and the New American Medical Association. J Am Med Assoc 266:1694
Ritzer G, Walczak D (1988) Rationalization and the deprofessionalization of physicians. Soc Forces 67:1–22
Rosengren WR (1967) Sociologists in medicine: contexts and careers. In: Abrahamson M (ed) The professional in the organization. RandMcNally and Company, Chicago, IL, pp 143–155
Ross J, Lackner JE, Lurie P, Gross CP, Wolfe SM (2007) Pharmaceutical company payments to physicians: early experiences with disclosure laws in Vermont and Minnesota. J Am Med Assoc 297:1216–1223
Rubinow IM (1925) Social case work: a profession in the making. Soc Forces 4:286–292
Schlesinger M (2002) A loss of faith: the sources of reduced political legitimacy for the American medical profession. Milbank Q 80:185–235
Sigerist HE (1960) The physician's profession through the ages. In: Marti-Ibernez F (ed) Henry E. Sigerist on the history of medicine. MD Publications, New York, pp 3–15
Spencer H (2002) The principles of sociology: in three volumes. Appleton, New York
Starr PE (1982) The social transformation of American medicine: the rise of a sovereign profession and the making of a vast industry. Basic Books, New York
Starr P (2004) Social transformation twenty years on. J Health Polit Policy Law 29:1005–1019
Steinman MA, Shlipak MG, McPhee SJ (2001) Of principles and pens: attitudes and practices of medicine housestaff toward pharmaceutical industry promotions. Am J Med 110:551–557
Stern D (2005) Measuring professionalism. Oxford University Press, New York
Sterrett JE (1906) The profession of accountancy. Ann Am Acad Pol Soc Sci 28:16–27
Straus R (1957) The nature and status of medical sociology. Am Sociol Rev 22:200–204
Sullivan WM (1999) What is left of professionalism after managed care? Hastings Cent Rep 29:8–13
Sullivan WM (2004) Can professionalism still be a viable ethic? Good Soc 31:15–20
Sullivan WM (2005) Work and integrity: the crisis and promise of professionalism in America, 2nd edn. Jossey-Bass, San Francisco, CA
Swick HM (2000) Toward a normative definition of medical professionalism. Acad Med 75:612–616
Talbott JA (2006) Professionalism: why now, what is it, how do we do something? J Cancer Educ 21:118–122
Tholhurst HM, Stewart SM (2004) Balancing work, family and other lifestyle aspects: a qualitative study of Australian medical students' attitudes. Med J Aust 181:361–364
Timmermans S, Kolker E (2004) Evidence-based medicine and the reconfiguration of medical knowledge. J Health Soc Behav 45:177–193
Vollmer HM, Mills DL (1966) Professionalization. Prentice-Hall, Englewood Cliffs, NJ
Wailoo K, Stoltzfus J, Schlesinger M (2004) Transforming American medicine: a twenty-year retrospective on the social transformation of American Medicine, vol 29(4–5). Duke University Press, Durham, NC
Waitzkin H (2001) At the front lines of medicine: how the health care system alienates doctors and mistreats patients. And what we can do about it. Rowman and Littlefield, Lanham, MD
Warren MG, Weitz R, Kulis S (1998) Physician satisfaction in a changing health care environment: the impact of challenges to professional autonomy, authority, and dominance. J Health Soc Behav 39:356–367

Wax M (1962) On public dissatisfaction with the medical profession: personal observations. J Health Human Behav 3:152–156
Wear D, Kuczewski MG (2004) The professionalism movement. Can we pause? Am J Bioeth 4:1–10
Whitcomb M (2005) Fostering civic professionalism in tomorrow's doctors. Acad Med 80:413–414
Wilensky H (1964) The professionalization of everyone? Am J Sociol 70:137–158
Wynia MK, Latham SR, Kao AC, Berg JW, Emanuel LL (1999a) Sounding board: medical professionalism in society. N Engl J Med 341:1612–1616
Wynia MK, Latham SR, Kao AC (1999b) Medical professionalism in society. N Engl J Med 341:1612–1616

Chapter 12
Medicine as a Family-Friendly Profession?

Ann Boulis and Jerry A. Jacobs

Over the past 3 decades, women have poured into the US labor force. Between 1970 and 2005, the percent of adult women working for pay increased from 43.3 to 59.3%. Women not only increased their participation in the labor force, they also increased their commitment to it. While 40% of employed women worked full-time year round in 1970, approximately 60% did so in 2004 (U.S. Bureau of Labor Statistics 2006).[1]

During this period, women not only increased their attachment to the labor force overall, they also significantly increased their presence among elite workers. In particular, women made significant progress in the US medical profession. Most notably, between 1970 and 2005, women's share of seats in medical schools increased from 11 to 48.9% (American Association of Medical Colleges 2004). During the same period, women's numerical representation among practicing physicians increased nearly ninefold, from 25,000 in 1970 to 225,000 in 2002, so that in 2006 women made up nearly 30% of all practicing physicians.

Although the growth of women in medicine has been profound, it is by no means unique. As women were pouring into US medical schools, they were also entering other heretofore male-dominated elite fields like law and business. In fact, between the late 1960s and 2001, women went from less than 5% to more than 50% of US law students. Currently, 33% of practicing attorneys in the USA are female (Rhode 2001).

Some have suggested that as the presence of women in medicine and other elite occupations increases, the prevalence of family-friendly working conditions for professionals who historically dedicated themselves entirely to work will also grow (Kotkin 2007). For example, in their editorial about the increasing number of women in medicine, Levinson and Lurie maintain that "women are changing the profession itself. The effects can be seen in the work–family balance." (Levinson and Lurie 2004; Croasdale 2004a; Wardrop 2004).

Women physicians, like other elite women workers, remain unlikely to have stay-at-home or minimally employed husbands (Boulis and Jacobs 2008).[2] As a result, these women rarely have the kind of family support system that allows some male physicians to work 70 or 80 h per week. This type of

---

[1] This essay draws on research presented in our book, The Changing Face of Medicine. Cornell University Press, 2009.

[2] In fact, there are extremely few stay-at-home fathers. In 2006, the Census estimated that there were only 143,000 married fathers with children under 15 who remained out of the workforce primarily so they could care for 245,000 children (U.S. Bureau of Census 2006).

A. Boulis (✉)
Department of Sociology, University of Pennsylvania, 217 McNeil Building,
3718 Locust Walk, Philadelphia, PA 19104, USA
e-mail: aboulis@sas.upenn.edu

single-minded devotion to a career is more challenging when both partners in a marriage are working full-time and are committed to their demanding careers. An exclusive focus on work can be even more challenging with the arrival of children, especially since evidence suggests that many women continue to feel guilty about combining paid work and mothering (Duncan et al. 2003; Jayson 2007). Consequently, the time demands of their family lives and the persistence of gendered ideas about parenting are likely to lead many women physicians to be interested in opportunities to dovetail their professional goals with their personal lives. As the number of women in medicine increases, it is reasonable to expect an increase in interest in family-friendly career options such as reduced work schedules, limited night call, and on-site child care.

Have elite professions, which have historically presumed exceptionally high levels of professional commitment, been responsive? There is some evidence of change in medicine and law. There has been growth in the number of hospitals with maternity leave policies, and the percent of physicians working part-time. In particular, results from AAMC surveys conducted in 1989 and 1994 indicated that the number of teaching hospitals with specified maternity leave policies increased from 52 to 77% in 5 years (Philibert and Bickel 1995). Further, evidence from a survey conducted by the American Academy of Pediatrics indicates that the number of practicing pediatricians who defined their position as part-time increased from 11% in 1993 to 15% in 2000 (Croasdale 2002). There is also increasing attention to the need for formalized reentry programs for physicians who take time off from medical work.[3]

In the legal profession, signs of reform are also surfacing. Most notably, in 1997, the American Bar Association adopted a resolution supporting alternative ways of working, including working from home and flexible hours (Kunde 1997). More recently, some evidence suggests that firms are abandoning billable hours in favor of flat fees that make more meaningful work–family balance possible (Belkin 1985).

In spite of the positive trends, we question the extent to which a family-friendly ethos has permeated the medical profession. In fact, the medical profession has not evolved as much as the popular and medical press suggests. Changes are clearly occurring, but they are not keeping pace with the growth of women physicians or the overall growth in demand for work–family balance. Further, in certain instances, such as the flexible tenure clock, the ultimate meaning of changes that have occurred is questionable. Moreover, the relative absence of reform in the medical profession does not stem from a lack of demand. Evidence from our research and others suggests that physicians of both genders are overworked. It also indicates that those who work reduced hours have higher professional satisfaction.

In this chapter, we examine how opportunities for work–family balance in medicine have evolved since women started entering the profession. The perspective that motivates our analysis focuses on structural change. The major idea here is that efforts to understand work–family balance must be understood within the context of a rapidly evolving profession that is confronting independent forces. This perspective suggests that although women and men physicians will continue to be affected by their gender, physicians' experiences over time will come to be defined more by the structure of the profession and less by the gender of the practitioner.

We find that women are seeking a more meaningful work–family balance for themselves, However, efforts to carve out time for personal endeavors are neither gender nor generationally

---

[3]The Federal Office on Women's Health convened the National Task Force on Reentry into Clinical Practice for Health Professionals in 2000 (Mark and Gupta 2002). This effort led to recommendations for a national reentry policy and to an updated compendium of physician retraining initiatives. The national task force was followed by the convening of an American Academy of Pediatrics sponsored Physician Reentry into the Workforce Project. The project is a collaborative effort that includes many medical institutions including the AMA, the VHA, the American Board of Medical Specialties, the American Academy of Family Physicians, the American Board of Surgeons, and the Council on Graduate Medical Education.

specific. Men and women in medicine are both seeking more manageable schedules. Similarly, while age and seniority is associated with enhanced control in many professions, we find that physicians of both genders at all stages of career development are finding it increasingly difficult to carve out meaningful time for family life or other personal pursuits.

We contrast our approach to three other views. The first perspective, which we refer to as personal choice, suggests that gender differences in the work-force stem primarily from differences in the choices that men and women make as they pursue education and paid employment. The most commonly cited theory encompassed by this perspective holds that gender differences in the status of male and female physicians reflect preferences and values that women bring with them into the medical profession (Hinze et al. 1997; Grant et al. 1990).

A closely related approach focuses on social change due to generational shifts among women physicians. It has been suggested that women who entered medicine during the 1990s and beyond may be seeking a fulfilling family life, along with the satisfactions of engaging professional work. As some have suggested, they may demand more flexible and part-time arrangements than did previous generations of women physicians (Bickel and Brown 2005). At the same time, it may be that work expectations are shifting for male physicians as well, as they are increasingly likely to find themselves in dual-career families.

A third perspective, which we refer to as the institutional discrimination thesis, suggests that specific industry and organizational characteristics and the behaviors of other key groups in the health services workforce are responsible for many of the disparities between male and female physicians. One of the most common theories in the discrimination group is the "structural difference" view (Kanter 1977). This theory holds that differences between men and women workers reflect gender differences in status and power in the organization or the profession.

Another aspect of the discrimination perspective is the "critical mass" hypothesis. Instead of focusing on women's presence in medical leadership, this view posits that critical change will occur in support of women's needs only after women make up a critical mass of the profession. This view would predict that part-time residencies and flexible schedules would be most common in female-dominated specialties like pediatrics and obstetrics and gynecology.

We find that although male and female physicians desire more manageable work lives, their ultimate capacity to create more workable schedules is greatly restricted by powerful countervailing pressures. These forces are evident in both the macrolevel environment, and in individual, or microlevel, decision making. That is, they permeate the broader institutional context of the profession and they also operate through the cost-benefit calculus of individual physicians. On the one hand, macro-level pressures from physicians' work environment, such as the need to pay for malpractice insurance and to meet productivity expectations, greatly limit opportunities for individual physicians and medical institutions to create work–family balance. On the other hand, concerns such as mounting educational debt also deter many physicians from taking advantage of flexible schedules when they are available. In short, reforms to date have fallen short because individuals' capacity to pursue family-friendly options is constrained.

At the same time, we suggest that many of the family-friendly reforms that are occurring in medicine stem from institutional developments that have little, if anything, to do with the representation of women in American medicine. One of the most obvious examples of such a change involves the relatively recent restrictions on resident work hours (Stanton 2007; Woodrow et al. 2006).

Family-friendly reforms in the medical profession have overall not resulted from significant organized efforts by physicians of either gender to reform their workplace. In fact, anecdotal evidence from resident union negotiations indicates that parking privileges, salaries, and access to interesting cases often takes priority over provisions for maternity leave. Our discussions also suggest that many residents are as concerned about finishing their training rapidly as they are about securing meaningful restrictions on work effort (Butterfield 2007). Although the number of organizations designed to represent female physicians is growing, reform efforts to date have not pushed an aggressive agenda of family-friendly institutional reforms. Policy makers and medical organizations are certainly aware of the increasing representation of women in the medical workforce, and many speculate about how women will change the profession.[4] Nonetheless, relatively few in the medical community or elsewhere are actively lobbying to increase family-friendly work environments such as available child care for physicians. When speaking about the panel to develop reentry regulations for physicians who have taken time off from practicing, one of the few recent concrete efforts to create a family-friendly work environment in medicine, an official at the AAMC said, "The panel has been around for years, but it never goes anywhere because no one is willing to put the time in to make those reentry regulations happen." (American Association of Medical Colleges 2006)

Furthermore, the family-friendly initiatives remain concentrated in a few corners of the profession. For example, primary care settings have made greater strides than other specialties, most notably surgery. These disparities not only reflect the number of women in a particular specialty or work environment, but also reflect broader institutional forces such as the disproportionate tendency for hospitals to employ primary care providers. Reforms to date have not principally reflected the concerted efforts of a united contingent of women doctors. If a unified group of female physicians could mobilize around issues of changes to the medical workplace, the medical profession could rapidly evolve in a much more family-friendly direction.

In this chapter, we compare trends in part-time employment with interest in this type of flexible career option. We find that there is a sizable gap between interest in part-time work arrangements and the availability of part-time opportunities. Many physicians express interest in reducing their work schedules, while the extent of part-time work is not increasingly rapidly. We explore the reasons for this mismatch.

We ask how women and men in the medical profession are balancing their work and family life in light of their surprisingly unresponsive workplace. For the overwhelming majority of women physicians, the answer does not appear to involve either a rejection of parenting or a rejection of the medical workplace. Instead, an increasing number of women and men in medicine are attempting to combine parenting with highly demanding professional commitments and inevitably enduring the stress that accompanies such a challenging and fast-paced life style.

The Medical Workweek: Kinder and Gentler or Crazier than Ever?

As we have documented elsewhere (Boulis and Jacobs 2008), although the data indicate that women physicians work less on average than their male peers, they still typically work well in excess of 40 h in an average week regardless of their personal status. The gender gap in the workweek exists only because male physicians work extremely long hours.[5]

It may be useful to examine trends in the extremes of work schedules, not just the average. For example, Jacobs and Gerson (2004) show that while the average workweek in the United States has not changed substantially over the last 30 years, more individuals are working long workweeks (50 h or more per week). In recent years, professionals and managers have logged the longest workweeks.

---

[4]In fact, the increasing relative and absolute presence of women in pediatrics was listed as the second most critical concern for the American Academy of Pediatrics' Committee on Workforce issues (American Association of Pediatrics 2005).

[5]It is also worth noting that the gender gap is specialty specific. While significant gaps exist between the average male and average female pediatrician work week, male and female surgeons and obstetrician-gynecologists log equivalent hours.

As shown in Table 3.1, female physicians are more likely to log more than 50 h per week on their jobs than was the case 20 years ago, while rates of long weeks have remained essentially constant for men. In 2000, nearly two-thirds of male physicians (64%) reported working 50 or more hours per week, down slightly from 65% in 1980. Among female physicians, nearly half (48%) worked 50 or more hours per week in 2000, up from 39% in 1980. Thus, the increased representation of women in the profession has not resulted in a general shift to more limited work schedules. Rather, both men and women in medicine have a high likelihood of working a long week.[6] Together these results suggest that the unique personal choices of female physicians are not transforming the health care system as many thought they might. They also suggest that differences in the work lives of male and female physicians which might create distinct workweeks are declining.

At the other end of the spectrum, the fraction of physicians working part-time should be revealing as well. Although many believe that the part-time medical workforce is growing in the USA (Croasdale 2002, 2004a), our findings from the US Census suggests otherwise. In fact, data from the Census suggest that rates of part-time work of 30 h or less for women has increased only slightly, from 13 to 15% between 1980 and 2000. In contrast to the 15% of female physicians who worked part-time in 2000, 8% of male physicians worked part-time, up four percentage points since 1980.[7] Thus, the vast majority of female physicians have been unable or unwilling to pursue part-time schedules.

Part-time employment is actually less common than it was during the 1970s when few physicians were women. In 1970, 20% of women physicians worked fewer than 35 h per week. Even recent research on pediatricians indicates that although the absolute numbers of women pediatricians working part-time increased during the 1990s, between 1993 and 2000 there was no change in the tendency for women pediatricians to work part-time. Further, growth in the percent of pediatricians working reduced schedules stems entirely from growth in the representation of women in the specialty (Cull et al. 2002).[8]

Data from the US Census indicate that over the last several decades, the work effort of female physicians is coming to more closely resemble the work effort of men who share their household composition. This trend is most pronounced for physicians over age 50. However, the trend toward parity does not imply a trend toward greater work–family balance. The average work effort of female physicians is increasing, while the average workweek of male physicians has remained relatively constant at a very high level. These trends fail to support either the personal choice or the social change perspectives on work–family balance. Ultimately, the trend is toward *less* work–family balance rather than more. This increase in work effort may signal increasing pressures on female physicians with regards to their lives outside of work.

How do conditions in the medical profession compare to conditions in other occupations? While all employed nonresident male physicians worked an average of 52 h per week, employed men

---

[6] Data from the Community Tracking Study physician surveys indicate that in 1996, 75% of men and 51% of women worked long weeks. By 2004, only 69.9% of men and 48.4% of women worked long weeks but the aging of the population between 1996 and 2004 might explain the decline in the tendency to work long weeks.

[7] Data from the 2004 CTS Physician Survey indicate that 16% of women and 6% of men physicians work less than 31 h in a normal week. Between the 1996 and the 2004 CTS Surveys, rates of part-time work increased slightly for men and women from 14.6 to 1% for women and from 4.1 to 5.9% for men. In contrast, between the 1990 and 2000 Census, the frequency of part-time work declined from 16 to 15%. The CTS survey involves only physicians who provide direct patient care at least 20 h per week and excludes radiologists, pathologists, and anesthesiologists. It also involves a survey of cities rather than a survey of the entire US population. Regardless of the data source, however, rates of part-time work for female physicians are remarkably stable.

[8] Data from the Physician Work Life Study indicates that 22% of US women respondents and 9% of US men respondents worked part-time (McMurray et al. 2005); however, this survey defines part-time as less than 40 h rather than less than 30 h.

overall work only 43.1 h per week and employed men in managerial and professional occupations work 45.6 h per week. (Jacobs and Gerson 2004: 34). The comparable numbers for employed women are 47 h for women physicians, 37.1 h overall and, 39.4 h for women in managerial and professional occupations (Jacobs and Gerson 2004: 34).

Further, according to the Census in 2000, only 26.5% of all male workers reported more than 50 h in their average workweek. Results from the 2004 American Community Survey reveal a slight decline in long workweeks for men overall. In 2004, 24.3% of male workers worked more than 48 h per week (Kuhn 2007). The comparable number for all male professional, managerial, and technical workers was 37.2%. Since 64% of male physicians work at least 50 h, on average male physicians are 1.7 times more likely then men in elite occupations overall to work long weeks.

Only 11.3% of the female workforce overall worked 50 or more hours. The comparable number for women in managerial, technical, and professional occupations was 17.1% in 2000. Since 48% of female physicians worked at least 50 h, in 2000, employed women physicians were 2.8 times more likely to work a long week than other women employed in elite occupations. Even married physician mothers were 2.5 times more likely to work a long week than their female peers in other elite occupations.

On the other hand, analysis of the 2000 Current Population Survey indicates that rates of part-time work in medicine are not too different from rates in other elite occupations. In 2000, 14.8% of women and 5.8% of men working in managerial, professional and technical fields logged less than 30 h per week (Jacobs and Gerson 2004: 34). The Hidden Brain Drain Task Force, a group of researchers and companies organized by Sylvia Hewlett helps to put conditions in medicine in perspective. As noted earlier, Hewlett's results indicate that 16% of highly qualified women work part-time. Thus, this result is very similar to results based on the Current Population Survey (Hewlett 2007). These patterns are broadly similar to the 15.1% of all employed female physicians and 7.8% of male physicians work part-time.

Today's Physicians: Workaholics or Overworked?

The growth of long workweeks and the limited expansion of part-time work are surprising in light of evidence indicating that huge portions of male and female physicians believe they work too much. While no doubt workaholics are well represented among physicians, there is a much larger and growing group that expresses interest in working fewer hours per week. For example, in the Young Physicians Survey, a nationally representative survey of physicians who finished training five or fewer years prior to the survey revealed that in 1987, 43% of male respondents and 42% of female respondents wished they could work less than they were working at the time. In 1991, 5 years after the initial survey, respondents' dissatisfaction with work hours had increased in this population such that 53% of men and 46% of women wished they could work less than their current professional schedule. After accounting for gender differences in hours worked, however, the gender gap in the desire to work less disappears. The desire to work less or to pursue part-time schedules has also been found in several studies of physicians in specific specialties including pediatrics and surgery (Fritz and Lantos 1991; Mayer et al. 2001). Interest in part-time opportunities goes well beyond physicians seeking more time for family. Many older physicians also seek reduced schedules. In fact, in 2005, 32% of physicians 50–64 years of age indicated that they were interested in part-time hours, but did not have that option in their current position (Harris 2007).

Like trends in work effort, data on physicians' interest in flexible or reduced work schedules belies the contention that the unique interests of female physicians are transforming the medical profession. It does not appear that the desire to work less or more flexibly is a uniquely female desire.

In fact, dissatisfaction with work hours is significantly more pervasive among physicians than among the general population. This is not surprising given the gap between physicians' work hours and those of their peers. Jacobs and Gerson report that roughly one-third of the workers in the United States labor force preferred to work fewer hours per week (2004:74).

The low rates of part-time work are even more surprising in light of recent research on the relationship between part-time work and physician satisfaction. According to analyses of the recent representative Physician Work Life Study, part-time US physicians of both genders felt better able to control their work hours, work interruptions and work hassles.

Part-time physicians were significantly more satisfied than full-time physicians with patient care issues, personal time, administrative issues, and their jobs overall, and they noted significantly less stress than full-time physicians (McMurray et al. 2005). A nationally representative study of members of the American Academy of Pediatrics found similar results. Limiting work hours enhances pediatricians' sense of work/personal balance. Part-time pediatricians are more satisfied with time for their children and other personal activities, and express similar or greater professional satisfaction (O'Connor et al. 2004).

The relationship between work effort and professional well-being is not simply about access to part-time work. Recent research reveals that the strongest predictors of whether physicians of both genders will experience burnout and career dissatisfaction are how much control they have over the total number of hours they work in a week and their work schedules.

In other words, statistics suggest that physicians of both genders are working more and feeling more overworked. Studies indicate that there is a growing belief that reduced hour work could address the problem and research suggests that such beliefs are grounded in reliable social research. Nevertheless, in spite of articles titled "Practices must cope as more physicians work part-time (Croasdale 2002)" and "Women physicians find ways to make part-time work (Croasdale 2004a)," a large scale trend toward part-time work has yet to occur.

The Culture of Unfettered Professional Commitment

What we have seen is a mismatch between the desire on the part of many physicians for more manageable work schedules and the increasingly long weeks many physicians regularly work. In seeking to understand the causes of this disconnect, it may be useful to put the dilemmas of today's physicians in historical context.

Before the large-scale entry of women, the traditional culture of the medical profession physicians expected a high degree of professional commitment. In this context, physicians worked long hours because of a culture that required total availability to patients (Adams 2004) because of a more established human connection with patients (Hobson 2005), because of a stronger association between work effort and reimbursement, because of a reluctance to rely on each other, and because of greater support at home via wives who did not work for pay outside the home.[9] Even as late as 1980, most physicians generally worked alone or with one other partner (Kletke et al. 1996), so they

---

[9] In 1968, Dr. Burch, then president of the American College of Cardiology, wrote in the American Journal of Cardiology: It is generally considered that there is too much to learn in medicine today. This is not true… Time is the premium, and how it is used is the important factor. The problem is not that there is too much to learn, but rather that there are too many distractions. The…physician devotes too much time to other interests…Such interests leave little time for medicine. The physician is often unable to resist these distractions and more often than not enjoys them more than he enjoys medicine…the devoted clinician obtains the greatest of pleasure from his work. He enjoys study, clinical practice and his patient more than anything else. He does not need to force himself to study and work with patients (Gerber 1983).

did not enjoy economies of scale. The small size of the average physician practice had an especially severe effect on the need to work at night and on the weekends. On-call hours have been greatly reduced as practice size has increased, and the effect of call time on physicians' lifestyles has been dramatically transformed by the development of reliable cell phones that enable physicians to take calls from where ever their lives take them.

Similarly, community-based physicians in the 1980s and earlier often established long-standing relationships with their patients. They not only knew them in the office, they also knew them in the community. This connection contributed to a larger incentive to create time for patients regardless of the physicians' schedule. During this era, it was more common for physicians to address patients' needs after hours even if they were not on call simply because their patients were members of their community. (It is worth emphasizing that our reference to time does not imply they were conducting longer visits. Instead, creating time involves the willingness to allow work to spill over into family life so that patients can see the same provider overtime rather than different members of the same group.) The obstetrician who himself delivered his pregnant patient will make a greater effort to be available to deliver his pregnant patient's child, than one who has only recently come to know his patient. This type of doctor–patient relationship is extremely rare for pregnant patients today since most obstetricians practice in a group and require patients to accept the services of whoever is on call when labor starts. Further, this type of doctor–patient relationship requires that obstetricians be completely unencumbered by family needs, an increasingly rare situation given the high numbers of women in the field. Similarly, the pediatrician, who sees his patients every time he goes to his child's sporting events, will feel a unique personal connection to them and may thus be more likely to offer medical advice when these children call the house or unexpectedly show up on the physicians' door step. Research indicates that both physician and patient enjoy greater satisfaction and trust when their relationship endures over time (Rodriguez et al. 2007). This enhanced satisfaction inevitably translated into greater physician availability and greater hours for physicians.

Finally, physicians prior to the 1980s arrived in the office early and worked late in part because they had the support at home to maintain this schedule. First, those with the support of a full-time homemaker spouse did not have to worry about being available for their children. And second, those with homemaker spouses may have felt greater responsibility to provide income to the family, so they had an extra incentive to provide additional services. Even today, male physicians with stay-at-home wives work more hours per week than do other physicians, although the difference is just a few hours per week.

Over time, although the factors keeping physicians work effort high before 1980 have dissipated, other forces have emerged that have maintained long workweeks. Connections between physicians and patients have weakened. Turnover is higher for patients because of insurance restrictions.[10] Access to unique physicians is more limited because practices have grown. So, even if a patient stays with one practice, they do not always see the same provider. Similarly, practice size has grown, so physicians can share responsibilities. And, physicians' spouses have begun to work at higher rates, so today's male medical professionals have somewhat less flexibility. Physicians are increasingly specialized so they are less likely to build relationships with families over time and more likely to see patients with isolated issues. As the availability of general practitioners declined, even primary physicians became less likely to handle everyone in the family and thus less likely to build relationships.

However, as the factors creating long weeks before 1980 dissipated, new structural forces have developed to take their place, and the new forces inevitably affect both male and female physicians.

---

[10] We suggest that as managed health care has become more common, continuity of care has declined. We base this on research by Flocke et al. (1997) who found in their analysis of 138 community-based providers that patients with IPA/PPO health insurance were four times as likely as patients with fee-for-service insurance to report a forced change in their primary care physician, and that these changes were strongly correlated with patient satisfaction and other health outcomes.

In particular, as health care technology and knowledge has improved and health care financing has evolved from a retrospective to a prospective model, the work of the average physician has become increasingly stressful and challenging (Schafermeyer and Asplin 2003). An astute observer of the medical scene, Charles Bosk has stressed the role of increased patient acuity in increasing the demands on physicians.

> Many of the changes of managed care have in essence been the operational equivalent of speeding up the assembly line. If hospital stays are shorter and if service size is constant, then those patients being treated are sicker as a group than they were twenty years ago… Sicker patients require more surveillance, more management, more worry, more coordination with nursing, more consulting with colleagues in other specialties, more scheduling of ancillary services and more communication with family members than do less sick ones. (Bosk 2003: 251)

It is important to emphasize that the increasing acuity of patients is occurring throughout the health care system rather than simply in the inpatient environment. Technological innovations have made it possible for patients with chronic illnesses like diabetes to survive significantly longer than they once did. Most of these patients need significant medical attention throughout their lives. Caring for sicker patients inevitably takes more time.

At the same time, it is no secret that the US health care delivery and financing systems are rapidly evolving. Historically, American physicians operated as a disorganized group of very independent professionals. Today, many are increasingly forced to practice within highly bureaucratized vertically integrated systems and to contend with increasingly powerful oversight from funders who often employ near monopsomy power. Together, these structural changes have resulted in declining reimbursements and increasing administrative hassles. A 2005 article in *U.S. News* entitled "Doctors Vanish from View: Harried by the bureaucracy of medicine, physicians are pulling back from patient care" captured the sentiments of many in medicine. In particular, according to Carl Getto, associate dean for hospital affairs at the University of Wisconsin Medical School:

> The hassle factors. The rewards – including satisfying relationships autonomy and high status are increasingly outweighed by… reams of time consuming paperwork, declining reimbursements and a loss of autonomy (Hobson 2005).

Bureaucratization assumes many forms. Although some enhance quality, many do not and almost all of these changes involve additional work for health care providers. For example, today, physicians must spend time seeking clearance to perform certain procedures and prescribe certain drugs. Physicians are also often expected to provide more proactive care to patients seeking relief from specific symptoms and to document all of their responses for multiple sources including private insurance and the government. So, while the average internist of past generations might simply treat a patient who presents with bronchitis symptoms for bronchitis, today's physicians are expected to offer that bronchitis patient care for his diabetes and counseling for his obesity. Yet, the visit is reimbursed at the same or even at a lower rate than it was in the past. In addition to providing more holistic care, they must also document these reforms more fully and more often for agencies attempting to enhance quality. Since this work is not reimbursed and since physicians' ability to set prices for their services has been severely restricted, these administrative hassles must either reduce physicians' pay or increase their work effort.

Further, physicians' stress is not limited to the increased acuity of their patients and the increased expectations of their bureaucracies. It also stems from increasing demands and knowledge of their clientele. David Mechanic tracks changes in patients' expectations in his 2003 article "Physician Discontent Challenges and Opportunities," He cites a 1957 study of ambulatory clinics that found patients to be poorly informed about their own illnesses and about common diseases and notes that they showed little evidence of demanding information. He then suggests that by the mid-1980s, as many as two-fifths of persons studied were behaving to some extent in a consumerist manner – seeking information exercising some independent judgment, showing cost consciousness, and demonstrating a reasonable level of knowledge. Those who demonstrated a consumerist orientation were on average better educated and reported less faith in and dependence on physicians (Roter and Hall 1992). Finally, mechanic cites a Community tracking Study by Tu and Hargraves (2003) which found that 38% of those surveyed in 2000–2001 had "looked for or obtained information about a personal health concern" from a source other than their physician. Those with a college education or higher were most likely to seek independent information and use the Internet. In addition to coping with better-informed patients, physicians also find themselves treating a growing population of misinformed patients. Since 1998, when the FDA relaxed guidelines surrounding direct to consumer pharmaceutical advertising, doctors have had to confront a growing population of patients who seek specific prescriptions after seeing pharmaceutical advertisements on television. Physicians complain that they must spend inordinate amounts of time negotiating with this population or provide the prescription inappropriately (Maguire 1999). Given changes in patients' knowledge and expectations, the average time a doctor spends per patient has actually been increasing (Mechanic et al. 2001). The increase in time per patient and the reductions in reimbursements together have contributed to the growing medical workweek.

Do these currents affect women as much as men? In general, the structural changes facing male physicians are also facing their female colleagues.[11] One female physician we interviewed who had achieved tenure at an elite medical school reflected on how things had changed in medicine. She said that when she finished one of her rotations as a resident, the patients had a going away party for her. Then she commented that such a party would be impossible today because patients who are healthy enough to have a party are not in the hospital.

The increasing representation of women in specialty fields that demand long workweeks is another contributing factor. As we have documented elsewhere (Boulis and Jacobs 2008), the level of gender differentiation across specialties has remained roughly constant since 1985. However, given the growing numbers of women in medicine, this means that the absolute numbers of women in fields that involve long and unpredictable hours like general surgery are increasing (see also Croasdale 2007).

Ultimately, the disconnect between the desire for work–family balance and the reality of medical work stems largely from structural pressures beyond the control of individual physicians. In some instances, those forces reside in the general labor market. As we suggest, our economy is constructed in a way that is increasing pressures on elite workers to work long weeks, and limiting meaningful part-time opportunities. In other respects, medicine remains unique. Pressures on modern physicians are creating work environments that are increasingly difficult to manage. While technological advances like personal computers, cell phones, and the internet have inevitably heightened expectations on professional workers overall, we suggest that technological and financial change has been even more pronounced in medicine. Thus, it is not surprising that physicians endure longer weeks than their professional peers. Although female physicians are more likely to seek and find part-time positions, their ultimate effect on the availability of part-time work within the profession will be greatly restricted by independent trends in American medicine.

Obstacles to Part-Time Work

Women entered a medical profession which took long workweeks for granted, and in recent years, powerful forces have contributed to an expansion of work commitment on the part of most physicians. The pursuit of part-time opportunities thus runs counter to these historical patterns.

---

[11] Under some circumstances, changes facing female physicians might be more severe since patients seeking specific drugs might expect female providers to be more accommodating of their requests.

Overall, there is a lack of viable part-time opportunities in many medical contexts. There are multiple barriers to part-time work in medicine. Some of these factors are unique to the profession but others occur in many elite occupations. In general, part-time work is lacking in the USA for professionals. Further, the part-time work that is available is clustered disproportionately in the lower tiers of the profession.

Barriers to part-time work include cultural and organizational obstacles. Many of these types of obstacles are not unique to medicine. In fact, they pervade professional work in the USA and may even be stronger in other professions (The Hidden Brain drain task force found that although rates of part-time work are limited for all elite women, it is lowest for women in business). However, there are also financial and patient-related factors that limit demand for part-time medical work, and in this arena obstacles are often unique to medical work. Many physicians who want to work less do not seek part-time schedules because such positions involve major sacrifices. Although many of the barriers to reduced schedules appear immutable, other barriers can be removed or reduced.

Cultural and Organizational Factors

Women physicians seeking reduced work hours have often encountered superiors who are willing to reduce their salaries and rewards but reluctant to reduce work-related expectations. This problem is evident throughout the profession, reflecting a long-standing view that devotion to medicine takes precedence over all other commitments (Adams 2004), but it is especially prominent in academic medicine. As the following quote from the MomMD Website suggests, those with authority in academic medicine can be reluctant to embrace part-time schedules for staff physicians and academic faculty.

> I have a similar experience in academic medicine (pathology). I asked my chair (a man) almost a year ago to be part-time. He was willing to cut my salary, but this did not come with a decrease in the work load. About a month ago, I informed him that I was not going to renew my contract as of July 1. I basically had to entirely quit my job to get more time for my family. There was no flexibility. Posted doski 04-24-2007

> I just have not figured out how to make it in my job only working 4 days. My boss has told me that in my area (mostly research) that women who "cut back" still wind up doing the same amount of work – they just get paid less for it. So she opposes part-time or "less time." She thinks that is made up for by the amazing flexibility that my job provides. All she says is "I don't care when or where you work, just get the job done." But really, I would like to just do 80% of the job for 80% of the money. 08-24-2006 *Conflicted*

The failure to reduce work-related expectations for part-time workers coexists with a trend to increasing expectations for full-time professional workers that is in part responsible for increases in the average workweek of the highly educated labor force.

This pattern is evident for many professional women outside the medical context as well. In a qualitative study of highly educated women who were out of the labor force, Stone and Lovejoy find that "upon becoming mothers, about half of the women in our sample expressed a desire to cut back on their work hours and/or to increase the flexibility of their schedules (Stone and Lovejoy 2004: 68)." Their efforts met with mixed results. However, one-third of the study sample cited workplace inflexibility as a major factor in their decision to interrupt their careers. The authors note that women spoke repeatedly about having full-time responsibilities on a part-time schedule, of doing a "job and half" when they were supposed to be doing half a job.

While workplace inflexibility is real in medicine, evidence suggests that women physicians are somewhat more likely than women in other elite careers to cope with the demands of family life by reducing their hours without accepting a formal part-time position. Results from the Hidden Brain Drain Task Force survey indicate that 38% of female physicians and 25% of elite workers in other occupations worked a reduced but nevertheless full-time job schedule (Hewlett and Luce 2005). Ultimately, the meaning of a reduced but full-time schedule is unclear, since physicians work so much more on average than others professionals.

The other side of this situation involves physicians who accept part-time positions and end up working full-time hours. One part-time internist we interviewed abandoned her position in favor of an oncology fellowship because she ultimately concluded that part-time work was not possible and that if she was going to work full-time, she preferred the type of work and the type of pay enjoyed by specialists.

Another critical problem limiting part-time work among professional workers overall involves the uniquely high sacrifices that part-time workers in elite occupations must endure. Physicians report facing both short-term disapproval and longer term career sacrifices for challenging time norms that expect them to work far more than 40 h a week so that they can spend time with their families.

Many physicians who seek better work and family balance share these experiences. As the following quotes from the MomMD Website suggests part-timers often feel they have to give up respect and a sense of professionalism:

> as a part-timer, i have had to continually advocate for myself. kpzr/9145 Plus Member Member # 4520 02-05-2007

> I have been part-time for 5 years now, and am probably quitting, mostly due to the treatment I get as a part-timer. I get considered last for the work schedule, don't get my name on the group prescription pads, don't get invited to any company social functions – all due to my part-time status. I have no benefits at all. I made it clear to my employer that I was limited to part-time due to family but that I was planning to commit to working there for the future as I live in that area and would even consider going full-time there when my kids were older. I am getting no credit toward partnership for these years. **Carole** 07-01-2005 08:39 AMJuly 01, 2005 08:39 AM Member # 3851

Physicians seeking better work–family balance sacrifice more than professional rewards like pay and promotion. They also incur the criticism of their colleagues. One survey of internal medicine specialists indicates that even in the Netherlands where rates of part-time work are generally high, physicians view part-time colleagues with suspicion (Lugtenberg et al. 2006). In the *Part-time Paradox*, Cynthia Epstein and her colleagues report a similar pattern among lawyers who sought out part-time work (Epstein et al., 1998). Further, the available part-time work is clustered disproportionately in the less prestigious aspects of the profession. According to the Physician Work Life Study, the highest proportions of part-time physicians were found in general pediatrics (20%) and in health maintenance organizations (22%). Although these results are in part related to the number of women in pediatrics and in health maintenance organizations, male pediatricians were significantly more likely to choose part-time practice than their family practice counterparts (16 vs. 7%; $P=0.05$) (McMurray et al. 2005). Here again, this pattern is reflected in other settings outside of medicine. Those professionals who do secure reduced schedules are often in the lower tiers of their industries (NALP 2006).[12]

One set of organizational constraints involves scheduling bottlenecks in hospital settings. Many physicians who desire flexible schedules must rely on hospitals and other institutions to provide their services. Hospitals have historically had a very difficult time allocating operating room time because assessing the length of an operation is very difficult. (Jarnberg et al. 2001). In an effort to cut costs and maintain fiscal solvency, hospitals are limiting staff anesthesiologists and operating

---

[12] In 2006, nearly all offices, 96%, allowed part-time schedules, either as an affirmative policy or on a case-by-case basis, but as has been the case since NALP first compiled this information in 1994, very few lawyers are working on a part-time basis, just 5% overall. Associates are more likely to work part-time (4.7%) than partners (2.8%), but other lawyers, such as counsel and staff attorneys, show the highest rate of part-time work, over 16% (NALP 2006).

room nurses, thus forcing surgeons and other providers who perform procedures with "add on" cases to wait until after the standard business day has ended in order to perform procedures that could theoretically be done during the standard workday if operating room staff were available (Matthias 1997). This is an especially prominent problem for cases that need prompt attention but are not life-threatening emergencies, like kidney stones.

Economic Constraints

Many physicians who would like to work less do not attempt to negotiate or find reduced work because of the inevitable financial penalty that part-time work involves.[13] Although physicians have high earnings prospects, there are several financial considerations that hit physicians harder than many other workers.

Like other Americans, physicians are increasingly too strapped financially to consider part-time work. Increasing tuition costs often leave medical students with considerable debt. Median debt in 2003 was 4.5 times median debt in 1984. By 2003, the median debt was $100,000 and $135,000 for public school and private school graduates, respectively (Croasdale 2004b).

As a result, part-time work is financially unrealistic for a growing portion of newly minted physicians. As mentioned earlier in the essay, research on pediatricians indicates that loans are a major obstacle to part-time work (Cull et al. 2002). Financial barriers are especially pronounced if, like the author of this MomMD post, physicians attempt to start their own practice:

> As far as payback, it is tough. I always wanted to work part-time, but I can't see cutting back at all anytime in the next several years. Right now, between my husband and myself, we are just barely covering our expenses, living paycheck to paycheck. We have no savings at all and have significant credit card debt because of all of those "emergencies" that pop up–like the cars breaking down, etc. At the moment one of our cars may be broken beyond repair and if that happens we'll have to take out yet another loan to buy a new (used) one. I'm not sure where we will come up with the money for that. 12-05-2006 06:35 AMDecember 05, 2006 06:35 AM rydys

However, it is misleading to think that financial stress is limited to those in the initial stages of establishing a practice. As this Mom MD quote suggests, reimbursements and overhead and making it increasingly difficult to make ends meet in some specialties:

> "One Family Practice physician recently complained that her net take-home pay after all expenses (including malpractice and student loans) is approximately $37,000 per year, less than her husband's salary as a Chief Petty Officer in the Navy." Now I really want to be a Dr bcuz I want to help people and I am challenged and interested by the field but the money part is somewhat important too. I mean, 11 years of school and tons of hard, hard work to make 37K/yr is ridiculous!! Is this realistic?!?!?! posted 04-07-2007 08:08 PM April 07, 2007 08:08 PM ALLALLY

> Yes, I personally know docs who have taken home less than 50K in a year. It has become extremely difficult to make a good living in private practice. 04-07-2007 09:40 PM AnnaM

Physicians' financial struggles are also seen in the general population. Although many workers indicated that they want to work less in general, answers shift markedly when issues of wages are added. When options are posed as trade-offs between time and money, working less becomes less attractive.

The fixed costs associated with a medical practice tend to encourage long workweeks. In other words, if there are costs that are present no matter how much work is done, the physician must

---

[13] Some have suggested that physicians dropping to part-time must be willing to take more than a proportional cut in take-home pay to make up for fixed expenses like overhead costs and health and malpractice insurance (Walpert 2002).

devote a considerable portion of the workweek recouping these unavoidable expenses. Malpractice insurance is an example of a large and growing cost of practicing medicine that endures whether the physician is employed 30 h per week or 60 h per week.

The limited availability of part-time work in medicine reflects these types of pressures, especially in those specialties of medicine and regions of the country where malpractice costs are high.[14] The experiences of one academic obstetrician capture this phenomenon:

> Creative options for balancing work and family are few. The recent escalation in the cost of malpractice insurance coverage has largely precluded options for part-time practice; the physician who delivers one patient per month pays just as high a rate as everyone else. At my academic medical center, premiums in my department increased by 68% last year, which brought the base rate to $100 000 per physician per year. (Some of my colleagues were assessed twice that.) A number of senior men, but interestingly enough, none of the women, promptly gave up obstetrics altogether and switched to a predominantly surgical gynecology practice. When I asked to cut back to a 4-day work week, I was told I couldn't possibly generate enough revenue to cover the expense of keeping me, what with salary, overhead, and liability insurance (Plante, 2004).

Although malpractice is a particularly severe barrier for high-risk specialists seeking work–family balance, malpractice premiums present a significant obstacle to any physicians seeking part-time work (Walpert 2002).

Practice ownership similarly tends to induce proprietors to put in long workweeks. Incentives among self-employed professionals involve a tradeoff between autonomy and control and the burden of fixed operating costs. On one hand, the self-employed ostensibly have more control over their work lives and should therefore be better able to strike a satisfying work and family balance. And there are instances when such control has actually helped women in medicine. For example, when Sandra Adamson Fryhofer, FACP, a general internist in Atlanta and the College's President-elect, gave birth to her twins, there was no maternity leave. But because she was in solo practice, she could choose not to schedule patients when she had a parent-teacher conference or another home-work conflict. The result may have been that she earned less that day, but it was her choice (Gesensway 1999).

On the other hand, the self-employed in medicine and other professions encounter severe pressures to work long hours both because they must personally shoulder all of the fixed costs associated with their businesses and because they often reap the financial rewards of additional work more directly than their professional peers who work for others and are often reimbursed with a fixed salary.

Ultimately, the pressures to pay the bills and earn the money appear to be winning out for self-employed physicians. Data from the 2000 Census indicate that male and female employed physicians between 30 and 50 who are self-employed owners or coowners of incorporated businesses work significantly longer hours than their peers. While women physicians work an average of 46.9 h per week, self-employed women physicians with incorporated businesses work 51 h per week. While men physicians work an average of 55.1 h per week, self-employed men physicians with incorporated businesses work 58 h per week.

The pressures on self-employed physicians to work long hours are inevitably stronger when physicians are part-owners rather than sole proprietors. Physicians who have partners must balance their desire for flexible schedules with their need to pay their share of the overhead. Since changes in health care are making solo practice increasingly difficult and unprofitable, fewer physicians are considering it as an option (Cook 2007), and those who do attempt private practice may have less control than Dr. Fryhofer because of the increasing bureaucratic demands on private practice physicians. Thus, while Dr. Fryhofer's solo practice seems like an ideal situation for a working mother, it is increasingly unrealistic to expect physicians of either gender to pursue self employment as an option (Cook 2007). Further, as we discussed above, today's young medical graduates may simply

---

[14] Not only do malpractice premiums vary by state and specialty, they also vary within state. In 2002, a family practitioner in Cincinnati is $12,650, according to insurer ProAssurance, whereas the rate is $21,375 in Cleveland (Hawkins 2002).

be unable to make the choice that Dr. Fryhofer made because of a radically different financial horizon. The odds are that they have loans which Dr. Fryhofer did not have, and the reality is that they will not be paid as well as Dr. Fryhofer was paid (Dolan 2006).

Practice Considerations

Cultural, organizational, and financial considerations are not the only barriers to flexible professional schedules. Physicians are often expected to be continuously available to their clients. While systematic data on client expectations are not readily available, we suspect that patients are even more likely than other types of clients to expect continuous access to services because of the essential nature of health problems. As this post on the MomMD Website suggests, some patients, including physician–patients, do not react well to part-time physicians:

> I know for one (and I hope that this does not piss anyone off) that if I had a pediatrician and my kid was sick and needed to see her/him and she was part-time and not available until X day…that would tick me off and we would chose someone else. I know this sounds bad and it is probably not the PC thing to say but it "is" how I feel for now. 08-27-2005 06:45 PM August 27, 2005 06:45 PM efex101.

In fact, studies of patient satisfaction with primary care suggest that satisfaction depends on access to care and care continuity, among a list of seven factors (Anderson et al. 2007; Fan et al. 2005). Thus, the perception that patients want their physicians to be available is grounded in some degree of reality.[15]

The need to be persistently available is equally present for specialists. However, as this MomMD quote indicates, for specialists, the issue often involves being available for referrals:

> I've been reading with interest about how physicians work part-time or job share, but I don't know how to cut back on my work hours. I am a general surgeon (with 2 young children) in a group practice, taking call every 4th weekend. Over the past 8 years, I have tried to limit my work hours and numbers of patients seen, but in a field where my business depends on *my availability for referrals* [emphasis added] as well as my desire to follow my patients postoperatively, I don't know how I can cut back any more without going out of business. I love surgery, especially the laparoscopy, and I want to "stay in the game" while still raising a family. http://www.mommd.com/ubb/ultimatebb.php/ubb/get_topic/f/2/t/000475

The issue involved with "availability for referrals" involves more than the absolute number of hours a specialist works. Ideally, specialist physicians must court primary care physicians in order to maintain referrals. This networking is normally done in the off hours and thus conflicts with the needs of physicians seeking a more realistic family life.

An additional force may pressure physicians to work long weeks in the near future. Health policy makers have suggested that there are not sufficient physicians to treat aging baby boomers and that access to care will be increasingly restricted because there are not enough physicians. Evidence from Massachusetts, the first state to adopt universal health insurance, indicates that the current supply of primary care physicians is already insufficient to meet demand (Ruiz 2008). Now that nearly all Massachusetts residents have health insurance, there is now a 3–4 week delay to see many specialists and a 10% increase in the number of family physicians who have closed their practices because they are so busy (Ruiz 2008). Although systematic evidence is lacking, it is reasonable to suspect that as the shortage persists and grows, many physicians will work more than they want to work because they do not want to turn sick or needy patients away.

---

[15]There is also limited evidence that continuity relates to positive health outcomes. In particular, research indicates that patients who see the same provider consistently are less likely to be hospitalized, are less likely to use emergency services, and are more likely to receive preventive services (Cabana and Jee, 2004).

Again, the need to be continuously available is a consideration not just for physicians, but in many other professions as well. Epstein et al. found that clients "stigmatize part-time lawyers by avoiding or refusing to work with them. Some attorneys reported that clients wanted to know why they have to work with someone who could be gone tomorrow" (Epstein et al. 1998: 32). Epstein's respondents reported being told that they needed to be available to take calls from clients on their day off.

A related problem that plagues many professionals seeking reduced schedules involves periods of high work load. As this MomMD post indicates, there is an expectation that part-time physicians will contribute additional time during periods of unanticipated high patient demand:

> I currently work part-time 2 days per week in a private pediatric office. My 2 days have been set for some time now, and I've therefore arranged my childcare around my schedule (don't have childcare on my off days). On multiple occasions over the past couple of years, my office mgr. has approached me to see if I could work "extra" days during busy winter months...I have firmly explained that I don't have childcare on those days, and that it would be impossible for me to add "extra" days... Now my office manager has approached me again to see if I could add a third day because the other docs are feeling so "slammed" this winter. I am very frustrated. I told her, once again, that I am unable to do this, and reviewed the reasons why. I might also mention that my contract specifies my days and hours. I wouldn't give it another thought, but I know that my office mgr's requests are coming from the other docs in the office, and it creates an aura that feels like I'm not "pulling my weight." I already feel this way, being the only part-time doc in the office. Does anyone have any suggestions for how to prevent these requests from continuing? 12-12-2006 kiddoc.

The immediate response to this part-time worker was a less than supportive MomMD post:

> While I can certainly understand where you are coming from, I can understand the other docs position as well. During the busy times of the year, everyone ends up working harder. For full time docs, that means staying later, working longer hours, and never having a day off. In the offices that I know the docs do not take vacation during holiday seasons and even if someone is usually off one day a week, they will often come in on that day to help out during the busiest weeks. There are a certain number of patients who need to be seen and the work just has to get done. During the busy seasons I often get out an hour or two later than usual and many docs I know will add extra evening hours.

The bottom line is that the part-time physician feels that since her hours are clearly stated in her contract she should not have to work late. The respondent suggests that although full-time is also clearly delineated, the expectation is that full-time physicians will work overtime to satisfy the need since they are professionals; so she reasons that a similar expectation should be placed on part-time professional workers. While this interaction may seem uniquely medical, we suggest that deadlines are common to many professional settings. A parallel situation inevitably exists, for example, for part-time accountants during tax season.

A final practice-related consideration concerns whether physicians working part-time can provide optimal care. The issues in this area differ for primary care and specialist physicians. Because primary care is often defined as continuous, coordinated, and comprehensive care (Gelb-Safran, 2003), some have inferred that continuous physician availability is important and that a traditional, full-time work schedule is optimal for patient care (Parkerton et al. 2003).

Although the reasoning seems sound, recent research calls the continuity-quality theory into question. For example, one study on part-time primary care physicians suggests that rather than demonstrating lower performance, primary care physicians working fewer clinical hours were associated with both slightly higher cancer screening rates and better diabetic management, and with patient satisfaction and ambulatory costs similar to those of full-time physicians (Parkerton et al. 2003).[16] Another study finds that although physicians working 65 h or more a week provided higher

---

[16] Research also suggests that part-time primary care physicians in an academic environment are more productive than their full-time counterparts. Most of these clinicians work full-time but limit their clinical responsibilities to attend to teaching and research (Warde 2001).

continuity of care, they also had significantly lower professional satisfaction, which ultimately may compromise their capacity to offer quality health care services (Muray et al. 2000).[17] In other words, while the patient continuity–physician work effort relationship is not debatable, the patient continuity-health care quality association is.

In light of the relationship between continuity and patient satisfaction, how can we explain the comparable satisfaction ratings of part- and full-time primary care physicians discussed earlier? One possibility is that the patients of part-time physicians tolerate the lack of continuity because they believe the higher quality of care provided by these physicians is worth the wait. This explanation jives well with the research that suggests that part-time physicians provide higher quality care, and suggests that although part-time medical work presents unique difficulties they are not insurmountable.

The issue for specialists has to do with the idea that "practice makes perfect." Thus, in some procedural areas, there is an association between case volume or surgical experience and patient outcomes for a variety of procedures (Gordon et al. 1999; Migliore et al. 2007; Dimick et al. 2003; Díaz-Montes et al. 2006; Hammond et al. 2003). In spite of this research, the leap between the volume-quality association and resistance to part-time surgical work may not follow as perfectly as it seems. At the very least, part-time workers could avoid the problem by limiting the range of procedures that they perform so that they can accrue sufficient volume. In fact, academic surgeons routinely specialize in this manner.

Further, while the research documenting a volume-outcome association is consistent and accepted, until recently, it has been limited in scope. Little effort has been made to follow surgeons over the course of their careers and to assess how total experience rather than annual volume relates to outcomes. One study on radical prostatectomy suggests that total experience plays a major role in outcomes. In particular, 5-year progression-free probabilities revealed a lifetime learning curve for the first 250-500 radical prostatectomies. This was true even after adjusting for positive surgical margins. The probability of recurrence decreased from 21% in the first ten cases to 12% after 250 prior cases. For every 11 men treated by an inexperienced urologist, one will relapse compared to those treated by an experienced surgeon (Vickers et al. 2007). If lifetime experience is a better proxy for skill then annual volume and the decisions to funnel patients to high volume surgeons should be rethought. Under such conditions, barriers to part-time surgical work might relax somewhat.

Further, research suggests that although high volume surgeons have better outcomes than low volume surgeons, there is significant variation in outcomes among the high volume population. These results suggest that volume may not entirely explain surgical outcomes. In fact, it is now thought that volume differences only proxy skill differences[18] and that a better approach to quality enhancement for surgical patients involves continuing education for surgeons, certification by procedure, and more frequent evaluation of health outcomes. Such improvements in outcomes research and surgical quality maintenance would inevitably enhance opportunities for part-time work among truly qualified surgeons.

---

[17] Research on the relationship between continuity of care and health outcomes for diabetes patients is mixed. Some studies fail to find an association (Guilliford et al. 2007), while others suggest an association exists.

[18] For example, evidence is mounting that surgeons can extend the survival of cancer patients by ensuring negative margins on their resections (Lange and Lin 2004). The theory is that the positive relationship between higher volume and outcomes for cancer surgery patients stems from the fact that surgeons who perform the case more often are more likely to ensure negative margins.

Residents and the 80-h-Per-Week Rule

One major step toward making medical training more family friendly has been the introduction of the 80-h rule for residents. As we will see, this development had less to do with women's entry into the profession and more to do with concerns about patient safety. Nevertheless, research suggests that residents of both genders are taking advantage of the 80 h work rule as much as they can (Jones and Jones 2007).

Until 2003, there was no official maximum on the number of hours per week that residents could spend in the hospital setting. Historically, residency training has been especially rigorous, with 70 h of work per week required in even the most lenient specialties. Before these regulations, most surgical residents worked a 36-h shift every third night, and routinely put in 12-h days on their "nights off." Residents always worked Saturday mornings. They often worked all day on Saturday and routinely spent at least one Sunday a month in the hospital. Residents in other fields normally had somewhat less demanding schedules that involved 36-h shifts every fourth night and less time on Saturday mornings, but routinely involved 12-h days.

The 80-h work rule was adopted primarily because of public concern about patient safety rather than about issues surrounding resident well-being (Woodrow et al. 2006).

Although the American Medical Student Association and the Council of Interns and Residents actively advocated for resident work hour restrictions, the well-being of residents of either gender was far from the major focus of the debates leading up to the adoption of work hour limits for US resident physicians. Indeed, the status of physician parents was hardly mentioned in these discussions. The initial public recognition of resident overwork came after Libby Zion died in 1984 as a result of the inadequate care provided by overworked and undersupervised medical residents. Her father, a writer for the *New York Times* worked to bring the issue to public attention. (Kwan and Levy 2006)

The Libby Zion case led the New York State Department of Health to convene a committee to review the state's residency training system. The committee recommended a series of reforms that were adopted by New York State in 1989. The regulations, often referred to as the Bell Code, stated that residents not work more than 24 consecutive hours and no more than 80 h a week, among a number of other provisions designed to enhance patient safety. While the Bell Code represented a milestone with respect to the regulation of residency training programs, these regulations were not uniformly implemented. Penalties for violations were limited and oversight was nearly nonexistent. So, many hospitals simply ignored the regulations.

A 1998 review conducted by the New York State Department of Health found that 60% of surgical residents worked more than 95 h per week (Kwan and Levy 2006). The investigation found violations at every single hospital it reviewed. As a result of this review, the state dramatically increased financial penalties for work code violations and hired an independent firm to monitor its hospitals.

As New York began to ratchet up its controls on resident work hours, national attention was drawn to the issue. In November of 1999, the Institute of Medicine released its report, *To Err is Human,* which suggested that medical errors result in 98,000 patient deaths and countless injuries every year. On the other hand, although the report focused public attention on patient safety, it had relatively little to say about residents work effort (Steinbrook 2002).

In April of 2001, the American Medical Student Association, the Committee on Interns and Residents and the nonprofit organization Public Citizen filed a petition with the Occupational Safety and Health Administration (OSHA) requesting that they restrict resident work hours to 80 h a week. The petitioners' main justification for their request involved the hazards sustained by student physicians. In November of 2001, Representative John Coyers (D-MI) introduced the Patient and Physician Safety and Protection Act of 2001 limiting resident work hours. However, the OSHA petition was denied and the federal legislation did not pass. Instead, the American Council on Graduate Medical

Education (ACGME) adopted its own regulations in July of 2003. But unlike the OSHA petition, the major impetus behind federal legislation involved efforts to improve patient care.

While the 2003 ACGME restrictions on resident work hours promise to limit the work effort of residents in the most challenging specialties, residency programs remain far from family friendly. Residents who become parents and seek to be meaningfully engaged in their children's lives will continue to face serious challenges. Even if the reforms are implemented accurately, and evidence suggests that they are still defied frequently (Landrigan et al. 2006), residents still must work 80 h a week and endure 24 straight hours of work periodically. Further, the regulations leave room for manipulation. In particular, at-home call is not subject to the same limitations as in-house call. Official regulations state that at-home call must not be "so frequent as to preclude reasonable rest and personal time." While the intent of the legislation is clear, there is ample room for abuse and interpretation. And research suggests that call duties vary significantly by specialty. One study found that residents in general surgery took call once every 6.9 min while residents in geriatric and general medicine took call once every 5 h (Chiu et al. 2006).

Further, as we noted earlier, changes in the technical content of American medicine are changing the nature of medical education. In particular, technological advances in medicine have increased the average morbidity of patients at all levels of care. Simply put, faced with more severe patient acuity, residents who are on-call at night have more to do, more procedures to complete, more tests to order, and more information to evaluate than was the case a generation ago. Residency programs remain very demanding temporally, physically, and mentally.

Residency programs are not only taxing but they can conflict with the peak period of family demands. Many, and perhaps most, female residents who become mothers do so during their residency training programs. Potee et al. (1999), who surveyed women who graduated from Yale University Medical School between 1922 and 1999, found that the overwhelming majority of these elite female physicians became mothers or intended to become mothers. The rate of having a first child during medical training was increasing for this group. Other studies confirm that more than one half of female physicians have their first child during residency (Seltzer 1999).

Accompanying the growing trend of child bearing during residency is increasing evidence of problem pregnancies for female physicians. Multiple studies show that pregnant residents endure higher rates of preterm labor, restricted fetal growth and preeclampsia than women of comparable age and socioeconomic status (Klebanoff et al. 1990; Gabbe et al. 2003).

Inadequate maternity leaves postbirth compound these problems. In separate studies of family practice and obstetrics – gynecology residents, the average length of maternity leave was between 4 and 8 weeks, derived from multiple sources including vacation, sick leave, and home-based electives. In other words, although residents took time off after child birth, most did not have a real maternity leave (Gjerdingen et al. 1995; Gabbe et al. 2003). And it is worth emphasizing that residents who returned to work so quickly usually did not do so in stages. Between 4 and 8 weeks after delivery, these women had the full responsibilities of a resident. So it is not surprising that many of them had difficulty arranging child care, guilt about being absent from their children, and difficulty continuing breast-feeding (Gjerdingen et al. 1995). In fact, recent research indicates that although many initiate breast-feeding, residents are often unable to continue because of their work schedules.[19]

Readers unacquainted with the specifics of medical training might find the results of these studies surprising, especially in light of the 1993 Family and Medical Leave Act. This Federal law requires that employees of firms with greater than 100 workers who have at least 1 year of firm specific experience be given at least 12 weeks of unpaid maternity leave. Since most residents do

---

[19] Healthy People goals suggest that 50% of mothers of 6-month olds should be breast-feeding. The rate for residents was only 15%. Residency work schedule was the most common reason cited for discontinuing breast-feeding (Miller et al. 1996).

not become pregnant during their first year and since most hospitals have at least 100 employees, residents should be eligible for 12 weeks of time that does not count against their vacation or sick leave. Yet, it appears that residents are not availing themselves of this opportunity.

This occurs, in part, because the status of residents is unclear, (residents are considered both employees and students). Their eligibility for maternity leave under the Family and Medical Leave Act is debatable. In other words, if residents are considered students, they are not eligible under FMLA. Only if residents are considered workers rather than students would they be eligible for FMLA coverage.

Second, although the number of teaching hospitals with established maternity leaves is increasing, (Surveys by the Council of Teaching Hospitals confirm this trend.), female residents know that much of the time they take after or before childbirth will have to be made up before they can graduate. They *also know* that other residents usually have to shoulder the additional work load whenever a resident takes any form of leave. Although practices may now be changing as a result of work hour restrictions, historically, replacement workers are almost never used to cope with resident absences. Third, because of their initially low salaries and high debts, residents are often not in a financial position to take unpaid maternity leave.

The obstacles are often logistical and financial. The structure of residency programs makes it logistically very difficult to incorporate women or men who wish to make up their leave time, especially if these individuals need to receive compensation during their make up period. Medicare pays hospitals for the residents they train and makes no allowance for temporary staff, so residents making up time and receiving pay are occupying the full-time slot of one of the potential next generation of residents. Needless to say, residency directors do not want to give up a training slot so that one student can work a few additional months.

Given these results, the availability of true flexibility for pregnant or nursing medical residents remains extremely low. Systematic research on residents in pediatrics revealed that only 43 of the 6609 pediatrics residents in 2003 completed all or some of their training on a part-time basis (Holmes et al. 2005). Data from the American Academy of Family Practice Website on family practice residency programs in the 2005–2006 training year indicate that of the 459 listed residency programs, only 45 of the 459 programs provide part-time or shared residency programs. If these opportunities are rare in family practice residencies, they are even less likely to exist in traditionally male residency programs such as surgery.

There is also some evidence that the female family practice residents are selecting those programs which offer family-friendly supports. We calculated the percent of residents in each program who were women in the 2003–2004 through 2005–2006 years. We then compared this 3-year average for the programs with part-time options to the programs without such flexible work schedules. In fact, programs with part-time schedules averaged 56% female, while programs without part-time options averaged 50% female. This evidence suggests that residency programs with part-time opportunities are more attractive to female residents.

The difference is less pronounced for on-site child care. Programs with this option were, on average, 52% female, while programs without this option were only 50% female. On the other hand, the existence of an on-site child care program does not ensure that resident parents can meet their child care needs since waiting lists often exist for these services and since they are often not available before or after standard business hours when residents are often working. As the number of female residents expands, these issues will become salient ones to larger and larger numbers of newly minted MDs.

Critics of the 80-h workweek might suggest that the solution to the resident mother problem is simple. Women in medicine, and perhaps other elite women, should simply wait until they have completed their training. Yet, many have suggested that graduate school is the ideal time to have children because work demands only increase after physicians enter practice. This is especially true for physicians entering research or management careers.

The Development of the 80 h Work Rules

Although an 80h maximum work rule offers some relief to physicians in training, the Bell Code and AGCME national rules that followed were not designed to make medicine more family friendly. As suggested earlier, the principal impetus instead was patient safety. The residency training period remains a physically demanding period, especially for physicians who are pregnant or nursing. Organizational and cultural barriers continue to inhibit the adoption of work structures that are truly conducive to a meaning work and family balance. It is not surprising that institutions have not acknowledged the need for paternal involvement in the lives of residents' children. There is little evidence that residents themselves consider such issues. One newly hired attending reflects on surgical residents' reactions to work hour regulations:

> You might expect that, as residents, we'd stand up and rejoice that these regulations have been passed. But I'll tell you, if you're the chief resident on the GI service and a case comes up that you may have one or two opportunities to do during your entire residency – well, many of us have to be dragged kicking and screaming out of the hospital (Gilbert and Miller 2004).

Although residents acknowledge that their lives are less stressed physically as a result of the regulations (Myers et al. 2006), many residents are critical of the regulations because the new policy can prevent them from gaining valuable experience and can prevent them from knowing their patients adequately (Cohen-Gadol et al. 2005).

The debate continues to center around whether 80 h is enough time to expose residents to the range of cases necessary to give them a thorough training and whether such regulations ultimately improve patient outcomes. Research on the effect of the new policy on residents' experiences is mixed. One recent study of internal medicine programs found that although hours allotted to inpatient clinical activity did not change, resident attendance at morning conference, a key didactic aspect of residents' training, declined. Further, residents' clinical elective time was reduced (Horwitz et al. 2006). Similarly, some studies suggest that operative experience did not change after work regulations were adopted (de Virgilio et al. 2006), and others suggest a different reality (Jarman et al. 2004). Still others suggest that the effect of regulations depends on the stage of the resident, with the fifth year residents getting sufficient operative experience (Ferguson et al. 2005). There is also a sense that the quality of medical students' experiences may be harmed by resident work restrictions (White et al. 2006). Further, studies of how the new policy influences patient outcomes have also yielded unclear results (Fletcher et al. 2004).

Thus, it appears that although the reforms were ultimately implemented, general resident well-being has not been prioritized in the health-care system and the well-being of resident parents is almost completely outside the purview of the public. Research indicates that resident well-being has improved since the implementation of work regulations, but there is no reason to believe that the success of these reforms stemmed from the residents themselves. On the other hand, the association between part-time residencies and the representation of women in family practice programs suggests that over time the collective power of women's individual choices might cause change in the profession. The change will be gradual, but it should ultimately occur because women's presence will ultimately be too significant. So, there is little reason to suspect that residents will actively promote more effective work–family balance, but perhaps the mere presence of women will result in small change.

In 2008, the Institute of Medicine released a report, "Resident Duty Hours: Enhancing Sleep, Supervision and Safety" that recommended revising the current regulations. In particular, it suggested providing 1 day off per week to residents, reducing the maximum number of hours a resident can work without rest and restricting the number of consecutive night float (graveyard) shifts to which residents are assigned. The current maximum shift length would be changed from 30 to 30 h with an uninterrupted 5-h break for sleep or a maximum of 16 h without a protected break (AMSA 2008).

While the American Medical Student Association officially supports the IOM recommendations (AMSA 2008), many individual medical students have expressed concern about how these revised regulations might effect their graduate medical education. One resident with whom we spoke suggested that the current regulations would either compromise the quality of her training or force her to extend her training for at least another year. As a result of her tremendous debt burden, she was not excited about the possibility of extending her training.

Further, many other medical organizations, like the American Association of Neurological Surgeons, have expressed concern about the IOM recommendations, suggesting that they will significantly harm patients and increase health care costs. For neurosurgeons concerns centered on the possibility that duty hours would increase mistakes related to patient handoffs and that work restrictions would limit the amount of experiences that residents receive (Jeffrey 2008).

Finally, there is concern if current reforms take effect without adequate oversight and funding, the burden of excessive work and accompanying fatigue may simply be shifted from residents to other providers. This sense was expressed in writing by the Committee on Bioethics of the American Academy of Pediatrics who issued comments on a draft version of the IOM report:

> ...there is a real danger in isolating resident hours from the rest of the system. It is doubtful that there will be additional resources available to the system to hire additional providers and there is no question that older physicians (i.e., attendings) are for the most part being asked to absorb the consequences of duty hour changes. The data are pretty clear that sleep deprivation and long hours are tolerated much less well by older individuals than by younger ones, so that shift can hardly be justified on the basis of patient safety (Tayloe 2009).

One attending physician suggested that the resident work regulations have effectively postponed the period in a physician's life when he or she must work extended hours. He suggested that because of work hour regulations, new attending physicians are being forced to handle middle of the night problems that used to be addressed by residents. Whereas the old system put the bulk of the burden on individuals in their twenties, the new system is forcing attending physicians who are older and thus even less capable of working all night to perform without sleep. Thus, ultimately, women and men in medicine may find that the work hour regulations only postpone the period of unreasonable hardship. Ultimately, middle of the night work is not conducive to family life at any point.

One hospitalist attending expressed a parallel concern. She recalled seeing several residents in the call room one evening who were ineligible to work because of current regulations, and a crowded emergency department being serviced by two physicians assistants. She suggested that health care quality would suffer without appropriate oversight of the extenders, who are hired to cover resident shifts.

Unlike previous reports, the current report dedicates an entire chapter to understanding how resident work schedules affect resident well-being.[20] On the one hand, the Institute's willingness to acknowledge residents' well-being reflects a dramatic change from prior publications on medical errors that focused primarily on health care quality. On the other hand, the discussion continues to be posed in terms of societal needs. According to the report, residents need sleep primarily so they can interact constructively with colleagues and patients. Ultimately, the attempt to understand the interface between work and well-being is woefully incomplete. This chapter considers how extreme work affects residents' physical and mental health as well as their capacity to relate to colleagues and patients, but it does not address work and family conflicts or consider how extreme work affects residents' personal relationships.

---

[20] The IOM describes research that suggests that extreme work schedules increase residents' risks of occupational injury through percutaneous needle sticks. It suggests that residents who endure long workdays are at significantly higher risks of traffic accidents, because they routinely drive in very fatigued states and it reviews research which indicates that extreme workweeks and limited sleep put resident physicians at risk for weight gain, depression, burnout, and other negative factors. The report even suggests that long workdays jeopardize resident physicians' professional relationships with other health care providers.

The Advent of "Convenient Care"

As restrictions in the resident work hour laws promise to make medical training more family friendly, the development of "convenient care" will increase opportunities for flexible work arrangements for primary care physicians. Convenient care clinics are health care facilities located in high-traffic retail outlets with pharmacies adjacent that provide affordable and accessible, episodic care to consumers who otherwise would have to wait for appointments with a traditional Primary Care Physician or Provider (PCP). Customers at these clinics are charged a flat rate of around $50.00 rather than a standard physician fee which is often over $100. Often, these clinics are staffed with physician extenders such as physicians' assistants and nurse practitioners rather than physicians. However, most clinics have a "collaborating" physician associated with them who oversees the work of the extenders. The exact hours of collaborating physicians vary, but many work only 12 h per week. According to staff we interviewed at flexdoc.com, an agency that recruits physicians for several convenient care organizations, the exact role of the collaborating physician varies in accordance with state-specific regulations, but many collaborating physicians can perform duties via teleconferencing. That is, they can work from home. While collaborating physicians have flexibility, they sacrifice a great deal in terms of benefits. Often, they are employed for an hourly wage rather than a salary.

Like the advent of resident work regulations, convenient care clinics were not developed with the needs of physicians in mind. Instead, companies like Walmart and Walgreens saw opportunities to make a profit and to capitalize on the convenience of their pharmacies. As we will show in section "Inflexibility in the Lives of Individual Male and Female Physicians", many physicians will be unable to consider working as collaborating physicians because of financial pressures. Staff at flexdoc.com emphasized that women are not the only ones taking these positions and that several are maintained by physicians who need extra work in order to make ends meet.

Inflexibility in the Lives of Individual Male and Female Physicians

In light of the significant limitations on family-friendly reforms in the profession, we consider how individual male and female physicians and physician organizations are coping. As we have discussed, since part-time work is available for only a select few, and since the percent of male physicians with full-time spouses is declining, physicians must consider alternative methods of work–family balance.

Those who attempted to balance work and family during the late 1970s and early 1980s did so largely on their own and inevitably endured extremely high levels of stress. Bonita Stanton reflects on her experiences as a young physician mother in 1978. She returned to work just weeks after her first daughter was born, including taking on-call responsibility every fourth night.

> My first night back on call was simply a disaster; I could not get back to my call room to nurse my hungry daughter. Patients kept arriving to be admitted and those already hospitalized demanded attention. As I hustled about, a cadre of students anxious for teaching were left as hungry as my child. Meanwhile, holed up in my hospital call room, my husband paged me repeatedly, eventually putting the phone next to our crying infant to emphasize the point that she was hungry. By the time I got to my room, my daughter was too overwrought to nurse. By the early light of day when a moment of quiet finally arrived, I was stunned with disappointment in the complete failure of my first foray into combining my roles as parent, physician, spouse, and teacher – and overwhelmed with the loneliness of the position in which I found myself. This was not how I had expected young motherhood to feel (Stanton 2007).

While this episode may well represent an extreme case, the obstacles to successful nursing as a physician remain very real. Statistics suggest that many resident (and attending) physician mothers react to them by weaning children earlier than other highly educated women rather than by delaying their children's feeding (Duke et al. 2007). Ultimately, the failure to provide residents with nursing opportunities reflects a severe hypocrisy in medicine since physicians are currently recommending that mothers breast-feed for the first year of their children's lives.

In addition to enduring severe physical stress, physician mothers of the 1970s and early 1980s had to endure social isolation. They lacked support from a broader community of working professional women. Gail Jacoby, who graduated from Jefferson in 1972, had her first child during the third year of residency. She worked until the day her daughter was born and returned 5 weeks later. A month before she and her husband finished their residencies they moved into a house. Gail comments that she was the only full-time working mother of an infant in the neighborhood. Similarly, Lori DePersia, a 1981 graduate, reflects on her efforts to balance work and family in a recent edition of the Jefferson Medical College alumni bulletin:

> What was the climate like for working mothers at that time? Most of the working moms had jobs to make ends meet. Being a new mom and working was frowned upon by much of society… Most of the other mothers at the schools did not work. It is different now, but back then most professional women took a few years off or went super part-time (one weekend a month or less) until their children were older (20–21).

Inevitably, women physicians of this era not only had to endure the grueling hours associated with medical work and the inevitable guilt associated with leaving young children, but they also had to endure the condemnation of their community.

Over time, it seems reasonable to expect that conditions would have improved for mothers in medicine. In some respects they have. Medical mothers not only encounter other physician mothers in the workplace, they are also more likely to encounter professional mothers in their neighborhoods because more women work. So, the sense of isolation that the early generation experienced inevitably has lessened.

Further, in some specialties, opportunities to pursue reduced schedules have increased so that women in those fields now encounter relatively more family-friendly work opportunities than professional women overall. Laura Weinstein, a 1994 graduate of Jefferson, comments that she went part-time after her youngest child turned three. She says that she reduced her hours so she could spend more time with her children now that "they're interactive humans." Another woman we interviewed, a 1994 graduate of Harvard medical school, dropped out of the labor force when her second child was born and then ultimately returned to work 15 h a week as the medical director of a public clinic.

Yet, as we suggested earlier, it would be premature to suggest that women entering the medical workforce today encounter a truly family-friendly environment. In many ways, the challenges that women physicians confront as they struggle to balance work and family closely parallel those experienced by all working mothers in two career families. For example, as we noted earlier, physicians struggle to continue breast-feeding after returning to work. One physician mother comments on her efforts to breast-feed in the late 1990s:

> When I breastfed in the late 90's, I worked in a small medical research institute. I am a physician. When I asked if there might be a private area where I may pump milk, I seemed to be looked at as if I had two heads. I was told no one there had ever pumped breast milk before, and though they did find me a nice quiet area, I felt as if I was causing a great disruption. Mind you, this is a medical research institute filled with pediatricians and internal medicine physicians. Even in such a place, at least as recently as a half-dozen years ago, breast-feeding was an anomaly (Kantor 2006).

Another woman commented on the lack of breast-feeding space in a recently built Harvard Medical School building:

> I'm at Harvard Medical School working in one of the newest and most spacious buildings on the campus, The New Research Building. Given that many of the young scientists and physicians and support staff are beginning families, you might think this building would include a room for breast-pumping. But in our new multi-million dollar beautiful building our "pump room" is simply a bathroom stall. This is just one of several ways in which Harvard remains hostile to women (Kantor 2006).

While these comments seem surprising, they are inevitably endured by many working women with infants. In this way, medicine is not unique. Only a third of large companies provide a private, secure area where women can express breast milk during the workday, and only 7% offer on-site or near-site child care, according to a 2005 national study of employers by the nonprofit Families and Work Institute (Kantor 2006)." Thus, for many women breast-feeding on the job involves breaking new ground.

Women in medicine, like other working women, endure criticism for pursuing paid work outside the home. One participant in the MomMD Website shared her surprise when she received this type of judgment from another physician:

> I recently had a strange email interaction with another mommy physician, and I am wondering if I will be in for more of it as I transition to my "first job". I belong to a local mother of twins group and we have an email group. One of the other moms noticed I was a physician, so she emailed, "Oh, how nice, another mommy who is a physician" type of email. I thought I had made a new friend. I replied to her and asked her if she had any tips on balancing career and family, and she replied, "I only moonlight occasionally on the weekend. I find that my twins' mental health is more important than fulfilling my own selfish goals of having a career." posted June 25, 2007 12:50 PM by Tsunami

Another MomMD participant complains about missing her children during the day when they are most energetic and positive, only to interact with them later on when they are tired and cranky:

> I always felt guilty and disappointed about this, that I couldn't be with the kids when they were their brightest. Be glad you are part-time so can enjoy them on your other days. I think it's very real – that we are tired and that our young children are tired by 5:30, and that we need more flexibility in the workplace to help us with our exhaustion (posted August 20, 2007 by sisriver).

Like other women with demanding careers, many women physicians cope with the demands of parenting and work by neglecting household duties. This can incur the judgment and disapproval of others and inevitably raises the stress of those struggling to balance. One woman described her domestic challenges in a post to the MomMD Website:

> We get nasty notes in our mailbox about our yard not being mowed and some of my kids' friends parents have stopped allowing their children to come to our house and play because our house is very lived-in and NEVER up to their standards. The only way to do it all is to give up doing some of it (the things that are least important) (posted August 11, 2006 by OBRN2MD).

Research on women physicians indicates that they spend almost no time gardening or doing yard work. This compares with 3 h per week for women overall (Robinson and Godbey 1997).

Like other women in the workforce, physician mothers struggle to focus their limited energy on bonding with their children. One participant in the MomMD Website commented on her experiences:

> It is MOST frustrating to get home "early" then spend time with unhappy kids/feeling guilty/exhausted. I agree with change of dinner plans if possible – kids will be much better off with cereal for dinner and attention from you in the long run. I also agree from personal experience that you need to eat before you play, too! My husband and I stock "healthy" cereal, snack bars, leftover salad to snack on if it's a "witching hour" night for the kids. For a while, I tried just making time to play before making dinner, but then the kids are tired by dinnertime and won't eat (even if happy). My husband's stomach also couldn't deal with the delay ;-) (posted August 20, 2007 by ohiomomMD).

Further, like other working mothers, women physicians with families struggle to achieve the ultimate efficiency. One physician mother recalls:

> When the kids were little, they slept in their clothes so I could shovel them from the car to the sitter's door without arousing them (quoted in Chin et al. 2002: 291).

Dr. Cabot is not alone. In a survey of 800 academic physicians in departments of medicine around the country, respondents were asked to provide coping strategies used to balance work and family life. More than 50% cited efforts to improve efficiency (Levinson et al. 1992). Inevitably, however, efficiency can only go so far without infringing on family life. Clearly, Dr. Cabot was not seeing her children when they were awake in the morning.

Another similarity between women physicians with children and other professional mothers involves spousal support. In general, mothers in elite occupations often suggest that supportive husbands are key to their success. Mothers in medicine are no exception:

> …I am really happy, but I think it's for exactly the reasons that have been already listed:…, and great husband who really IS involved and very supportive. I wonder if we did a survey and correlated "happiness" with "supportive husband who actively participates in child and house care" whether that would explain most of the variance?… (posted march 14, 2003 by psych).

In reality, however, like other working women, physician mothers often assume the bulk of the child care responsibilities. This is especially true for women physicians with physician spouses. One midlife female physician with a physician spouse complained that she often had to reject speaking opportunities during the early years of her career because she could not arrange adequate child care, but that her husband accepted speaking invitations without ensuring that child care was available. He simply assumed that the children would be handled by his wife. Another complained that her husband can, "Clip an aneurysm without breaking a sweat, but a poopie diaper makes him cry like a baby."

On the other hand, it also appears that because of their earning potential, and their increasing willingness to marry men outside of medicine, that there is an increasing cadre of women physicians who honestly share household chores equally and/or who have more supportive spouses. Two MomMD participants shared their experiences:

> My husband had a very involved dad, and I think that has really shaped him in being a very involved dad himself. He took over as primary parent during my first 1 and a 1/2 yrs of residency (when my son was 1) until my schedule got reasonable again. When I had my daughter, I stayed home for 8 months, but I went back to work 2 evenings and Sat afternoon from 2 months on, and guess who took care of the baby and our 5 year old? My husband! I am so glad we talked about all of this before we got married. Posted by psyc posted April 11, 2003 7:12 PM

> My call is endocrinology (my specialty) and medicine shared and is 1 in 10. When I am off, I am OFF. I work in the office 8:30–4:45 with Wednesday afternoon off. My husband is home all day on Thursdays. We have evening meals together. My husband [who was a lawyer] has a gourmet kitchen store. He can cook, clean, wipe babies at either end. He does windows, does my taxes, reviews my contracts, and is a consistent, persistent force in my life. I am so sorry there aren't any available brothers. Posted by enddoc April 16, 2003 10:11 PM April 16, 2003 10:11 PM

One woman physician whom we interviewed admitted being seriously involved with a retina surgeon, but ultimately ending the relationship because she knew that the marriage would have required her to sacrifice her career. The woman is now the head of a hospital department and the mother of two children. Her husband is a part-time chaplain at the hospital where she works. Increasingly, women physicians find themselves in more balanced marriages. Here again, there experiences parallel those of other high earners. Research by Julie Brines finds that men take "men tend to share more housework as their wives' incomes approach theirs (McNeil 2004)" Another woman we interviewed has four children and a husband who stays at home to maintain her house and care for them. She commented that they made this decision because his earning potential as an engineer was ultimately lower and less stable than hers was as a primary care physician.

On the other hand, the essential nature of physicians' work makes the challenges faced by physician parents somewhat unique. Since it is not possible for many physicians to stay home with sick children, they have to make alternative arrangements. On the other hand, many of the physicians in this category, earn enough to hire in-house child care. One anesthesiologist addressed this issue in her recent comments on the MomMD Website:

> I (anesthesiologist) will be going back to work in Jan 2008 for 2 days of the week- after taking a year + off. My husband is returning from an Iraq deployment soon and is an ER doc. Our son will be 15 months old when we start work in Jan 2008. Between both of our jobs, I don't forsee either one of us being able to leave immediately or even soon to get him if he is in daycare- how do other people work this esp if no family is in the area. we don't live in a neighborhood with extremely friendly people – I think that is just part of living in DC- and everyone we know works full-time. Anyone been in this situation. We'd like to avoid paying an agency for back up care esp as I only work 2 days per week. (posted October 7, 2007 by bpt).

This woman was quickly advised to seek in-home nanny care so that she did not have to confront the possibility of leaving work for a sick child, and the woman seemed very receptive to the idea, not mentioning the possibility that such services would be costly compared with 2 days of earnings.

Another discussion on the MomMD Website involved the struggle to get housekeeping and child care services simultaneously. Prior research on working women physicians indicates that they typically spend about one half hour a day cooking and another half hour per day on housework (Frank et al. 2000). A nationally representative survey indicates that working women in general spend on 1 h and 10 min per day on cooking and only 40 min per day on housework (Robinson and Godbey 1997). Women physicians appear to make up the gap by relying more on domestic services. One recent woman participant on the MomMD Website discusses how she solved her need for household help by hiring two nannies.

> but my experience and that of my friends who have worked with nannies in the past, it's difficult to find a nanny who wants to both take care of your child and do the housework and do the cooking. I started with one nanny for my twins at 8 weeks. All we asked of her was to prepared meals for the kids and pick up after them and do their laundry as needed (though we frequently did it ourselves). We also had someone come clean our house once a week for a few hours. As they got older and more mobile, she asked that we hire someone part-time to help her. Also, the nanny and housekeeper did not get along so we had to get rid of the housekeeper. Well, in the end, we have one full-time live-out nanny (7–6 pm M-F) and another nanny/housekeeper (9-6 M-F) who helps with the kids and picks up the house, cleans bathrooms, kitchens, etc. She's not the best housekeeper and we end up doing more stuff on the weekends ourselves, but it keeps our house from looking like a war zone and she's great with the kids and gets along with our primary nanny (posted August 6, 2007 by Pulpo).

Another couple we interviewed, who was expecting their fourth child, turned to the two nanny solution when the wife decided to quit a part-time primary care internal medicine job and pursue an oncology fellowship. The wife commented that her entire fellowship salary would not cover their child care costs. While the two nanny solution discussed in this post may seem extreme, it must be increasingly common throughout the medical workforce as the number of two physician, two career marriages grows. As we have seen, 95% of female physicians with physician spouses are in two career marriages and 50% of these couples work an average of 100 h or more collectively in an average week. So, these couples are facing extreme pressures on their time and increasingly they have significant additional income. Since many of these couples have children, they must seek the additional help. For some, two nannies is an attractive solution.

Although efforts to promote greater work–family balance remained limited, there is some evidence that the critical mass of women in medicine began having a small effect on the structure of the profession during the 1980s and 1990s. One of the first major reforms that occurred involved the couples match. Prior to 1983, physician couples seeking residency spots had to either limit their selections to one city or rely on the poorly known and rarely used option 7, which allowed physician couples to negotiate their residencies outside of the match system. Apparently, the few who attempted to use option 7 encountered significant resistance from hospitals who preferred single residents or residents with a supporting spouse. Nevertheless, the critical mass of women in medicine and the growing number of two physician couples forced the system to evolve so that couples can now match together (Belkin 1985). Between its inception and 2004, the number of two physician couples taking advantage of the couples match increased continuously. It has declined only slightly since then.

Further, there is limited evidence that conditions are improving for women in the medical education system. One woman we interviewed who graduated in 1985 told the story of a classmate who was pregnant with her first child during their first year in medical school. At the time, the woman gave birth 2 days before her final exams. She was not granted an extension and was told that she needed to take the test or get a zero. She took the test standing because she couldn't sit on her episiotomy. She got a D. Although this story appears draconian, there is every reason to believe that relatively little changed throughout the 1990s. The following 2006 letter to editor of the New York Times captures the experiences of one physician mother struggling to breast-feed:

> To the Editor:
>
> I am a mother of four and a pediatrician. My first child was born when I was in medical school, and my second and third during my residency. Returning to work after only 10 weeks (12 weeks was the maximum maternity allowed), I struggled to breast-feed my babies while working nights, weekends, 15-h days and 24-h shifts. I was forced to pump breast milk in bathrooms, call rooms, wherever I could find an outlet and a place to sit. I would struggle with engorgement through rounds that lasted for hours, or E.R. shifts that were too busy to take a break from. If the very profession that is supposed to be the largest supporter of breast-feeding treats its own mothers in this way, who are we to put such pressure, guilt and expectation on all new mothers? Until this society is structured to support and nurture those women who are lucky enough to be able to breast-feed, we can only expect any mother to do the best she can.
>
> Dr. Kimberly Fahey Brown
Sands Point, N.Y.

Today, in contrast, a Massachusetts appeals court recently ruled in favor of Sophie Currie. As a result, Ms. Curie will be granted additional break time when she takes Step 2 of the U.S. Medical Licensing Exam so that she can pump milk for her young infant.

It also appears that medical specialty societies like the American Academy of Pediatrics and the American College of Physicians have acknowledged the increasing demand for flexible schedules. In particular, the American Academy of Pediatrics; Committee on the Pediatric Workforce has a section dedicated to women's issues. They have helped to fund significant survey research to understand the scope of part-time work in their specialty and have drafted written resources for those in their field who are seeking flexible schedules.

Nevertheless, it is worth reiterating that women physicians failed to unite even during the 1990s over work and family issues. Instead, the growing number of women in medicine has continued to face motherhood alone. One woman obstetrician reflects on her experiences trying to combine work and family as a fellow during the 1990s:

> When, at age 37, I delivered my firstborn 1 week to the day after beginning a fellowship in high-risk pregnancy, I was devastated to have him admitted to the neonatal intensive care unit. On my way out the door, I ran into the senior fellow, who said to me, "Too bad about what happened. When can I put you back on the call schedule?" I seriously considered skipping my 4 allotted weeks of maternity leave, since if both my son and I were at the hospital, I could arrange to see him more. Little has changed since then: Our residents get a few weeks off for maternity leave, after which they must either resume their 12-h days (and every third or fourth night in the hospital) or add extra time to their 4 years of residency training (Plante 2004: 840).

The efforts that women physicians must make to balance work and family do not end with their children age out of infancy. They continue to make hard choices and ultimately they seriously limit their time for parenting.

Conclusion

Although relatively little has been done to promote family-friendly work environments, we remain cautiously optimistic and acknowledge that even in the absence of a large-scale transformation of medical work, women's presence in the profession is having effects. Over time, there has been little change in the tendency for men and women in medicine to work part-time. Nevertheless, the stability of trends in part-time work ultimately suggests that women's presence in medicine will have an effect on the structure of the profession simply because more women work part-time, and more physicians are women. So, ultimately, as the representation of women in the profession grows, the intensity of medical work effort per provider should decline and in the absence of increases in physician supply, the availability of medical care should decrease. This structural change has already been noted by many in medical policy. Further, as we noted earlier, structural changes in the profession of medicine may be increasing opportunities for some physicians, like residents and primary care providers to maintain more family-friendly schedules.

We emphasize, however, that declines in the supply of medical services are driven almost exclusively by demographic changes rather than by structural reforms prompted by women's presence. Further, we reiterate that increases in the total number of part-time physicians must be understood in the context of increasing diversity in work effort. On the one hand, the feminization of medicine will cause declines in the average medical workweek in the short term. On the other hand, trends suggest that more female physicians are working long weeks. So, in the absence of change, over time the initial declines in work effort will dissipate. The increasing numbers of women in all aspects of the medical profession will inevitably enhance the possibilities for meaningful change. Mary Lou Schmidt, an Associate Professor of Pediatrics and a contributor to Eliza Chin 2002 anthology on the experiences of women physicians reflects on her friend Becca and "her six girlfriends who created their own private OB/GYN practice where everybody works four days a week, everybody has at least one or two kids and everybody shares the profits equally (Chin 2002: 280)." And Becca is not alone. The number of all female practices is inevitably increasing, especially in specialties where women are well-represented. Health care institutions are also slowly increasing their response to the growing need for family-friendly support. One neonatologist we interviewed said that she had negotiated a position that involved nearly continuous work 1 week out of every month, but that during that week, her child would receive 24-h care in a hospital center. There is even an advocacy organization, Child Care in Health Care, designed to encourage the development of child care options for health care workers. The questions are whether a critical mass of women physicians will be able to take medicine in a new direction, and how many women it will take to create a critical mass.

Agenda for the Future

As we write this, some form of national health insurance seems on the horizon, but we cannot say what form it will take. How will this impact women physicians? This is a key area for future research. The role that women physicians play in the future of the medical profession and the potential of the profession to adopt more family-friendly work schedules will inevitably depend on the structure that health care reform takes.

In previous generations, women physicians have opted to pursue primary care medicine more than their male colleagues. The current generation of physicians is not adopting this traditional gender gap. As we discuss elsewhere (Boulis and Jacobs 2008), the rate at which new physicians opt to pursue primary care is declining at an alarming rate, regardless of medical student gender, and the future supply of foreign medical graduates is not stable. So, an increasing number of primary care visits are now handled by nurse practitioners and physicians assistants. Yet, as we discussed earlier, the evolution of primary care is not completely eclipsing the need for primary care physicians. In the absence of legal reforms, physicians are still needed to supervise nurse practitioners and physicians assistants providing primary care.

Future research needs to explore how the evolution of primary care will affect the profession. On the one hand, in the absence of government intervention, the shift toward physician extenders might increase opportunities for family-friendly work schedules among physicians. As we discussed earlier, the development of convenient care has resulted in more opportunities for part-time work. On the other hand, the widespread adoption of the primary care home might increase pressure on physicians to adopt more continuous hours because one of the primary premises of the primary care home is that patients need a continuous relationship with their provider (Champlin 2007).

Future research could also focus on the specialties that have, heretofore, offered greater opportunities for family-friendly work. According to the Community Tracking Study Physician Survey, the percent of psychiatrists and pediatricians who currently work reduced schedules is significantly higher than in other specialties. Research efforts could explore how and why these fields have evolved and consider if they will evolve further in the face of health care reforms.

A third issue to consider in future investigations involves how the cost of medical school and physician salaries influences physicians' work efforts. In the absence of change, physicians will continue to accrue substantial debt and face declining reimbursements. These realities will make the possibility of family-friendly schedules increasingly unrealistic unless something is done.

Finally, efforts should explore how physicians' family structures will affect the profession's family-friendly opportunities. As we discuss elsewhere (Boulis and Jacobs 2008), the number of two physician marriages is increasing. Although women in these relationships continue to assume the bulk of responsibilities for domestic life, the willingness of male physicians to sacrifice work hours and work location for family life should increase as their spouses' commitment to the labor force increases.

References

American Association of Medical Colleges (2006) Women in U.S. Academic Medicine Statistics and Medical School Benchmarking 2005–2006. Association of American Medical Colleges. Washington DC: AAMC. http://www.aamc.org/members/wim/wimguide/wim6.pdf

Adams D (2004) Generation gripe: Young doctors less dedicated, hardworking? In: http://www.amednews.com, American Medical Association News. February 2

American Academy of Pediatrics (2005) Pediatrician workforce statement. Pediatrics 116(1):263–269

AMSA (2008) Medical students react to IOM Report: resident work hours reexamined. December, 2, 2008. Retrieved July 7, 2009 from http://www.amsa.org/news/release2.cfx?id=363.

Anderson R, Barbara A, Feldman S (2007) What patients want: a content analysis of key qualities that influence patient satisfaction. J Med Pract Manage 22:255–61

Belkin L (1985) A group for dual-doctor families. New York Times. June 16

Bickel J, Brown AJ (2005) Generation X: implications for faculty recruitment and development in academic health centers. Acad Med 80(3):205–210

Bosk C (2003) Forgive and remember: managing medical failure. University of Chicago Press, Chicago, IL

Boulis A, Jacobs J (2008) The changing face of medicine: women doctors and the evolution of health care in America. Cornell Press, Ithaca, NY

Butterfield, S. 2007. Resident's Union Celebrates Golden Anniversary. ACP Internist. July–August

Cabana M, Jee S (2004) Does continuity of care improve patient outcomes? J Fam Pract 53(12):974–980

Champlin L (2007) Principles establish basis for health system reform. AAFP News Now; March 6

Chin E (ed) (2002) This side of doctoring: reflections from women in medicine. Sage, Thousand Oaks, CA

Chiu T, Old A, Naden G, Child S (2006) Frequency of calls to "on-call" house officer pagers at Auckland City Hospital, New Zealand. NZ Med J 119(1231):U1913

Cook, Bob (2007) Finances driving physicians out of solo practice. In: http://Amednews.com, September 10

Croasdale M (2002) Practices must cope as more physicians work part-time hours. AMA News, October, 21

Croasdale M (2004a) Women physicians find ways to make "part time" work. The trend toward fewer hours is gaining momentum as men join in. AMA News November 15

Croasdale M (2004b) High medical school debt steers life choices for young doctors. http://www.amednews.com, May 17

Croasdale M (2007) More women choosing surgical residencies. http://www.amednews.com, September 17

Cull WL, Mulvey HJ, O'Connor KG, Sowell DR, Berkowitz CD, Britton CV (2002) Pediatricians working part-time: past, present, and future. Pediatrics 109:1015–1102

Cohen-Gadol AA, Piepgras DG, Krishnamurthy S, Fessler RD (2005) Resident duty hours reform: results of a national survey of the program directors and residents in neurosurgery training programs. Neurosurgery 56:398–403

de Virgilio C, Yaghoubian A, Lewis RJ, Stabile BE, Putnam BA (2006) The 80-hour resident workweek does not adversely affect patient outcomes or resident education. Curr Surg 63:435–9

Díaz-Montes TP, Zahurak ML et al (2006) Uterine cancer in Maryland: impact of surgeon case volume and other prognostic factors on short-term mortality. Gynecol Oncol 103(3):1043–7

Dimick JB, Cowan JA Jr, Stanley JC, Henke PK, Pronovost PJ, Upchurch GR (2003) Surgeon specialty and provider volumes are related to outcome of intact abdominal aortic aneurysm repair in the United States. J Vasc Surg 38:739–44

Dolan PL (2006) MGMA: Doctors on "unsustainable course". http://www.amednews.com, November 6

Duke PS, Wanda MF, Parsons L et al (2007) Physicians as mothers. Can Fam Physician 53(5):887–891

Duncan S, Edwards R, Reynolds T, Alldred P (2003) Motherhood, paid work and parenting. Work, Employment Soc 17(2):309–330

Epstein C, Senon C et al (1998) The part time paradox: time norms professional life, family and gender. Routledge, New York, NY

Fan V, Burman M et al (2005) Continuity of care and other determinants of patient satisfaction with primary care. J Gen Intern Med 20:226–33

Ferguson C, Kellogg K et al (2005) Effect of work-hour reforms on operative case volume of surgical residents. Curr Surg 62:535–38

Fletcher K, Davis S et al (2004) Systematic review: effects of resident work hours on patient safety. Ann Intern Med 141(11):851–57

Flocke SA, Stange KC et al (1997) The impact of insurance type and forced discontinuity on the delivery of primary care. J Fam Pract 45(2):129–35

Fritz N, Lantos J (1991) Pediatrician's practice choices: differences between part-time and full-time practice. Pediatrics 88:764–69

Frank E, Harvey L et al (2000) Family responsibilities and domestic activities of U.S. women physicians. Arch Fam Med 9:134–40

Gabbe SG, Morgan MA, Power ML, Schulkin J, Williams SB (2003) Duty hours and pregnancy outcome among residents in obstetrics and gynecology. Obstet Gynecol 102(5):948–951

Gelb-Safran D (2003) Defining the future of primary care: what can we learn from patients? Ann Intern Med 138(3):248–55

Gerber L (1983) Married to their careers: career and family dilemmas in doctor's lives. Tavistock, New York, NY

Gesensway D (1999) Changes in medicine's mommy track. ACP Internist, December

Gilbert P, Miller ME (2004) Out of time. Hopkins Medicine Winter 2004

Gjerdingen DK, Chaloner KM, Vanderscoff JA (1995) Family practice residents' maternity leave experiences and benefits. Fam Med 27:512–518

Gordon TA, Bowman HM, Bass EB, Lillemoe KD, Heitmiller RF, Choti MA, Burleyson GP, Hsieh G, Cameron JL (1999) Complex gastrointestinal surgery: impact of provider experience on clinical and economic outcomes. J Am Coll Surg 189:46–56

Grant L, Simpson LA, Rong XL, Peters-Golden H (1990) Gender, parenthood, and work hours of physicians. J Marriage Fam 52(1):39–49

Guilliford MC, Naithani S, Morgan M (2007) Continuity of care and intermediate outcomes of type 2 diabetes mellitus. Fam Pract 24(3):2

Hammond JW, Queale WS, Kim TK, McFarland EG (2003) Surgeon experience and clinical and economic outcomes for shoulder arthroplasty. J Bone Joint Surg 85:2318–2324

Harris S (2007) Solutions sought on predicted oncologist shortage. AAMC Reporter April

Hawkins J (2002) Recruiting physicians to states with high malpractice insurance premiums. Recruiting Physicians Today, N Engl J Med 10(5):1

Hewlett SA (2007) Off-ramps and on-ramps: keeping talented women on the road to success. Harvard Press, Boston, MA

Hewlett S, Luce C (2005) Off-ramps and on-ramps keeping talented women on the road to success. Harvard Business Review 83(3)

Hinze SW, Chirayath HT, Sobecks N, Landefeld CS (1997) MD2 Couples in the nineties: the his and hers of medical marriages. In: Presentation at the American Sociological Association Meetings. Toronto, ON, Canada

Hobson K (2005) Doctors vanish from view blamed by the bureaucracy of medicine, physicians are pulling back from patient care. USNews.com

Holmes A, Cull W et al (2005) Part-time residency in pediatrics. Description of current practice. Pediatrics 116:32–27

Horwitz LI, Krumholz HM, Huot SJ, Green ML (2006) Internal medicine residents' clinical and didactic experiences after work hour regulation: a survey of chief residents. J Gen Intern Med 21:961–965

Jacobs JA, Gerson K (2004) The time divide: work, family, and gender inequality. Harvard University Press, Cambridge, MA

Jarman BT, Miller MR et al (2004) The 80-hour work week: Will we have less-experienced graduating surgeons? J Surg Educ 61(6):612–615

Jarnberg P-O, Hicks JS, Quint Gaebel BA (2001) Scheduling of call and operating room staffing: A Nationwide Survey of Academic Anesthesiology Centers. Anesthesiology 95:1110

Jayson S (2007) Attitude gap widens between working and stay at home moms. USA Today; July 12

Jeffrey S (2008) Neurosurgery associations push back on IOM resident work-hour report. Medscape Medical News. December

Jones AM, Jones KB (2007) The 88-hour family: effects of the 80-hour work week on marriage and childbirth in a surgical residency. Iowa Orthop J 27:128–33

Kanter RM (1977) Men and women of the corporation. Basic Books, New York

Kantor J (2006) On the job, nursing mothers are finding a 2-class system. The New York Times. September 1

Klebanoff MA, Shiono PH, Rhoads GG (1990) Outcomes of pregnancy in a national sample of resident physicians. N Engl J Med 323:1040–1045

Kletke PR, Emmons DW, Gillis KD (1996) Current trends in physicians' practice arrangements: from owners to employees. JAMA 276:555–560

Kotkin S (2007) Opening the on-ramp for women. New York Times. August 5

Kuhn P (2007) The expanding work week understanding trends in long work hours among US Men 1979–2006. University of California Press, Santa Barbara, CA

Kunde D (1997) Family friendly work: lawyers plead for flexible time to handle job, home. Daily News, Los Angeles, CA

Kwan R, Levy R (2006) A primer on resident work hours. American Medical Student Association, Reston, VA

Landrigan CP, Barger LK, Cade BE, Ayas NT, Czeisler CA (2006) Interns' compliance with accreditation council for graduate medical education work-hour limits. J Am Med Assoc 296:1063–1070

Lange PH, Lin DW (2004) Does the who and how of surgery in bladder cancer matter? J Clin Oncol 22(14):2762–2764

Levinson W, Kaufman K et al (1992) Women in academic medicine: strategies for balancing career and personal life. J Am Med Womens Assoc 47:25–28

Levinson W, Lurie N (2004) When most doctors are women. Ann Intern Med 141:471–475

Lugtenberg M, Heiligers PJ et al (2006) Internal medicine specialists' attitudes towards working part-time: A comparison between 1996 and 2004. BMC Health Serv Res 6:126

Maguire P (1999) How direct to consumer advertising is putting the squeeze on physicians. American College of Physicians-American Society of Internal Medicine Observer March.

Mechanic D, McAlpine D, Rosenthal M (2001) Are patients' office visits with physicians getting shorter? N Engl J Med 344(3):198–204

Mark S, Gupta J (2002) Reentry into clinical practice. J Am Med Assoc 288:1091–1096

Matthias J (1997) Surgeons decry OR layoffs of nurse managers. OR Manager 13:1

Mayer K, Ho H et al (2001) Childbearing and child care in surgery. Arch Surg 136:649–55

McMurray J, Heilingers P et al (2005) Part-time medical practice: where is it headed? Am J Med 118(1):87–92

McNeil D (2004) Culture or chromosomes? New York Times. New York City

Migliore M, Chong CK, Lim E, Goldsmith KA, Ritchie A, Wells FC (2007) A surgeon's case volume of oesophagectomy for cancer strongly influences the operative mortality rate. Eur J Cardiothorac Surg 32:375–380

Miller NH, Miller DJ, Chism M (1996) Breastfeeding practices among resident physicians. Pediatrics 98:434–7

Muray A et al (2000) Physician workload and patient-based assessments of primary care performance. Arch Fam Med 9:327–332

Myers JS et al (2006) Internal medicine and general surgery residents' attitudes about the ACGME duty hours regulations: a multicenter study. Acad Med 81:1052–8

National Association for Law Placement Inc (NALP) (2006) "Few lawyers work part-time 2006." Retrieved May 20, 2009 from http://www.nalp.org/2006fewlawyersworkpart-time?s=staff%20attorney%20AND%20part%20time

O'Connor, Karen G, Katcher A, Sherman H, Cull WL (2004) Balancing work and personal life: perceptions of part-time and full-time pediatricians. In: Paper presented at the Pediatric Academic Societies Meetings, San Francisco, CA

Parkerton PH, Wagner EH, Smith DG, Straley HL (2003) Effect of part-time practice on patient outcomes. J Gen Intern Med 18:717–724

Philibert I, Bickel J (1995) Maternity and parental leave policies at COTH teaching hospitals. Acad Med 70:1056–1058

Plante L (2004) Obstetricians wanted: no mothers need apply. Ann Intern Med 140:840–841

Potee R, Gerber A et al (1999) Medicine and motherhood shifting trends among female physicians from 1922 to 1999. Acad Med 74:911–919

Rhode D (2001) The unfinished agenda. In: Report prepared for the ABA Commission on Women in the Profession.

Robinson J, Godbey G (1997) Time for life: the surprising ways Americans use their time. Pennsylvania State University Press, State College, PA

Rodriguez H, Rogers W et al (2007) The effects of primary care physician visit continuity on patients' experiences with care. J Gen Intern Med 22(6):787–793

Roter DL, Hall JA (1992) Doctors talking with patients/patients talking with doctors: improving communication in medical visits. Auburn House, Westport, CT

Ruiz R (2008) What doctor shortages mean for health care. Forbes December 2

Schafermeyer RW, Asplin BR (2003) Hospital and emergency department crowding in the United States. Emerg Med 15(1):22–27

Seltzer VL (1999) Changes and challenges for women in academic obstetrics and gynecology. Am J Obstet Gynecol 180(4):837–848

Stanton B (2007) Family friendly workplaces as a foundation for the future of pediatrics. Arch Pediatr Adolesc Med 161:511–514

Steinbrook R (2002) The debate over residents' work hours. N Engl J Med 347:1296–1302

Stone P, Lovejoy M (2004) Fast track women and the 'choice' to stay home. Ann Pol Soc Sci 596:62–86

Tayloe D (2009) Letter from American Academy of Pediatrics to Institute of Medicine, March 24

Tu HT, Hargraves JL (2003) Seeking health care information: most consumers still on the sidelines. Washington, DC: Center for Studying Health System Change. March 2003. Issue Brief 61.

U.S. Bureau of Census (2006) Facts for features: Father's day: June 18. Washington, DC, U.S. Census Bureau

U.S. Bureau of Labor Statistics (2006) Women in the labor force data book

Vickers AJ et al (2007) The surgical learning curve for prostate cancer control after radical prostatectomy. J Natl Cancer Inst 99:1171–1177

Walpert B (2002) Working part time: can it fit into your practice? American College of Physicians Observer. July/August. Accessed online at: http://www.acponline.org/journals/news/jul-aug02/part_time.htm

Warde C (2001) Work-family balance. Ann Intern Med 134:343

Wardrop T (2004) As more women enter medicine, cultures will change. Managed Healthcare Executive, February 1

White C, Haftel H et al (2006) Multidimensional effects of the 80-hour work week at the University of Michigan Medical School. Acad Med 81(1):57–62

Woodrow SI, Segouin C et al (2006) Duty hours reforms in the United States, France, and Canada: is it time to refocus our attention on education? Acad Med 81:1045–1051

Chapter 13
Clash of Logics, Crisis of Trust: Entering the Era of Public For-Profit Health Care?

Carol A. Caronna

Introduction

Who is responsible for providing Americans health care and health insurance? What practices create the best health care system? Can the US health care system deliver high-quality care with controlled costs and equitable access? Historically these questions have been answered in ways that incorporate, in varying degrees, four broad logics specifying the optimal sectors and organizational forms suitable to meet the challenges of the health care field: public, private, nonprofit, and for-profit. At the beginning of the twenty-first century, we stand at the edge of an ideological battle over the government's responsibility for providing health insurance for all Americans. The future is uncertain, as the clash of private and public logics plays out in political campaigns and legislative efforts. At the same time, the health care system faces a crisis of trust (Schlesinger et al. 2005). At the micro level, whether or not patients trust their providers seems like an issue that is the luxury of the insured, with the nation facing more pressing problems of access to care and rising costs. But the issue of trust is multilayered, including the trust individual providers place in health care organizations and the trust Americans have in the health care system as a whole.

The trust is embedded in a nonprofit vs. for-profit comparison is well known, with nonprofits considered inherently more trustworthy due to certain market failures and a lack of conflict of interest (Arrow 1963). But how is trust embedded in a public vs. private comparison? Do we trust the government to provide health insurance and leadership? Or do we trust the private sector more? The intersections of these four logics raise additional pressing questions. To support universal health insurance implies a public agenda, but is it necessarily a nonprofit agenda? To refute the need for universal health insurance implies that the responsibility for insurance should be kept in the private sector, but does that mean the for-profit sector or the nonprofit sector? Does a private agenda necessarily follow a for-profit logic? Does a public agenda necessarily follow a nonprofit logic?

To explore these questions, this chapter examines issues of trust and the varying dominance of the four logics in the health care field. Institutional logics are sets of "material practices and symbolic constructions which constitute [a field's] organizing principles and which are available to organizations and individuals to elaborate" (Friedland and Alford 1991, p. 248). Institutional theory (DiMaggio and Powell 1983; Scott 2001) places logics within the domain of the cognitive "pillar" of the institutional environment, as logics are "shared conceptions that constitute the nature of social reality and the frames through which meaning is made" (Scott 2001, p. 57). Logics also influence

C.A. Caronna (✉)
Department of Sociology, Anthropology, and Criminal Justice, Towson University, Towson, MD, USA
e-mail: ccaronna@towson.edu

the normative and regulatory pillars of the institutional environment (Caronna 2004), as they shape professional norms, values, and governance structures. In previous studies, specific logics found to shape the health care field included quality, equity, and efficiency (Scott et al. 2000; see also Kitchener and Harrington 2004), managerialism (Kitchener 2002), and medical professionalism and business-like health care (Reay and Hinings 2005).

Importantly, the types of organizations that exist in the field over time, and the actual distribution of health expenditures, may not reflect the dominant logics. As Mechanic (2004, p. 83) points out, "while 60% of all health expenditures are from government through health programs, tax subsidies, and coverage of health benefits for government employees (Woolhandler and Himmelstein 2002), we maintain the illusion of a private health care system..." In addition, the health care field has always been characterized as a mixed market (Needleman 2001; Schlesinger and Gray 2006), with the presence of both nonprofit and for-profit entities (although the nature of the for-profit entities has changed, from small proprietary organizations to large investor-owned corporations; see Schlesinger and Gray 2006). The degree to which nonprofit or for-profit organizations exist in the health care field, and the degree to which their behavior differs, depends upon the subfield, including the specific service being offered as well as the stage of the subfield's life cycle (Schlesinger and Gray 2006). The prevalent type of organizations may not imply the field's dominant logics.

At the same time, the simple fact that the health care field has always had a mix of public and private involvement and nonprofit and for-profit organizations does not mean that broad-based meaning systems have not leaned toward public over private or for-profit over nonprofit, at various points in time. These types of involvements and organizations exist within institutional contexts that define values, symbolic meanings, and beliefs, and these cultural-cognitive elements construct perceptions, opportunities, and constraints (Scott et al. 2000; Scott 2001). The solutions to problems of access, quality, and cost have been embedded in the dominant combinations of the public, private, nonprofit, and for-profit logics, and the ease with which solutions are found has depended on the resonance or conflict of these combinations. Examining the role of these logics in shaping our field illuminates the past, but also may lead to an understanding of where we stand in the twenty-first century, and where our health care system may be headed in the future. In addition, these logics demonstrate the role of social forces in health, illness, and healing – the social forces of broad-based motives, understandings, and beliefs – and the need for medical sociologists to incorporate macro-institutional conceptions into the full range of our studies.

The Multiple Layers of Trust

The health care system involves a complex set of actors and stakeholders – providers, purchasers, intermediaries, and governance structures (Scott et al. 2000) – with multiple potentials for trustworthy relations or crises of trust. The dominant logics as well as prevalent organizational forms of a time period influence the trust purchasers have in providers and intermediaries, individual providers have in organizational providers, and providers, purchasers, and intermediaries have in governance structures. At the microlevel, the trust between patients and providers depends on the providers' avoidance of deception, lack of exploitative practices, and full disclosure of all information needed for patients to understand illnesses and make decisions about treatments (Schlesinger et al. 2005). The complexity of the health care system facing patients and the lack of full information about providers led Arrow (1963) to explicate the need for nonprofit health care organizations. In addition, providers in for-profit organizations experience a potential conflict of interest between meeting patients' needs and serving investors' interests.

But do consumers differentiate between nonprofit and for-profit intermediaries and providers, and do they perceive nonprofit providers to be more trustworthy than for-profits? Mechanic (2004) claimed that patients value being able to trust their health care systems and providers. However, Needleman (2001, p.1118), citing surveys from the late 1990s, argued that "trust and agency issues do not dominate individual patient or consumer decision making." In part, consumers often cannot correctly identify the ownership status of specific providers, and consumers see advantages and disadvantages of both nonprofit and for-profit models (Needleman 2001). Thus, does the patient–provider relation of trust necessitate a nonprofit logic? Can patients trust providers who work for for-profit organizations? Is patient–provider trust an issue best solved by the public or private sector?

The issue of trust between individual and organizational providers seems more straightforward. Using data from a 1998 American Medical Association study of physicians, Schlesinger and colleagues found that physicians trust nonprofit organizations more than for profits and local organizations more than multistate plans (Schlesinger et al. 2005). The lower trustworthiness of for-profits was "limited to for-profit plans that (were) affiliated with large national corporations" (Schlesinger et al. 2005, p. 607). Although consumers may not be aware of many issues of trust, physicians paid attention to "cream skimming," the steering of sick patients to other hospitals, shorter hospital stays, and the conflict of interest between meeting patient and budget needs (see also Gray 1997). Their findings led Schlesinger and colleagues to advocate for the preservation of a substantial nonprofit presence in health care. But should this nonprofit presence be private or public? And can issues of trust between providers be solved in a field dominated by for-profit logics?

In the twenty-first century, a third issue of trust is salient: the trust patients, providers, and intermediaries have in the health care system as a whole. In the age of managed care and for-profit insurers, Americans worry about the rationing of care and the limits on their choices of treatments and providers. As the ranks of the uninsured grow and include more and more middle class, employed Americans, the expectation of being insured becomes an uncertainty. Although the poor, the elderly, and many employed Americans still have health insurance, media coverage of the health care field paints a picture of "the sheer cruelty and injustice of the American health care system – sick people who can't pay their hospital bills literally dumped on the sidewalk, a child who dies because an emergency room that isn't a participant in her mother's health plan won't treat her, hardworking Americans driven into humiliating poverty by medical bills" (Krugman 2007, p. 17). General issues about Social Security and America's safety nets for the poor, the elderly, and the unemployed reveal a lack of trust in current policies and practices. But how are these large-scale issues of trust resolved? Who or what is responsible for ensuring that the health care system, as a whole, is trustworthy? Can trust be restored by the private sector or must the public sector step in? Is a nonprofit logic the only solution, or can a for-profit logic generate trust? To answer these questions about the multiple layers of trust requires further exploration of these logics and their implications.

Institutional Logics: Public, Private, Profit?

The four institutional logics of public, private, nonprofit, and for-profit are more commonly implied by three sectors: government/public, nonprofit, and for-profit (Steinberg and Powell 2006; Steinberg 2006). In this triad, both the nonprofit and for-profit sectors are assumed to be private. In his "three failures" theory, Steinberg (2006) describes how each sector responds to the other two sectors' failures. In contract failure, the public and nonprofit sectors step in to resolve failures of the market. In this case, the solution to private market failure could either be public or private. In government failure, the government's attention to the majority becomes a failure for the minority, who turn to the private sector for services or benefits. Thus, the response to government failure involves the private sector, either nonprofit or for-profit. Voluntary failure involves the shortcomings of nonprofit, philanthropic enterprises, with either the public sector or the private for-profit sector providing resolution. Applying these three sectors to the health care field begs the question, why does a for-profit logic currently dominate the health care field, which by the nature of information asymmetries involves contract failure? In simple terms, the health care field should involve both the public sector and the private nonprofit sector in response to contract failure, yet the degree to which the public sector has been involved in health care financing and planning has varied over time. Understanding how and why different sectors respond to different failures requires parsing these three sectors into four logics and examining the interplay of these logics in the health care field over time.

Before defining the four logics and examining their historical trajectories, a few points must be made about logics themselves. First, logics do not simply exist but are created and reinforced by various stakeholders. For example, Quadagno (2004) documents physicians' role in protecting the private sector involvement in health care, while Schlesinger and colleagues (2005) describe the role of public policy in encouraging the development of for-profit health maintenance organizations. Purchasers, providers, intermediaries, and agents of governance are all involved in the maintenance and transformation of prevailing logics. Second, in the health care field, institutional logics may be loosely coupled from the existing mix of organizational forms. Since different types of health care organizations are in different stages of a competitive life cycle (Schlesinger and Gray 2006), the mix of nonprofit and for-profit organizations may change, while the overarching logic governing the field may remain the same. For example, the fact that the majority of US hospitals are nonprofit organizations does not negate the fact that a for-profit logic dominates the contemporary health care field. Looking to the organizational structures of existing providers may or may not lead to a correct interpretation of prevailing logics.

Third, the logics of public, private, nonprofit, and for-profit in the health care field exist in the even broader context of American cultural preferences. As Mechanic (2004, p. 77) explains, "basic to the backlash against managed care is the underlying American cultural preference for independence, autonomy, choice, and activism, and the view shared by many Americans that there should be no barriers to their access and choices in seeking and receiving medical care." Attempts to change dominant logics in the health care field must contend with the larger meanings of government, capitalism, the private sector, and the role of nonprofits in American lives. Finally, institutional logics, as well as organizational forms, are interpreted and perceived. Schlesinger and Gray (2006) note that certain factors in the health care field persistently distort the way nonprofit and for-profit ownership are understood to matter. For example, at the time of much publicity about the investor-owned health care system Columbia/HCA, more Americans surveyed thought Columbia/HCA was nonprofit than for-profit. Thus, they may have interpreted Columbia/HCA's unethical behavior as representative of the voluntary sector (Schlesinger and Gray 2006). Of course, perceptions can vary across all the elements of the health care field, with various interpretations of logics held by purchasers, providers, intermediaries, and agents of governance.

The Private Logic

Given these complexities, what does each broad logic mean in the health care field? Beginning with the private sector, a private logic implies that the state is not trusted to finance and organize health care. Limited governmental involvement allows liberty (Quadagno 2004), which resonates with American values. Privatization also allows the government to be more flexible with subsidizing health care than paying for health care directly (Bloom and Brown 2003). One of the issues surrounding the private logic is that it can be interpreted as for-profit. For example, in a book about the future of public health, Bloom and Brown wrote (2003, p. 146): "most people perceive that privatization is increasing across America's health care institutions...But the perception is mistaken. In fact, the proportion of the hospital industry that is operated for profit has stayed roughly the same since the end of the Second World War." To make the private logic useful analytically, it must allow for both nonprofit and for-profit private interests. Thus, the private logic in the health care field could be expressed as follows:

> The Private Logic in the Health Care Field: The government plays a limited role in health planning, promotion, and provision. Purchasers select from an array of privately held health plans and providers. Private entities, such as professional associations, govern and regulate individual and organizational providers and intermediaries.

The Public Logic

The role of the government in shaping the health care field falls in the domain of the public logic. The sphere of public health, for example, includes investment and work for the common good, such as providing care for the uninsured, funding medical research, and subsidizing the education and training of health professionals (Lawrence 1997). In the "three failures" model, the government steps in when the private sector fails. This failure could be due to problems in the health care market or the inability of nonprofits to provide community benefits. In the health care field, the public logic could be expressed as follows:

> The Public Logic in the Health Care Field: The government is responsible for health planning, promotion, and provision. The government dominates purchasing due to its role as the primary provider of health insurance. The government oversees and regulates individual and organizational providers and intermediaries.

The Nonprofit Logic

In the last 20 years, much attention has been paid to nonprofit organizations and the nonprofit sector (Powell and Steinberg 1987, 2006; DiMaggio and Anheier 1990; Powell and Steinberg 2006). Definitions of nonprofit organizations vary, often focusing on the types of services nonprofits are expected to deliver in exchange for tax exemption (Bennet and DiLorenzo 1997). Steinberg and Powell (2006, p. 1) provide a definition based on returns on investment: "a *nonprofit organization*...is precluded, by external regulation or its own governance structure, from distributing its financial surplus to those who control the use of organizational assets." In these definitions, nonprofit organizations are presumed to be in the private sector. In theory, nonprofits are expected to have different incentives than investor-owned firms and therefore more community level connections and constraints on untrustworthy behavior (Needleman 2001; Schlesinger et al. 2005). In the health care field, these constraints benefit both patients and donors (Bennett and DiLorenzo 1997). In line with traditional American values of independence and liberty, if the nonprofit sector can provide community benefits, the government will not have to become involved in the health care field. Thus, nonprofit organizations receive a tax benefit for providing public services that would otherwise have to be provided by the government. Based on all these factors, the nonprofit logic in the health care field could be expressed as follows:

> The Nonprofit Logic in the Health Care Field: Providers are responsible for broadening access to care, promoting community health, supporting research and training, and participating in field leadership. No financial return is expected for capital investments. Professional norms protect consumers and providers, intermediaries, and governance structures work together for the common good.

The For-Profit Logic

In contrast to the nonprofit logic, the for-profit logic resonates with the common American belief that commercial enterprise is the preferred alternative (Quadagno 2004). Market-based competition and accountability to investors encourage efficiency and effectiveness, potentially driving down prices and eliminating incompetent or unethical providers. Although for-profit organizations in the health care field come in two forms, "locally owned proprietary organizations and facilities of investor-owned corporations that own multiple facilities" (Schlesinger and Gray 2006, p. 395), a more general understanding of the for-profit logic is that profit maximization prevails. As noted above, for-profit health care organizations are considered susceptible to serving dual and conflicting interests – the needs of the patients, and the expectations of the shareholders. Thus, the nonprofit logic is less controversial than the for-profit logic, which could be expressed as follows:

> The For-Profit Logic in the Health Care Field: Providers have no expected responsibility to provide community benefits. Financial return is expected for capital investments. Providers, intermediaries, and agents of governance seek to control costs and maximize efficiency.

The Private Nonprofit Logic

These four logics can stand alone in their influence on the US health care field, but they are best examined further in pairs (see Table 13.1). In doing so, the historical changes from one pair to another may lead to an understanding of our current dominant logics and where our health care system may be headed in the future. We begin with the pairing of the private and nonprofit logics. Historically, this pair of logics characterized the health care field after World War II until the mid-1960s, the time period Scott and colleagues (2000) termed the era of professional dominance. In general, following the war, the US government funded the growth of the private nonprofit sector and depended on it to perform pubic services, create policy, and generate research, ideas, and analysis (Hall 2006). In the health care field, government subsidies from the Hill Burton program prompted the development of nonprofit hospitals (Starr 1982; Needleman 2001). Individuals and their employers were expected to purchase or provide health insurance. Health plans were privately held and primarily nonprofit. Most hospitals were nonprofit, and for-profit hospitals were small proprietary businesses typically owned by physicians. The federal government provided health care funding for veterans, but other vulnerable populations were served by a safety net funded by private charities, foundations, and nonprofit health care organizations. The government played a limited role in health planning and leadership, with the era's governance dominated by the American Medical Association and other professional providers (Starr 1982; Scott et al. 2000).

The dominant logics of this era resonated with American values of freedom and liberty. Private providers were free to deliver health care in the manner they desired, allowing for both moral and religious freedom for patients and providers. In matters of trust, the nonprofit ethos and organizing principle protected patients from exploitative providers. Individual providers worked either for nonprofit organizations or small proprietary firms, which fostered their trust in their workplaces. As long as private organizations and professional associations could ensure the care of vulnerable populations and provide necessary field-level leadership and investment in research and training, Americans could trust the private, nonprofit health care system. As we see below, the private, nonprofit sector in the mid-century could only meet some of these expectations, leading to a call for change.

By integrating the key elements of the nonprofit logic and the private logic, and based on the historical description, the combined private nonprofit logic could be expressed as follows:

> The Private, Nonprofit Logic in the Health Care Field: The proper place for health planning, promotion, and provision is the private sector. Private organizations allow the government to maintain a limited role in the

field, which is desirable. Nonprofit organizations are legitimate providers because they are not motivated by profit. Nonprofit organizations can be trusted to protect consumers and raise enough funds to fulfill their missions. Individuals are responsible for acquiring health insurance, aided by employers. Trust is centered on nonprofit mission and provider ethics.

As a generic description taken out of the historical context, this combined logic raises a number of questions. First, when community benefits, such as indigent care and research funding, rely on nonprofit fundraising, what happens to community benefits when contributions run dry? Would either the public or for-profit sector have to respond to this voluntary failure? Are all employers able and willing to purchase and/or broker insurance plans, and what happens when they cannot afford to provide health benefits to their employees? Are all providers ethical, and can we rely on professional norms and associations to enforce professional ethics? What secondary mechanisms exist, if any, to enforce ethical behavior? In addition, when responsibility for health planning and leadership lies in the private sector, is there a role for public policy? And what happens when the government decides to take a larger role in health planning? Is there room for government in a private, nonprofit world?

Table 13.1 Four dominant logics in the U.S. health care field

	Nonprofit	For-profit
Private	Private sector is the proper place for health planning, promotion, and provision.	Private sector is the proper place for health planning, promotion, and provision.
	Limited government role in field desirable.	Limited government role in field desirable.
	Nonprofit organizations are legitimate due to lack of profit-motive.	Health care field requires corporate control and market competition.
	Nonprofits can be trusted to protect consumers and raise enough funds to fulfill missions.	Consumers and system benefit from market efficiencies.
	Individuals responsible for acquiring health insurance, aided by employers.	Investor ownership preferred method of raising capital. Taxes paid by for-profits return to the community.
	Trust centered on nonprofit mission and provider ethics.	Individuals responsible for acquiring health insurance, aided by employers.
		Trust centered on market's ability to eliminate ineffective and unethical providers through competition.
Public	Public sector is the proper place for health planning, promotion, and provision.	Public sector is the proper place for health planning, promotion and, provision.
	Government must do what private sector cannot do adequately.	Government must correct market failures.
	Nonprofit organizations are legitimate due to lack of profit-motive.	Health care field requires corporate control and market competition.
	Nonprofits can be trusted to protect consumers but have limited resources and may not be able to fulfill mission.	Consumers and system benefit from market efficiencies.
	Government and nonprofits must work together to provide insurance.	Investor ownership preferred method of raising capital. Taxes paid by for-profits return to the community.
	Trust centered on public mission, nonprofit mission, and government oversight.	Government and for-profits must work together to provide a cost-effective, efficient health care system.
		Trust centered on market's ability to eliminate ineffective and unethical providers through competition, combined with public oversight and protections.

The Public Nonprofit Logic

In 1965, the Social Security Act and Medicare and Medicaid programs ushered in a new era in the health care field, the era of federal involvement (Scott et al. 2000). One of the main failures of the voluntary sector was its inability to provide health insurance and financing for the elderly, the poor, and people with long-term disabilities. The Johnson Administration's response was to institute a federally funded system of financing health care for these vulnerable populations. In addition, the federal government became heavily involved in health care regulation and health planning (Starr 1982; Scott et al. 2000). In part, the rising costs of care brought on by the guaranteed reimbursement of the Medicare and Medicaid programs necessitated this larger role in health planning.

In the early 1970s the federal government's involvement went all the way down to community-level issues, such as the purchasing and utilization of equipment for hospitals. The federal government's involvement also concerned the macrolevel issues of shaping health care logics and the creation of new organizational forms, such as the health maintenance organization. In all, this era was characterized by the replacement of the private logic with a public logic. This is not to say that private providers and intermediaries no longer existed; in fact, with the nonprofit logic intact, providers were still expected to provide community benefits and sector leadership, and employers were still expected to provide health insurance for their employees. But the federal government had stepped in to respond to both voluntary failure and gaps in coverage for the unemployed. This era of public, nonprofit logics turned out to be a transitory time in the history of the American health care field, as guaranteed federal reimbursements for care prompted the growth of investor-owned health care organizations, and rising costs led to a search for new logics and organizational forms. In terms of trust, this turbulent time placed the onus of regulatory responsibility on the federal government, weakening the need for professional self-enforcement of provider ethics. However, providers and purchasers generally trusted the primarily nonprofit health care system, and the federal government's new role increased the number of sectors involved in building a better health care system. The health care system of this era was more cumbersome and turbulent than before, but it would be difficult to argue that it was less trustworthy.

Based on the combination of the public logic and the nonprofit logic, as well as historical trends during the era of federal involvement, the public nonprofit logic could be expressed as follows:

> The Public Nonprofit Logic in the Health Care Field: The proper place for health planning, promotion, and provision is the public sector. Government must do what the private sector cannot do adequately: protect consumers, provide insurance, conduct or fund research, and/or train practitioners. Nonprofit organizations are legitimate providers because they are not motivated by profit. Nonprofit organizations can be trusted to protect consumers. But nonprofits have limited resources and may not be able to fulfill all parts of their missions at all times. The government and nonprofit organizations must work together to provide health care and insurance. Trust lies in public mission, nonprofit mission, and government oversight.

Paired together, the dual public and nonprofit missions raise questions of redundancy. If the public sector takes responsibility for the common good, what benefit can nonprofits provide in exchange for tax-exemption? This blurring of missions is reflected in Steinberg and Powell's comment that a "challenge in some cases is distinguishing private nonprofit organizations from public government agencies" (Steinberg and Powell 2006, p. 2). In terms of funding a public nonprofit health care field, what is the key source of funding – contributions to nonprofit organizations, or taxes? If both, which source pays for what aspects of health care and health planning? How is responsibility for community benefit divided between two sectors intent on, if not responsible for, providing community benefit? Given historical developments, does a public nonprofit logic lead to rising health care costs? In addition, if the government steps in to provide oversight and regulate the health care field, what are the roles of professionals, professional expertise, and professional ethics? Is the nonprofit ethos necessarily overshadowed or possibly weakened by the involvement of the public sector?

The Private For-Profit Logic

In the early 1980s, the Reagan administration dismantled public involvement in many industries, including health care. This wave of privatization ushered in what Scott and colleagues call the era of managerial control and market mechanisms (Scott et al. 2000). The health planning and regulatory activity of the 1970s was curtailed, and in 1983 Medicare was restructured to introduce a prospective payment system, limiting reimbursements to providers. Broad-based market logics grew in influence over the field; providers were expected to be efficient and cost effective, regardless of ownership status (Scott et al. 2000). Cost-shifting to private insurers in order to make up losses from federal insurance and charity care led, in part, to the rise of managed care insurance plans, many of which were for-profit. In the 1980s and early 1990s, managed care plans held down the costs of insurance premiums, making them attractive to employers and individual purchasers. As health plans competed for business and required capital investment, the late 1990s saw a wave of conversions of nonprofit health plans to investor-owned status (Gray 1997). Although the health care field retained its mix of nonprofit and for-profit organizations, by the twenty-first century "much of the American public believe(d) that the health-care system ha(d) become dominated by for-profit enterprise" (Schlesinger and Gray 2006, p. 381).

Several scholars argue that the rise of market logics did not merely replace a nonprofit logic in the health care field but undermined the nonprofit logic. Estes and colleagues (Estes et al. 2001) point to eight distinct shocks to the nonprofit sector that occurred during the 1980s and 1990s, including cuts to the federal budget during the Reagan administration; the increase of privatization, competition, cost constraints, and unbundling of services; corporate mergers and conversions to for-profit status; the rising intensity of labor conflict in the nonprofit system; attempts to silence nonprofit entities through congressional proposals; and the impact of the expense of information technology. They argue, "from the mid-1960s to the 1980s, a major legitimating rationale for the (nonprofit sector) was that it could contain the size of the state while also dealing with the nation's social ills. With the newly energized market ideology reemerging during the Reagan era..., the (nonprofit sector) was, for the first time, redefined as a negative competitive force and perhaps redundant" (Estes et al. 2001, p. 67). Needleman (2001, pp. 1118–1119) cites a Blue Cross/Blue Shield publication justifying nonprofit to for-profit conversion, that "cited research showing 'that the vast majority of consumers either did not know the difference between for-profit and nonprofit insurers, or did not care. The vast majority of business decision-makers who bought health insurance had decidedly negative impressions of the nonprofit form' (Orloff 1997, p. 290)."

Despite the fact that the federal and state governments continued to finance health insurance for the elderly and poor, the private logic was reinforced again and again during this era. After the demise of the Clinton Health Security Act, "health policy making moved toward shoring up the private health insurance system by tightening regulations to make private insurance less insecure" (Quadagno 2004, p. 38). The Health Insurance Portability and Accountability Act of 1996, for example, kept insurance in the hands of employers, not the government, and created incentives for individuals to purchase private long-term care insurance (Quadagno 2004). Even the long-awaited Medicare prescription drug benefit, put in place in 2003, supported the private sector. The federal government was prohibited from negotiating drug prices (Quadagno 2004), which allowed the market to set prices and placed no constraints on the investor-owned pharmaceutical industry. In addition, the Medicare prescription drug benefit (Medicare Part D) contains a gap in coverage, the "donut hole," in which individuals with high prescription costs are liable for nearly four thousand dollars in out-of-pocket payments (per year) before they reach the status of catastrophic coverage. In the 1980s and 1990s, and some would argue the twenty-first century as well, the health care field had a "uniquely American system of health care financing (that) involve(d) social legislation that defer(red) to market principles and federal sponsorship of private sector alternatives to public programs" (Quadagno 2004, p. 27).

The dominant for-profit and private logics raise a whole host of issues regarding trust. At the micro level, patients who see providers working for for-profit organizations, receive care from for-profit provider organizations, or are enrolled in for-profit insurance plans cannot trust that their providers or insurers have their best interest in mind. The turn of the twenty-first century was characterized by a cultural backlash against managed care, with numerous horror stories about unethical and inappropriate care played out in the media (Mechanic 2001). In addition, managed competition implies that managers are more trustworthy than physicians, undermining physicians' ability to make medical decisions in the best interest of patients (Light 2004). As discussed above, an American Medical Association survey taken in the late 1990s showed that physicians were less trusting of for-profit provider corporations (Schlesinger et al. 2005). At the macro level, the general sense that the US health care system is a "mess," or "something must be done," shows a lack of trust in the system as a whole.

Given the private and for-profit logics individually and the discussion of this era's trends and issues, the combination of a private and for-profit logic might be expressed as follows:

> The Private For-Profit Logic in the Health Care Field: The proper and most desirable place for health planning, promotion, and provision is the private sector. Private organizations allow the government to maintain a limited role in the field, which is desirable. The health care field, like other sectors of the economy, requires corporate control and market competition, which the nonprofit sector cannot provide. Market governance forces organizations to minimize costs and maximize efficiency, which benefits the consumer and the system as a whole. Investor ownership is the preferred method of raising capital, and taxes paid by for-profit organizations return to the community, providing a community benefit. Individuals are responsible for acquiring health insurance, aided by employers. Trust is centered on the market's ability to eliminate ineffective and unethical providers through competition.

The private for-profit logic raises a number of questions, many of which our society is struggling with in the twenty-first century. In highly privatized system, who or what provides a safety net for people who are unemployed, retired, and/or poor? Although the federal government has retained its commitment to financing health insurance for the elderly and indigent, health insurance for the unemployed and the underemployed is a pressing issue. The complexity of the health care field makes it difficult to definitively answer the question of whether the for-profit motive interferes with the provision of care, but a more specific question can be raised: who or what protects consumers from ineffective and unethical providers, prior to their elimination from the market? In today's society, the answer points to the courts, in the form of costly malpractice lawsuits, and for individual providers, malpractice insurance. In the last few years another question has become pressing: Are all employers able and willing to purchase and/or broker insurance plans? As the ranks of the uninsured swell with employed individuals and their families, we know the answer is sometimes no. With out- of- control profits for pharmaceuticals, razor- thin margins for most providers, and a severe lack of services for many Americans, we know this private for-profit logic shapes, at the least, a dysfunctional health care system, and for many, an exploitative one. Thus, the most salient question raised by the private for-profit logic is: where do we go from here?

The Public For-Profit Logic

The last combination of logics, pairing a public logic with a for-profit logic, seems the most unusual, yet potentially this combination governs the health care field in the twenty-first century. To examine if the dominant logics of the era of managerial control and market mechanisms have changed, first we must ask if the private logic remains in the field or if it has been replaced by a public logic. There are a number of indicators that, if a public logic does not prevail in the twenty-first century, at the very least there is increasing tension between the public and private sectors' roles and responsibilities in the health care field. In the mid-1990s, federal and state governments enacted a number of consumer protection laws in response to market failures, including the 1996 Newborns' and Mothers' Health Protection Act and the 1996 Mental Health Parity Act. By 2002, all but three states had patients' bills of rights (Sloan and Hall 2002). In 1997, for the first time since 1965, the federal government expanded insurance coverage through S-CHIP to a new population of Americans: low-income children living above the poverty level. In addition, in 2003 Medicare benefits were expanded to provide prescription drug coverage.

Taken together, these governmental actions demonstrate some renewed public responsibility for health care leadership and financing, but on the whole these actions were limited responses to specific market failures. These actions did not comprehensively deprivatize the heath care field and reintroduce motivations such as community benefits and equitable access present during the era of federal involvement. As the controversy in 2007 over renewing S-CHIP demonstrated, these governmental actions were no "natural" step toward a public ethos but a reactionary and forced response to a series of problems stemming from the for-profit logic governing health care. The fight over S-CHIP renewal, in which President Bush threatened to veto legislation that would increase the income ceilings for low-income families with children insured by S-CHIP, was a fight "about the government's place in providing health care" (Covering More Children 2007, p. A18). To the Bush administration, S-CHIP was a threatening program because it recognizes that the market has failed to insure individuals at lower income levels through their employers. If employment-based health insurance is no longer a given, who will insure uninsured working Americans? If the answer remains "no one" for adults, at the very least Americans expect the government to save the children. S-CHIP reinforces, depending on one's point of view, the celebrated renewal of the public logic, or the encroachment of the public logic on the private.

The impact of the growing influence of the public logic has not necessarily undermined the for-profit logic. Medicare Part D, for example, essentially pats the pharmaceutical industry on the back for making so many expensive medications and helps the elderly afford their medications, so that they will keep taking their medications. With the donut hole in place, the government does not even have to pay very much for these prescriptions. Consumer protection laws address specific market corrections but do not override the market's ultimate responsibility for the governance of the health care field. At the same time, the public logic paired with the for-profit logic undermines the nonprofit system: "one solution to the crisis tendencies of capitalism is the restructuring of the nonprofit health and social services to expand the for-profit sector financed by the state at the expense of traditional NPS services" (Estes et al. 2001, p. 74). With the state taking a larger community service role and addressing issues of access, "the historic ability of nonprofit health plans to address these goals has already been seriously eroded and partly replaced by Medicaid expansions, state high-risk pools, and other state mechanisms" (Needleman 2001, p. 1125).

Issues of trust abound in a public for-profit field. Can we trust the government to step in to restore a nonprofit ethos to the health care system, or should community benefits be left to the private sector? Can we trust for-profit organizations if they are regulated by the government? If health care providers are held to the for-profit logics of containing costs and maximizing efficiency, then a public logic would do little to address information asymmetries and potentials for exploitation. Physicians may not be any more likely to trust for-profit corporate providers operating under a public logic than a private logic. In terms of the field as a whole, the mix of public and for-profit logics seems the most uneasy of the pairings. A private nonprofit logic sits well with American traditions of limited government involvement, freedom of choice, and liberty. A public nonprofit logic creates synergy with its undeniable focus on community benefits and the common good. A private for-profit logic resonates with Americans' faith in the capitalist economy and the free market, but a public, for-profit logic seems to pit regulation against competition, state responsibility against individual responsibility, and individual rights against the common good.

Combining the two logics of public and for-profit, the public for-profit logic could be expressed as follows:

> The Public For-Profit Logic in the Health Care Field: The proper place for health planning, promotion, and provision is the public sector. The government must correct market failures. These corrections may involve consumer protection regulation, government- financed insurance, and/or grants for research and professional training. At the same time, the health care field, like other sectors of the economy, requires market competition. For-profit organizations minimize costs and maximize efficiency, which benefits the consumer. Investor ownership is the preferred method of raising capital, and taxes paid by for-profit organizations return to the community. The government and for-profit corporations must work together to provide a cost-effective, efficient health care system. Trust lies in the market's ability to eliminate ineffective and unethical providers through competition, combined with public oversight and protections.

The public for-profit logic raises a number of issues. Although many industries in the American economy are governed by regulated markets, is a regulated market an appropriate model for the health care field? What is the appropriate balance of governmental and corporate controls, and how willing is the state to step into the corporate domain? What is the key source of funding in a public for-profit health care field – investor capital, or taxes? If both, which source pays for what? In addition, who is to blame when things go wrong? Is it the government for not regulating enough or the market for not weeding out incompetent or unethical providers? Can a regulated market eliminate inefficient and inappropriate providers? Or will the state's governance impede market competition, at the expense of consumers? And can a government that values the free market and encourages or allows a for-profit logic to dominate the health care field do enough to ensure equal access to affordable care?

Restoring Trust? Issues for Medical Sociology

This chapter demonstrates the necessity of addressing institutional logics in medical sociology research. From the micro to the macro levels of analysis, understandings of individual choices, provider forms, and public policies are incomplete without a consideration of under what broad-based systems of belief health care purchasers, providers, intermediaries, and agents of governance are operating. These broad-based systems should include both the prevailing logics about the role of the government versus the private sector and the appropriate forms of ownership and financial returns on investment. Analyzing all four logics helps prevent some typical and limiting assumptions, such as that "private" means for-profit, and that "public" automatically supports nonprofit logics. In the era of public management, this latter assumption is particularly problematic. These four logics also are important when considering the issue of universal health care coverage. If the goal of universal health care is that everyone has some form of insurance coverage, purchased by a variety of agents including individuals, employers, and governments, then a public for-profit logic might accommodate this system. But if universal health care means a single-payer system and government ownership of health care facilities, then the for-profit logic cannot persist. If our historical progression has indeed led us to the prevalence of a public for-profit logic, then is a single-payer system even cognitively possible?

A key issue concerns the relationship between logics and the behavior and ownership of organizational providers. For-profit corporations may not conform to for-profit motivations and norms when nonprofit logics are salient. Schlesinger and colleagues (2005, p. 607) found that "the frequency of untrustworthy practices among for-profit plans is much reduced when they operate in markets in which 20% or more of their competitors are nonprofit plans." Notably, a market in which 20% of the for-profits' competitors are nonprofit means that for-profit corporations (and for-profit logics) are still dominant, yet a significant minority of nonprofit organizational forms can change behavior. For-profits also may behave like nonprofits if market conditions sort more vulnerable consumers to nonprofits and well-informed consumers to for-profits (Schlesinger et al. 2005). Examining for-profits more generally, Campbell (2006) predicted that investor-owned organizations would be likely to engage in corporate social responsibility when influenced by a number of internal and external factors, such as self-regulation; state regulation, monitoring, and enforcement; coverage from the media; lobbying by social movement organizations; the expectations of non-profit organizations, and so forth.

In a similar vein, nonprofit organizations do not follow nonprofit norms uniformly. Involvement in charity care, for example, differs depending on state regulations and demand (Needleman 2001). The markets in which both for-profits and nonprofits operate have a large effect on their structures, strategies, and behavior (Needleman 2001), as does the life cycle stage of the health service (Schlesinger and Gray 2006). These findings and arguments imply that simply identifying the overarching logics creating meaning in an organizational field is not enough to understand organizational behavior, but more importantly, a prevalence of for-profit logics and organizations does not necessarily mean that the health care field cannot incorporate community benefits and work for the common good.

This chapter also raises the question: Is a public for-profit logic inevitable, based on the historical development of health care in the twentieth and twenty-first centuries? Whether or not a renewed emphasis on public responsibility is upon us, it seems apparent that the nonprofit logic of the past has been undermined and weakened (Estes et al. 2001; Schlesinger and Gray 2006). With a weakened nonprofit sector, the "three failures" model (Steinberg 2006) predicts that the government and the market step in to correct for voluntary failure. A public for-profit logic thus resonates with this model. But if the nonprofit sector is so weakened that it can no longer respond to failures in the other sectors, then the "three failures" model becomes a "two failures" model, in which only the market can respond to government failure and only the government can respond to contract failure. Ironically, relying on the for-profit sector ends up involving the state more in health care: as health care costs rise in the private sector, "the most difficult (and least profitable) clients…are dumped on the public sector as too costly for either the nonprofits or for-profits to treat or serve" (Estes et al. 2001, p. 75). As market mechanisms lead to employed individuals losing their health insurance, the state steps in to protect them or at least their children. Could it be that privatization, in the form of encouraging managerial control and market competition, set our country on a path to 1965 redux? If so, "universal insurance would virtually eliminate the need for private provision of (charitable and unprofitable) services" (Needleman 2001, p. 1126) – and possibly the value of the nonprofit sector in health care.

A prevailing public for-profit logic may lead to increased health insurance coverage for vulnerable populations, but how does it address the multiple layers and issues of trust? In the descriptions of the various logics and pairings, the nonprofit logic is the most inherently trustworthy. Under a nonprofit logic, patients trust that their providers will give them appropriate and necessary treatments, individual providers trust that organizational providers will not force upon them conflicts of interest, and the system as a whole incorporates norms of community benefits and the common good. Some researchers argue that "preserving a substantial market niche for nonprofit plans… should be considered by policymakers as a strategy for restoring trust in the health care system" (Schlesinger et al. 2005, p. 606), as other solutions, such as stronger professional norms, consumer empowerment, and enhanced regulation would be less effective. Presumably, this market niche would be both nonprofit and private.

Is such a solution viable when a private nonprofit logic has not prevailed in over 40 years? And given the intangible nature of trust and the intangible nature of logics, can trust be regained by returning to a nonprofit logic, rather than sustaining nonprofit organizations? Would a consumer or an individual provider trust an investor-owned organizational provider if that organization conformed to nonprofit-oriented norms? Where does the trust lie – in the organizational form, or in the field's broader organizing principles? If returning to a nonprofit logic is unrealistic, is a public logic substitutable? Can the government buffer the health care market to an extent that trust is restored to the system? And can the public logic and for-profit logic coexist, or must the tension resolve toward either the public nonprofit or the private for-profit logic? At any rate, at the beginning of the twenty-first century, if we do not trust the government, and we do not trust the market, then we are headed into even choppier waters than we have experienced before.

Potential Directions for Future Research

This chapter suggests several directions for future research on issues of trust and the influence of institutional logics on the US health care field. A first step would be to assess if the USA has indeed entered a new historical era framed by a public, for-profit logic. One approach to this analysis would be to update key variables that Scott and colleagues (2000) used to trace the presence of and changes across historical eras, and then determine if these variables have changed significantly since the mid- or late-1990s (when the Scott et al. project ended). The areas Scott and colleagues studied included (but are not limited to) five populations of organizations (hospitals, home health agencies, health care systems, HMOs, and end-stage renal disease centers); trends in regulatory policy and health planning; types of insurance coverage and expenditures by insurers and government; membership in professional associations; and the presence or absence of key words in medical and health policy journals.

Because the era of managerial controls and market mechanisms (beginning in 1983) emphasized deregulation and market competition, a comparison of old and new data would need to determine if a faith in market competition still governs the field (for-profit logic), while at the same time the government is becoming increasingly involved in regulating and structuring the health care field (public logic). Indicators of change might include a growth in the number or market share of government-owned health care delivery organizations; increased state and federal regulation of health care providers and purchasers; a shift in Medicare and Medicaid enrollment from private insurers back to public plans; and/or an increase in medical and health policy journals of the presence of key words such as "public responsibility," "public management," and so forth. A new era or logic also might be marked by new types of health care providers, new organizational forms, novel partnerships between organizations, and/or changes in the focus and culture of professional associations (such as the American Medical Association).

Following Reay and Hinings (2005), shifts in belief systems and logics could emerge from an in-depth study of the language used in government documents, legislative debates and testimonies, and newspaper articles about health care reform. The questions that opened this chapter could be used as a frame for this exploration. For example, the researcher could look for answers to the question "who is responsible for health care and health insurance?" to see if the discourse on this subject is shifting from pinpointing individuals and the private sector to targeting the government. A different spin on this question, which also would be fruitful to ask and study, would be, "who is accountable for failures of the health care system?" Are the answers to "who is responsible" and "who is accountable" the same?

In terms of "what practices create the best health care system," the language in government documents, legislative debates, and news articles might indicate which actors in the twenty-first century get to define "best" and determine "best practices" – practitioners, organizations, professional associations, the government, and/or the market? Examining the question "can the US health care system deliver high quality care, control costs, and ensure equitable access" might reveal the presence, absence, or strength of dominant institutional logics, as well as if quality care, cost control, and equitable access are valued. For example, a researcher might examine discussions of who or what is responsible for cost control – market forces, patients, individual providers and delivery organizations, the federal government, or a lack of a profit motive in the field? Who or what should promote equitable access to care – the government, nonprofit and charitable organizations, or for-profits? And who or what is responsible for monitoring quality of care – the professions, the government, or market competition? Studying the use of language in responses to these questions could help tease out not just the presence of a public, for-profit logic, but also the differences in logics adopted and articulated by key actors and power shifts in the health care field.

A second direction for future research would be to incorporate the presence and influence of macroinstitutional logics into studies of trust in the health care field. For example, it would be useful to explore if patients' trust in providers, health care organizations, and insurers is influenced by broad-based meaning systems and how they are employed by providers and purchasers. Would a public logic create an extra layer of trust in a field dominated by nonprofits? Or would a fear of government incompetence weaken trust in nonprofit organizations? Could a public logic soften concerns about for-profit malfeasance? In a field dominated by for-profit logics, do patients still trust nonprofit organizations?

Similar questions could be examined with regard to physicians' trust of health care delivery organizations, purchasers, and the government. Building off the Schlesinger et al. (2005) study of physicians' perceptions of for-profit health plans' trustworthiness, another research direction might be to assess if the presence of public plans has the same influence on for-profits as the presence of nonprofit plans. In other words, will physicians perceive that for-profits engage in more trustworthy behavior if the for-profits are competing with, or located near, public organizations? Do non-profits and/or public hospitals have a similar effect on physicians' perceptions of for-profit hospitals?

At a macro level, research on trust in the US health care system should incorporate an understanding of the historical trajectory of public, private, nonprofit, and for-profit logics and their different pairings over time. As this chapter demonstrates, trust in the system as a whole can stem from a number of diverse sources: a nonprofit mission, a public mission, professional ethics, government oversight, government regulation, and market forces. Which combinations of these factors in the health care field have led to the highest and lowest trust over time? How have combinations of these factors affected trust levels in other industries and fields, such as utilities, transportation, and education? Is there any historical evidence of trust emerging under a public, for-profit logic? Or are we on new institutional ground, not just in health care, but in other industries as well?

As the scope of these directions for research indicates, incorporating institutional logics into studies of trust would yield a wide range of new and potentially insightful analyses of the sociology of health, illness, and healing. In addition, a nuanced and improved understanding of the effects of institutional logics on health policy and health care could reframe the debates, sharpen the issues, and shape the direction of our health care future.

References

Arrow K (1963) Uncertainty and the welfare economics of medical care. Am Econ Rev 53:941–973
Bennet JT, DiLorenzo TJ (1997) Commercialization of America's health charities. Society May/June:67–72
Bloom BR, Brown P (2003) America's health system and how to make it more effective. In: Brown P, Bloom BR (eds) The future of public health. Harvard School of Public Health, Cambridge, MA, pp 145–155
Campbell JL (2006) Institutional analysis and the paradox of corporate responsibility. Am Behav Sci 49:925–938
Caronna C (2004). The Mis-alignment of institutional 'pillars': consequences for the U.S. health care field. J Health Soc Behav 45(Extra Issue):45–58
Covering more children: The administration balks at the expansion of a healthcare program that works (2007, July 17). The Washington Post, p. A18
DiMaggio PJ, Anheier HK (1990) The sociology of nonprofit organizations and sectors. Annu Rev Sociol 16:137–159
DiMaggio PJ, Powell WW (1983) The iron cage revisited: institutional isomorphism and collective rationality in organizational fields. Am Sociol Rev 82:147–160

Estes CL, Alford RR, Egan AH (2001) The transformation of the nonprofit sector: systemic crisis and the political economy of aging services. In: Estes CL et al (eds) Social policy and aging: a critical perspective. Sage, Thousand Oaks, CA, pp 69–94

Friedland R, Alford RR (1991) Bringing society back in: symbols, practices, and institutional contradictions. In: Powell WW, DiMaggio PJ (eds) The new institutionalism in organizational analysis. University of Chicago Press, Chicago, IL, pp 232–263

Gray BH (1997) Conversion of HMOs and hospitals: what's at stake? Health Aff 16(2):29–47

Hall PD (2006) A historical overview of philanthropy, voluntary associations, and nonprofit organizations in the United States, 1600–2000. In: Powell WW, Steinberg R (eds) The nonprofit sector: a research handbook, 2nd edn. Yale University Press, New Haven, CT, pp 32–65

Kitchener M (2002) Mobilizing the logic of managerialism in professional fields: the case of academic health centre mergers. Organ Stud 23(3):391–420

Kitchener M, Harrington C (2004) The U.S. long-term care field: a dialectical analysis of institution dynamics. J Health Soc Behav 45(Extra Issue):87–101

Krugman P (2007, July 9) Health care terror. The New York Times, p. 17

Lawrence D (1997) Why we want to remain a nonprofit health care organization. Health Aff 16(2):118–120

Light DW (2004) Ironies of success: a new history of the American health care 'system'. J Health Soc Behav 45(Extra Issue):1–24

Mechanic D (2001) The managed care backlash: perceptions and rhetoric in health care policy and the potential for health care reform. Milbank Q 79(1):35–54

Mechanic D (2004) The rise and fall of managed care. J Health Soc Behav 45(Extra Issue):76–86

Needleman J (2001) The role of nonprofits in health care. J Health Polit Policy Law 26:1113–1130

Orloff MA (1997) A perspective from the national blue cross and blue shield organizations. Bull NY Acad Med 74(2):286–291

Powell WW, Steinberg R (1987) The non-profit sector: a research handbook. Yale University Press, New Haven, CT

Powell WW, Steinberg R (2006) The non-profit sector: a research handbook, 2nd edn. Yale University Press, New Haven, CT

Quadagno J (2004) Why the United States has no national health insurance: stakeholder mobilization against the welfare state, 1945–1996. J Health Soc Behav 45(Extra Issue):25–44

Reay T, Hinings CR (2005) The recomposition of an organizational field: health care in Alberta. Organ Stud 26(3):351–384

Schlesinger M, Gray BH (2006) Nonprofit organizations and health care: some paradoxes of persistent scrutiny. In: Powell WW, Steinberg R (eds) The nonprofit sector: a research handbook, 2nd edn. Yale University Press, New Haven, CT, pp 378–414

Schlesinger M, Quon N, Wynia M, Cummins D, Gray B (2005) Profit-seeking, corporate control, and the trustworthiness of health care organizations: assessments of health plan performance by their affiliated physicians. HSR: Health Serv Res 40:605–645

Scott WR (2001) Institutions and organizations, 2nd edn. Sage, Thousand Oaks, CA

Scott WR, Ruef M, Mendel PJ, Caronna CA (2000) Institutional change and healthcare organizations: from professional dominance to managed care. University of Chicago Press, Chicago, IL

Sloan FA, Hall MA (2002) Market failures and the evolution of state regulation of managed care. Law Contemp Probl 65:169–208

Starr P (1982) The social transformation of American medicine. Basic Books, New York

Steinberg R (2006) Economic theories of nonprofit organizations. In: Powel WW, Steinberg R (eds) The nonprofit sector: a research handbook, 2nd edn. Yale University Press, New Haven, CT, pp 117–139

Steinberg R, Powell WW (2006) Introduction. In: Powell WW, Steinberg R (eds) The nonprofit sector: a research handbook, 2nd edn. Yale University Press, New Haven, CT, pp 1–11

Woolhandler S, Himmelstein DU (2002) Paying for national health insurance – and not getting it. Health Aff 21:88–98

Chapter 14
Health Care Policy and Medical Sociology

Jennie Jacobs Kronenfeld

Health Care Policy and Medical Sociology

Health policy concerns are important, but to some extent, understudied within medical sociology, particularly at the overall broadest system level. Even in smaller studies that look at specific aspects of health care and health behavior issues, sociologists have not paid much attention in the past few decades to drawing out the implications of the research being done for policy questions within health and health care. Some people have viewed policy as more in the purview of political scientists, and, to some extent, the presence of a journal such as *Journal of Health Care Politics, Policy and Research* (JHPPPL) and its closer connections with political scientists and historians than with sociologists have reinforced that feeling. In addition, for the last 35 years, studies of the health care delivery system have broadened into many areas of social and administrative sciences and public health. Increasingly, these types of research have become part of an interdisciplinary effort often known as health services research. This chapter argues that sociologists must become concerned with policy issues if we are to remain relevant to some of the most important issues relating to health and health services delivery in the population. To help sociologists apply their research in the future to broader policy concerns and to raise awareness among medical sociologists of the importance of paying attention to policy concerns, this chapter first discusses what we mean by policy and reviews some of the past emphases and attempts to look at the relationship between medical sociology and health policy. Next, the chapter discusses issues about how policy is made in the USA, and presents a quick review of aspects of the policy-making process with a focus on the broader system level, not because sociologists should be in the forefront of this research, but because a better understanding of these issues will help sociologists to broaden the applicability of their more focused research and to better understand its potential to have some impact on policy issues. Then the chapter discusses some of the most important themes in health services research (cost, access, and a bit on quality) and focus more on a review of issues of access, health insurance, and cost. At the end, I return to discussion of some of the kinds of questions that are important in health policy and for which medical sociology can help broaden the way in which policy issues are addressed in the USA and help the research of medical sociologists to be important in the formulation of health policy broadly as well as in smaller, more specific ways. An important theme is that sociologists should not surrender the application of research to policy concerns to other disciplines but should also think about ways their own work can be applied to ongoing issues of policy and public concern.

J.J. Kronenfeld (✉)
Sociology Program, School of Family and Social Dynamics, Arizona State University,
873701, Tempe, AZ 85287-3701, USA
e-mail: jennie.kronenfeld@asu.edu

What is health policy? According to Gray and O'Leary in the *Handbook of Medical Sociology* (Bird et al. 2000) although people most generally think of policy as the product of governmental actions, health policy can also be a part of the efforts of private entities and can encompass decisions made by employers on the details of provision of health insurance to employees (Gray and O'Leary 2000). More often, however, people do focus on public policy and that is more of the focus in this chapter, although the issue of private decisions and the role of administrative agencies in smaller policy decisions is also discussed at the end of the chapter. Not all health policy decisions occur at the national level; however, the national level is the more important level. Medicare, the program to provide health care services to the elderly and disabled, is a federal program. Medicaid and SCHIP (state child health insurance program), both of which provide health services to the poor or near poor, are joint federal–state efforts, as are federal welfare programs overall. In joint federal–state welfare programs, such as Medicare, the federal government sets certain requirements that states must meet, often relating to a minimum set of services that must be provided, and sometimes the federal level also sets limits about how many services can be provided or some aspects of eligibility for the programs. Generally, the funding of these programs is a shared responsibility between the state and federal level, with poorer states often receiving a higher proportion of federal dollars toward the overall costs of the program. These programs are generally administered at the state level, and there are variations in programs from state to state. Because of variations in these types of programs from state to state, states have sometimes been described as laboratories for testing new federal programs in the labor, welfare, and health areas. During the New Deal in the USA in the 1930s, a number of the welfare and labor programs enacted had first been state level programs.

Recently, some states are taking leadership roles in trying to expand health insurance coverage to all citizens. Recently, Massachusetts has enacted such a plan which builds on its private health insurance system and its current high rates of coverage, but also includes the presence of Medicare as a federal program and Medicaid as a shared program. On April 12, 2006, Chapter 58 of the Acts of 2006 in Massachusetts became law. This plan established ambitious goals for health care reform, with the overall goal that Massachusetts would achieve nearly universal coverage for its residents. As part of this overall goal, the state was to help create new, low-cost plans for individuals and small businesses and expand public programs for people without access to employer-sponsored health insurance. After a year, the number of Massachusetts residents covered by MassHealth, the state's Medicaid program, and Commonwealth Care, the new, publicly subsidized insurance program for low-income residents, increased by 122,000 (Raymond 2007). California has also discussed a plan. These are ways in which states are currently innovating in health policy and are trying out approaches that may later be broadened to include other states or become federal policy. Medical sociologists in these states may be able to have a more direct impact on public policy questions, especially if their research involves use of state-based data. As the debate about health care reform at the national level is likely to be renewed with the election of Obama as President, there may be more issues about health policy reform for medical sociologists to discuss.

Medical Sociology and Health Policy

Earlier Ideas About Medical Sociology and Health Policy

As Gray and O'Leary (2000) point out in their review of the evolving relationship between medical sociology and health policy, health policy was not seen as an important enough topic for medical sociology to be explicitly included in the earliest (1963) edition of the Handbook of Medical Sociology (Freeman et al. 1963), although it was implicitly addressed in some ways in one of the book's important themes about the problems of the biological paradigm that was at the heart of the biomedical research effort of that era. Others who have reviewed the early history of medical sociology as a field (Bloom 1986, 2002) also did not view health policy as important to medical sociology throughout the 1950s. Bloom argued that one of the reasons for the lack of interest in health policy in the development of medical sociology prior to the 1960s and 1970s was the tension between applied and basic approaches to research in sociology and the implicit lower value placed on applied research. After the passage of Medicare and Medicaid in 1965, the role of the federal government in health care policy grew and continued to expand as extensions to the Medicare program were passed in 1972 (Kronenfeld 1997, 2002). By the second edition of the Handbook (Freeman et al. 1972), Medicare and Medicaid had been passed, and this began a transition that has made the federal government the most powerful force in the American health care system (Gray and O'Leary 2000). This change, however, was not that well reflected in the second edition, with the index having neither policy nor government as part of the subject index.

In the third (Freeman et al. 1979) and fourth (Freeman and Levine 1989) editions of the Handbook, there was more coverage of health policy topics, in various ways. In the third edition, there were chapters looking at community variables and a chapter examining technology and medical care. There was also a chapter on health politics; however, this chapter had a nonsociologist author (Daniel Fox, a historian), also illustrating the tendency at some points within medical sociology to turn more explicit considerations of health policy and politics topics over to other social science disciplines. By the fourth edition, policy concerns relating to various topics were often covered in specific chapters, and there was more consideration of issues such as health care for the poor in the introduction to the volume.

A special issue of the *Journal of Health and Social Behavior* included an article that reviewed the impact of medical sociology on health care policy concerns (Gray and Phillips 1995). Referring mostly to policy issues that pertain to the organization and financing of the health care system, Gray and Phillips (1995) argue that although there is potential interest among policy makers in sociological contributions to health policy issues, the policy impact of medical sociologists has been limited by the ambivalence of sociologists as regards policy, academic career considerations, and the separate development of health research as a distinct field of research. The 2000 edition of the Handbook (Bird et al. 2000) included an explicit chapter on the relationship between medical sociology and health policy (Gray and O'Leary 2000) and a concluding chapter (Pescosolido et al. 2000) that discussed the place of medical sociology in research and policy in the twenty-first century. Gray and O'Leary (2000) argue that the creation of a separate field of policy research and health services research means that medical sociologists who pursue policy-oriented research often end up in a different career path than medical sociologists who remain in sociology departments. Pescosolido and colleagues (2000) argue that medical sociologists of the future will need to reach across disciplines and integrate ideas from medical sociology into policy-relevant areas as well as into the larger overall sociological concerns.

Health Services Research and Medical Sociology

Parallel to the addressing of health policy interests within the scholarly literature in medical sociology is the growth of interest within parts of the federal government in an improved understanding of the impact of federal policy changes on the use of health care services and health. This interest within the federal government led to the creation of NCHSR (National Center for Health Services Research, Department of Health, Education and Welfare). The role of some sociologists such as Arlene Daniels, Robert Ehrlich, and Jack Elinson both as researchers and project officers in the new institute and as grantees increased the interest of medical sociology in the policy process and the interests of federal government policy personnel in medical sociology specifically and the social sciences more generally (Ebert-Flateau and Perkoff 1983). During that time frame, some funding for graduate training programs in medical sociology at Brown University, Boston University, Purdue University, University of Chicago, and Columbia University, for example, also were a part of the efforts of NCHSR, following the establishment of the agency in 1968.

Health services research is generally described as a "field of inquiry, both basic and applied, that examines the use, costs, quality, accessibility, delivery, organization, financing, and outcomes of health care services to increase knowledge and understanding of the structure, processes, and effects of health services for individuals and populations" (Wholey and Burns 2000, p. 220). Medical sociology, medical anthropology, and health economics became involved in the development of the field over time, as did researchers from a public health perspective, especially those involved with medical care-related research. Some statisticians and epidemiologists from schools of public health also became involved. One of the early applications of health services research cited in some sociological publications was the Wennberg and Gittelsohn (1973) finding that health services utilization varied dramatically across small areas (Wholey and Burns 2000). Looking at variation in rates of tonsillectomy within Vermont, Wennberg and Gittelsohn (1973) found that a person living in the area with the highest rates had a 66% chance of having the procedure by age 20, while people living in neighboring areas had only a 20% chance. Studies of issues related to utilization of health care, unequal access to health care services, and quality of life became topics that medical sociologists studied that were also linked to health services research during the 1970s and 1980s (Levine 1987; Aday et al. 1980).

In 1989, the health services research agency became the Agency for Health Care Policy and Research, and that title change reflected a growing interest in explicit policy considerations. Some have argued that health services research has now become "so imbued with policy as to be indistinguishable from health-policy research" (Gray and O'Leary 2000, p. 268). The more recent new name for the agency is now AHRQ, the Agency for Healthcare Research and Quality – the Nation's lead Federal agency for research on health care quality, costs, outcomes, and patient safety located within the Department of Health and Human Services. While this agency's budget has not grown as rapidly in recent years as have budgets of the National Institutes of Health agencies, it is nevertheless a major funding agency in the area of health policy and health services research, especially for research that does not fit within the disease or age-specific emphases of some of the NIH institutes. That agency's greater emphasis in recent years on topics such as costs, quality, and patient safety have also been important, since topics of costs and patient safety has not been as related to sociological interest as have concerns about access to health care services. For example, a major effort of the agency in the late 1980s and early 1990s was a greater focus on health care outcomes, evidence-based practice, and the development of clinical guidelines and disease management protocols (Grimshaw and Russell 1993). These efforts have led to an increase in the numbers of clinicians and public health specialists working with the agency, but not sociologists. The specific applied nature of some of these areas and the integration of clinical concerns and education have not drawn upon the strengths of sociologists.

For sociologists, there are some concerns now as costs and quality have become more important concerns of the agency. Both the focus of the agency on cost and quality and the expansion of the study of the health care delivery system across the social sciences with a greater role for economists as well as researchers in schools of public health have been factors in the role of sociologists having diminished in this agency over time. Some of the efforts of the agency in funding basic data collection efforts in recent years have also, on the surface, reflected the concerns of cost and financing more heavily than the concerns of sociologists. Examples of data and survey efforts include MEPS, the Medical Expenditure Panel Survey, and HCUP, the Healthcare Cost and Utilization project, and these efforts do not lend themselves to the types of research questions of interest to sociologists as easily as to those of economists and researchers interested in health care financing questions. However, with some creativity in applying broader more policy-oriented terms to the topics of study, the areas that many sociologists are researching could fit within the policy concerns of AHRQ, as well as growing policy concerns of other federal research-based agencies also. In an era of diminished dollars for funding for research and greater pressure by universities for scholars to have funded research, sociologists need to stay involved with agencies such as AHRQ as a potential funding source because sociologists have important insights about access and quality that differ from other approaches.

In addition to federal agencies and health services research, there has been a growth of other professional associations that study these topics. The Association for Health Services Research has become Academy Health and is now one of the major professional associations that hold conferences on these topics. While there is a perception that Academy Health is dominated by health economists, and they are certainly very important in the organization, the current chair of the board is a medical sociologist. Again, medical sociologists may need to increase their involvement in some of these broader organizations as a way of increasing their credibility in the policy arena.

To increase the involvement of sociologists in these efforts in the future, sociologists also need to understand the policy making process in the USA, some of the issues of reforms and health policy, and some of the issues of access, cost, and health insurance, which are topics addressed in the next two sections.

The Policy Making Process in the USA and Incremental Reform

Policy analysts in the USA have argued for a number of years that change in US policy in many areas, and especially in areas of social and health policy, is characterized by a process of incremental reform. This argument states that the political process in the USA is not one of broad, bold movements but rather is characterized by policy changes occurring in small steps (increments). This approach argues that rarely in the USA does policy become modified in dramatic ways (Lindblom 1959; Wildavsky 1964). The presence of a chief executive (President) who may be from a different political party than the legislative branch and the presence of two different legislative branches, the Senate and the House of Representative, each of which can be controlled by a different political party, also contribute to making reform and passage of policy more difficult in the US political system than is true in a parliamentary system such as in Great Britain in which the executive is always a member of the political party in power.

The incremental model has been developed further by decision theorists. Within sociology, one of its best known applications to health care was developed by Alford (1975), who described three different approaches to reform: market reformers, bureaucratic reformers, and a structural interest type of reformer. The first two approaches each lead to incremental reform. One contrast between the two is that market reformers prefer an end to government interference in health care delivery and therefore are in favor of greater market competition, whereas bureaucratic reformers prefer increased administrative regulation of health care to deal with inequities in market competition. Both approaches are limited and represent a type of incremental reform. At some points over the past 40 years of reform in health and social policy in the USA, the market approach has been more typical of Republican policy and the bureaucratic reform approach more typical of Democratic policy, although parties in the USA do not represent pure ideological groups, and therefore reforms proposed do not fit so neatly into theoretical classifications. Alford (1975) argues that these two approaches are more readily accepted by Americans than the structural interest perspective, which does raise more fundamental questions about who benefits from current arrangements in health care and the social welfare system in the USA.

Analysts of health reform efforts in the USA have argued that an excellent example of the success of an "incremental" strategy for health care reform was the enactment of Medicare legislation in 1965 (the same year and debates that also produced the Medicaid legislation) and that this success can be traced back to President Harry Truman's failed campaign for national health insurance in 1948–1950 (Hacker and Skocpol 1997). Recently, Jacobs (2007) has pointed out that Medicare was actually an "accomplishment born of defeat" and understood by reformers at the time it passed as an approach to reform, not just one program but with the exception of expansion to those with chronic kidney disease and perhaps the recent drug benefits addition to Medicare, attempts to use Medicare as an approach and not just a specific program were not successful. The attempted passage of the Health Security Act by President Bill Clinton during 1993 and 1994 can be viewed, using Alford's terms, as a structural interest-type reform, which sought to enact comprehensive changes that would have simultaneously controlled medical costs and ensured universal coverage for health insurance (Hacker 1997; Steinmo and Watts 1995). Once Clinton won election to the Presidency in November, 1992, his administration started a discussion of health care reform with a goal of improving access to health care for all while containing costs. To accomplish this, a special task force was created. While the creation of such a task force could have been productive, most experts now agree that the task force became problematic, with the attempt at openness and discussion backfiring (Kronenfeld 1997; Blendon et al. 1995; Starr 1994). The public became confused, the initial momentum needed to push the reform was lost, and negative ads by some interest groups further lowered the chances of the reform plan passing (Johnson and Broder 1996). Some sociological analysts focus on budgetary and political exigencies as part of the reason for failure (Skocpol 1997), while others focus more on the impact of powerful stakeholders (Quadagno 2005). Skocpol (1997) argues that the political situation was a very important factor in the defeat of the Clinton health care plan, and that the large deficits inherited from the Reagan administration made the political situation more difficult. In addition, health reform became target for conservative political enemies, and they distorted the presentation of the plan and the image of the plan as viewed by the public. Quadagno argues that powerful stakeholders have defeated health care reform a number of times in US history, but that the specific stakeholders change over time. She particularly focuses on the impact of the Health Insurance Association of America and small businesses as organized groups that led the opposition to the Clinton plan.

The failure of the Clinton reform attempts led to a backing away from a more comprehensive reform agenda and a return to incremental changes, some of which (SCHIP – the State Child Health Insurance Program) were the largest increases in public financing of health care in the USA since Medicare/Medicaid. SCHIP has been successful in increasing the number of children with health insurance, but the program is part of a series of developments in health policy changes for children that are small, incremental steps (Kronenfeld 2006). The program did not deal with a major overhaul of either child health policy or overall health policy. Similarly, the passage of the Medicare Drug Benefit is another example of a small, incremental reform, a modification to Medicare that is an example of incremental change, rather than a well-thought out major change in the system. Policy experts have argued that drug costs for the elderly need to be covered, especially since prescription drug costs now represent the fastest growing segment of health care spending. The reform represented a compromise between Republicans and Democrats in Congress and was pushed so that each party could claim a political success in that year's Congressional elections. The enacted plan, however, is quite complicated, with a variety of different plans in each state and variation in costs of the plan depending upon the income of the elderly. In the initial sign-up period, many elderly were confused about options and upset about the complexity of choosing a plan, although most elderly are now enrolled in and using these benefits. The 2008 Presidential election has led to discussions about the need for reform in health care, and the election of the Democratic party's candidate, Obama, to the Presidency and the election of a majority Democratic Congress make it more likely that health care reform may again be a major discussion at the national level, although the economic and financial crises at the end of 2008 may limit the ability to address major health care reform initially.

Important Themes: Access, Cost, Health Insurance, and Quality

Within health services research in the past three decades, issues of access, cost, and quality of care have become major foci of attention. Access to health care is increasingly understood to be a function both of overall costs of health care and the availability of insurance to cover those costs. While most middle-class Americans has health insurance coverage, the rates of coverage for the population under 65 years of age has fluctuated around 16–18% between 1994 and 2004 (Centers for Disease Control 2006). Many people under age 65, particularly those with low incomes, do not have health insurance coverage consistently throughout the year. In 2004, about 20% of people under age 65 reported that they had been uninsured for at least part of the previous 12-month period (Centers for Disease Control 2006). As costs of care have increased, even people with middle-class incomes cannot afford health care unless they have health insurance coverage. The role of the federal (and state) governments in providing health insurance to selected groups (first the elderly with Medicare, then some of the poor with Medicaid, and most recently children of the working poor with SCHIP) has increased and so has the role of the federal government as a payer for health care services. If sociologists are to become more involved in the inclusion of their work and its implications within the health policy community, they need to have both a basic appreciation of these important themes and be convinced that publication of their work in more policy-oriented journals that are more likely to be read by policy groups, Congressional staff, and picked up by journalists and thus read as news stories by the general public is important and valued within the discipline. The rest of this section discusses access, cost, and health insurance and briefly reviews some issues of health care quality, to help medical sociologists improve their basic understanding of these issues.

Health Care Costs and Expenditures

National health care expenditures have grown at a rate substantially outpacing the gross national product for most of the years since 1940. Prior to World War II, only 4% of the nation's overall wealth each year was spent on health care. By 1960, this figure had increased only to 5.1% of the gross domestic product (GDP). Expressed in per capita terms, the growth in health expenditures appears much larger, partially because this was a period of rapid economic growth. Per capita expenses increased from 30 dollars per capita in 1940 to 143 in 1960 (Waldo et al. 1986; National Health Expenditures Tables 2001). These trends continued and accelerated in the next 30 years, as the percent of gross domestic product spent on health care increased to 8.8% in 1980 and 12% in 1990 (Waldo et al. 1986; National Health Expenditures Tables 2001; Levit et al. 1991).

Costs continued to increase from 1990 to 1993. Since 1993, national health expenditures as a percentage of GDP remained relatively stable through 1999, ranging from 13.4 or 13.3%t in 1993, 1994, 1996, and 1998, with a small decrease to 13.0% in 1998 and 1999 (National Health Expenditures Tables 2001; Cowan et al. 2001). One explanation for the small decrease in the percentage of GDP spent on health care in the late 1990s is the large increase in the GDP during that time period, a period of expansive economic growth. Other factors that helped to stabilize costs in that time period were one-time effects of managed care and some impact of federal legislation, such as the Balanced Budget Act of 1997 which limited growth in some of the government health spending programs. Per capita health expenditures have continued to increase in the decade of the 1990s, going from 2,738 dollars a person figure in 1990 to 4,402 in 1999 (National Health Expenditures Tables 2001; Cowan et al. 2001; National Health Expenditures Aggregate Per Capita Amount 2004).

After 6 years of slower growth, estimates are that total national health care expenditures are now increasing as much as 7–10% from 2000 to 2002 (Gardner 2001). For the fourth consecutive year, health spending grew faster than the overall GDP, reversing the trends of the late to middle 1990s.

By 2004, the health care share of GDP increased to 16% and per capita expenditures were up to 6,280 dollars a person (National Health Expenditures Aggregate Per Capita Amount 2004; CMMS data 2006). The USA generally is the highest on these figures in the world, and one of the issues raised by health researchers and sociologists is whether the USA ends up receiving good value for those expenditures, since the USA is at the top of spending but not at the top of comparisons across countries on health outcome measures (Budrys 2001; Kronenfeld 2002). Long-term projections of rising costs, especially in terms of per capita expenses, are of even greater concern. As the large baby boom population begins to age, the pressures of care for that large group will help create increased costs, probably overall and most definitely on a per capita basis since the proportion of the population in the age groups that tend to be high users of health care will grow. It is important to incorporate changing population and demographic trends, such as the aging of the baby boomers, into analyses and projections of health care costs in the future, and this is one way that sociologists can contribute to research that is dominated by health economists.

Another way to understand health care expenditures in the USA as a backdrop to exploring issues of health insurance is to understand where the nation's health care dollars come from (the sources of funds) and where the dollars went (types of expenditures). While in 1960, only 24 cents out of every health dollar came from government programs, by 2004, government programs of all types covered 46 cents out of every health care dollar. About 17 cents is being spent for Medicare, 16 cents for Medicaid and SCHIP, and 13 cents for all other public programs such as worker's compensation, public health activities, and health programs sponsored by the Department of Defense for active duty military personnel, the Veteran's Administration, and the Indian Health Service. The next largest source of the health care dollars by 2004 was private health insurance, accounting for 35 cents of every health care dollar, an increase from 22 cents in 1960. Far and away, the largest source of the health care dollars in 1960 was out-of-pocket payments (i.e, costs not reimbursed to the consumer). This category was 49 cents, or almost half of all the health care dollar in 1960 but was only 13 cents by 2004 (Levit et al. 1991; Office of National Cost Estimates 1990; Cowan et al. 2001, 2004). Understanding these broad trends in where funds in health care come from and the increasing role of the federal government can help sociologists consider the importance of incorporation of these factors into studies of health care, whether focused on utilization of individuals or studies about changes in health care professions and professional autonomy.

A comparison of where the health care dollar actually went in 1960 and 2004 reveals much greater similarities over the roughly 40-year period. Hospital care was the largest single category of expense at both points in time and took up 34 cents of the health care dollar in 1960 and 30 in 2004, reflecting a small decline in the importance of expenditures in hospitals, with the growth of outpatient care. The next largest category in 2004 is the catch-all category of other spending (25 cents), which covered such services as dental, other professional services, home health, and durable medical products and over-the-counter medicines for 20 cents. In earlier years, the categories were not identical, but the category of personal health care services was the second largest in 1960 (31 cents) and included dental, home health care, drugs, and other non-durable products. The third largest category is physician and clinical services, now 21 cents out of every health care dollar. This category has been increasing over the last ten or so years. Nursing home care is one category that doubled over the 30 years from 1960 to 1990, taking only 4 cents of the health care dollar in 1960, 8 cents in 1990, and then beginning to drop to 7 cents in 2002 and 6 cents in 2004, the reduction being due to the growth in home health-based services (Levit et al. 1991; Office of National Cost Estimates 1990; Cowan et al. 2001, 2004). The importance of prescription drugs is indicated by its being given a separate category in the 1990s, accounting for 8 cents of the national health dollar in 1999 and 10 cents of the national health dollar in 2004. Understanding these broad trends in where expenditures in health care are going will help sociologists interested in policy-relevant research to consider more studies looking at issues such as long-term care and prescription drugs, both areas with limited research in medical sociology at this point.

Access to Healthcare and Healthcare Insurance

Because the costs of health care are increasing, the costs of health insurance are increasing and more Americans are either losing coverage at their workplace or paying much higher costs for health care insurance. In 2000, about 40 million Americans did not have health insurance, a figure that increased to 45 million by 2004 and to 46.6 million people in 2005 or about 18% of the population under 65 (almost all people 65 and over have coverage through the Medicare program). As a percentage of the overall population, the percentage without health insurance increased slightly from 2004 to 2005, from 15.6 to 15.9% (US Census Bureau 2006; Denavas-Valt et al. 2006). The percentage of people with employment-based health insurance continues to decline a bit each year, and it was 59.5% in 2005. Ethnicity plays an important role in variation in health insurance coverage, with one-third of Hispanics and one quarter of Native Americans uncovered. About 21% of African Americans are uncovered versus only 11% of white Americans (Denavas-Valt et al. 2006; Holohan and Cook 2006). Rates of coverage also vary by state, partially because Medicaid (the program that covers some of the poor) is more generous in some states than in other states. People in the south and southwest are twice as likely to be uninsured as those in better-covered regions such as the Upper Midwest.

One of the reasons nationally behind these trends of increased rates of uninsurance is the rising cost of health insurance and the premiums that most working Americans pay for such insurance. Costs of health insurance have started to have double digit increases since 1999 in some parts of the USA During the economic expansion of the late 1990s, many employers absorbed health insurance cost increases. As the economic downturn began in late 2001, many employers passed along such price increases, which ranged from 12 to 14% in large companies and 18–20% for small businesses.

Results from the 2004 Annual Employer Health Benefits Survey and the 2006 data help to demonstrate some of the current concerns in health care insurance coverage and rising costs both to employees and employers (Gabel et al. 2004; Clemens-Cope et al. 2006). Employee-sponsored health insurance premiums have been continuing to increase, although the rate of increase has moderated over the last three years. In 2004, premiums increased an average of 11.2. The rate of increase was 9.2% in 2005 and 7.7% from 2005 to 2006. Thus, there is some improvement in the rate of increase each of the last 3 years, but there remains a continued sign of problems with rising health insurance rates. While the rate of increase is down from the double digit rates of increase from 2000 to 2004, this has been a period of low overall inflation in the US economy (Gabel et al. 2004). Premiums have continued to increase much faster than overall inflation (3.5 %) and wage gains (3.8 %) (Clemens-Cope et al. 2006). Another way to view this trend is that from 2001 to 2004, health insurance premiums have increased 59%, employee contributions have increased 57% for single coverage and 49% for family coverage, and the percentage of workers covered by their own employer's health insurance plan has decreased from 69% in 2000 to 61% in 2006.

One trend is that the employer providing all the costs of health insurance as a benefit to employees is decreasing. For the insured worker, the percentage of plans where the employer covers 100% of the premium has been falling from 34% in 2001 to 23% in 2006. For family coverage, the percentage of plans where the employer paid for all the coverage decreased from fourteen to 9%. While these figures indicate that employees are paying more, it is important to understand just how much of a benefit the provision of health insurance is to employed people. In 2004, employees paid an average 16% of the cost of single coverage and 28% of the cost of family coverage (Gabel et al. 2004).

These facts and figures help to demonstrate the growing issues about the availability of health care insurance and the access to health care services that health insurance allows that are important issues for everyone in the USA. These issues lead to calls for reform in the health care delivery system. One important fact about health insurance in the USA in the most recent decades is that the uninsured are not only low-income people who work for small employers or in temporary jobs or the temporarily unemployed. While among all people under 65 without health insurance, the majority (about 70%) have lower income, the number of uninsured has been growing over the past 25 years, and the likelihood that a middle-class person will be uninsured has been increasing. Now, about one in ten working age adults from 23 to 64 years old with an annual income above the median household income in the USA are uninsured, while only 6% fitting this income definition were uninsured in 1979 (Swartz 2006).

Why are more middle-income people now without health insurance and why are more workers of all incomes uninsured? Swartz (2006) argues that there are three main factors. The first is significant shifts in employment; the second is rising costs of medical care; and the third is insurer avoidance of people likely to have high health expenses. There have been three important shifts in employment in the past 25 years. Manufactoring employment has continued to decline, and there has been major loss of unionized blue collar jobs that tended to provide good health insurance benefits. As late as the early 1980s, 22% of all workers were in manufacturing jobs. Now it is only 11%. This decline in manufacturing jobs has led to the second employment shift, the rising share of workers employed in small firms. Around 50% of firms with three to nine employees offer health insurance versus 99% of large companies with 200 or more employers. The third shift in employment is the growing use of self-employed workers. This change is less straightforward, because some of these self-employed people "appear" to work in companies. They go to offices and work with groups of people. Many companies now hire workers as independent contractors to avoid the costs of benefits and to avoid state laws that provide employment protection to workers. The third major factor as to why more middle-income people are now uninsured is insurer avoidance of people likely to have high expenses. This issue becomes especially important as people are not in large work groups or at a job with health insurance, because a person with a serious health problem will have a very difficult (and expensive) time trying to buy a private health insurance policy.

Quality of Care

Quality of care is inextricably intertwined with societal, professional, and patient expectations concerning the role of health care in the society. Over the last 20 years, there have been several critical periods of more detailed attention to what quality means and how to define it. In 1990, the Institute of Medicine defined quality as "the degree to which health services for individuals and populations increase the likelihood of desired health outcomes and are consistent with current professional knowledge" (Lohr and Schroeder 1990). Major concerns about quality of health care are not new. In the first six months of 1988, four different public agencies released reports about issues in quality of health care (Belcher and Chassin 2001). This initial concern led to research on the effectiveness of health care services and the development of practice guidelines to assist providers in improving quality, efforts in which sociologists were not very much involved.

In the past decade, several major new reports have been issued relating to quality of care concerns. A number of recent articles have tried to summarize the new quality concerns in the USA, incorporating especially the critiques of the Institute of Medicine (2001) report that argued that physicians, nurses, and other health professionals are doing their best to provide good-quality care but that the current system does not reward innovation and communication. The 1999 report *To Err Is Human* (Institute of Medicine 1999) found that more people die each year from medical mistakes than from highway accidents, breast cancer, and AIDS. This report created enormous concern among the public and controversy among US physicians and physician organizations, many arguing that the public was becoming unnecessarily panicked about such problems. The more recent report has been received more favorably from within the medical profession and is raising among experts a number of questions about how to best think about quality issues.

One way to think about quality issues is that patients may suffer harm from three different types of quality problems (Belcher and Chassin 2001). The first type of harm is if patients do not receive beneficial health services. The second is when patients undergo treatments or procedures from which they do not benefit. The third situation is when patients do receive appropriate medical services but the services are provided inappropriately. A simple way to summarize these three types of problems is as underuse, overuse, and misuse. Health services research literature demonstrates that, on average, half of Americans do not receive recommended preventive care, 30% do not receive recommended care for acute conditions, and 40% for chronic conditions. Similarly high rates of overuse have been demonstrated, about 30% for acute conditions and 40% for chronic (Schuster et al. 1998). These types of studies are important places for connection between more traditional work in medical sociology and quality, much of which has focused on quality of life concerns, rather than on quality of care concerns (Lerner and Schwartz 2000) and health policy concerns. Within medicine, these efforts and the 2001 IOM report have led to calls for greater teamwork among health professionals, greater use of information technology and evidence-based medical practice. Quality concerns are not new to the health policy arena nor are issues of access, health insurance coverage, and cost. Issues of quality, cost, and access are intertwined and will continue to receive attention as among the most important issues facing the health care system of the US.

Health Policy, Health Reform, and Medical Sociology

Health Disparities and Sociological Interests

The time for again increasing the role for medical sociologists in health policy may be approaching. One of the major policy initiatives in the past decade has been concerns about health disparities and health inequalities. In 2000, Congress established the National Center on Minority Health and Health Disparities (NCHMD) (NCHMD 2007) and a strategic plan and budget to eliminate health disparities (National Institutes of Health 2002). Reports on this topic have been published by the federal government in more recent years also (Agency for Healthcare Research and Quality 2005). Now, major foundations in health also have efforts in addressing inequalities in health, such as the Robert Wood Johnson Foundation and the Kaiser Family Foundation, both foundations that are important sources of funding for sociological researchers. As an outgrowth of these federal efforts, a number of recent research articles have dealt with these topics, some with sociologists as authors and many others written by physicians and other researchers (Basky 2000; Dunlap et al. 2002; Hargraves and Hadley 2003; Rosenbaum 2003; Bloche 2004; Gamble and Stone 2006; Read and Emerson 2005). Many of these articles deal with racial/ethnic disparities but add in issues of gender (Dunlap et al. 2002), insurance coverage (Hargraves and Hadley 2003), and immigration (Read and Emerson 2005).

Several recent articles have discussed ways to advance health disparities research by having broader conceptual frameworks. Kilbourne et al. (2006), writing from a public health perspective, argue for a need to focus more on determinants that underlie disparities and use that knowledge to apply to interventions to address disparities. Dealing with determinants and more complex understandings of factors that link to health disparities draws on the strengths of medical sociology, but medical sociologists must be willing to engage the issues in these terms. Malat (2006), in a medical sociology journal, deals explicitly with ways to incorporate ideas from sociology into expanded research on racial disparities. She argues that medical sociologists need to use the disciplinary tradition of studying inequalities to broaden the study of racial disparities in medical treatment. She believes that incorporation of concepts such as cultural capital, social networks, and social distance can all be ways that medical sociology contributes to this discussion within the health sciences and the policy community. Scambler (2007), in a journal focused on social theory and health, argues that the concept of social structure, which has been an important part of classical sociology, has been neglected in contemporary sociological studies of health inequalities. This neglect is also true in public health research looking at health inequalities and could be another important way that medical sociology can bring more explicit sociological concepts into the study of health inequalities. The long tradition in medical sociological research of concerns about access and use of care needs to continue, and sociologists need to incorporate the health inequalities framework that is now so important in the health care field into their own discussions of these types of work.

Public Opinion Research

Another area of research in which sociologists have been leaders in the past has been public opinion research, drawing upon the long tradition in sociology of survey research in general as well as survey research applied to studies of physical and mental health, health services utilization, and health care issues (Anderson 1966, Andersen and Newman 1973; Andersen et al. 1982; Kronenfeld 1978; Wolinsky 1978; House 1981; Pescosolido et al. 2001). There are now some well-established studies of public opinion and the health care system. These studies of public opinion have shown for more than two decades that Americans are dissatisfied with the current health care system. More detailed examinations of public opinion reveal more conflicting opinions. On Election Day, 2004, voters ranked health care as the fifth most important issue, and those who voted for President Bush ranked it as sixth (Blendon et al. 2006a). When asked about five major different systems in the USA, people rated the health care system lowest, behind the tax system, Social security, and the legal and educational systems (Pew Research Center For the People and the Press Poll 2005). When looking at a survey question that has been asked since 1982 about satisfaction with the health care system, Americans in 2006 were more dissatisfied than in 1987 but less dissatisfied than in 1991 (Blendon et al. 2006a). In a different study looking at views about health care for children and the elderly, Americans felt that the needs of both groups are not being met and there was widespread support for a government role in ensuring adequate health care when placed in the contexts of these specific groups (Berk et al. 2004). About 59% of adults did not believe that the health care needs of children were being addressed, and 67% did not believe that the health care needs of the elderly were being met.

In a democracy, at some point, public opinion and public attitudes should result in public policy changes, but the movement from public concern about an issue to new legislation is not simple, sure, or fast. Another place to bring some sociological content into this topic is for medical sociologists to integrate material by sociologists that has pointed out that studies may overestimate the effect of public opinion on issues because some past studies have focused on issues on which governments are most likely to be responsive (Burstein 2006). In looking at a random sample of proposals addressed by the US Congress, Burstein (2006) found that public opinion had considerably less impact in the random sample. Moreover, on many issues, the public may have conflicting or weak opinions, making it easier for organized interests to override public opinion sentiments (Burstein 2003). Some more recent public opinion data indicate that this is often true about public opinion and health care. Blendon and colleagues (2006b) reported that health care is an important, but second-tier issue for most Americans when asked to rank issues in terms of government priorities. The top health care concerns of Americans are linked to economic insecurity and focus on rising costs of health care and problems of the uninsured. The public does continue to favor more rather than less health care spending in the aggregate, and these attitudes may create an atmosphere that will be supportive of change in health care in the future. The inclusion of more critical sociological approaches that link public opinion research and policy making may be one way that medical sociologists can add a different approach to studies of public opinion research and health care, a research area that has been dominated in the last decade by public health researchers. Sociologists need to increase their involvement in these types of studies and provide a more nuanced, complex, and sociological vision to help to explain the meaning of variation in public opinions about issues linked to health and health care services.

Politics, Sociology, and Policy Concerns

Many political experts do believe that the issue of health care reform has again emerged on the public agenda as part of the 2008 Presidential election. Important public commentators such as David Brodie writing in newspapers such as the Washington Post have argued that there is a swelling momentum for health reform (Hiebert-White 2007). Both Obama as a Democratic candidate and McCain as a Republican candidate addressed health care changes, with quite different solutions. With the election of Obama and Democratic majorities in both houses of Congress, the possibility of major health reform at the national level is more likely, although the economic crises of the financial and banking industries, the decline of the stock market, and the growing recognition that both the US economy and many economies in other countries are entering a recession may limit the initial proposals for health care reform. While it is difficult to predict at this point what types of reform might eventually become enacted, especially because the financial and banking problems that emerged in the last 2 months of the campaign meant that economic issues became the major focus of discussion, it is important that medical sociologists remain involved in health policy issues and become involved in public statements about these issues. In the last few years, there has been great discussion within the American Sociological Association about the need for public sociology and for sociologists to take a public role in policy debates (Clawson et al. 2007). At the 2004 American Sociological Association meeting, Burawoy speaking as the President of the Association, called for more "Public Sociology" and a need for sociologists to speak beyond the university and engage with social movements and efforts for social reform. Certainly, it is important for medical sociologists to do this in public discussions of health care reform, and while some sociologists such as Paul Starr and Theda Skocpol were involved in the failed health care reform effort in the first Clinton administration, hopefully more will become engaged in future public debates and reform efforts, especially since the support for involvement of sociologists in the public arena has been receiving more disciplinary attention in the last few years.

Medical sociologists have written books and articles recently focused on the topic of overall reform of the health care system and why the US has no national health care system, although these topics are not generally a major topic in most of the medical sociology journals. Mechanic (2004), in an exploration of the rise and fall of managed care from a sociological perspective, has provided both a sociological perspective on that issue and also a critique concerning the relative absence of research on this topic by medical sociologists. He argues that one of the most important explanations for the rise and fall of managed care is the middle class's rejection of explicit rationing at the point of service. He links this to an underlying fault in the US health care system, the failure to introduce a rational system of universal health care. He does point out, however, that with some notable exceptions, sociologists have not been that important in research on managed care or research on the transformation of health care. This is not a new theme for Mechanic, since in a 1993 article he also pointed out that at that point in time sociologists had receded in importance in research on health care delivery and allowed health economists, health administrators, and health services researchers to dominate (Mechanic 1993). In his 2004 article, he points out that political science and law are now fields in which there is more research on health care delivery. He analyzes a special issue of the *Journal of Health Politics, Policy and Law* as an illustration of that critique. Twelve of the contributors were from political science, 15 from economics, 7 from business and management, 5 from law, and 10 from a variety of other fields including one sociologist (Mechanic 2004).

Other examples of recent important books and articles by medical sociologists that have provided a sociological framework to major policy questions such as why the USA has no national health insurance are those by Quadagno (2004, 2005). She proposed a theory of stakeholder mobilization as the primary obstacle to national health insurance and has published parts of this analysis in major journals such as the *Journal of Health and Social Behavior* and, following that, in a more detailed book. Other sociological researchers have looked at some issues related to health services research and health policy, such as Caronna (2004) who used an institutional perspective to analyze both the history and current state of health care in the USA through a consideration of the alignment of normative, cognitive, and regulatory issues. Other sociological researchers have used survey data to examine issues of the extent to which health insurance coverage and the source of that coverage impact adult health (Quesnel-Vallee 2004). Although some earlier studies (Hahn and Flood 1995; Ross and Mirowsky 2000) found an inverse association between public insurance and health status, Quesnel-Vallee (2004) does not find that to be true and finds that it is the uninsured who suffer from the least access to health care services and that the lack of health insurance coverage has a strong negative impact on adult health. Mechanic (2005) has also recently published a book that he describes as a broader, less academic treatment of the issue of how to improve health care and problems of the uninsured in the USA. While continuing to address issues of rationing and American approaches to that topic, he also has specific chapters on narrower health care concerns, such as chapters on diseases in general, mental health, long-term care, and quality concerns.

In general, sociologists need to apply some of their unique areas of expertise to matters of public policy and public concern. Some of the same issues that have been pointed out as reasons why medical sociology has not been as involved as one might expect in issues of bioethics may also apply to medical sociology and policy approaches or at least may help us to broaden our thinking and scholarly writing to include interpretations that link to public policy. Conrad (1994) discusses the fundamentally different worldviews that he believes have limited the interaction between sociological researchers and bioethics researchers. Philosophers concerned with ethical actions focus on what ought to be, while sociologists focus on what is. This is also true at times about policy research as conducted in public health and health services research. The goals of greater equity, holding down cost increases, and improving quality are clear in policy research. Medical sociologists view themselves as critical researchers, questioning the validity of data, analytical approaches, and goals of research. Public policy personnel need to read critical approaches, and this is one important contribution of medical sociologists. There are some recent examples, however, of medical sociologists conducting research on many topics that have important policy applications and often drawing out the implications of that work for broader policy concerns. One area discussed at the beginning of this chapter was the issue of health care inequalities and social class and racial/ethnic variations in health and health care. This is a topic that has long been a central concern within medical sociology. In recent years, sociologists have been addressing some of these concerns in new ways related to increased rates of immigration and changing patterns of immigration in the USA. The expertise of sociologists on immigration and the complexities which that topic added to a discussion of health care inequalities need to be included in public and public health discussions, and there are a few recent examples of that type of work (Lopez-Gonzalez et al. 2005). This recent article examines the complexity of issues of immigrant acculturation and health behaviors such as smoking and alcohol use and points out how the acculturation process may be different for men and women. Some of these complexities as linked to health care have not yet reached the level of public policy and debate, but sociologists are in a good position to help improve the quality of these discussions and the data brought to bear on the consideration of these issues. Often, the research from a public health perspective focuses on levels of coverage of health insurance and variations in rates of coverage. Research in prevention and substance abuse has pointed out how immigrant cultures may be protective of the adoption of negative health habits, at least initially, and that the composition of neighborhoods and schools as related to race/ethnicity and immigration may also make a difference in how adolescents learn to resist negative health habits (Kulis et al. 2004, 2007a, b). Research on use of complementary and alternative health care has pointed out that immigrants may continue to use CAM approaches that were common in their countries of origin, and that only in later generations do patterns become more similar to other groups in the society (Ayers and Kronenfeld 2007).

Sociologists need to make this research accessible in more public forums and as part of expanded policy discussions. Some medical sociologists have conducted research that links to health behavior issues in the past, and some are now beginning to do this with some of the newer concerns of obesity, diet, and immunization (Kim et al. 2007). In addition to studies that look at the health care delivery system and broader issues, another important way that sociologists can contribute to health policy discussions is through empirical work that addresses the complex interplay of social structural factors, health behaviors, and the health care delivery system. If major health care reform is passed, there will be important lines of research developed to examine the impact of those reforms on access to care and utilization of health care services, and these would be areas of study in which medical sociologists have a rich past tradition and in which it would be good for sociologists to be in the forefront of these types of studies if major reforms are passed.

In a recent article discussing US health system performance and providing a national scorecard for health care reform, Schoen and her coauthors (2006) argue that the overall picture is one of missed opportunities in health care reform with room for improvement in the US health care system. The indicators focus on the USA lagging behind other countries on indicators of mortality and healthy life despite high expenditures. They also point out the substantial spread between top and bottom groups of states, health plans, and hospitals in these indicators. They argue that there is a need to improve access, quality, and efficiency of care in the USA and that the USA needs better data and better research to understand how to improve these aspects of health and health care in the USA. Many of these topics are those that sociological researchers can help explore or have explored some in the past. This article helps to provide background in broader policy issues that sociologists can pursue. In the future, medical sociologists may incorporate more policy-relevant factors into their more focused research on health and the health care system, so that medical sociology will also be a part of public sociology and public policy debates about health care changes, health care reform, and the impact of health care reform (if passed) in the twenty-first century.

References

Aday L, Andersen R, Fleming G (1980) Health care in the U.S.: equitable for whom? Sage, Beverly Hills, CA

AHCPR (Agency for Healthcare Research and Quality) (2005) National Healthcare Disparities Report. http://www.ahrq.gov/qual/nhdr05/nhdr05.htm

Alford RR (1975) Health care politics: ideological and interest group barriers to reform. University of Chicago Press, Chicago, IL

Andersen R, Fleming GV, Champney TF (1982) Exploring a paradox: belief in a crisis and general satisfaction with medical care. Milbank Mem Fund Q 60(2):329–354

Andersen R, Newman J (1973) Social and individual determinants of medical care utilization in the United States. Milbank Mem Fund Q Health Soc 51(1):95–124

Anderson O (1966) Health services research – Influence of social and economic research on public policy in the health field. Milbank Mem Fund Q XLIV(3, Part 2, July):11–54

Ayers S, Kronenfeld JJ (2007) Does philosophical congruence theory explain racial and ethnic differences in use of CAM? American Sociological Association Annual Meeting (New York)

Basky G (2000) Socioeconomic status at the heart of health inequality. Can Med Assoc J 162:253a

Belcher EC, Chassin MR (2001) Improving the quality of health care: who will lead? Health Aff 20:164–179

Berk ML, Schur CL, Chang DL, Knight EK, Kleinman LC (2004) Americans' view about the adequacy of health care for children and the elderly. Health Aff (September):w336–w454

Bird CE, Conrad P, Fremont AM (eds) (2000) Handbook of medical sociology, 5th edn. Prentice-Hall, Upper Saddle River, NJ

Blendon RJ, Brodie M, Benson J (1995) What happened to Americans' support for the Clinton health plan? Health Aff 14:7–23

Blendon RJ, Brodie M, Benson JM, Altman DE, Buhr T (2006a) Americans' view of health care costs, access and quality. Milbank Q 84:623–657

Blendon RJ, Hunt K, Benson JM, Fleischfresser C, Buhr T (2006b) Understanding the American public's health priorities: a 2006 perspective. Health Aff (July–November):w508–w530

Bloche MG (2004) Health care disparities – science, politics, and race. N Engl J Med 2004:1568–1570

Bloom S (1986) Institutional trends in medical sociology. J Health Soc Behav 27:265–276

Bloom SW (2002) Word as scalpel: a history of medical sociology. Oxford University Press, New York

Budrys G (2001) Our unsystematic health care system. Rowman and Littlefield, Lanham, Md

Burstein P (2006) Why estimates of the impact of public opinion on public policy are too high. Soc Forces 84:2273–2290

Burstein P (2003) The impact of public opinion on public policy: a review and an agenda. Polit Res Q 56:29–40

Caronna CA (2004) The misalignment of institutional "pillars": consequences for the US health care field. J Health Soc Behav 45(Extra Issue):45–58

Centers for Disease Control, Department of Health and Human Services (2006) Health US, 2006 with chartbook on trends in the health of Americans. www.cdc.gov/nchs/data/hus/hus06.pdf#tocfigures

Center for Medicare and Medicaid Statistics (2006)

Clawson D, Zussman R, Misra J, Gerstell N, Stokes R, Anderton D, Burawoy M (2007) Public sociology: fifteen eminent sociologists debate politics and the profession in the twenty-first century. University of California Press, Berkeley, CA

Clemens-Cope L, Garrett B, Hoffman C (2006) Changes in employees' health insurance coverage, 2001–2005. Kaiser Commission on Medicaid and the Uninsured, Issue Paper. ww.hff.org/uninsured/upload/7570.pdf

Conrad P (1994) How ethnography can help bioethics. Bul Med Ethics 98:13–18

Cowan CA, Lazenby HC, Martin AB, McDonnell PA, Sensenig AL, Smith CE, Whittle LS, Zezza MA, Donham CS, Long AM, Stewart MW (2001) National health care expenditures, 1999. Health Care Financ Rev 22:77–110

Cowan C, Catlin A, Smith C, Sensenig A (2004) National health expenditures, 2002. Health Care Financ Rev 25:143–166

Denavas-Valt C, Proctor BD, Lee CH (2006) Income, poverty and health insurance coverage in the United States, 2005. Current Population Reports. U.S. Census Bureau, P60-231, www.census.gov/prod/2006pubs/p60.231.pdf

Dunlap DD, Manheim LM, Song J, Chang RW (2002) Gender and ethnic/racial disparities in health care utilization among older adults. J Gerontol Soc Sci 57B:s221–s233

Ebert-Flateau P, Perkoff GT (1983) The HSR force in the US. Med Care XXI:253–265

Freeman H, Levine S, Reeder LG (eds) (1963) Handbook of medical sociology. Prentice Hall, Englewood Cliffs, NJ

Freeman H, Levine S, Reeder LG (eds) (1972) Handbook of medical sociology, 2nd edn. Prentice Hall, Englewood Cliffs, NJ

Freeman H, Levine S, Reeder LG (eds) (1979) Handbook of medical sociology, 3rd edn. Prentice Hall, Englewood Cliffs, NJ

Freeman HE, Levine S (eds) (1989) Handbook of medical sociology, 4th edn. Prentice Hall, Englewood Cliffs, NJ

Gabel J, Claxton G, Gil I, Pickreign J, Whitmore H, Holve E, Finder B, Hawkins S, Rowland D (2004) Health benefits in 2004: four years of double-digit premium increases takes their toll on coverage. Health Aff 23(5):200–209

Gardner J (2001) The 800 pound gorilla returns. Mod HealthC 12:5–15

Gamble VN, Stone D (2006) U.S. policy on health inequities: the interplay of politics and research. J Health Polit Policy Law 31:93–126

Gray BH, O'Leary J (2000) The evolving relationship between medical sociology and health policy. In: Bird CE, Conrad P, Fremont AM (eds) Handbook of medical socioloy, 5th edn. Prentice-Hall, Upper Saddle River, NJ, pp 258–270

Gray BH, Phillips SR (1995) Medical sociology and health policy where are the connections? J Health Soc Behav 45(Extra Issue):170–181

Grimshaw JT, Russell IT (1993) Effect of clinical guidelines on medical practice: a systematic review of rigorous evaluations. Lancet 342(8883):1317–1322

Hacker JS (1997) The road to nowhere: the genesis of President Clinton's plan for health security. Princeton University Press, Princeton, NJ

Hacker JS, Skocpol T (1997) The new politics of U.S. health policy. J Health Polit Policy Law 22:315–338

Hahn BA, Flood AB (1995) No insurance public insurance, and private insurance – do these options contribute to differences in general health? J Health Care Poor Underserved 69:41–59

Hargraves JL, Hadley J (2003) The contribution of insurance coverage and community resources to reducing racial/ethnic disparities in access to care. Health Serv Res 38:809–829

Hiebert-White J (2007) Health reform and the political agenda. Health Aff Blog February 5. http:/healthaffairs.org/blog/2007/02/06health-reform-and-the-political-agenda

Holohan J, Cook A (2006) Why did the number of uninsured continue to increase in 2005? Kaiser Commission on Medicaid and the Uninsured. Issue Paper. www.kff.org/uninsured/upload/7571.pdf

House JS (1981) Work, stress and social support. Addison-Wesley, Reading, MA

Institute of Medicine (2001) Crossing the quality chasm: a new health system for the 21st century. National Academy of Sciences, Washington, DC

Institute of Medicine (1999) To err is human. National Academy of Sciences, Washington, DC

Jacobs LW (2007) The Medicare approach: political choice and American institutions. J Health Polit Policy Law 32:159–186

Johnson H, Broder DS (1996) The system: the American way of politics at the breaking point. Little, Brown and Company, Boston, MA

Kilbourne AM, Switzer G, Hyman K, Crowley-Matoka M, Fine MJ (2006) Advancing health disparities research within the health care system: a conceptual framework. Am J Public Health 96:2113–2121

Kim SS, Frimpong JA, Rivers PA, Kronenfeld JJ (2007) The effects of maternal and provider characteristics on up to date immunization status of children aged 19–35 Months. Am J Public Health 97:259–266

Kronenfeld JJ (1997) The changing federal role in US healthcare policy. Praeger, Westport CT

Kronenfeld JJ (2006) Expansion of publicly funded health insurance in the United States: the children's health insurance program and its implications. Lexington Press, Lanham, Md

Kronenfeld JJ (2002) Health care policy: issues and trends. Praeger, Westport, CT

Kronenfeld JJ (1978) Provider variables and utilization of ambulatory care services. J Health Soc Behav 19:68–76

Kulis S, Yabiku ST, Marsiglia FF, Nieri T, Crossman A (2007a) Differences by gender, ethnicity, and acculturation in the efficacy of the keepin' it REAL model prevention program. J Drug Educ 37(2):123–144

Kulis SK, Marsiglia FF, Nieri T, Sicotte D, Hohmann-Marriott B (2004) Majority rules?: the effects of school ethnic composition on substance use by Mexican heritage adolescents. Sociol Focus 37(4):373–393

Kulis S, Marsiglia FF, Sicotte DM, Nieri T (2007b) Neighborhood effects on youth substance use in a southwestern city. Sociol Perspect 50(2):273–301

Lerner D, Schwartz CE (2000) Quality of life in health, illness and medical care. In: Conrad P, Fremont AM, Bird CE (eds) Handbook of medical sociology, 5th edn. Prentice-Hall, Upper Saddle River, NJ, pp 298–308

Levine S (1987) The changing terrains in medical sociology: emergent concerns with quality of life. J Health Soc Behav 28:1–6

Levit KR, Lazenby HC, Cowan CA, Letsch SW (1991) National health care expenditures, 1990. Health Care Financ Rev 13:29–54

Lindblom CE (1959) The science of muddling through. Pub Adm Rev 14:79–88

Lohr KN, Schroeder SA (1990) A strategy for quality assurance in Medicare. N Engl J Med 322:707–712

Lopez-Gonzalez L, Aravena VC, Hummer RA (2005) Immigrant acculturation, gender, and health behavior: a research note. Soc Forces 84:581–593

Malat J (2006) Expanding research on the racial disparity in medical treatment with ideas from sociology. Health 10:303–321

Mechanic D (1993) Social research in health and the american sociopolitical context: the changing fortunes of medical sociology. Soc Sci Med 36:95–102

Mechanic D (2004) The rise and fall of managed care. J Health Soc Behav 45(Extra Issue):76–86

Mechanic D (2005) The truth about health care: why reform is not working in America. Rutgers University Press, New Brunswick, NJ

National Health Expenditures Aggregate Per Capita Amount (2004) http://www.cms.hhs.gov/statistics/hhe/historical/tables.pdf

National Health Expenditures Tables (2001) http://www.hcfa.gov/stats/nhe-oact/tables

NCHMD (National Center on Minority Health and Health Disparities) (2007)

NIH (National Institutes of Health) (2002) Strategic plan and budget for eliminating healthcare disparities. http://ncmhd.nih.gov/our_programs/strategic/pubs/VolumeI_031003EDrev.pdf

Office of National Cost Estimates (1990) National health expenditures, 1988. Heath Care Financ Rev 11:1–54

Pescosolido BA, McLeod JD, Alegria M (2000) Confronting the second social contract: the place of medical sociology in research and policy for the twenty-first century. In: Bird CE, Conrad P, Fremont AM (eds) Handbook of medical sociology, 5th edn. Prentice-Hall, Upper Saddle River, NJ, pp 311–426

Pescosolido BA, Tuch S, Martin J (2001) The profession of medicine and the public. J Health Soc Behav 42:1–16

Pew Research Center For The People and the Press Poll (2005) Storrs, Ct: Roper Center for Public Opinion Research, January 5–9

Raymond AG (2007) The 2006 Massachusetts health care reform law: progress and challenges after one year of implementation. http://masshealthpolicyforum.brandeis.edu/publications/pdfs/31- May07/MassHealthCareReformProgess%20Report.pdf

Quadagno J (2005) One nation uninsured: why the U.S. has no national health insurance. Oxford University Press, New York

Quadagno J (2004) Why the United States has no national health insurance: stakeholder mobilization against the welfare state, 1945–1996. J Health Soc Behav 45(Extra Issue):25–44

Quesnel-Vallee A (2004) Is it really worse to have public insurance than to have no insurance at all? health insurance and adult health in the United States. J Health Soc Behav 45:376–392

Read JG, Emerson MO (2005) Racial context, black immigration and the u.s. black/white health disparity. Soc Forces 84:181–199

Rosenbaum S (2003) Racial and ethnic disparities in health care: issues in the design, structure, and administration of federal health care financing programs. In: Smedley BD, Stith AY, Nelson AR (eds) Unequal treatment: confronting racial and ethnic disparities in health care. The National Academy Press, Washington DC

Ross CE, Mirowsky J (2000) Does medical insurance contribute to socioeconomic differentials in health? Milbank Q 78:291–321

Scambler G (2007) Social structure and the production, reproduction and the durability of health inequalities. Soc Theory Health 5:297–315

Schoen C, Davis K, How SKH, Schoenbam SC (2006) U.S. health system performance: a national scorecard. Health Aff Web (July–November):w457–475

Schuster MA, McGlynn EA, Brook RH (1998) How good is the quality of health care in the United States? Milbank Q 76(4):517–563

Skocpol T (1997) Health care reform and the turn against government. W.W. Norton, New York

Starr P (1994) The logic of health care reform. Penguin Books, New York

Steinmo S, Watts J (1995) It's the institutions, stupid! why comprehensive national health insurance always fails in America. J Health Polit Policy Law 20:329–372

Swartz K (2006) Reinsuring health: why more middle-class people are uninsured and what government can do. Russell Sage Foundation, New York

U.S. Census Bureau (2006) Health Insurance Coverage (2005) www.census.gov/hhes/www/hlthins/hlthin5/hltho5asc.html

Waldo DR, Levit KR, Lazenby HC (1986) National health expenditures, 1985. Health Care Financ Rev 8:1–21

Wennberg J, Gittelsohn A (1973) Small area variations in health care delivery. Science 182:1103–1108

Wildavsky A (1964) The politics of the budgetary process. Little Brown and Company, Boston, MA

Wholey DR, Burns LR (2000) Tides of change: the evolution of managed care in the United States. In: Bird CE, Conrad P, Fremont AM (eds) Handbook of medical sociology, 5th edn. Prentice-Hall, Upper Saddle River, NJ, pp 217–237

Wolinsky F (1978) Assessing the effects of predisposing, enabling, and illness-morbidity characteristics on health service utilization. J Health Soc Behav 19(4):384–396

Part IV
Connecting To the People:
The Public as Patient and Powerful Force

Chapter 15
The Consumer Turn in Medicalization: Future Directions with Historical Foundations

Anne E. Figert

The concept of medicalization is one of the most successful and enduring contributions to the field of medical sociology (Bird et al. 2000). Early thinking and empirical studies of medicalization focused primarily upon the notions of deviance and social control by the institution of medicine (Szasz 1974; Zola 1972; Conrad and Schneider 1980). Since then, the concept of medicalization has successfully migrated out of the sociological literature and into the mainstream public press (Nye 2003). For example, medicalization has its own Wikipedia entry, and there are YouTube sites on the medicalization of childbirth, circumcision, and autism.[1] Public use of sociological terms is not new. Medicalization follows the path of other "successful" sociological concepts such as anomie, focus groups, social networks, and gender. Like all things academic, there is a need to continually shape and refine our concepts and techniques to keep them current and relevant. In order for medicalization to remain an important concept in the twenty-first century, sociologists need to continually adapt the concept in relationship to structural and cultural changes in society.

Some of this debate is already taking place in the medical sociology literature (Clarke et al. 2003; Conrad 2005) and is proving to be fruitful. However, what appear to be missing from the debate are the people, both in their role as individual consumers of health and medical care and as organized political participants in social movements for change. In this chapter, I highlight the role of individuals in the medicalization process and their redefinition from patients into consumers and to argue for the continued expansion of the research agenda in this field. Future directions for medicalization studies necessarily need to include the individual, whether we conceive of this person as a patient, a client, a consumer, or part of a larger health social movement (distinctions which are important and described later in the paper).

In order to do this, I first examine how medicalization has been analyzed and studied in the past. Since there is ample evidence to suggest that ideas about medicalization are widely accepted among the public and in scholarly communities, what can we do as sociologists to help guide the discussion and to contribute to scholarly understanding of it? In addition to understanding concepts such as biomedicalization, we can also recover older concepts in sociology and medicalization studies (such as social class and professions); methodologically, we would take the perspective of ordinary or

---

[1] See the Wikipedia entry at http://en.wikipedia.org/wiki/Medicalization and examples of YouTube videos at http://www.youtube.com/watch?v=f4unKTMpBGA, http://www.youtube.com/watch?v=H9Av4hBNsW8, and http://www.youtube.com/watch?v=f15JexiQt4U.

A.E. Figert (✉)
Department of Sociology, Loyola University Chicago, Coffey Hall 421, 1032 W. Sheridan Road, Chicago, IL 60660, USA
e-mail: afigert@luc.edu

everyday actors as the unit of analysis using illness narratives, surveys, or interviews; and finally we can extend our analytic focus to newer ideas/concepts such as intersectionality and expertise (in particular, the negotiation between lay experts and professional experts).

Medicalization in Sociological Perspective

Medicalization has traditionally been analyzed as an issue about the authority of medical professionals to define, treat, and control individuals. As numerous texts and reviews of the term point out, the notion of medicalization has its roots in Parson's concept of the sick role (1951). At one level, the sick role is about the individual and the social control of deviance. However, it is also about a relationship rooted within the larger social structures of the institution of medicine and physicians' authority to diagnose and treat the person seeking "technically competent" help (Freidson 1970). A substantial portion of sociological work on medicalization has focused exactly upon the technically competent power and authority of physicians in modern society. Freidson's discussion of the social organization of illness provides a framework for thinking about the "medical consumer," but he more consistently calls individuals "laymen" and "patients" (1970). In Freidson's framework, however, there is more emphasis on the reasons and means by which people enter "the medical consulting room" and thereby seek professional help. By virtue of having the authority and professional power in modern society to define and control what is formally recognized as a disorder, sickness, or deviance, physicians have played an important role in the medicalization process (Freidson 1970; Zola 1972; Illich 1976; Conrad and Schneider 1980).

Studies examining and exposing the power and authority of science and medicine to medicalize conditions will also continue to be an important contribution of sociology. My own work on PMS (1996) and recent books by Horwitz and Wakefield (2007) and Lane (2007) have explored in depth the relationship between psychiatry, pharmaceutical companies, and the medicalization process on people's lives. These works analyze this relationship using a macro level focus. Even Conrad's recent exhortation (2005) to move from the social constructionist approach and use a political economic approach to medicalization still retains the focus on the power of the professions and mediating organizations such as pharmaceutical companies and government regulations and less emphasis on individuals. This structural perspective has thrived over the last 30 years in the sociology of the professions, critical or Marxist sociology of health care, and medical sociology in general. This top–down perspective about the definition and control of individuals by the scientific and medical professions is an important aspect of the medicalization process, but it is beginning to be contested in more contemporary studies of medicalization and the professions.

Shifting Engines and Biomedicalization

Conrad has written extensively on the history of the concept of medicalization, its roots in theories of the professions and deviance, and its changes over time (1992, 2005, 2007). Most scholars recognize (as Conrad and others have outlined) that "medicalization is a process" and not just an outcome, and that individuals play an important role in that process. Certainly, Conrad is still trying to do this in his re-thinking about medicalization and its "shifting engines" of "biotechnology (especially the pharmaceutical industry and genetics), consumers, and managed care" (2005, p. 3). Most discussions about medicalization need to take seriously what he has written and the pivotal role he has played in shaping the field. After almost 30 years of writing about the subject, Conrad suggests that: "[t]he key to medicalization is definition. That is, a problem is defined in medical terms, described using medical language, understood through the adoption of a medical framework, or 'treated' with a medical intervention" (2007, p. 5). In his demarcation of the definitional issues about medicalization, Conrad is focusing not just upon the medical professionals but also in the way that individuals experience and fight for/against medical labels alone or in lay groups. This approach and focus on the definitional aspects of medicalization implies more of a top–down focus even when the analytic eye is focused upon consumers.

Both Conrad's recent writing (2005, 2007) and that by Clarke et al. (2003, 2010) identify the new scientific and genetic challenges posed to both individuals, organizations, and the institution of medicine that create a fertile site for examining (bio) medicalization. In what has resulted in a very important body of work in biomedicalization and covered in a separate chapter of this volume, Clarke and her collaborators argue, however, that the generally accepted concept of medicalization in sociology may be outdated and should be replaced with the newer concept of "biomedicalization" that reflects the changing "technoscientific" reality of people's lives (Clarke et al. 2003; Clarke and Shim 2011). This is an important contribution to our theoretical and empirical understanding by redefining medicalization into biomedicalization highlighting the "…. increasingly complex, multisided, multidirectional processes of medicalization that today are being reconstituted through the emergence of social forms and practices of a highly and increasingly technoscientific biomedicine" (2003, p. 162).

Clarke and her collaborators go further than Conrad to argue that what has changed is new and emerging forms of organization and new practices of modern medicine (or biomedicine) and technoscience (science/technology) in the twenty-first century. Like Conrad's recent work, biomedicalization re-focuses our analytic gaze from the power and authority of the medical profession and extends it to include the individual as an active participant in the medicalization process. Particularly relevant for this discussion are the areas in their 2003 early statement in which they focus on the large scale but also say we should also look at the details of how biomedicalization informs and transforms knowledge and its users. The "patient/consumer/user" is transformed from an object of the medical professional's gaze and control (in terms of both expertise and knowledge) into a more active and informed participant in the world (Clarke et al. 2010; Mamo 2005, 2007; Shim 2005).

Epstein highlights that one of the agreed-upon areas stemming from the debate about "biomedicalization" versus the "shifting engines" is a move to the micro and meso level approaches to the study of medicalization processes and outcomes focusing upon the individual patient/user/consumer (2008). He affirms this new direction in the study of medicalization into the biomedicalization perspective such that "new biomedical developments cannot be understood only in top down fashion, we must simultaneously be on the lookout for 'new forms of agency, empowerment, confusion, resistance, responsibility, docility, subjugation, citizenship, subjectivity, and morality' that emerge from dispersed social locations in response to such changes" (Epstein 2008, p. 503 quoting Clarke et al. 2003, p. 184).

Eliot Freidson (best known for his studies of the professions) also conceded in his final book that in the U.S. health system today there are two dominant logics of bureaucracy and markets ("in which consumers control the work people do") that have come to overrule the logic of professionalism (Freidson 2001, p. 12). He concludes by foregrounding individual agency in that "[m]edicalization is as often a process initiated by those desiring the benefits of being classified and treated as ill or disabled as it is the outcome of medical imperialism" (Freidson 2001, p. 193).

In spite of mentioning individuals, patients, and consumers as important agents of active change in the medicalization process and highlighting their importance, there is still more room for more fully developing our thinking. In their thorough review of medicalization and biomedicalization for this volume, Clarke and Shim specifically mention consumers as a site for future research (2011). They write: "Future directions for research might include using the now nicely honed lenses of consumption studies per se to examine the modes and consequences of patients becoming consumers and biomedicine using the language and sales strategies of other consumer products and services (e.g., advertising)" (Clarke and Shim 2011). So how would the inclusion of consumers specifically change our thinking about medicalization?

Part of moving forward with studies of the place of individuals, consumers, and SMOs and medicalization studies involves recovering useful concepts and perspectives in mainstream sociology such as professions, social movements, and social class and using them in new ways. In looking at medicalization from below (with the focus on the individual or social movement organization) instead of the top down, then these concepts and theories can be useful or reformulated to be more inclusive of a focus on individuals and consumers. This is not to say that we should hang on to outdated concepts or studies. As developed in this chapter, the concept of professions, professional knowledge, and control are still useful but we need to adapt them to the material and cultural circumstances of what we are studying. Both medicalization and biomedicalization are useful terms and we do not have to decide if one term is more useful or supercedes the other. If the concept of biomedicalization is more useful as a heuristic and methodological concept than medicalization, then we should use it where it applies and vice versa. Although both sides seem to be staking out oppositional turfs, I think that they are more similar than different and that medical sociology will benefit from increased development of both concepts under the larger umbrella term of medicalization studies.

We also need to extend our ideas about professional control to include studies of expertise. If the days of physician control and dominance are over (Light 2000), how does medicalization occur within the increasingly complex health care system? Who are all the actors/interested parties? How does professional knowledge interact with bureaucratic control in health care system? How does the expert knowledge claimed by the consumer/patient/client interact with and confront professional control and bureaucratic control? As Fischer writes:

> The fundamental argument to emerge from these critiques of expertise is put forth in the following terms: if citizens are to participate in the development of the policy decisions that affect their own lives, the standard practitioner-client model must give way to a more democratic relationship between them. (Fischer 2000, pp. 39–40)

If, as Collins and Evans (2007) suggest, we need to shift our analysis to study authority and expertise by both professionals and lay persons, then how can we use these ideas to more fully develop a model of medicalization related to the individual patients/users/consumers?

Patients, Clients, Consumers, and Health Movements

As suggested, the earlier writings in the medicalization and professions literature only briefly addressed the role of individuals and even more rarely used the term "consumers" but did not really expand or make consumers a central focus of the work. An important direction for the field of medicalization studies is to more fully address and develop the role of individuals and consumers in the medicalization process in the twenty-first century.

Definitions

The term "consumer" and the increased use of the term in the medical literature invite definition and further exploration. Clarke and Shim (2011) and Henderson and Peterson (2002) point out that not all medical sociologists and analysts willingly embrace the term. I start with the general definition offered in the Oxford English Dictionary that a consumer is "[o]ne who purchases goods or pays for service; a customer, purchaser" (OED Online). As Henderson and Peterson argue about today's health care situation: "[i]ncreasingly, health is viewed as a 'commodity' and individuals are defined as health care 'consumers'" (2002, p. 1). Although the word may evoke notions of buyers and purchasers of goods and services in the economic sense, the use of the word "consumer" has come into a more sustained and broader use in the medical context.

In the traditional heath/medical relationship, a patient/client is distinguished from a "mere consumer" as someone who uses "the services of a professional" (OED online). This definition says more about the context of the services and the person supplying those services than about the individual. It also leads us back to the issue of authority and definition of a profession (see Abbott 1988 for a more elaborate discussion of the client–professional relationship). However, managed care, utilization review, and the impact of technological devices and pharmaceutical interventions in the late twentieth century all had an enormous impact on redefining the client–medical professional relationship. For example, Winnick, Werum, and Pavalko found that the diagnostic criteria found in the DSM-III and innovations by pharmaceutical companies had a major influence on treatment recommendations in family practice journals and that by the 1990s, "articles began to remind practitioners to not forget the importance of interacting with their patients" instead of just prescribing medication (2001, p. 199). The increased use of research and diagnostic criteria used by government agencies and insurance companies and the decreased time spent with patients in order to increase efficiency and increase output have created a situation in which patients are viewed as customers and clients, both by professionals and by the patients themselves.

Moreover, in wealthy, developed post-industrial capitalist economies, medical knowledge and information is ubiquitous. Whether we are actively seeking goods or services, we are bombarded through the mass media with advertisements about medical studies/findings and products. Recent articles have shown that television shows and news are the primary means by which Americans receive medical information (Brodie et al. 2001). In the "potential consumer" category, anyone who is living or breathing, has a headache, or a family history of certain disease is "at risk" of disease alongside those who are already sick (Scott et al. 2005). The news media (e.g., television, the Internet, and print media) play an important role not only in informing the public but also in possibly exaggerating the prevalence of disease and the need for treatment. In a study of the media representation of restless legs syndrome, Woloshin and Schwartz argue that the media seemed to be co-opted by pharmaceutical companies engaged in "disease mongering" to solicit more potential customers or consumers of their medication/product (2006). Viewed in this framework, we are all actual or potential consumers of medical products or services which have significant implications for medicalization.

Situating the Medical Consumer

In the context of understanding medicalization, the notion of "consumer" subsumes the concept of the "client" or "patient" and exposes the economic nature of the medical professional enterprise. Whereas client or patient is conceptualized within the professional relationship, the word consumer highlights and locates a person within a larger economic system. Where and when did this shift of using the term consumer instead of patient and client occur? Policy makers and health economists began talking or referring clients and patients as consumers in the last 30 years. Lupton locates the shift toward a "consumerist" approach toward the medical profession and encounter as having both liberal and conservative underpinnings in Western societies (1997). From a liberal humanist approach, the use of the word consumer has emphasized equitable access to health and medical care and the empowerment of individuals in the medical encounter. From a more conservative and free market approach, the individual is encouraged to embrace a consumerist approach to health care that involves evaluating physicians as providers of services like other types of providers, health care as just another commodity bought and sold in the free market and thus "to refuse to accept paternalism or 'medical dominance' on the art of the doctor, to 'shop around', to actively evaluate doctors' services and to go elsewhere should the 'commodity' be found unsatisfactory" (Lupton 1997, p. 373). In terms of its implications for medicalization and professional authority, both perspectives on the political spectrum have emphasized lay people as post-modern "rational actors" who are skeptical about expert knowledge (explored later in the paper).

Consumerism and Patient Expertise in Health and Medical Care

Medical sociologists and health policy scholars in the United Kingdom have been at the forefront of research in this area. The emphasis on consumerism in UK health policy is related to what Fox, Ward, and O'Rourke describe as the emergence of the "expert patient" (2005). In their study of participants in an Internet forum on obesity, the authors document the effects of a government program promoting the concept of expert patients. They found that people share knowledge and information with each other and use this information in the medical encounter with physicians who prescribe their weight loss drug. These "expert patients" were able to manage their own illnesses and conditions "by developing knowledge relevant to maintaining health and countering illness" (2005, p. 1299). This suggests that using the consumer model of asking individuals to educate themselves and to be more responsible for their own bodies and health outcomes can have a transformative effect on the nature of the doctor–patient relationship. However, in spite of the fact that some people became "technically competent experts" about their own health/bodies, the users still reinforced cultural and biomedical standards of body shape and size in the Internet forum. The authors end on a hopeful note for a consumers in that "the growth of a consumerist approach to health care may, however, offer an alternative basis for an informed 'patient,' who resists biomedical formulations of health and illness, and uses the kinds of community [internet] described in this paper to develop expertise that empowers rather than constraints" (Fox et al. 2005, pp. 1307–1308).

In documenting the field of mental health services and social movements to resist psychiatry in the U.K., Crossley (2006) presents a more structural history of the shift to consumerism by the National Health Service and also points out that the consumer model does not have to be portrayed in an entirely critical or negative fashion for people and health activist groups. He writes that although the consumer model of refashioning patients into "consumers" was started within the Thatcher administration, it was continued as a policy by both Tory and Labour governments. Although it was criticized by both medical practitioners and patient groups, some patient groups found ways to work effectively and in new ways within the new system. Crossely writes:

> Moreover, they claim that the introduction of a language and philosophy of consumerism, whilst flawed in some respects has helped to tip the balance of power slightly in their favour, improving their bargaining power within the system. The customer, so the saying goes, knows best, and these particular customers endorse that view (2006, p. 67).

In the U.S. context, the reorganization and structure of health care and regulations as more market driven and corporately controlled have also helped to shape the rise of the word consumer over the term patient or even client. Kaufmann historically locates the emergence of mental health consumers as a direct consequence of the massive deinstitutionalization of mental health patients first into clients of community health centers and then into consumers since the 1980s (1999). She writes: "[a]lready preferred among activists in the disability rights movements, the consumer rubric trades on issues of choice and freedom in an ideal market for mental health services. The mental health consumer as a social role is based on experiential knowledge developed through interactions with the mental health treatment and welfare systems" (1999, p. 495). Similar to the U.K., the consumer language and focus in the U.S. can create knowledgeable consumers who can successfully navigate a system whose rhetoric and emphasis is on efficient service provision. Alternatively, it can create consumers who negotiate a market place without sufficient knowledge or resources to make informed medical decisions.

The consumerist model can also provide roadblocks for other parts of the health care system. Take for example, health insurance. In the consumer model, health insurance is a service or product that is to be bought or sold in the free market. The consumer model has also minimized the political and policy debate and possibility for change. Employers may provide some or all of the cost to their employees as a benefit and the U.S. government may provide some health insurance to the elderly or poor through Medicare and Medicaid. But for more than 30 million people in the U.S. who are not currently insured, it is still a product or service that they cannot afford. Indeed, sociologist and policy analyst Jill Quadagno argues that: "[u]ntil we view health insurance as a social right, not a consumer product, we will never receive the coverage we need" (2005, p. 6).

Perhaps the most symbolically significant indicator of the trend toward a consumerist policy in U.S. medical history (which reflects this "free market" emphasis on consumer choice) occurred in late 1990s when the Food and Drug Administration first allowed pharmaceutical companies to use "direct to consumer advertising" (DTCA) for their products. Both Conrad (2005, 2007) and Clarke et al. (2003, 2010) point to direct to consumer advertising as a key site in which the "shifting engines of medicalization" and increased biomedicalization occur. In a series of slide presentations on the effects of this advertising at the FDA website, Aiken (an FDA staff member) presents data from a random sample of 500 physicians who indicated an increased interest on the part of their patients asking about specific drugs and in their overall interest in treatment options (Aiken 2003). The physicians also noted some of the other benefits of increased consumer awareness as a result of this type of advertising such as asking better questions about their health and potential health problems. Problems created as the result of DTCA include an increase in tension or second guessing diagnoses, anxiety about potential diseases or side effects, and confusion about the overall benefits of certain drug effectiveness (Boden and Diamond 2008).

As more researchers pay attention to issues about the rhetoric and reality of consumerism in the medical market place, we will need to fully develop our thinking about individuals as consumers in the medical context. As I have briefly shown, we can learn a lot about individuals successfully negotiating the health care system to their advantage using the consumer framework, the need to change attitudes about health insurance as a right and not a consumer product and direct to consumer advertising using this consumer framework.

"What Does the Term "Consumer" Do in/for Medicalization?"

The governmental policy shift toward a consumer or the expert patient is not always fully embraced by medical professionals and is seen as a threat to their professional authority (Fox et al. 2005; Crossley 2006). For example, Dingwall's recent essay in memory of Eliot Freidson highlights some of the new professional tensions about medical licensing which have arisen in the consumerist perspective. Dingwall echoes and extends Freidson's and Parson's thinking about professions and the sick role when he describes the tensions between the health care system and government regulations to ensure that consumers "get what they think they are paying for rather than wondering whether the society can afford for them to get it at all?" (2008, p. xv). Further, he warns that if "physicians are merely suppliers of a consumer good, then the case for licensing is one of consumer protection rather than of a socially accountable control agent" (Dingwall 2008, p. 140).

The consumerist model creates demand and expectations for health care delivery that cannot always be met. The 1980s and 1990s gave rise to a "market ideology" in which the market was used to reform the public health sector. There were some unintended consequences. For example, when governments label citizens as "customers" or "consumers," they shaped and influenced the behavior and attitudes of people requesting services. In turn, the citizens exerted pressure on health care professionals in these systems (Duyvendak et al. 2006) with very negative effects for professional authority and trust. Ironically, Kremer and Tonkens found that when "[c]lient movements embraced the market as savior, hoping it would provide them with the rights of bureaucratic logic without the inconvenience of slow procedures. ....but the market has instead brought authority, trust, knowledge, and the public good into disarray" (Kremer and Tonkens 2006, p. 129). But instead of serving to help consumers to challenge professional authority by educating and empowering themselves, Kremer and Tonkens point out that the free market system limits the authority and knowledge of consumers because "competition is not based on expertise and skills, but merely on prices" (2006, p. 129).[2]

Pescosolido effectively argues that the use of the term consumer exposes has not served to end the professional dominance of physicians in the medical market place (2006). In spite of all these mediating effects and impacts of the changing health care system, Pescosolido states that "[t]here has never been a point in time when the worldview of the ability of medical science to provide answers to health, and even social problems has been more pervasive" (2006, p. 21). Lupton (1997) affirms this point in showing that indeed sometimes even knowledgeable consumers want "the expert to tell me what to do" in the medical encounter (1997). In an article exploring the contribution of Foucault to the medicalization critique, Lupton asserts that critics of medicalization: "Fail to acknowledge the ambivalent nature of the feelings and opinions that many people have in relation to medicine or the ways that patients willing participate in medical dominance and may indeed seek 'medicalization'" (1997, p. 98). Even the physicians surveyed by Aiken about the effects of DTCA indicated that even though patients asked about particular drugs and they felt some pressure to prescribe, only a small percentage of patients "tried to influence the course of treatment in a way that would have been harmful to him or her" (Aiken 2003). Patients still will listen to what their physicians have to say and actively seek out their advice.

This "paradox of consumerism" in the medical context as outlined by Henderson and Peterson (2002) highlights the "complex 'double-edged' character" of consumerism. On the one hand, it can obscure a need for societal change of the health care system by focusing upon individual consumers (being responsible for their own health and health outcomes) and, on the other hand, it can be useful to mobilize groups to advocate for change in the system (2002). Thus, it is not just "the consumer" that is involved in consumerism but also the consumer groups, organizations, and social movements. The study of consumers and medicalization needs to go beyond the micro or individual level of analysis.

Self-Help and Advocacy Groups

Often demarcated or seen as the province of scholars working in the fields of social movements or political processes (couched in terms of expert knowledge versus democratic process), the study of patient groups, lay groups, and patient advocacy groups has recently garnered more attention from

---

[2] This theme is echoed elsewhere in the biomedicalization literature when Clarke and Oleson point out that "[s]urveillance medicine and genomics together have already begun to impose new burdens on health care consumers. There are incredible burdens of knowledge expectations—what lay people are expected to know and do about our health, especially in terms of prevention and especially if we have risk factors. As best we can determine, we all are at greater risk for something" (1999, p. 23).

within medical sociology and increasingly medicalization scholars. As early as Freidson (1970), lay groups were mentioned as the impetus for the medicalization process and outcomes. However, Freidson's "special lay interest groups" were unique organizational creatures "sometimes led by physicians but always including at least one prominent physician" (1970, p. 254) seeking to medicalize, demedicalize, or redefine an illness to make it less stigmatizing in society (alcoholism, leprosy, and epilepsy).

As recently explored in depth by Epstein (2008), the study of patient groups and health advocacy organizations now occupies a central role and poses crucial questions in both the fields of medical sociology and science and technology studies. In trying to answer the question why there is now scholarly emphasis on patient groups and health movements, Epstein points to the success that such groups have had in changing health care policies, in challenging the professional and epistemologically privileged knowledge of doctors and scientists, and in being a part of a larger rights-based movement for change since the 1960s. Beyond this success, patient and health movements are central to the "processes by which bodies, diseases, and life itself are being remade by the biomedical revolutions of recent years" (2008, p. 502).

This area of study is consistent with Kelleher's argument that self-help groups are not necessarily antithetical to the institution of medicine and actually address some of the shortcomings of institutional medicine to meet the expressive needs of people (1994). Such groups "enable a range of concerns to be kept alive, rather than being distorted by expert systems and the discourse of the market, and a form of non-coercive talk becomes possible" (1994, p. 116). Groups can work together with physicians or governments to create change. However, this type of model may not work effectively because it can lead to an "elitism" which would effectively block or impede democratic participation by all members (Fischer 2000).

Much of this literature has come from the feminist and women's health research in sociology and other disciplines (Inhorn 2006; Epstein 2008). Feminist scholars were among the first to explicitly connect lay group participation with both the political and epistemological challenge to modern physician-dominated medicine (e.g., Ruzek 1978; Martin 1987; Davis 2007). Within this area, there is a substantial and growing body of scholarship which explicitly examines lay groups and especially lay knowledge and expertise as challenges to professional expertise and authority with both gender and social class implications for the study of individuals and medicalization.

The creation of groups such as the Boston Women's Health collective and the publication of *Our Bodies, Ourselves* (1973) are related to feminist awareness and to scientific and political changes in the way that research on women is conceptualized and conducted (Auerbach and Figert 1995; Inhorn 2006). Riska argues that after an initial non-gendered history of medicalization studies, feminist scholars in the mid-1970s began "to unravel the history of modern medicine" and critique the male bias in the diagnosis, treatment, and delivery of health care. The notion of individuals and consumers of health care is rooted in the women's health movement of the 1970s where "women would emancipate themselves from victimization by medicine and become actors who would promote their gender-specific health needs and health services" (Riska 2003, p. 67).

Drawing upon a developing literature in feminist scholarship on women's health, Riessman's article on the central role of gender in the process of medicalization was one of the first articles in medical sociology to point out the gendered implications of medicalization (1983). This article is often cited because of its early focus on gender and the important role it plays in the medicalization process. However, a key point that is often lost in her analysis is that even though women and women's bodies are susceptible to medicalization, consumers (in her case women) are not always "duped" by the medical establishment and played a very active role in the medicalization of childbirth and other medical conditions specific to women (1983). Riesman suggests that individual women and women's groups (particularly white middle-class women) were active participants in the medicalization process of women's bodies such as reproduction (abortion, birth control, and birth) and menstruation (menopause and PMS) issues. Finally, Tomes highlights the complexity of issues such as consumerism and the dynamic relationship between women and health professionals in which women are "neither irrational, easily manipulated tools nor all powerful sovereign shoppers" (2001).

Feminist and women's health scholars have drawn extensively on a feminist and gendered framework to further analyze conditions such as PMS, menopause, childbirth and parenting, and fibromyalgia (Bell 1987; Figert 1996; Litt 2000; Houck 2006) and the agency of women as active consumers either as individuals or as part of organizations or movements. In her work about women and fibromyalgia, Barker writes: "As patients, we sometimes actively participate in or demand the medicalization of our experiences as we earnestly seek meaning for our suffering" (2005, p. 12). One way in which individuals (as patients) seek meaning of their lives is to participate in social movements for change based upon their shared illness experience.

Embodied Health Movements

As indicated in the vast body of feminist scholarship in this area, in terms of medicalization, patient groups and advocacy groups may be very active proponents of the medicalization process. They fight for or they work with professional organizations to get their lived or bodily experience labeled or diagnosed. These are "the illness you fight to get" (Dumit 2006) and include such recently "discovered" or "labeled" conditions such as PTSD, Gulf War Syndrome (Scott 1990; Zavestoski et al. 2004), and fibromyalgia (Barker 2005). But, patient groups or advocacy groups can also work with or fight professional organizations to demedicalize conditions (Figert 1996). Epstein explores the relationship of patient groups and social movements to medicalization and the demedicalization processes and concludes that "it may be wise to be skeptical of the idea that any single, unidimensional typology adequately can capture the variation of patient groups and health movements" (2008, p. 509). Epstein further argues that attempts to classify and define patient groups and health movements may be helpful but not in all cases or particularities because "medicalization" and "demedicalization" capture something of what these various groups are up to, but the terms should be used with caution in dealing with lay groups (2008, p. 511).

The complexity of these issues involved with lay groups and social movements have been thet specific focus of the subfield of health social movements. Brown and his collaborators have been major contributors to the development of this subfield and the subfield of "popular epidemiology." They define health social movements (HSMs) as:

> collective challenges to medical policy, public health policy and politics, belief systems, research, and practice that include an array of formal and informal organizations, supporters, networks of cooperation, and medial (Morello-Frosch et al. 2006, p. 245).

Using this definition, they have developed three ideal types of these movements which serve to guide both the empirical case studies and theoretical contributions to medical sociology: *health access movements* which work for the equitable provision of health care services; *constituency-based movements* which focus on health along lines of a shared characteristic such as gender, race, ethnicity, sexuality, or other defining variable; and *embodied health movements* which "address disease, disability or illness experience by challenging science on etiology, diagnosis, treatment and prevention" (Brown et al. 2004, pp. 52–32).

Embodied health movements as a more recent form of health social movements are important to the discussion of consumers and medicalization because they politicize illness "by making the socioeconomic drivers of health explicit and central to their struggle" (Morello-Frosch et al. 2006, p. 265). In doing so, they engage and challenge medical professionals and policy makers with the explicit goal of changing the way in which medical research and treatment is conducted. Whether at the local level of individual experience or through collective action, "embodied health" often takes place within the economic framework of the consumer or consumer advocacy groups fighting to get the services wanted and needed and making "expert" claims based upon the embodiment of the illness or disease. Such claims often challenge professional authority of medical experts in terms of knowing how to define, diagnose, and treat certain embodied conditions. The demand for effective diagnosis and treatment is often couched within a consumer framework of not getting the services needed both by medical professionals and from the insurance companies and government agencies. In terms of medicalization, the arguments can be both for (PTSD or Fibromyalgia) or against (PMS) diagnosis of certain conditions, but there is a high degree of activism on the part of groups organized around the conditions.

What Is Old Is New Again

So, what happens if medical sociologists take consumers' role and political economic factors in medicalization processes and outcomes seriously? The paradox of consumerism in health care as outlined by Henderson and Peterson (2002) suggests that there is a double-edged sword to using a consumer terminology. In looking at issues of patient groups and embodied health movements, scholarship by sociologists is pivotal in highlighting the positive features surrounding lay advocacy and movements to create social change. Sociological scholarship has also been successful in exploring the loss of physician authority both to diagnose and to treat people as a result of mediating factors such as health insurance coverage and government control. What has not been developed as adequately is an exploration of the negative features surrounding a language requiring individuals to be in charge and responsible for the care and treatment of their own bodies. These issues highlight two major issues that make room for recovery and expansion in the consumer turn in medicalization studies: social class and expertise.

Social Class and Intersectionality

Although historians of medicine (Peterson 1978; Porter 1985), anthropologists (Martin 1987), and some sociologists (Brown 1979; Berlant 1975; Larson 1977) have long argued that class has mattered in the way that the medical profession controls and maintains its authority, sociologists have been slower to embrace this focus in terms of the medicalization process. As argued earlier in this chapter, some of the initial scholarly work about the medicalization process came out of a structural framework focusing on the issues of the power and authority of the medical profession to diagnose, label, and control the individual. The medical encounter become one in which the individual was essentially stripped of any power and agency (Illich 1976; Zola 1972; Waitzkin 1993). There are exceptions. An important aspect of Riessman's (1983) essay on women and medicalization that has not been developed as much in medical sociology concerns the role and difference that social class plays in the medicalization processes. Riessman states:

> Although medicalization theory has emphasized power, it has tended to minimize the significance of class. Historically…the medicalization of certain problems was rooted in specific class interests. Physicians and women from the dominant class joined together – albeit of very different motives – to redefine certain human events into medical categories. Women from other class groups at times embraced and at other times resisted these class-based definitions of experience (1983, pp. 49–50).

This point is echoed in Riska's more recent review of gender and medicalization which stresses the role of the consumer but criticizes the middle-class nature of much of the women's health movement (2003). Riska states:

> Underlying the endeavor was a notion of a middle-class consumer with purchasing power and a belief that the market was the right location for offering the best service to women. Poor women without purchasing power got less attention and political support for the provision of family planning and health care services in the public sector. Rather than demedicalizing women's health needs, as the feminist health advocates originally had envisioned, the middle-class character of the movement resulted in a confirmation of the trend towards medicalization (2003, p. 68).

In her review of ethnographic contributions to women's health, anthropologist Inhorn disagrees with Riska's analysis and points out the ways in which a class analysis has been subsumed into an intersectional approach of feminist scholarship to highlight the "interlocking nature of various oppressions" such as gender, race, class, and sexuality (Inhorn 2006). Class is an important part of the analysis, but it does not stand alone as the only important factor which is a point that gets lost in Riska's critique.

Much of the recent work in biomedicalization also echoes this intersectional approach as Clarke and others working within this framework are mindful of these interlocking oppressions and the way in which people and their bodies are differentially affected by biomedicalization. The intersectionality approach in medicalization is already proving to be useful. With a renewed focus on the intersection of class with other variables, other medicalization scholars have also expanded their gender focus to analyze the unique nature of masculinity men's bodies in relationship to the medicalization process (Riska 2003; Loe 2004; Conrad 2007). Riska notes that unlike the middle-class nature of the medicalization of women's bodies, the medicalization of men's bodies focuses upon "men of color, men of low income, rural and inner-city men" (2003, p. 75).

The re-focus on social class (whether it is solely focused on class or as part of an intersectional approach) is pivotal for any re-examination of the role of consumers within medicalization studies and medical sociology in general. Scholars are beginning to re-examine the role that social class has played in medicalization and power in the knowledge and authority of institutionalized medicine (Pescosolido and Martin 2004). Recent work by Conrad and his colleagues (Conrad and Leiter 2004; Conrad 2007) is also suggestive of this turn toward examining the role of consumers but has not fully developed the agenda for this century.

Knowledge: Power, Authority, and Expertise

In addition to incorporating more issues about social class back into our studies of consumers and medicalization, we also have to *more fully* examine and develop the role that knowledge, power, authority, and expertise play in the medicalization process. I say more fully not because power and authority have been ignored in the medicalization literature. In fact, the literature has traditionally been about the power and the authority of the medical profession to medicalize. However, as indicated in the above quotation by Riessman, most of the existing studies of medicalization have tended to be very top–down models of the medical profession and its authority/power to medicalize or make human problems under the definitional and jurisdictional control of medicine. To quote Riessman again: "Women were not simply passive victims of medical ascendancy" (1983, p. 3).

Do patients redefined as "consumers" in the ideology of a free market inherently challenge professional expert knowledge? As suggested earlier in this essay, when the consumer label is adopted by individuals and embodied health movements, there is often an emphasis on self-knowledge or "lay expertise" on the part of the person experiencing the condition. Claims to embodied expertise and knowledge are used to negotiate, agitate, or challenge professional knowledge. These issues have been explored in the context of individual experiences of health and illness. Whereas most of the sociological scholarship on lay/professional expertise is at the macro level (what is power, what do various groups do to get it), Lupton (1997) and Popay et al. (1998) talked to people about how they use knowledge to negotiate issues of health and illness. Individuals have agency and that it is important in the power/expertise dynamic. They state:

> Lay knowledge may stand not just as a different kind of knowledge but as knowledge which takes issue with the way in which media or experts characterise the relationships between events or the nature or needs and/or identity – on occasions forming what Nancy Fraser (1989) has described as 'oppositional discourses' (1998, p. 640).

Lupton writes: "[m]ost critics also advocate the 'empowerment' of patents (often renamed 'consumers'), encouraging people to 'take back control' over their own health by engaging in preventative health activities, assuming the role of 'consumer' by challenging the decisions and knowledge of doctors in the medical encounter, joining patient advocacy groups and eschewing medicine by seeking the attentions of alternative practitioners" (1997, p. 97). These issues about expertise are front and center in ways that medical sociologists need to re-think our ideas about scientific and medical knowledge and the medicalization process. Who controls what counts as expertise? Truth? How does that get negotiated? What are the effects and consequences?

How can we begin to do this? Collins and Evans (2007) offer insights from their study of scientific expertise that are applicable to the study of medicalization and medical expertise. Collins and Evens treat expertise as "real and substantive" and not just in a relational manner to other people (such as that found in the professions literature). In developing a "periodic table of expertises," Collins and Evans explore the range of knowledge and expertise ranging from ubiquitous tacit knowledge (the everyday knowledge employed to negotiate the world, such as reading a map) to specialized expertise (writing a topographical map). People can acquire real expertise through group membership and not just from the attributions of expertise from others. The implications of the new sociology of expertise model for medical sociology is that the medicalization is analyzed specifically as an interactional, multidirectional process that involves intersecting or mediating factors such as race, class, and gender within specific sociohistorical settings. Consumers and lay expertise are just as important in the analysis of medicalization as professions or corporations or governments.

In medical sociology, we have competing views about the issue of lay experts. On the one hand, there are scholars who argue that "for the most part, lay people are not experts" because "lay thinking is experiential and therefore limited, but that it can also be in error (Prior 2003, p. 45, 49). On the other hand, there are sociologists who are documenting that ways in which lay activists and consumers can be co-creators of scientific and medical knowledge and this is an important area for future study. Scholars working in the health movement area are well versed in the science and technology studies area that has more fully developed the study of expertise in the last couple of decades (Epstein 2008; Brown et al. 2004; Shim 2005). These and other scholars suggest that these movements "blur the boundary between experts and lay people" (Brown et al. 2004, p. 64) and can change science by valuing the embodied knowledge of illness sufferers.

Conclusions

The purpose of this volume is to address the major issues facing medical sociologists and to set part of the research agenda for the twenty-first century. Medicalization and biomedicalization include technological innovations, cultural shifts, and institutional changes in health care and the larger society. Medicalization studies have always highlighted the role of individuals (usually as the object of medicalization) but only recently have we begun to explore their agency (both as individuals and as members of lay groups/movements) in the process of medicalization. I have argued that we need to be more expansive in our thinking about individuals and their relationship to medicalization processes and outcomes. We need to focus on the definition and role of consumer in a specific economic health markets as both active agent and recipient of medicalization process. We need to further document how individuals form relationships, social networks, and health social movements related to health or medical conditions.

How do we accomplish this re-thinking: In many ways, we can continue the models examining the "shifting engines," biomedicalization, and embodied lay health movements that already exist in scholarly work of Conrad (2005), Clarke et al. (2003), Brown et al. (2004), and Epstein (2008). What these scholars share is a model that treats medicalization studies along a bisecting continuum with level of analysis and expertise within existing political economic systems. The benefit of this thinking is that it firmly roots our studies within historical context while at the same time providing more explanatory power beyond the case study approach in social constructivist studies of medicalization. It is also critical of the use of the term consumer while at the same time acknowledging its real potential to change the nature of relationships within the health care system and society.

There are also methodological implications for future studies of medicalization. We need to move beyond or figure out how to more effectively use case studies of diseases, disorders, or conditions that have been medicalized. Conrad recently argued that we need to move beyond social constructionist studies of medicalization and focus on political economy issues (2005). The inclusion of class into our medicalization studies will help to achieve this in part but we also need to develop a more local and nuanced understanding of the meanings that medicalization or embodied health movements have in people's lives. For example, embodied health movement studies are about specific health movements, but they are also about the everyday experience of people's bodies and how they claim and use this "embodied" knowledge to make their own expert claims and negotiate with physicians, insurance companies, government officials, and other entities. How do individuals and consumer health groups rely upon and use their embodied health experience to make sense of diagnoses? How do they negotiate a shared meaning?

Feminist scholars in medical sociology and anthropology are showing us the way (Inhorn 2006; Epstein 2008). Bell's extensive body of work with DES survivors shows how individuals see themselves as consumers/participants in the medicalization process and not just as the embodied outcome, e.g., DES daughters (Bell 1999). Barker's interviews with people with fibromyalgia syndrome or FMS go beyond the story of the social construction or contestation of the disease between lay people and embodied health movements to allow the women to speak about their illness experience and how they make sense of it (2005). Loe's analysis of the drug Viagra includes the historical, political, and economic medicalization of "erectile dysfunction" to include both men and women's relationships to the drug and sex as consumers or members "of the marketplace with an investment in Viagra" (2004, p. 202). The complexity of the stories highlights the myriad ways in which gender, race, and social class play roles in the way in which people's experiences are shaped. Likewise, Litt uses interview data from her study of African–American and Jewish women who raised children in the 1930s and 1940s to show that "medicalization held different meanings for people of different social-class and ethnoracial positions" and how "medicalization of birth and child care was something only the privileged could afford to reject" (2000, p. 15).

The consumer turn in medicalization studies that has already begun is ultimately important because it involves questions of both epistemology and methodology which are central to medical sociology. In terms of epistemology, there are definitional aspects in the debate about shifting engines of medicalization versus biomedicalization that shape ways of thinking about medicalization. The use of the term "consumer" instead of patient could just be a semantic shift, but it has also played a part in shifting our thinking about the doctor–patient relationship in the medical encounter. In terms of methodology, by its very nature, the term consumer extends medicalization studies from top–down (institutional and professional control) studies to bottom–up (ethnographic, situated) studies of meaning and expertise. The consumer turn extends the multiple ways and relationships the individual has in negotiating the medicalization process that both Conrad (2007) and Clarke et al. (2003) recommend.

Finally, the consumer turn re-focuses medical sociology back to some very basic and integral concepts in sociology: economic class, gender and professions, and authority as medicalization is experienced and negotiated in new ways. Using our skills as medical sociologists, we can use a more comparative analysis to examine the intersecting roles of gender, race, class, and sexuality in the medicalization process. We can begin to be more international in our focus and move beyond the Western world to understand the perspectives from the global South.

References

Abbott A (1988) The system of professions. University of Chicago Press, Chicago, IL
Aiken K (2003) Direct-to-consumer advertising of prescription drugs: physician survey preliminary results. http://www.fda.gov/cder/ddmac/globalsummit2003/
Auerbach J, Figert A (1995) Women's health research: public policy and sociology. J Health Soc Behav (Special Issue):115–131
Barker K (2005) The fibromyalgia story: medical authority and women's worlds of pain. Temple University Press, Philadelphia, PA
Bell S (1999) Narratives and lives: women's health politics and the diagnosis of cancer for DES daughters. Narrative Inq 9(2):347–389
Bell S (1987) Changing ideas: the medicalization of menopause. Soc Sci Med 24(6):535–542
Berlant J (1975) Profession and monopoly: a study of medicine in the United States and Great Britain. University of California Press, Berkeley, CA
Bird C, Conrad P, Fremont A (eds) (2000) Handbook of medical sociology, 5th edn. Prentice Hall, Upper Saddle River, NJ
Boden WE, Diamond G (2008) DTCA for PTCA – Crossing the ine in consumer health education? N Engl J Med 358(21):2197–2200
Boston Women's Health Book Collective (1973) Our bodies, ourselves. Boston Women's Health Book Collective, Boston, MA
Brodie M, Foehr U, Rideout V, Baer N, Miller C, Flournoy R, Altman D (2001) Communicating health information through the entertainment media. Health Aff 20(1):192–199
Brown ER (1979) Rockefeller medicine men: medicine and capitalism in America. University of California Press, Berkeley, CA
Brown P, Zavestoski S, McCormick S, Mayer B, Morello-Frosch R, Altman RG (2004) Embodied health movements: new approaches to social movements in health. Sociol Health Illn 26(1):50–80
Clarke A, Oleson V (1999) Revising, diffracting, acting. In: Clarke A, Oleson V (eds) Revisioning women, health, and healing. Routledge, New York, pp 3–4
Clarke A, Shim J (2011) Medicalization and biomedicalization revisited: technoscience and transformations of health and illness. B.A. Pescosolido et al. (eds), Handbook of the Sociology of Health, Illness, and Healing: A Blueprint for the 21st Century, Spring.
Clarke A, Shim J, Mamo L, Fosket JR, Fishman JR (2003) Biomedicalization: technoscientific transformations of health, illness, and U.S. biomedicine. Am Sociol Rev 68(2):161–194
Clarke A, Shim J, Mamo L, Fosket J, Fishman J (eds) (2010) Biomedicalization: technoscience and transformations of health, illness and U.S. biomedicine. Duke University Press, Durham, NC
Collins H, Evans R (2007) Rethinking expertise. University of Chicago Press, Chicago
Conrad P (1992) Medicalization and social control. Ann Rev Sociol 18:209–232
Conrad P (2005) The shifting engines of medicalization. J Health Soc Behav 46:3–14
Conrad P, Leiter V (2004) Medicalization, markets, and consumer. J Health Soc Behav 45:158–176
Conrad P, Schneider J (1980) Deviance and medicalization: from badness to sickness. Mosby, St. Louis, MO
Conrad P (2007) The medicalization of society: on the transformation of human conditions into treatable disorders. The Johns Hopkins University Press, Baltimore, MD
Crossley N (2006) Contesting psychiatry: social movements in mental health. Routledge, London and New York

Davis K (2007) The making of our bodies, ourselves: how feminism travels across borders. Duke University Press, Durham, NC
Dingwall R (2008) Essays on professions. Ashgate Publishing, Hampshire
Dumit J (2006) Illnesses you have to fight to get: facts as forces in uncertain, emergent illnesses. Soc Sci Med 62(3):577–590
Duyvendak J, Knijn T, Kremer M (eds) (2006) Policy, people, and the new professional: de-professionalisation and re-professionalisation in care and welfare. Amsterdam University Press, Amsterdam
Epstein S (2008) Patient groups and health movements. In: Hackett E, Lynch M, Amsterdamska O, Wajcman J (eds) The handbook of science and technology studies, 3rd edn. MIT, Cambridge, MA
Figert A (1996) Women and the ownership of PMS. Aldine de Gruyter, Hawthorne, NY
Fischer F (2000) Citizens, experts and the environment: the politics of local knowledge. Duke University Press, Durham, NC
Fox N, Ward K, O'Rourke A (2005) The 'expert patient': empowerment or medical dominance? The case of weight loss, pharmaceutical drugs and the Internet. Soc Sci Med 60(6):1299–1309
Fraser N (1989) Unruly practices: power, discourse and gender in contemporary social theory. Polity Press, Cambridge
Freidson E (1970) Profession of medicine: a study of the sociology of applied knowledge. Dodd, Mead and Company, New York
Freidson E (2001) Professionalism: the third logic. University of Chicago Press, Chicago, IL
Henderson S, Peterson A (2002) Consuming health: the commodification of health care. Routledge, London
Horwitz A, Wakefield J (2007) The loss of sadness: how psychiatry has transformed normal sadness into depressive disorder. Oxford University Press, New York
Houck J (2006) Hot and bothered: women, medicine, and menopause in modern America. Harvard University Press, Cambridge, MA
Illich I (1976) Medical nemesis. Pantheon, New York
Inhorn M (2006) Defining women's health: a dozen messages from more than 150 ethnographies. Med Anthropol Q 20(3):345–378
Kaufmann C (1999) An introduction to the mental health consumer movement. In: Horwitz AV, Scheid TL (eds) A handbook for the study of mental health: social contexts, theories, and systems. Cambridge University Press, Cambridge, pp 493–506
Kelleher D (1994) Self-help groups and medicine. In: Gabe J, Kelleher D, Williams G (eds) Challenging medicine. Routledge, New York, pp 104–117
Kremer M, Tonkens E (2006) Authority, trust, knowledge, and the public good in disarray. In: Duyvendak J, Knijn T, Kremer M (eds) Policy, people, and the new professional: de-professionalisation and re-professionalisation in care and welfare. Amsterdam University Press, Amsterdam, pp 122–134
Lane C (2007) Shyness: how normal behavior became a sickness. Yale University Press, New Haven, CT
Larson M (1977) The rise of professionalism. University of California Press, Berkeley, CA
Light D (2000) The medical profession and organizational change: from professional dominance to countervailing power. In: Bird C, Conrad P, Fremont A (eds) Handbook of medical sociology. Prentice-Hall, Upper Saddle River, NJ, pp 201–216
Litt J (2000) Medicalized motherhood: perspectives from the lives of African-American and Jewish women. Rutgers University Press, New Brunswick, NJ
Loe M (2004) The rise of Viagra. New York University Press, New York
Lupton D (1997) Consumerism, reflexivity and the medical encounter. Soc Sci Med 45(3):373–381
Mamo L (2005) Biomedicalizing kinship: sperm banks and the creation of affinity-ties. Sci Cult 14(3):237–264
Mamo L (2007) Queering reproduction: achieving pregnancy in the age of technoscience. Duke University Press, Durham, NC
Martin E (1987) The woman in the body: a cultural analysis of reproduction. Beacon Press, Boston, MA
Morello-Frosch R, Zawestoski S, Brown P, Altman RG, McCormick S, Mayer B (2006) Embodied health movements: responses to a 'scientized' World. In: Frickel S, Moore K (eds) The new political sociology of science: institutions, networks and power. University of Wisconsin Press, Madison, WI
Nye R (2003) The evolution of the concept of medicalization in the twentieth century. J Hist Behav Sci 39(2):115–129
Oxford English Dictionary (2008) Oxford, UK http://dictionary.oed.com
Parsons T (1951) The social system. The Free Press, Glencoe, IL
Pescosolido B (2006) Professional dominance and the limits of erosion. Society 43(6):21–29
Pescosolido B, Martin J (2004) Cultural authority and the sovereignty of american medicine: the role of networks, class and community. J Health Polit Policy Law 29(4–5):735–755
Peterson MJ (1978) The medical profession in mid-Victorian London. University of California Press, Berkeley, CA

Popay J, Williams G, Thomas C, Gatrell A (1998) "Theorising inequalities in health: the place of lay knowledge. Sociol Health Illn 20(5):619–644

Porter R (1985) The patient's view: doing medical history from below. Theory Soc 14:175–198

Prior L (2003) Belief, knowledge and expertise: the emergence of the lay expert in medical sociology. Sociol Health Illn 25(3):41–57

Quadagno J (2005) One nation uninsured: why the U.S. has no national health insurance. Oxford University Press, New York

Riessman CK (1983) Women and medicalization: a new perspective. Soc Policy (Summer):3–18

Riska, Elianne (2003) "Gendering the Medicalization Thesis." Advances in Gender Research: Gender Perspectives on Health and Medicine, edited by M. Segal and V. Demos. London: Elsevier 7:59–87

Ruzek S (1978) The women's health movement. Praeger, New York

Scott W (1990) PTSD in the DSM-III: a case in the politics of diagnosis and disease. Soc Probl 37(3):294–310

Shim J (2005) Constructing 'race' across the science-lay divide: racial formation in the epidemiology and experience of cardiovascular disease. Soc Stud Sci 35(3):405–436

Scott S, Prior L, Wood F, Gray J (2005) Repositioning the patient: the implications of being 'at risk'. Soc Sci Med 60:1869–1879

Szasz T ([1961]1974) The myth of mental illness: foundations of a theory of personal conduct, Revisedth edn. HarperCollins, New York

Tomes N (2001) Merchants of health: medicine and consumer culture in the United States, 1900–1940.J Am Hist <http://www.historycooperative.org/cgibin/justtop.cgi?act=justtop&url=http://www.historycooperative.org/journals/jah/88.2/tomes.html> (16 Oct. 2008)

Waitzkin H (1993) The politics of medical encounters: how patients and doctors deal with social problems. Yale University Press, New Haven

Winnick T, Werum R, Pavalko E (2001) Managing mental illness: trends in continuing mental health education for family doctors, 1977–1996. In: Kronenfeld JJ (ed) Research in the sociology of health care. JAI, Greenwich, CT, pp 179–203

Woloshin S, Schwartz L (2006) Giving legs to restless legs: a case study of how the media helps make people sick. PLoS Med 3(4):e170. doi:10.1371/journal.pmed.0030170

Zavestoski S, Brown P, McCormick S, Mayer B, D'Ottavi M, Lucove JC (2004) Patient activism and the struggle for diagnosis: Gulf War illnesses and other medically unexplained physical symptoms in the U.S. Soc Sci Med 58(1):161–175

Zola I (1972) Medicine as an institution of social control. Sociol Rev 20:497–504

Chapter 16
Mundane Medicine, Therapeutic Relationships, and the Clinical Encounter: Current and Future Agendas for Sociology

Carl May

Introduction

Since the 1950s, a long period of peace and steady economic growth in advanced economies has permitted the diversion of capital into both coordinated taxation or insurance based health services and a concomitant expansion in educational and professional infrastructures for health professionals. Sociological writings over the past 40 years have shown how these have provided a foundation for large scale developments in health services and massive R&D networks. These, in combination with increasing affluence, have meant major improvements in population health (Moran 1999; Starr 1982).

Almost all developed countries now have a substantial and sophisticated institutional apparatus for delivering healthcare. But the rapidly rising relative costs of that healthcare provision have combined with radical changes in the epidemiological landscape – a steadily expanding number of people with chronic illnesses (Holman 2006), and a steadily expanding remit of medicalized explanations for personal problems (Conrad 2007) – to make healthcare a major political problem. There is need for this to be *managed* simultaneously at the macro-level of policy formation and the micro-level of interactions between healthcare providers and consumers. This is a major problem for policy makers (Rosenman et al. 2006). In all of these shifts, experiences of illness have ceased to be a private matter; instead they are not only to be diagnosed and treated, but also to be recorded, managed, organized, costed, and paid for.

Illnesses are not only experienced, but are measured, classified, coded, and treated according to categories and algorithms that belong to insurers, electronic health record designers, researchers, governments, and evidence makers. The discovery of diseases and their effects is similarly a corporate effort, involving large programs of research, bureaucratically organized, with complex relationships with government and mechanisms of governance and processes of *biomedicalization* (see Clarke and Shim 2009). For, as chronic illness has been constituted as a political and fiscal burden (Hacker 2004), there have been regulatory interventions, in central policy response, that attempt to control costs either by shifting the burden of care from healthcare providers to healthcare consumers, or by restructuring healthcare provision through corporate providers. Also included is bureaucratic interventions that place socio-political constraints on the experiences and actions of people with chronic illness and those who work with them. Chronic illness raises problems of *costs* at every turn.

C. May (✉)
Institute of Health and Society, Newcastle University, 21 Claremont Place,
Newcastle upon Tyne, NE2 4AA, UK
e-mail: c.r.may@ncl.ac.uk

In the light of these changing structural features of health and healthcare, sociologies of medicine, health, and illness need to attend more closely to the *work* that stems from illness – and the technologies and organizational interfaces (May 2007) – through which this work is configured. This in turn leads, to important questions that will inform future sociological research. It also raises important theoretical questions about how to understand the relationship between the interactional conduct of healthcare and its organizational contexts.

If we are to balance the interactional conduct of healthcare with its organizational contexts, we must start with a reconsideration of the very units of analysis with which we are sociologically concerned. Elsewhere (May 2007) I have argued that to understand the impact of these shifts, sociology needs to reconsider one of its central units of analysis – the Parsonian vision of the autonomous clinical encounter between doctor and patient. The Parsonian paradigm draws its continuity and strength from the notion of the clinical encounter as a dyadic system (Henderson 1935). It is more rigorously developed in Parson's analysis of medicine in *The Social System* (Parsons 1951) in which professional and patient roles are conceived in terms of privatized and proximal relations, and in which the moral qualities of these roles rest on the capacity of doctors to maintain the direction and boundaries of the clinical encounter itself. Parsons points to the way in which the "segregation of the context of clinical practice from other contexts" (1951, p. 457) underpins this analysis. In the Parsonian paradigm, the clinical encounter rests not just on a division of labor, but also on a labor of division. Medicine's practices are seen to be organizationally and professionally located, but these locations are secondary to the privatized – mainly dyadic – social *relations* through which they are mobilized and enacted in the clinic.

Since the 1960s, Parsons' concept of the clinical encounter has been criticized by sociologists concerned with chronic illness (Gerhardt 1989), and its continuing effects have been argued to represent under-theorization from within sociology itself (Scambler and Britten 2001). Nevertheless, it has continuously sedimented into sociological research and practice. It finds expression across a range of theoretical perspectives ranging from microscopic studies of professional–patient interaction (Heritage and Maynard 2006), to critiques of the social construction of medical knowledge and institutions (Morris 2003). Indeed, as William Cockerham (2005) has observed, Parsons' theoretical position on the clinical encounter represents a continuous point of engagement for medical sociology – to which we could add that it contributes significantly to both sociological theorizing about medicine and health, and medical theorizing about practice.

A renewed perspective on the sociology of professional practice in healthcare needs to focus critical attention on its relationships with the corporate terrain on which it is set. This is not an appeal for an organizational sociology of healthcare. It does, however, recognize that the clinical encounter is now penetrated systematically by corporate mechanisms of reciprocal regulation and surveillance. Parsons (1951, 1965) acknowledged this tendency (1951, p. 426), but characterized it as a product of improvements in technologies of *treatment* rather than the amplification of governance and management. The latter have now become critical to the production and mobilization of clinical practices. This means that sociological understanding of the clinical encounter needs to be framed explicitly in relation to the organizing impulses that run through it. In what follows, I am going to argue that in the future, sociological research will need to take more seriously the technologies and practices of therapeutic relationships that are currently constituted in the ecological spaces of healthcare.

One implication of these shifts is, as I have hinted above, the problem of theorizing the problems of health and health care. A focus on constructedness and identity is a consequence of the so-called "narrative turn" in social science of the 1980s and 1990s (Rosenau 1992), and its consequence for contemporary medical sociology is the great emphasis that is laid on socially constructed identities, the narratives through which these identities are expressed, and the lived experiences of belonging that stem from them. Interrogating identity, however, can only carry us so far. The problem of the hard *work* of chronic illness, and the practices of its *management*, raises questions about *action* – both individual and collective – that open up important terrain for future sociological research. The shift that I propose here is from a sociology of the discursive constitution of chronic illness (focused on lived experiences of identities and narratives of (dis) integration with the lifeworld), to a sociology of enacting chronic illness (focused on the work of managing and exchanging material and symbolic resources and mechanisms for (re)integration with the lifeworld). This draws health inequalities and health care organization into the frame of analysis not only as problems of policy, but as fields of action for ordinary citizens in everyday life. Although I cannot pursue the question here, the business of enacting and managing chronic illness also raises a core problem of intra and inter-disciplinary research, which is to consider the relative contributions of individual differences and social factors in achieving the outcomes of healthcare innovations and interventions.

In what follows, I consider the changing terrain of the work through which chronic illness is *enacted* using Normalization Process Theory (May and Finch 2009) My aim is (1) to show how this process of normalizing the *work* of managing chronic illness itself accords with four generative mechanisms: *coherence*; *cognitive participation*; *collective action*; and *reflexive monitoring*; and (2) to show how these mechanisms are made visible in the tendencies or impulses that can be observed in the changing social organization of chronic illness.

The Chronic Disease Epidemic and the Problem of Mundane Healthcare

Sociological analysis in the area of chronic illness has been conducted against a backdrop of the seismic shift in the epidemiological landscapes of the U.S., UK, and other advanced economies. Much of this research has been conducted against the background of dedicated policy structures that apply models for the long term management of this problem (Gately et al. 2007; Holman 2006; Rosenman et al. 2006; Solberg 2007). In the UK, for example, the so-called Kaiser triangle (Fig. 16.1), named after the Californian HMO, Kaiser Permanente, has made frequent appearances in health policy (Conrad 2007). It divides the population into three groups:

- *Case management* is for patients with multiple, complex conditions, involving intensive, proactive care to avoid complications and admissions.
- *Disease management* is for patients at some risk and involves supporting patients with chronic conditions through guideline-based programs in primary care, facilitated by new financial incentives.
- *Self-management* is for low risk patients (and is estimated at 70–80% of those with a chronic condition).

These attributions are important. At the beginning of this chapter, I pointed to the ways in which the problems of costs are crucial, and frameworks such as these function as tools by which those costs are to be divide, equally, and by which eligibility for expenditure is to be decided. Once again, they draw our attention to the problem of management and the labor of division. In this context, for example, recent work on medicalization of personal problems (Conrad 2007) draws attention to only one side of the story. It is true that elements of everyday life are steadily medicalized, but it is also the case that there are reciprocal relations and counter-relations that seek to relocate or blur the boundaries of the formal responsibilities of healthcare agencies. The politicization of disease categories, through the activities of social movements and interest groups as clinical knowledge and social policy become increasingly integrated through evidence-based medicine and health policy is one expression of this. The bureaucratization of medicine as a mechanism for regulating and governing health professionals, services, and decisions about coverage, is another. The Kaiser triangle is exactly such a device: it specifies the focus of expenditure, the thresholds of service provision, and the boundaries of personal responsibility. It fits well with ideas about the threats posed by

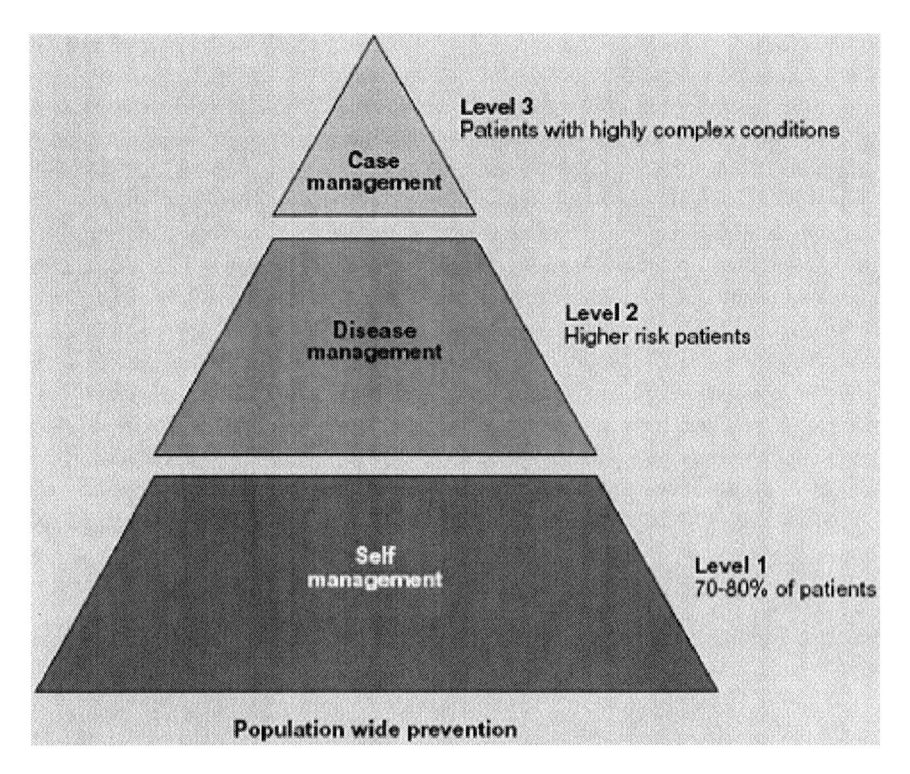

Fig. 16.1 The Kaiser Permanente triangle (Department of Health, 2004, p. 36)

chronic illness. Elsewhere (May 2005), I have characterized these threats through three propositions:

- *Many chronic illnesses are related to an aging and relatively affluent society.* This may be characterized by multiple and complex co-morbidities, and a variety of social problems. These include organic *systems failures*: Type 2 diabetes; some cardiovascular diseases; some respiratory diseases; and some cancers. In older age these diseases also include neurodegenerative diseases (e.g., the dementias), some gastro–intestinal disorders (including constipation, diverticulitis, and incontinence), more cardiovascular diseases (e.g. chronic heart failure), and cancers.
- *Many chronic illnesses are related to a society that experiences particular kinds of social problems around personal agency, capacity, and mobility.* Biomechanical incapacities which are explicable in medical terms include arthritis and its variants, along with musculo–skeletal strains, injuries and architectural failures (e.g., prolapsed discs); while those which have a poor medical explanation include chronic lower back pain, fibromyalgia, chronic fatigue syndrome, and most obviously of all, medically unexplained symptoms.
- *Many chronic illnesses are related to experiences of existential alienation, disengagement and dismay,* often in the face of fractured or decaying life-chances. Personal psychosocial problems which are explicable in medical terms include addiction, depression and anxiety, and other mental health problems ranging from eating disorders to schizophrenia. Personal psychosocial problems which seem less easily medicalized include chronic unhappiness and stress.

These are clearly not the "families" of pathologies that are found in the *International Classification of Diseases,* or the *Diagnostic and Statistical Manual of the American Medical Association* . This links disease categories to the bureaucratic systems of insurance and research (Bowker and Leigh-Star 1999) but they are of sociological relevance because they shape chronicity in ways that are fundamentally *social* in their production, mediation, and effects. In doing so, they raise problems and questions around professional knowledge and practice, and each leads to the therapeutic problems of persons, as well as some pathological process. These therapeutic problems are formed around, for example, the psychological sequelae of chronic pain (Eccleston et al. 1997); quality of life factors, such as obstructive airways in diseases like asthma (Lagerlov et al. 1998); and as emotional obstacles to patients' or professionals' understanding, action and adherence to treatment regimens in diabetes (Bissell et al. 2004).

One way of looking at this explosion of personal factors that frames chronic illness is by representing a process of medicalization – human experiences, identities, and personal problems are colonized by knowledge and practice from the clinical sciences, and come to be routinely defined (Conrad 2007). However, there is an alternative to medicalization perspectives. This is to see the extension of "clinical" definitions of personal experience in chronic illness as the product of a reciprocal interaction between medicine and society. This is, at least in part, because it reflects the extent to which social factors have penetrated the biomedical world-view. In the light of the cultural and political shifts of the 1960s onwards, patients – and increasingly, professionals – began to complain about what they saw as the *objectification* of experiences of illness (May 1992a). As objects of clinical procedure and practice, patients began to see themselves as alienated, not simply from decisions about the trajectories of their treatment, but also from their own bodies and lives. The root of this was seen to be in a kind of biomedical paternalism, which separated personal experiences from medical knowledge (Turner 1995). These political complaints about the experience of medicine, rather than the experience of disease, fit well with internal shifts within medical discourse – and were co-opted and harnessed by clinical proponents of biopsychosocial models of health, holistic medical practice (Engel 1977), and person-centered care (Mead and Bower 2002). Most recently, they have run through criticisms of "evidence-based" medicine (Summerskill and Pope 2002).

Whatever the clinical, moral or political impulses that drive it, clinical acknowledgement of the individuality of patients' experiences is problematic. First, just as the Parsonian Paradigm in medical sociology focused on the dyadic relations between patient and doctor, so too have the clinical proponents of holism. "Individual care" is a problem because it no longer refers to bounded social relations: in chronic illness, specific temporal episodes of disease are displaced by lifetime careers and co-morbidities. Similarly, the sick role (Parsons 1951) expressed by doctor and patient in intensive experiences of disease, has been displaced by "biographical disruption" (Bury 1982). In this context, the emergence of ideas about patient-centeredness in medicine and nursing (May 1992a), and a concern with the quality of communications (Heritage and Maynard 2006), are elements of the breakdown of the processes of objectification that drove medicine through the first great wave of scientific reconstruction between 1850 and 1950 (Armstrong 1983). The strange bifurcation between acute disease and chronic illness that has subsequently formed around both changes in the epidemiological landscape, and the organization of healthcare, is reflected in the routine embedding of work to manage or palliate signs and symptoms in the community, rather than to engender the cure of disease. Indeed, one reason why the lived experiences of people with chronic illnesses have become so important to the clinical and social sciences is that they are increasingly concerned with "managing" these experiences themselves. This leads us to the first of the mechanisms that I signaled at the beginning of the chapter:

- *Coherence*: Healthcare work that defines and organizes patients and their problems as objects of clinical attention; and micro-level practices that ensure the sick person's *contextual integration* with healthcare systems and services.

At a micro-level, the acknowledgement of individuality is central to making the work of managing chronic illness coherent, it defines the rationale for its component practices in relation to the person who must perform them, and in relation to the resources that they can call upon to complete them.

At a macro-level, work around the production of a coherent field of practice specifies the expectations of its inhabitants, and frames the ways that these are defined and understood. Individualization is crucial to healthcare systems because it makes sensible the idea that sick people are "consumers," and enrolls them in processes of choice, satisfaction, and quality control (Sullivan 2003). It is important not to over-estimate these historical changes in professional attitudes, or to assume that patients' preferences are central to medical knowledge and practice. Sociological and anthropological research consistently emphasizes that medical students learn that "real" medicine is about organic disease and biological dysfunctions, and that patients' social experiences and social contexts are more or less irrelevant to their deliberations (Good 1994; Sinclair 1997). Their subsequent challenge, then, is to fit together the understanding of the social and emotional with the biological. Hunter (1991) has shown just how hard, in practice, it is for young doctors and how difficult it is to integrate knowledge about the *experiences* of sick people into the *institutional* worldview of the clinic. Although the choices and preferences of "consumers" may not always be important to the practice of medicine, they can matter very much to healthcare *systems* as these seek to define their operational relations with people who are simultaneously dependent clients and discerning customers.

Routinizing the Work of Patient-Hood

The emergence of work to *manage* chronic illness in contemporary healthcare does not simply revolve around the individualization of patients, and integrating the experiential aspects of patient-hood within the clinic. The work of management itself makes new kinds of works, and impacts powerfully the division of labor in healthcare. It affects the structure of labor processes themselves (Harrison 2002) because the efforts of the workers involved (who need not be professionals) are invested in care rather than cure. This becomes evident when we look at three further propositions about the social organization of chronic illness.

- *Chronic illness demands surveillance of the stability and trajectory of illness states* (through routine tests and examinations, and by the use of remote monitoring systems) and impact on gross workload (May et al. 2005). There is now so much chronic illness encountered in the community that it can no longer be solely medically managed.
- *Chronic illness produces routine and highly determinate patterns of professional labor* that extends over a lifetime of illness careers. This leads to Fordist models of task centeredness (Braverman 1974) – reducing work to its simplest components and delegating these downwards to aides and home care workers, while retaining key complex assessments and treatment decisions within medicine and nursing (Hanlon et al. 2005).
- *Chronic illness produces forms of professional work which are more amenable to external regulation and governance*. Here, the professional labor which is involved in the management of chronic illness is increasingly bureaucratic in form, because of the pressures to control costs, to meet the demands of clinical governance (Castellani and Wear 2000; Snooks et al. 2008), and to standardize care around "evidence" (Berg et al. 2000).

To say that social processes of *routinization* are an important part of the ways that healthcare systems have responded to the epidemiological transition from acute to chronic illness is in no way to assume that these illnesses – for example, diabetes, asthma, and heart failure – have an inferior moral status to their episodic counterparts, or that they are less dangerous to their sufferers. Put bluntly: people with asthma can die horribly from suffocation; diabetes can cause people to lose their sight or limbs; while people with heart failure sometimes drown on dry land (Nuland 1994). These are sometimes horrible diseases. But they demand different kinds of *work* than their acute counterparts, and as I have suggested above, they demand a different kind of division of labor. Central to this is the notion not of an integrated professional workforce, but of a distributed division of labor. That includes not only the different categories of healthcare, workers but also the patient and a local network of others – who might include close or extended family members – that blurs the divisions in the division of labor.

The division of labor in the management of chronic illness is a complex one, and involves not only variations in knowledge and practice, but also significant differences in the degrees of dependence that stem from them. But from this analysis of the business of *dividing* and *doing* mundane healthcare, and normalizing chronicity into everyday practice, we can derive a second mechanism:

- *Cognitive Participation*: Healthcare work that defines and organizes the allocation and performance of tasks implicated in the management of chronic illness; and micro-level practices that are defined by their *skill-set workability* within formal and informal divisions of healthcare labor.

The heterogeneous relations along which these tasks are arrayed, and the divisions of labor that are formed around it, are illustrated in Fig. 16.2, which maps the range of actors that have coalesced around a person with diabetes. Some of these actors are formally defined in direct relation to the *disease* of diabetes, because they primarily work to test and assess its physiological processes and their effects, and then to act upon those processes with drug treatments that deal with the primary problem and its co-morbidities (physicians and nurses). Others are formally defined as *intermediaries*, either in a professional services capacity (the dietician), as intermediaries like the call center operative who gathers data about blood sugar levels, and the pharmacist, who acts as one in a chain of intermediaries between the person with diabetes and the pharmaceutical companies that sell drugs. These formally defined relations offer clinical and related services through which the routine trajectory of the disease is managed. With each of them the diabetic person can enter into a degree of therapeutic negotiation – and they may reciprocate with notions of patient centered or client

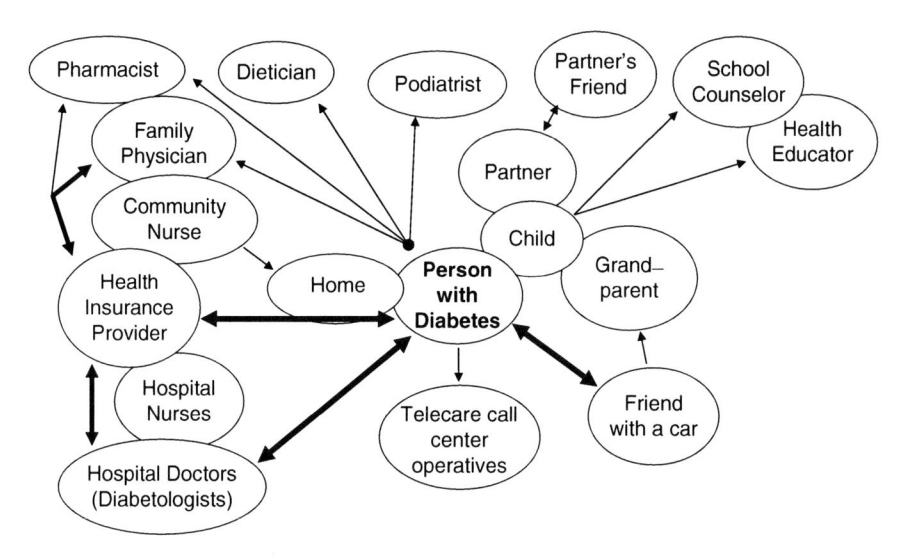

Fig. 16.2 Mapping the hard work of managing chronic illness

centered practice (Epstein et al. 2002). Their work can, again, be defined through three propositions:

- *The management of chronic illness requires both the surveillance of the body to maintain stability* (e.g., diabetes or ischemic heart disease); and acting on the body to palliate organic decline (e.g., chronic heart failure or COPD).
- *The management of chronic illness requires attempts to palliate longstanding symptoms* (e.g., arthritis) or to conceptualize the often poor "fit" between revealed organic pathology and expressed symptoms (e.g., chronic low back pain) with a view to restoring independence and mobilization.
- *The management of chronic illness requires attempts to resolve problems stemming from the interaction between the sufferer and the social world* (e.g., anxiety) or to palliate existential pain and personal crises (e.g., depression), with a view to restoring personal and social engagement.

Professional intermediaries have therapeutic relationships with patients that are organized around norms of membership (what it takes to be a doctor or a nurse), behavior (how professional patient interaction should be accomplished, and the boundaries that should be placed on it), and distribution (how resources and rewards are organized and allocated). This normative approach (Therborn 2003) helps us understand the structure as well as the content of professional–patient relations. But these normative relationships are made meaningful by ideas about the importance of *relationships*. The professional–patient relationship has, of course, a legal as well as a moral meaning (Jacob 1999). But as the professions have struggled with individualization – the process by which experiencing subjects can be integrated within the clinical domain – so to have they struggled with the notion that these integrative interactions have personally integrative qualities (May 1992b). Ideas about patient centeredness in medicine (Mead and Bower 2000), and phenomenological theories of practice in nursing (Fawcett 2000), provide a framework for the work of controlling (and sometimes palliating) chronic disease. This work also seeks to effect the patient's mobilization and engagement with the life-world. Further, this relationship-building lubricates – for both parties – the incivilities of the healthcare system itself. "Good" personal relations, "knowing the patient" and "being known" by professionals have positive effects for all parties, imbuing a sense of community and common purpose (Solberg 2007).

It is also clear from Fig. 16.2 that there are other actors with strong ties to the person with diabetes who make it possible for the routine work of being ill to be accomplished. Families and friends carry a significant burden on behalf of people with chronic illness, managing and organizing medications and coordinating interactions with services (Dovey-Pearce et al. 2007) (for example, a car is a practical necessity in an environment where there is no public transport). Indeed, just as the divisions of labor amongst healthcare workers are often blurred, so too is the identity of the "patient" in chronic illness, when many actors also benefit from the services not only of professionals, but also from the family and friends who support them. In consideration of these factors, we can find a third mechanism:

- *Collective Action*: Healthcare work that defines and organizes the enacting of practices of care in the management of chronic illness; and micro-level practices that are defined by their *interactional workability* within a set of everyday social relations.

In Fig. 16.2, there is a further actor upon whom the person with diabetes is dependent, who delegates the routine office work of establishing eligibility and maintaining coverage, and who decides the care that professionals can give to their patients (Gask 2004; Harrison and Dowswell 2002). That is, the agency that funds all or part of the business of being sick.In the US, it is the health insurance corporations, Medicaid or the Veterans' Administration, and in other countries, it is the government – such as the National Health Service in the UK or trade union funded health services in Germany or the Netherlands (Moran 1999). At the time of writing, around 47 million Americans have no health insurance (Benoit 2003).

Shared Decisions and the Mobilization of Patient-Hood

So far, we have seen that the *management* of chronic disease depends on cognitive participation and collective action, as a set of processes that "fit" mainly routine practices to the skill-sets of patients and professionals, and that further makes these practices interactionally workable in the clinical encounter. I want to turn now to one set of specific mechanisms, by which management is embedded in experiences of patient-hood – shared-decision-making tools. These are means by which the perspective of the sick person can be accommodated in decisions about how to manage the trajectory of their illness. They may include computer software (Robinson and Thomson 2001; Thomson et al. 2007) that structures decisions according to preferences, protocols for embedding "evidence" in clinical practice though leaflets (so called "bibliotherapy"), video, or audio, and structured workbooks that guide professionals through the process of engaging patients in choices about medication and other clinical interventions (O'Connor et al. 1999, 2007). Elsewhere, with colleagues, I have outlined three "impulses" of *technogovernance* (May et al. 2006) that seem to be implicated in the drive towards these new systems of clinical practice. In keeping with the focus of this chapter, these are recast here as a set of three propositions:

- *The codification and representation of "evidence" is a possible point of departure for shared decision-making.* Evidence itself is embedded in "soft" and "hard" technologies that routinize and simplify complex management strategies (Bloomfield and Vurdubakis 1999).
- *The incorporation of decision-management technologies in the clinical encounter threatens to decouple subjective experience from clinical action.* New technologies (in the form of guidelines, protocols, and decision-making tools) act to structure the range of possible decisions in the clinical encounter itself. The patient's (and to a lesser degree, the professional's) subjective experience is therefore separated from decisions about the proper management of a problem (May et al. 2006).
- *Decision-management technologies begin to distribute accountability beyond the clinical encounter*, and frame the patient as both self-manager and the source of a minimum data-set about clinical condition. The first of these firmly relocates subjectivity in the life-world of the patient. The second abstracts from the life-world only those data that are necessary to determine the trajectory of a chronic illness, analyses this within parameters that objectively define the point at which health care interventions might be required, and alerts an appropriate authority (May et al. 2005).

I have argued that clinical interaction cannot be seen as an autonomous or privatized encounter, but needs to be seen as representing the organizing interfaces of corporate forces (May 2007). Inevitably, this structure leads to a set of tensions. This is primarily between the production of individual identities and qualities in the clinical encounter (about which, of course, the professional retains medico-legal responsibility), and the production and mediation of facts about groups and populations, which in recent years have come to be called "evidence-based" medicine. This forms a commonly noted key impulse (May 2007), between *individualization* (the *patient-centred* clinical practices in which patients' experiences and perspectives of ill-health are *qualitatively* engaged in decisions about the management of illness trajectories); and *aggregation* (the mobilization of evidence about populations revealed through *quantitative* knowledge about populations that is enrolled to guide the management of illness, and is mediated through clinical guidelines).

Questions about evidence and evidence-based medicine have become central to debates about the institutional and political relationship between "medicine" and "patients," and have focused on the problems of simultaneously working out both individualised and aggregate knowledge about patients in the clinical encounter. The focus on the production, mediation, and effects of *evidential* facts about individuals and about populations are key elements of healthcare work that act to categorise and discipline the routinization of *management*. Just as Weber (1947) observed that rule-bound bureaucracies rationalized social relations, so too the bureaucratization of clinical decisions controls the calls that chronic sickness can place on systems of healthcare by returning responsibilities for interpretation and action to the sick person. For healthcare funders it holds out the possibility of ironing out special pleading for spending, and controlling the clinical decisions of professionals. But more than this, these technologies provide a framework for individualization that mitigates its most disruptive effects not on *medical* authority, but on the protocols and procedures of *corporate* healthcare systems. We can define this according to a fourth mechanism:

- *Reflexive Monitoring*: Healthcare work that defines and organizes mechanisms for he organization of social knowledge around which the management of chronic illness is formed; and micro-level practices that ensure the *relational integration* of lay and professional knowledge with clinical practice.

Corporate healthcare systems depend on such mechanisms to rationalize and organize the activities of all of their participants. We are used to seeing these extend to professionals and service providers, through governance systems (Rhodes 1997), performance measurement, data-sharing, and information management (Mor 2005). However, they increasingly extend to sick people themselves. Telecare systems, for example, offer means to monitor physiological indicators such as blood sugar in diabetes (Gomez et al. 2002), or blood oxygenation in obstructive airway disease (Hibbert et al. 2004). Web-based interfaces call upon sick people to enter data and manage assessments themselves (Celler et al. 2003; Glykas and Chytas 2004). These innovations go beyond self-care, but integrate the *work* of routine data collection and management across the formal boundaries of the healthcare provider and the informal boundaries of the home. They do one other thing. The individualized, managed (and managing) sick person's narrative of subjective experience, and negotiated field of therapeutic relations with health professionals, is to be put in second place. What *is* brought forward are the objective thresholds of disease measures. Eligibility for care is defined in population terms, and is offered in exchange for the work of individual data entry (May et al. 2005). Being "known" is displaced by meeting measures.

Conclusion: Reconfiguring the Parsonian Paradigm

So far, I have argued that the Parsonian vision of the clinical encounter as a privatized set of practices has been overwhelmed by the corporate impulses that now run through healthcare systems. Further, I have argued that practices and technologies of management are now central to the production of clinical problems and the ways that these are worked through in the lives of people with chronic illnesses, their families, and the various professionals and paraprofessionals that work with them. This argument has implications for one of Parsons' key contributions to understanding health behaviors – the "sick role" – which is discussed on pp 436–437 of *The Social System*.[1]

Parsons argued that the sick role represented far more than a condition, and that it should be seen as a "set of institutionalized expectations" and that these are "relative to the nature and severity of the illness." There are four of them. The sick person is exempted from normal social role responsibilities, and is also exempted from responsibility for the sickness itself. By the same token, the sick person is obliged to want to be well, and is also obliged to seek technically competent help. This vision of rights and obligations has been criticized because it fails to deal adequately with the problem of chronic illness (Gerhardt 1989). Parsons himself was well aware of this problem (Parsons 1975), which can be explained in part by his concentration on *acute* hospital medicine in the detailed fieldwork that led up to the elaboration of the sick role (Parsons 1977), and also in part by

---

[1] Page numbers refer to the English edition published by Routledge and Kegan Paul (London, 1951)

the longstanding illness (panic disorder and major depression) of his daughter Anne which led to her suicide in 1968 (Orr 2006).

Most importantly, Parsons' account of the sick role should not be assumed to be an *individualizing* account of the moral standing of sick people. It is rather more complicated than that, since what Parsons seems to be doing is to pointing to the ways in which roles are articulated to (socialized) action, and given Parsons' interest in Freud (Parsons 1977; Rocher 1974), to (unconscious) motivation. The discussion of the sick role in *The Social System* is in this sense a prolog to the much more detailed discussion of formal and informal roles and situations that is then developed. In this context, Parsons has important things to say about how doctor and patient are positioned *in relation* to each other – and these seem to be oriented towards securing independence of each other. The physician is objective and detached, and does not become caught up in sentimental relations with the patient; the patient is seeking technical help, and is motivated to want to be well.

Motivation remains crucial to the management of chronic illness. Work that is organized around mechanisms of coherence, cognitive participation, collective action, and reflexive monitoring, depends on a set of attitudinal expectations of the sick person. Normalizing practices of management require that sick people seek to meet four conditions. They need to be:

- *Prudent* (willing to minimize the load that they place on formal healthcare provision)
- *Resourceful* (with the capacity to operationalize knowledge and link it to existing patterns of service provision)
- *Agentic* (actively engaged in decision-making and treatment processes)
- *Expert* (in possession of the knowledge and skills for appraising management advice and self-care outcomes)

These attitudinal expectations are much less concerned with securing independence and much more concerned with the organization of *interdependence*, and they specify very particular kinds of engagement with the hard work of being ill. Earlier, I observed that the "sick role" has been displaced by "biographical disruption," and these attitudinal expectations are, of course, congruent with those qualities that support not "adjustment" or "coping" with the disruptions that chronic illness brings in its wake, but with actively engaging them. In Table 16.1, these qualities are connected with the four theorized mechanisms outlined in the course of the chapter. This links the moral status of the sick person with the kinds of work they are now expected to do in the managed economy of chronic illness. It is governed in important ways by their capacity and motivation – so that susceptibility to disease has its counterpart in culpability for failure to engage with organizational objectives.

My thesis, simply put, is that the tremendous epidemiological explosion in chronic illness since the 1950s has brought in its wake not only major changes in the distribution and experience of illness and ill-health, but also major changes in the *work* of being ill and managing illness. These need to form the focus of a sociological agenda at the beginning of the twenty-first century. The nature of much clinical care is increasingly stabilized and routinized as it focuses on managing symptoms across lifetime illness careers, but it is also shared. Boundaries between formal (professional) and informal (lay) systems of practice are blurred by changing patterns of eligibility and definitions of personal responsibility. At the same time, this routinized clinical work is increasingly aimed at creating conditions to secure stable disease trajectories and palliate symptoms, and new technologies that enable these to be monitored are coming into play. One of the aims of this chapter has been to show how this leads us to a set of expectations of ideal organizational qualities of sick people.

In this context, there is nothing ironic in drawing a parallel between the management of workers and the management of patients, for such an approach offers a fruitful set of questions for future work in the sociology of health and healing. Both processes share the same concerns with rationalization of skills and costs, the struggle to define rights and responsibilities, and hegemony and

Table 16.1 Factors that promote the normalization of systems of 'management' for chronic illness

Domain of work (Macro level)	Everyday practices (Micro level)	Expectation of the patient
Coherence: Work that defines and organizes patients and their problems as objects of clinical attention.	Practices that ensure the sick person's *contextual integration* with healthcare systems and services.	*resourcefulness* (capacity to operationalize knowledge and link it to existing patterns of service provision)
Cognitive Participation: Work that defines and organizes the allocation and performance of tasks implicated in the management of chronic illness.	Practices that are defined by their *skill-set workability* within formal and informal divisions of healthcare labor.	*agency* (active engagement in shared decision-making and treatment processes)
Collective Action: Work that defines and organizes the enacting of practices of care in the management of chronic illness,	Practices that are defined by their *interactional workability* within a set of everyday social relations.	*prudence* (willingness to minimize the load that they place on formal healthcareprovision).
Reflexive Monitoring: Work that defines and organizes mechanisms for social accountability and confidence in the professional knowledge around which the management of chronic illness is formed.	Practices that ensure the *relational integration* of lay and professional knowledge with clinical practice.	*expertise* (possession of the knowledge and skills for appraising management advice and self-management outcomes)

resistance to authoritative knowledge and practice. Michel Foucault argued in *The Birth of the Clinic* that the history of modernity is imbued with struggles about the boundaries of subjects and subjectivities (Foucault 1973), but he also noted that the discourse of subjectivity was one of the means by which power was implicated as a quality of relations between persons and institutions. The strategic discourses of management that run through policy responses to chronic illness on both sides of the Atlantic blur the boundaries between health workers and, increasingly, incorporate sick people and their families in the processes of organizing and delivering care. Foucault's dictum, that "discourse constitutes its own objects" (Foucault 1986) hints at the ways that the process of institutionalization is formed around ways of characterizing and organizing ideas about the *work that we do*.

I gratefully acknowledge a personal research fellowship awarded by the UK Economic and Social Research Council (Grant RES 0002 700 84) that supported the work leading up to this chapter, which builds on a contribution to the inaugural seminar for the journal *Chronic Illness* (May 2005). I thank Chris Dowrick, Catherine Exley, Tracy Finch, Linda Gask, Catherine Exley, Frances Mair, Chris May, Tiago Moreira, Tim Rapley and Anne Rogers for their helpful comments on this work at various stages of its development.

References

Armstrong D (1983) Political economy of the body. Cambridge University Press, Cambridge
Benoit C (2003) The politics of health care policy – The United States in comparative perspective. Perspect Biolo Med 46:592–599
Berg M et al (2000) Guidelines, professionals and the production of objectivity: standardisation and the professionalism of insurance medicine. Sociol Health Illn 22:765–791
Bissell P et al (2004) From compliance to concordance: barriers to accomplishing a reframed model of health care interactions. Soc Sci Med 58:851–862
Bloomfield BP, Vurdubakis T (1999) The outer limits: monsters, actor networks and the writing of displacement. Organization 6:625–647

Bowker G, Leigh-Star S (1999) Sorting things out. Classification and its consequences. MIT, Cambridge, MA
Braverman H (1974) Labor and monopoly capital: the degradation of work in the twentieth century. Monthly Review Press, London
Bury M (1982) Chronic illness as biographical disruption. Sociol Health Illn 4:167–182
Castellani B, Wear D (2000) Physician views on practicing professionalism in the corporate age. Qual Health Res 10:490–506
Celler BG et al (2003) Using information technology to improve the management of chronic disease. Med J Aust 179:242–246
Clarke A, Shim J (2009) Medicalization and biomedicalization revisited: technoscience and transformations of health and illness. In: Pescosolido BA, McLeod J, Martin JK, Rogers A (eds) The handbook of the sociology of health, illness, and healing. Springer, New York, p XX
Cockerham WC (2005) Medical sociology and sociological theory. In: Cockerham WC (ed) The Blackwell companion to medical sociology. Blackwell, Oxford, pp 3–22
Conrad P (2007) The medicalization of society: on the transformation of human conditions into treatable disorders. Johns Hopkins University Press, Baltimore, MD
Dovey-Pearce G et al (2007) The influence of diabetes upon adolescent and young adult development: a qualitative study. Br J Health Psychol 12:75–91
Eccleston C et al (1997) Patients' and professionals' understandings of the causes of chronic pain: blame, responsibility and identity protection. Soc Sci Med 45:699–709
Engel GL (1977) The need for a new medical model: a challenge for biomedicine. Science 196:136
Epstein RM et al (2002) Hearing voices: patient-centered care with diverse populations. Patient Educ Couns 48:1–3
Fawcett J (2000) Analysis and evaluation of contemporary nursing knowledge: nursing models and theories. FA Davis, Philadelphia, PA
Foucault M (1973) The birth of the clinic: an archaeology of medical perception. Tavistock, London
Foucault M (1986) Afterword: the subject and power. In: Dreyfus HL, Rabinow P (eds) Michel Foucalt: beyond structuralism and hermeneutics. Harvester, Brighton, pp 208–226
Gask L (2004) Powerlessness, control and complexity: the experience of family physicians and a group model HMO. Ann Fam Med 2:150–155
Gately C et al (2007) Re-thinking the relationship between long-term condition self-management education and the utilisation of health services. Soc Sci Med 65:934–945
Gerhardt U (1989) Ideas about Illness: an intellectual and political history of medical sociology. Basingstoke, London
Glykas M, Chytas P (2004) Technological innovations in asthma patient monitoring and care. Expert Syst Appl 27:121–131
Gomez EJ et al (2002) Telemedicine as a tool for intensive management of diabetes: the DIABTel experience. Comput Methods Programs Biomed 69:163–177
Good BJ (1994) How medicine constructs its objects. In: Good BJ (ed) Medicine, rationality and experience. Cambridge University Press, Cambridge, pp 65–87
Hacker JS (2004) Review article: dismantling the health care state? Political institutions, public policies and the comparative politics of health reform. Br J Polit Sci 34:693–724
Hanlon G et al (2005) Knowledge, technology and nursing: the case of NHS direct. Hum Relat 58:147–171
Harrison S (2002) New labour, modernisation and the medical labour process. J Soc Policy 31:465–485
Harrison S, Dowswell G (2002) Autonomy and bureaucratic accountability in primary care: what English general practitioners say. Sociol Health Illn 24:208–226
Henderson LJ (1935) Physician and patient as a social system. N Engl J Med 212:819–823
Heritage J, Maynard DW (2006) Problems and prospects in the study of physician-patient interaction: 30 years of research. Annu Rev Sociol 32:351–374
Hibbert D et al (2004) Health professionals' responses to the introduction of a home telehealth service. J Telemed Telecare 10:226–230
Holman HR (2006) Chronic illness and the healthcare crisis. Chronic Illn 1:265–274
Hunter KM (1991) Doctors' stories: the narrative structure of medical knowledge. Princeton University Press, Princeton, NJ
Jacob JM (1999) Doctors and rules: a sociology of professional values. Transaction, London
Lagerlov P et al (1998) The doctor-patient relationship and the management of asthma. Soc Sci Med 47:85–91
May C (1992a) Individual care? Power and subjectivity in therapeutic relationships. Sociology 26:589–602
May C (1992b) Nursing work, nurses' knowledge, and the subjectification of the patient. Sociol Health Illn 14:472–487
May C (2005) Chronic illness and intractability: professional-patient interactions in primary care. Chronic Illn 1:15–20
May C (2007) The clinical encounter and the problem of context. Sociology 41:29–45

May C, Finch T (2009) Implementation, embedding, and integration: an outline of normalization process theory. Under review
May C et al (2005) Towards a wireless patient: chronic illness scarce care and technological innovation in the United Kingdom. Soc Sci Med 61:1485–1494
May C et al (2006) Technogovernance: evidence, subjectivity, and the clinical encounter in primary care medicine. Soc Sci Med 62:1022–1030
Mead N, Bower P (2000) Patient-centredness: a conceptual framework and review of the empirical literature. Soc Sci Med 51:1087–1110
Mead N, Bower P (2002) Patient-centred consultations and outcomes in primary care: a review of the literature. Patient Educ Couns 48:51–61
Mor V (2005) Improving the quality of long-term care with better information. Milbank Q 83:333–364
Moran M (1999) Governing the health care state: a comparative study of the United Kingdom, the United States and Germany. Manchester University Press, Manchester
Morris DB (2003) Illness and culture in the postmodern age. University of California Press, Berkeley, CA
Nuland SB (1994) How we die. Chatto and Windus, London
O'Connor AM et al (1999) Decision aids for patients facing health treatment or screening decisions: systematic review. Br Med J 319:731–734
O'Connor AM et al (2007) Toward the 'tipping point': decision aids and informed patient choice. Health Aff 26:716–725
Orr J (2006) Panic diaries: a genealogy of panic disorder. Duke University Press, Durham, NC
Parsons T (1951) The social system. Routledge and Kegan Paul, London
Parsons T (1965) Social structure and personality. Free Press, New York
Parsons T (1975) The sick role and the role of the physician reconsidered. In *Action theory and the human condition*. Free Press, New York, pp 17–34
Parsons T (1977) On building social system theory: a personal history. In: Parsons T (ed) Social systems and the evolution of action theory. Free Press, New York, pp 22–77
Rhodes RAW (1997) Understanding governance: policy networks, governance, reflexivity and accountability. Open University Press, Buckingham
Robinson A, Thomson RG (2001) The potential use of decision analysis to support shared decision making in the face of uncertainty: the example of atrial fibrillation and warfarin anticoagulation. Qual Health Care 10:128
Rocher G (1974) Talcott parsons and American sociology. Thomas Nelson and Sons, London
Rosenau P (1992) Postmodernism and the social sciences: insights, inroads and intrusions. Princeton University Press, Princeton, NJ
Rosenman MB et al (2006) The Indiana chronic disease management program. Milbank Q 84:135–163
Scambler G, Britten N (2001) System, lifeworld and doctor-patient interaction: Issues of trust in a changing world. In: Scambler G (ed) Habermas, critical theory and health. Blackwell, London, pp 45–67
Sinclair S (1997) Making doctors: an institutional apprenticeship. Berg, Oxford
Snooks HA et al (2008) Real nursing? The development of telenursing. J Adv Nurs 61:631–640
Solberg LI (2007) Improving medical practice: a conceptual framework. Ann Fam Med 5:251–256
Starr P (1982) The social transformation of American medicine: the rise of a sovereign profession and the making of a vast industry. Basic Books (a division of HarperCollins), London
Sullivan M (2003) The new subjective medicine: taking the patient's point of view on health care and health. Soc Sci Med 56:1595–1604
Summerskill WSM, Pope C (2002) 'I saw the panic rise in her eyes, and evidence-based medicine went out of the door' – An exploratory qualitative study of the barriers to secondary prevention in the management of coronary heart disease. Fam Pract 19:605–610
Therborn G (2003) Back to norms! On the scope and dynamics of norms and normative action. Curr Sociol 50:863–880
Thomson RG et al (2007) A patient decision aid to support shared decision-making on anti-thrombotic treatment of patients with atrial fibrillation: randomised controlled trial. Qual Saf Health Care 16:216–223
Turner BS (1995) Medical power and social knowledge. Sage, London
Weber M (1947) The theory of social and economic organization. Free Press, New York

Chapter 17
After 30 Years, Problems and Prospects in the Study of Doctor–Patient Interaction

John Heritage and Douglas W. Maynard

Introduction

In the 1970s, two major studies established the systematic study of doctor–patient interaction as a viable research domain. The first, conducted by Korsch and Negrete (1972) at the Children's Hospital of Los Angeles was based on observations of 800 pediatric acute care visits and used a modifield version of Bales' (1950) Interaction Process Analysis to code the data. The results were striking. Nearly a fifth of the parents left the clinic without a clear statement of what was wrong with their child, and nearly half were left wondering what had caused their child's illness. A quarter of the parents reported that they had not mentioned their greatest concern because of lack of opportunity or encouragement. The study uncovered a strong relationship between these and other communication failures and nonadherence with medical recommendations, showing that 56% of parents who felt that the physicians had not met their expectations were "grossly noncompliant."

On the other side of the Atlantic, *Doctors Talking to Patients* (Byrne and Long 1976), based on some 2,500 audio recordings of primary care encounters, anatomized the medical visit into a series of stages and developed an elaborate characterization of doctor behaviors in each of them. Drawing on Balint's (1957) proposal that the primary care visit has therapeutic value in its own right, Byrne and Long focused on the ways in which its therapeutic possibilities were attenuated by the prevalence of doctor-centered behaviors in the encounters they studied. The study documented the overwhelming prevalence of doctor-centered behavior and was also conceived as an intervention: physicians were invited to use its coding framework to evaluate their own conduct and to modify it in a more patient-centered direction. Not surprisingly, given these goals, *Doctors Talking to Patients* was itself somewhat doctor-centered. The authors had much less to say about patients' contributions to the encounter or the sociocultural context of social interaction in primary care. Here, we consider approaches to the medical interview that, developing from these initiatives, have a primary focus on observable features of doctor–patient interaction. Within this orientation, we consider literature dealing with social, moral, and technical dilemmas that physicians and patients face in primary care, and the resources that they deploy in solving them. This literature embodies a steady evolution towards a more balanced focus on the conduct of doctors and patients together.

J. Heritage (✉)
Department of Sociology, University of California, Los Angeles, CA 90024-1551, USA
e-mail: heritage@ucla.edu

D.W. Maynard (✉)
Department of Sociology, University of Wisconsin, Madison, WI, 53706-1393
e-mail: maynard@ssc.wisc.edu

Sociological Approaches to the Physician–Patient Relationship

Although the sociology of medicine predates Parsons' (1951) theoretical analysis, *The Social System* contains an account of the doctor–patient relationship that is classic in every sense. Parsons conceptualizes the institution of medicine as a social system's normative mechanism for assisting those who fall ill and returning them to their regular work-related contributory capacities. Medical practitioners treat patients according to generalized technical standards of treatment (universalism), rather than standards that are adjusted to the social characteristics of the patient (particularism); they enact a specific technical focus on medical care (specificity) rather than a general "wise counselor" role (diffuseness); they treat patients without extensive emotional involvement (affective neutrality) rather than the reverse (affectivity); and they put patient welfare above their personal interests (a "collectivity" rather than "self" orientation). Complementary to the practitioner's role is the "sick role" for the patient, which means exemption from responsibility for the illness itself and from normal duties, but it also requires sick persons to be motivated to get well, rather than languish in a state of illness, and to pursue this end by seeking help from a competent physician and following a prescribed therapeutic path.

There were, of course, significant difficulties with this analysis. Parsons (1951:440) himself notes that his formulation of the patient's situation is highly abstract because it was designed to offer a general picture of the physician–patient relationship, without particular regard to the range of illnesses that patients can experience. Almost immediately, Szasz and Hollender (1956) observed that the extent to which patients will be passive recipients of medical expertise and authority will vary with the character and severity of their illness, whether it is severe and requiring physically intrusive intervention (such as surgery), or chronic and only necessitating unsupervised self-medication (diabetes or hypertension, for example).

Other voices expressed reservations about the Parsonian emphasis on the functional significance of institutionalized patterns in medicine, the benign treatment of the complementarities of the physician–patient relationship, and bland endorsement of medical authority. Foucault's (1975) critique of the normalizing and control functions of medical disciplines has found concrete extension in treatments of the medicalization of social problems (Conrad and Schneider 1992). Parsons' analysis emerged at a time – the "golden age of doctoring" (McKinlay 1999) – when medical authority reached its zenith (Freidson 1985; Shorter 1985; Starr 1982). The so-called "modern doctor" (Shorter 1985:75–106) worked within a "sovereign profession" (Starr 1982) and serenely dispensed both medication and authoritative judgment. During the period 1945–1965 US medicine, Freidson (1988:384) comments, "was at a historically unprecedented peak of prestige, prosperity and political and cultural influence – perhaps as autonomous as it is possible for a profession can be."

Subsequently, Medicare and Medicaid legislation, the growth of third party payers and for-profit medical service corporations (Gray 1991; Waitzkin 2000, 2001), rising health care costs, and the growth of medical consumerism have created conditions that are erosive of not only the political and economic influence of the profession but also the cultural authority (Starr 1982) and technical autonomy of medicine (Freidson 1988). While the practice of medicine has never been free of complex financial incentives (Rodwin 1993), managed care organizations have built incentive structures that reward minimized care (Waitzkin 2001) and designed review processes that regulate the exercise of clinical judgment, reaching deeply into the citadel of medical autonomy (Light 2000). As Potter and McKinlay (2005:467–8) suggest, a corporatist metaphor, in which patients become clients and physicians become providers, "came to define the doctor–patient relationship at the beginning of the 21st century." In short, as Light (2000) argues, the well-known notion of *professional dominance* (Freidson 1970) needs to be supplanted by the concept of *countervailing powers*.

Even as we recognize that health care has undergone big changes in recent decades, rather less is known about its effects on the particulars of the doctor–patient encounter (Waitzkin 2000:272).

There is no stable conceptual framework for the analysis of the doctor–patient relationship as realized in situ, and few historical benchmarks against which to evaluate evolution and change. Yet it is important to recognize how much of the doctor–patient relationship is realized interactively in the here and now. Abstract statements about this relationship almost universally gloss the complexity and specificity of the actions and responses that make up the medical interview. Sociological theory and research on the doctor–patient encounter tend to opt for generalized characterizations rather than dealing with concrete particulars. In short, there has been sparse attention to interaction as it is conducted in real-time, and to "the study of life as it is experienced by those who are living it" (Pescosolido et al. 2000:413). The result is that theoretical formulations of the physician–patient relationship are insufficiently responsive to the specific elements of talk and action through which it is constituted. Conversely, lacking an empirical baseline founded in recordings and explication of the range and extent of the proceedings between physician and patient, it is difficult to evaluate current relationships, explicate processes of historical change, and determine the impact of specific factors such as the rise of managed care or the impact of internet-based information on the contemporary practice of primary care.

The Physician–Patient Relationship: The View from Medicine

Reflection on the physician–patient relationship is undoubtedly as old as medicine itself, and recognition of its therapeutic power goes back to Hippocrates who, in his Precepts (VI), observed that "some patients, though conscious that their condition is perilous, recover their health simply through their contentment with the goodness of the physician." Modern investigation of the relationship stems from the psychoanalytically inspired revival of this insight that has issued in the movement for patient-centered medicine (McWhinney 1989). In an influential critique of traditional biomedicine, Engel (1977) called for a *biopsychosocial* approach, which considers interpersonal and social aspects of patients' lives along with biological processes, to supplant it. Since that critique, physicians and social scientists jointly have sought to evaluate the significance of interaction in shaping medical outcomes (Frankel et al. 2003). Related to Engel's model is research on relationship- or patient-centered care. This research suggests that patients who receive such care are enhanced in their program attendance, smoking cessation, glucose control, long-term exercise, weight loss, and adherence to treatment regiments, and other aspects of physical as well as mental health (Williams et al. 2000). Both quantitative and qualitative studies show that when physicians listen fully, exhibit care and compassion, and engage in other prosocial behaviors, patients' psychological status, physiological symptoms, and functional outcomes all improve (Stewart 2003).

The unifying conception of patient-centered medicine is a critique that contemporary scientific medicine has become preoccupied with disease and its evaluation, at the expense of patients and their concerns. Its objective is to reverse this process:

> The essence of the patient-centered method is that the physician tries to enter the patient's world, to see the illness through his or her eyes. In the traditional doctor-centered method, physicians try to bring the patient's illness into their world and to interpret the illness in terms of pathology. The transformed method will, of course, include this process, but it will no longer have the dominance it now enjoys. (McWhinney 1989:34)

Patient-centered practice is now widely taught through well known American Academy of Physician and Patient three-function model of the medical interview (Cohen-Cole 1991; Cohen-Cole and Bird 1991). The three-function model, for example, explicitly sets the biomedical/diagnostic objectives of the medical interview within the context of (a) the patient's psychosocial context – "why this person has become a patient, what the disease (or perceived disease) means to him or her, and how he or she is behaving in the role of a patient" (Lazare et al. 1995:5), (b) the construction of a therapeutic relationship in which the physician builds an alliance with the patient, and (c) education of the patient – not only recommending and negotiating therapeutic measures to treat disease but also determining any areas of conflict between clinician and patient and working with social and psychological consequences of the illness.

In making the nature of the interview explicit across types of diagnosis, clinical settings, and temporal nodes in the illness or the doctor–patient relationship, the three-function model provides a normative baseline for researchers, clinicians, and students to assess the success of the interview (Carroll 1995; Lazare et al. 1995) according to whether physicians treat the patient, rather than just the disease. It invites an approach that prioritizes skills in communication and in empathy, and a more involved and less authoritarian pattern of interaction between doctor and patient.

As a normative baseline, the three-function approach is a work of advocacy, designed to influence medical practice. To evaluate practice, Emanuel and Emanuel (1992) provide an influential conceptualization. They suggest these dimensions by which to measure the medical visit: (1) which person sets the goals of the visit (the physician, patient or both in negotiation); (2) the status of the patient's values (assumed by the physician, jointly explored, or unexamined); and (3) the functional role of the physician (guardian, advisor or consulting technician). In a *mutual* relationship where the power and symbolic resources of each participant are broadly balanced, the visit's agenda is negotiated, the patient's values are explored, and the physician adopts an advisory role with regard to the patient's goals and decisions. In a *paternalistic* relationship, where the physician's power and symbolic resources outweigh those of the patient, physicians control the visit's agenda, goals, and outcomes. The physician tends to adopt a more narrowly biomedical stance and acts as a guardian in the best interests of the patient, though those interests are not explicitly explored, but rather assumed to be congruent with the physician's. In a *consumerist* relationship, patients set the goals and agenda and make decisions on treatment and other outcomes. Patient values are explicit but not discussed, and the physician becomes a technical consultant in a "market" relationship.

Most contributors to the medical literature are advocates for, and working towards, the mutual model. However, the literature on patient attitudes suggests that the kind of patient autonomy and patient-centeredness that the model advocates are not universally desired (Ende et al. 1989; Frosch and Kaplan 1999). A large scale study of routine (chronic care) visits by Roter et al. (1997) suggests that only about 20% of such visits approximate a mutual model in which both parties contribute, and the discussion embraces the psychosocial context of the patient's concerns along with its biomedical content. In their analysis, 8% of the visits emerged as predominantly "consumerist," while the majority (66%) were largely physician driven in terms of narrowly biomedical, or "expanded biomedical" concerns. Not surprisingly, the narrowly biomedical visits were rated least satisfying by physicians and patients alike. Because contemporary measures of patient-centeredness in the medical visit are far from stable (Epstein et al. 2005; Mead and Bower 2000), it is difficult to evaluate the extent to which the beneficial effects of mutually founded medical visits vary according to patient preferences and medical conditions. The three-function model, with its normative approach, needs a robust empirical component that has strong implications for clinical practice.

Studies of Doctor–Patient Interaction: A Methodological Dichotomy

Research on doctor–patient interaction has increased greatly since its inception in the late 1960s, and it has resulted in a large literature ranging over many medical settings and illness conditions (Roter and Hall 1992). While a number of medical and social scientific disciplines have converged in this literature, two main approaches have emerged: process analysis and the microanalysis of discourse (Charon et al. 1994).

Process Analysis

As already noted, process analysis was introduced into medicine in a series of pathbreaking studies by Korsch and Negrete (1972) on interaction in a pediatric acute care hospital context. Their findings made a powerful case for the study of physician–patient interaction. They showed that systematic study in the field is achievable and that the results can be significant for patient health outcomes. Roter (1977) extended the Korsch studies, showing that training patients to be more proactive in the medical interview led to improved health outcomes. Further studies developing this approach to encompass patients with chronic conditions showed significant improvements in physiological and functional outcomes (Greenfield et al. 1988; Greenfield et al. 1985; Kaplan et al. 1989). Related studies showed that eliciting the patient's view of the illness increased recall, understanding, and commitment to following physician advice (Brown et al. 2003; Stewart 1995).

We also noted that the original Korsch studies quantified interaction using Bales' (1950) interaction process analysis. This classified role behavior in task-oriented small groups in terms of a contrast between task oriented and socio-emotional behaviors. The Bales scheme had real strengths, including the attempt to be exhaustive and to facilitate administration so that a trained Bales researcher can code interaction in real time, without the need even of a tape recorder. As an approach to doctor–patient interaction, however, the scheme also had significant weaknesses. Its categories are exceedingly general, yielding a picture of the physician–patient encounter that is fuzzy at best. Nor are they adapted to the specificities of doctor–patient communication and the phases of the medical encounter. Moreover, the Bales system's strict dichotomization of behaviors into task-focused and socio-emotional categories forced coders to make awkward judgements. For example, as Wasserman and Inui (1983:286) noted, when a patient says "Doctor, am I going to die?," is the coder to treat this as category 8 (asks for opinion) or category 11 (shows tension)? Few researchers would want to make this call, yet it was mandated by the system.

As a result, coding schemes have undergone progressive refinements over the years to address these problems, tailor them to dyadic interaction, and accomodate the specific content of physician–patient interactions (Inui and Carter 1985; Inui et al. 1982; Roter and McNeilis 2003; Roter et al. 1988; Wasserman and Inui 1983). By far, the most influential of the emergent schemes has been developed and refined by Roter and colleagues. The current Roter interaction analysis system (RIAS) contains 39 categories broadly subdivided into socioemotional (15 categories) and task focused (24 categories) (Roter and Larson 2002). Like the Bales system, RIAS is designed to implement an exhaustive classification of the events of the medical visit using categories that are compatible with the three-function model of the medical visit described above (Roter and Larson 2001, 2002). Coders can do so without the necessity for transcription, thus conserving costs and enabling analysis of large numbers of interactions required for intervention and evaluation studies. With the use of additional codes, RIAS also accommodates a wide range of contents and circumstances beyond primary care, including oncology, obstetrics and gynecology, end of life discussions, well-baby care, and specific diagnostic categories such as asthma, hypertension, and diabetes (Roter and Larson 2002).

The RIAS framework has opened up the physician–patient relationship to a significant degree. Shown by comparative studies to be superior to other coding systems (Inui et al. 1982; Thompson 2001), it has revealed important differences in how men and women (both physicians and patients) interact in the medical visit and how these interaction patterns are related to physician and patient satisfaction (Hall et al. 1994a, b; Roter and Hall 1992). It has formed the basis for a valuable empirical specification of the main styles of primary care visit (Roter et al. 1997) described above. And it has been used in nearly 100 empirical investigations of a wide variety of medical contexts (Roter and Larson 2002).

Although the Roter system has served as the backbone for the study of the physician–patient relationship over the past 20 years, it is not without controversy. Criticisms of the RIAS system have focused on the very features that have contributed to its success – its capacity to deliver an exhaustive and quantified overview of the medical encounter.

As Charon et al. (1994) note, process models take little account of the context or content of medical visits, sacrificing this for an overview across medical encounters in which the interactivity – the capacity for one party to influence the behavior of another or to adjust behavior in response to another – becomes invisible (Stiles 1989). Hence "because the content or context of the interview is not assessed, these methods implicitly assume no connection between how people talk and either what they talk about or why they talk" (Charon et al. 1994:956). Further, the focus on medical outcomes as the primary object of research – typical outcomes being patient satisfaction, physician satisfaction, patient compliance, and functional status of patient (Charon et al. 1994) – can generate awkward choices because they commit researchers to substantive positions on the goals of medicine. For example, when physicians use a consumer model in making decisions about prescriptions and attempt to meet perceived patient preferences, this can result in inappropriate treatment outcomes (Kravitz et al. 2005; Mangione-Smith et al. 1999). Patient satisfaction may improve, and clinical outcomes may deteriorate. Finally, general patient preferences may well vary in relation to illness conditions: a "consumerist" patient in the context of upper respiratory infections may look for a more "paternalist" stance from a physician in the context of a cancer diagnosis.

Microanalysis

At the opposite pole of the analytic continuum lie studies that focus on the microanalysis of medical discourse. Originating within anthropology and sociology, these studies deploy an essentially ethnographic and interpretive methodology to disclose the background orientations, individual experiences, sensibilities, understandings, and objectives that inhabit the medical visit. In sociology, microanalytic studies have a heritage that includes the "Chicago School" of ethnography. Those studies that draw on Hughes' work focus primarily on medicine as an occupation, and for these studies, an astute observation by Fox (1989:38) still holds true: "Sociologists have written more about health professionals – especially about physicians – than they have about patients." However, other ethnographic work in the tradition of Goffman has concentrated less on the sociology of the profession and contributed more to the study of the physician–patient relationship per se.

Strong's (1979) comparative study of pediatric clinics in the USA and Scotland introduces the notion that a "ceremonial" order of the pediatric encounter can emerge in different formats. In particular, a bureaucratic format – involving formality, politeness, and control of emotions – predominates as compared with clinical, charity, and private formats. Although Strong agrees with Parsons and Freidson that the technical expertise of the physician is a source of medical control, he adds a dimension documenting how the ceremonial order and bureaucratic format of clinical encounters enable expression of medical authority. His study is complemented by Emerson (1970) who, in a symbolic interactionist study of the gynecological exam, demonstrates the existence of "counter-themes" to the traditional medical model and resistances to the authority relations embedded within it.

Throughout the 1980s, British ethnographers drew on Strong's fusion between ethnographic observation and discourse analysis. Significant contributions by Bloor (1976, 1997), Silverman (1987), and Atkinson (1995, 1999) represent a convergence between field observation and the systematic use of recorded data in the medical arena, which is a feature of discourse studies of the medical visit. In the USA, Anspach's (1993) distinguished investigation of interactions between pediatricians, nurses, and the parents of children in the intensive care unit detailed the ways in which the medical professionals preconstructed end-of-life decisions for which parent assent was required.

In recent years, ethnographers have included discourse analysis as part of their investigation of doctoring. Their analyses of patients' experiences, sensibilities, understandings, and objectives suggest that patients' subjectivity resides, like an iceberg, mainly below the surface of talk. It is maintained in this submerged condition by a combination of patient diffidence and self-censorship (Strong 1979), and practitioner disattention and obfuscation. Practitioner suppression of patient experience, investigators argue, is due to status and authority as built from educational, socioeconomic, ethnic, gender, and other differences between patients and physicians (Atkinson 1995; Clair and Allman 1993; Davis 1963; Fisher 1984; Todd 1989; Zola 1964, 1973). Ethnographic research in this vein has also drawn on the perspective of social constructionism (Miller and Holstein 1993; Spector and Kitsuse 1977). For example, Brown (1995:37) argues for an approach to the social construction of diagnosis and illness in which an understanding of social and political contexts informs the analysis of "interpersonal communication" between doctor and patient.

Medicine as Discourse

Mishler's (1984) *The Discourse of Medicine* is a compelling implementation of microanalysis. In an analysis focused on history taking, Mishler observes that physician and patient often pursue distinct, and sometimes conflicting, agendas in the medical visit: the doctor's medical agenda focuses on biomedical evaluation and treatment, and the patient's "lifeworld" agenda concentrates on personal fears, anxieties, and other everyday lifeworld circumstances. Enforcing a medical agenda through questioning, physicians recurrently suppress the patient's concerns, even though they can be important sources of evidence and further medical problems.

Mishler's observations were expanded in Waitzkin's (1991) *The Politics of Medical Encounters*. In a nutshell, Waitzkin's (1991:231–2) proposal is that the underlying, and largely unrecognized, structure of medical discourse militates against the expression of personal troubles including "difficulties with work, economic insecurity, family life and gender roles, the process of aging, the patterning of substance use and other 'vices,' and resources to deal with emotional stress" (Waitzkin 1991: 231–2). Instead, the medical management of patients' contextually generated problems focuses on technical solutions, reinforces ideologically dominant outlooks and prohibitions, and contributes to social control by reinforcing the patient's accommodation to the social contexts from which illness arises. As described in Waitzkin (1985), this pattern of medical management and social control is pursued through all phases of the medical encounter and is richly documented for a wide variety of the personal problems previously listed. Waitzkin (1991:231–2) observes that the dysfunctional features of the medical visit emerged in 70% of the cases he examines.

Similar findings are reported in microanalytic studies involving women's reproductive choices (Fisher and Todd 1986, 1993; Todd 1989), which also address a wide variety of aspects of the medical visit. In a persuasive discussion, Todd (1989) documents several patterns by which "women's voices and medical care all too often pass each other by."

While the mechanics through which these miscommunications emerge are various (West and Frankel 1991), West (1984) observes several gender-based communication patterns in physician–patient interaction that are strongly associated with dominance and subordination. The most fundamental of these is interruption – the verbal interdiction of another's talk – which is associated with social dominance, regardless of whether that involves gender or not (Kollock et al. 1985). West found that physicians interrupt patients more than the reverse, except when the patient is male and the physician is female where, it appears, gender trumps occupational role as a co-variate of interruptive behavior. In research on the same data set, West (1984) also showed that patients asked fewer questions than physicians and were less likely to receive answers to them than physicians were.

Taking Stock

It is now time to take stock of these two traditions of interaction research: the Bales-based RIAS coding model and the microanalytic approach. In principle, the strengths and weaknesses of the two approaches are complementary, and combining them should result in a greatly enhanced view of the medical encounter (Roter and Frankel 1992; Waitzkin 1990). In practice, this has not come about (Roter and McNeilis 2003) and it is instructive to consider why this is the case. Process approaches have resulted in findings about the medical encounter that are systematic and replicable. The most robust findings have centered on relationships between interaction variables and patient and provider characteristics, and to a lesser extent with patient satisfaction and adherence outcomes. Process approaches have not developed associations between interaction variables and medical decision making (surely one of the core areas of medical practice), nor in relation to patients' treatment preferences or physicians' perceptions of those preferences. In short, there is a lack of systematic investigation of the relationship between process variables and the *content* of medical practice and patient concern.

This deficiency is clearly associated with the kinds of coding categories used in process analysis. In the effort to generalize across practice contexts, coding categories are pitched at a very general level; they hence lack detail and specificity. This is a familiar criticism of process analysis (Inui and Carter 1985; Mishler 1986; Pendleton 1983; Tuckett et al. 1985; Tuckett and Williams 1984), and it is associated with two related problems. The first of these is that, in the course of coding, the *content* of the medical encounter is largely washed out. What the physician and patient were talking about is lost, often irretrievably when the original tapes are destroyed and the coded material rather than the actual interaction on which it is based effectively becomes "the data" (Charon et al. 1994; Mishler 1984). A second problem is that coding expunges the *context* of utterances and actions – their location in a phased activity within the encounter such as history taking or counseling, and their placement in a specific and authocthonously intelligible sequence and course of action. It is precisely these aspects of context that give utterances and actions the meaning they have.

On the other side of the ledger, microanalytic approaches have retained crucial elements of medical sense making. Moreover, where process techniques such as those of Roter concentrate on what is present in medical conversations, the microanalytic discourse approach, in highlighting absences in the dialog, imparts a strongly critical edge to appraisals of medical practice. Nevertheless, many small-scale quasi-ethnographic studies of discourse have not been able to establish a noninterpretive evidential base for associations between meaningful conduct on the one hand and social context or medical outcomes on the other. They retain vulnerabilities to objections in terms of what Mishler (1986), following Katz (1983), terms the four R's: representativeness, reactivity, reliability and replicability. Granted the insight of observer and the compelling nature of the observations, how can we be sure that the same phenomena obtain elsewhere and that another observer would come up with similar observations? To these insistent difficulties may be added another. What kinds of systematic patterns can be extracted from so little data that is also very particular in terms of time, place, participation, medical condition, payment, and other circumstances? If the objective is that of the cautionary tale, to describe ways in which physicians should not conduct themselves, then the message is often plain enough. Or if the objective is to identify the generics of interactional methods by which doctor and patient communicate, there are recommendations to be made that enhance that communication. But the message may go awry if physicians and others can find in the examples some exceptional element that makes their application to other circumstances moot.

In sum, neither coding nor microanalytic perspectives have resulted in the kind of data that permits us to extract clear conclusions about how physicians (or patients) should conduct themselves in specific moments in the flow of the medical encounter. This is not because there are no normative principles of patient care to guide the application of research. Rather, it is because neither perspective has connected with the data of doctor–patient interaction in ways that permit results that are *both* specific *and* generalizable. By the same token, it has not been possible to establish many clear connections between exogenous factors that putatively impact physician–patient interaction and the details of medical encounters, nor relationships between conduct in medical encounters and the outcomes of those encounters. Finally, it has not as yet been possible to find a meeting point between the two methodologies. Progress in research on physician–patient interaction, as several prominent researchers (Roter and Frankel 1992; Roter and McNeilis 2003) have attested, is seriously weakened by the lack of reconciliation between the two approaches.

Clearly the same interactional conduct, addressed in such very different ways in the two research traditions, is the source both of individual meaning, shared understanding, interactional obfuscation, and the rest, and of systematic outcomes that can be subjected to quantitative investigation. An analytical framework is required that is responsive to very granular, individual moments in the physician–patient encounter, but that simultaneously supports coding at a higher level of abstraction sufficient to reach beyond individual cases to generate findings at a statistical evidential standard. Such a framework requires an analysis of interaction, grounded and validated in the direct analysis of the conduct of participants, and application to the medical encounter that is illuminating at both qualitative and quantitative levels.

Conversation Analysis as an Approach to Physician–Patient Interaction

During the past 20 years, conversation analysis has become a substantial presence in studies of physician–patient communication. Beginning with pioneering work by Frankel (1983, 1984), Heath (1982, 1986), and West (1984), it now spans the gamut of activities that make up physician–patient interaction in primary care (Heritage and Maynard 2006; Maynard and Heritage 2005) and has a growing presence in many more specialized aspects of medicine from AIDS counseling (Peräkylä 1995; Silverman 1997) to surgery (Koschmann et al. 2005; Maynard and Hudak 2008; Mondada 2003) to diabetes care (Lutfey 2004, 2005). We review this literature as a kind of model for other approaches that aim for close analysis of interaction and that may also want to codify and relate practices of talk to measureable outcomes in the medical interview.

In its application to medical care, CA begins from the perspective that much of what goes on in the medical encounter is *conversation* and that this involves the importation of the interaction order (Goffman 1983) – together with ordinary methods of commonsense reasoning (Garfinkel 1967) – into the very heart of medical encounter. This point of view has several important implications. First, interactional practices through which persons conduct themselves elsewhere are not abandoned at the threshold of the medical clinic. That is, the organization of interaction described in CA studies of ordinary conversation, for example, turn taking (Sacks et al. 1974) and repair (Schegloff et al. 1977), is largely carried forward from the everyday world into the doctor's office. Second, practices for effecting particular kinds of actions, for example, describing a problem or trouble (Jefferson 1980, 1988) or telling bad and good news (Maynard 2003), are also carried across the threshold of the doctor's office and affect how doctors and patients go about addressing particular interactional tasks. Third, the organization of interaction is fundamentally geared to the joint management of self-other relations (Brown and Levinson 1987; Goffman 1955; Heritage and Raymond 2005; Maynard and Zimmerman 1984). Departures from this organization, as in the interruption of one speaker by another, often represent violations of this joint management process. Within this perspective, CA begins from the presumption that physician and patient, with various levels of mutual understanding, conflict, cooperation, authority, and subordination, jointly construct the medical visit. This is a point of view that mandates a departure from the physician-centered approaches previously described because the contributions of the patient, no matter how minimal, are unavoidably implicated in the co-construction of the medical encounter.

The CA perspective has been extensively described elsewhere (Clayman and Gill 2004; Drew and Sorjonen 1997; Goodwin and Heritage 1990; Heritage 2005; Hutchby and Wooffitt 1998; Maynard and Clayman 1991; ten Have 1999; Zimmerman 1988). In what follows, we will identify some of the main ways in which CA offers a distinctive perspective on physician–patient interaction.

Primary Care Interaction Comprises an Overall Structure of Component Activities

Unlike many forms of interaction, physician–patient encounters have a discernable overall structure. For example, the acute primary care encounter ordinarily manifests itself as an ordered structure of component activities, beginning with an opening sequence, progressing through problem presentation, history taking, physical examination, diagnosis, and treatment recommendations, to a closing sequence (Byrne and Long 1976; Heritage and Maynard 2006; Robinson 2003) (other types of medical visit – follow-up, routine maintenance, and physical check-ups – have distinctive, but equally patterned, structures). This structure is institutionalized in a fully sociological sense: it is taught in medical school, patients are repeatedly trained by exposure to it from childhood (Stivers and Majid 2007), and both parties to the interaction orient to the internal boundaries in this structure with considerable exactness (Robinson and Heritage 2005; Robinson and Stivers 2001). The importance of overall structure is that it is a source of endogenously generated order that is realized in doctor–patient interaction. As such, it is also an important baseline for comparisons. While analysis of the contributions of doctors and patients without reference to the structural sub-components of medical visits can lead to results that are vague and difficult to interpret, analyzing the conduct of the parties in different phases of the interview yields clearly meaningful findings. Inquiry into medical openings, for example, or problem presentation, or diagnosis, or treatment recommendations readily yield patterns that permit comparisons across such dimensions as gender, race, specialty, payment system, national culture, and all of these across historical time (Stivers and Majid 2007; Tates et al. 2002).

Activities in Primary Care are Constructed as Interaction Sequences

The activities that make up the medical encounter are transacted through sequences of interaction. In general, sequence organization is the engine room of interaction. It is the primary means by which interactional context is generated and, in turn, through which context-bound utterances achieve their sense, and interactional identities and roles (story teller, news deliverer, sympathizer) and larger social and institutional identities (woman, grandparent, latino, physician, patient, etc.) are established and maintained. Sequential structure is a robust form of interactional organization, subject to sanction and amenable to manipulation, as when patients subtly pressure physicians for particular diagnoses, treatments, or tests and physicians work to handle such pressure (Gill 2005). We will illustrate the relevance of sequence organization by reference to studies of sequences in which physicians offer diagnoses and make treatment recommendations.

A substantial body of CA research has shown that physicians and patients treat the management of diagnosis and treatment discussions in sequentially distinctive ways. Diagnoses tend to be offered and accepted "on authority" and ordinarily do not attract significant overt acknowledgement or "acceptance" by patients (Heath 1992; Peräkylä 1998, 2002, 2006; Stivers 2005a, b); although when diagnostic news is bad, silence also may be a patient's exhibit of stoicism (Maynard 2003).

Moreover, patients may view the diagnosis as a precursor to treatment proposals (Freidson 1970) and tend to withhold response in light of that consideration (Robinson 2003). In sequential terms, this manifests itself in little or no patient responsiveness to clinician's diagnostic statements. Treatment proposals, by contrast with diagnostic announcements, tend to receive some form of acknowledgement, most often in the form of a fully overt acceptance (Heritage and Sefi 1992; Stivers 2005a, b, 2006). Underlying this sequential variation are profound differences in the social, epistemic, and interactional foundations of the two actions. Diagnoses are produced and recognized as actions performed by an expert who is licensed to perform medicine and render authoritative judgments about the nature of medical conditions. Nevertheless, when the diagnosis is favorable, patients and other recipients may produce a positive evaluation, while as recipients of adverse diagnoses, they regularly refrain from evaluative assessment in part to avoid any appearance of self-pity (Maynard 2003). However, in orienting to treatment recommendations as *proposals*, participants understand the sequences in which they appear as complete only when, normatively speaking, some exhibit of *acceptance* is produced. The contrasting properties of diagnostic announcements and treatment proposals offer different affordances to patients who wish to resist diagnoses, by comparison with those who wish to resist treatment recommendations (Stivers 2002a, 2005a, b). Diagnoses that, from the patient's point of view, are adverse must be resisted *actively* (e.g. "You don't think it's strep?"). Treatment recommendations, by comparison, can be resisted *passively*: patients, by withholding acceptance to a treatment recommendation, can pressure clinicians into elaborate justifications of a recommendation and, not infrequently, to alter or reverse it (Stivers 2005a, b).

Before leaving the topic of sequence organization, it is also relevant to note that physicians often systematically and strategically manipulate sequence structures to achieve rather specific objectives. For example, in a series of papers, Maynard (1991a, b, 1992) has identified practices involved in the perspective display sequence (PDS) whereby clinicians prepare recipients for the delivery of adverse medical diagnoses. In presequence fashion, patients are invited to describe their own view of the medical problem before clinicians present their own diagnostic conclusions. At one level, the use of these practices can seem like a grotesque manipulation of medical authority: what possible value can the lay person's view be in a context where a professional medical judgment is about to be expertly rendered? But Maynard shows that, among other things, the PDS facilitates "forecasting" the news, not only preparing the patient for the difficult information they must receive but also establishing an auspicious interactional environment in which the professional can build on the patient's perspective through agreement rather than confrontation. The patient's perspective is *co-implicated* in the diagnostic presentation. The PDS does involve a strategic manipulation of the asymmetric relations between doctor and patient, but in a displayed benign way and with consequences that are often beneficial to the patient's understanding and acceptance (Maynard, 1996).

The Turns Making up Sequences Have Significant Variability

Thus far, we have treated the actions that compose sequences as if they were uniform and monolithic, but of course, these actions are anything but uniform. Much conversation analytic research focuses on the ways in which similar actions-within-sequences are distinctively designed, both as motivated by local contingencies of the interaction and more broadly in terms of the causes and consequences of variation. This analysis is often comparative, and comparisons can be performed at a wide variety of levels. For example, at the level of word choice, it is possible to evaluate the impact of the word "any" (as in "Do you have any other concerns?") by comparing it with similar questions using the word "some" instead of "any" (Heritage et al. 2007). Alternatively, the scope of a question's agenda and presuppositions can be compared: for example, in soliciting a patient's problem one could contrast the import of a question like "What can I do for you today?" with "Not feeling so good, huh?" (Heritage and Robinson 2006b), and with "How are you feeling" (Robinson 2006).

Or, more broadly, it is possible to compare questions that invoke collegial relationships with others with those that evoke bureaucratic ones (Boyd 1998), or physicians' questions that are "optimized" with those which are not (Boyd and Heritage 2006).

Moving beyond question design, conversation analysts have examined problem presentations, comparing those that offer candidate diagnoses with those that do not (Stivers 2002b), or examining the ways in which problem presentations defend the legitimacy of medical visits (Halkowski 2006; Heritage and Robinson 2006a). There are parallel studies of how and when patients introduce their own diagnostic or etiological theories into the encounter (Gill 1998; Gill and Maynard 2006). Similarly, research on diagnostic announcements shows fascinating variations in the extent to which different constructions can invite or inhibit response (Byrne and Long 1976; Heath 1992; Maynard 2004; Peräkylä 1998). Yet again, patients' difficulties with "no problem" diagnostic results and their associated residues of unexplained symptoms are explored by Maynard and Frankel (2006).

The CA studies described in the preceding were developed using the qualitative methods that have been the stock in trade of CA research for the past 30 years. In each case, investigators, by analyzing conduct on a case by case basis, identify structures and their significance as resources to which the participants are oriented and in terms of which they act. This CA research has opened a bright window into how participants in doctor–patient interaction strategize, structure, interpret, and derive meaning from structured sequences of action that are located at specific junctures of the medical visit. This research is interpretively valid "at the level of meaning" as Weber (1947:11) put it. It gives rise to new social scientific understandings of how doctor–patient interaction works. To the extent that it can be developed into valid quantitative analyses of the medical encounter, and thus bridge the extant qualitative–quantitative divide, CA research is also a decisive advance on the methods described earlier.

Interaction, Contexts, and Outcomes

In this section, we argue that because CA results are descriptions of the organization of conduct that are validated qualitatively by reference to the participants' own actions in situ, it is possible to integrate CA findings into quantitative analyses that incorporate normal survey and outcome data to yield a more complete picture of a particular dimension of medical practice. Although the question of quantification has been controversial in CA (Drummond and Hopper 1993; Guthrie 1997; Schegloff 1993; Zimmerman 1993), it is clear that a number of questions about the relationship between talk, its contexts, and its outcomes cannot be answered without the statistical analysis of results.

We begin by noting that a number of studies suggest that specific interactional choices can have surprisingly large effects both on the interaction itself and its outcomes. For example, responses to the question "What can I do for you today?" are on average four times as long as responses to the question "Sore throat and runny nose for two days, huh?" (Heritage and Robinson 2006b), and the choice has a significant influence on patients' satisfaction with their physicians regardless of how long they actually spend in presenting a medical problem (Robinson and Heritage 2006). Similarly, in the earlier-mentioned choice between "some" and "any" in the question "Do you have some/any other concerns you want to address today?," the choice of "some" will reduce the incidence of patients' unaddressed concerns in the visit by up to 50%, while the choice of "any" will not make a statistically significant impact on the reduction of unaddressed concerns (Heritage et al. 2007).

The consequences of interactional choices also reach well beyond immediate responses. For example, in a study of utilization review in which pediatric patients' medical records were being reviewed by insurance companies to determine whether they were eligible for tympanostomy tube surgery (Heritage et al. 2001; Kleinman et al. 1997), Boyd (1998) looked at interactions in which board-certified physicians call attending physicians who are proposing surgical procedures, interview them about the details of the case, and approve or disapprove insurance reimbursement for the procedure. The decisions of these reviewers were, formally at least, controlled by a set of explicit clinical criteria that cases must meet to merit reimbursement (Kleinman et al. 1997). Reviewers open the review according in one of three ways – "bureaucratic," "consensus building," or "collegial" (Boyd 1998). In the bureaucratic opening, the reviewer stresses a need for specific missing information, while in the collegial style, the reviewer asks for information in an open-ended fashion, as if consulting a colleague on a case. Boyd found that, although these openings initiate a review process intended to implement explicit criteria, the question designs predicted the outcome of the review. Controlling for individual differences and other factors, the odds of collegially opened reviews resulting in approval were three times greater than their bureaucratic counterparts, a finding that remained robust in more complex regression models incorporating all the variables predicting decisions that departed from the reviewing organization's explicit criteria for surgery, and a number of additional, potentially confounding, variables.

Researchers have conducted similar studies concerned with prescribing decisions in pediatric medical visits, finding that inappropriate antibiotic therapy (for viral conditions) is linked to physicians' belief that parents expected an antibiotic prescription for their child. In a substantial study, Mangione-Smith et al. (1999) showed that this perception was the only significant predictor of inappropriate prescribing: When physicians thought the parent wanted an antibiotic for their child, they prescribed them 62% of the time versus 7% when they did not think antibiotics were desired. Actual parental expectations for antibiotics (as reported in a pre-visit survey) were not a significant predictor of inappropriate antibiotic prescribing after controlling for covariates. Additionally, when physicians thought parents wanted antibiotics, they diagnosed middle ear infections and sinusitis much more frequently (49% and 38% of the time, respectively) than when they did not think antibiotics were desired (13% and 5%, respectively).

Given that overt requests for antibiotics were rare in the data (Stivers 2002a), Stivers (2002b) examined parents' opening descriptions of their child's medical condition and distinguished between "symptoms only" descriptions and those descriptions that included (or strongly implied) a candidate's bacterial diagnosis. She argued that the "symptoms only" descriptions assert a medical problem but are agnostic on whether the problem can be treated with an antibiotics prescription. By contrast, the parent's candidate diagnoses (found in references to "ear infections," "strep throat," or "bronchitis") assert the treatability of the child's complaint and may imply that the treatment should be antibiotic. Quantitative analysis showed that physicians are significantly more likely to perceive parental expectations in favor of antibiotics when they are presented with a candidate diagnosis rather than a "symptoms only" presentation. On the other hand, the data also indicate that parents do not systematically discriminate between these problem presentations: equal numbers of those who indicated prior to the consultation that they expected to get an antibiotic prescription for their child used each type of problem presentation (Stivers et al. 2003). The researchers found similarly significant results from the examination of physician conduct. For example, when physicians asserted that children did not need antibiotics, parents were more likely to question the treatment plan (Mangione-Smith et al. 1999) and to passively resist physicians' proposals (Stivers 2005a, b). When, by contrast, physicians engaged in reassuring online commentary (comments contemporaneous with the physician examination [Heritage and Stivers 1999]), fewer antibiotics were inappropriately prescribed (Mangione-Smith et al. 2003; Heritage et al. 2010), and parents were less likely to resist nonantibiotic treatment proposals for viral conditions (Heritage et al. 2010).

The studies described above demonstrate robust and sizable relationships between interactional conduct on the one hand and various kinds of interactional, relational, and medical outcomes on the other. These results hold promise for the idea, promoted by Goffman (1983) in his Presidential Address to the ASA, that interaction is a significant element in the linkage between sociological variables such as gender, race, ethnicity, and SES on the one hand and medical decision making and outcomes on the other. Unfortunately, much less is known about the relationship between these determinants and the details of interactional conduct in medicine.

However, in the pediatric data described previously, which comprised a large multiethnic sample, Stivers and Majid (2007) have shown that patient/parent ethnicity and parent education levels influence whether a child will be included in the talk of the medical visit (and thereby undergo "hands on" in situ training in becoming a competent patient). These same factors do not influence children's success in participating in the visit when actively included (Stivers 2007). These results are a clear harbinger of what CA may be able to deliver in multivariate analyses of race, gender, and class in relation to the doctor–patient relationship, a domain of research that will certainly repay sustained investigation in the next wave of research.

Although the introduction of CA research into a multivariate framework is still in its infancy, these and other results are very encouraging. The CA observations, introduced into several analyses as coded variables, have proved strikingly robust in the multivariate context. This may be less surprising than it seems. The CA variables have been painstaking validated in the most direct way possible – by examination of the unmediated behavior of recipients of the conduct in question. If this conduct has significance on a case-by-case basis, it should survive and enrich multivariate analysis. And this validation has a further pay-off: empirical findings have direct interpretations in the conduct of the participants and are thus transparent as well as robust (Maynard and Frankel 2006).

Conclusion

In this overview, we have sketched the main perspectives and lines of development that have emerged in 30 years of studies of recorded doctor–patient interaction. This is a large field that has been extensively supported by the National Institutes of Health and other funding agencies in the United States and elsewhere. Its complexities are enhanced by disciplinary, methodological, and ideological divisions that are relatively enduring features of the field, by the changing structure of health care provision in many societies and by the sheer multiplicity of health contexts and types of health care service in which social interaction plays a pivotal role. Amid these contingencies, it has been difficult to anchor generalizations in repeatedly observable particulars of medical interactions. Neither the Parsonian nor the three-function models as normative approaches have come to grips with the empirical process and content of doctor–patient interaction, and critiques that emphasize authority and dominance have done only somewhat better. Recent ethnographic, discourse analytic, or other qualitative inquiries have needed more disciplined or systematic approaches to counter the charge that findings are interpretive and idiosyncratic. While efforts to adapt Bales' interaction process analysis to the medical context have provided a basis for a substantial number of studies, they are pitched at a level of abstraction entailing a considerable cost of its own: the loss of concrete content that interaction in the interview comprises.

Bifurcation of the field of doctor–patient interaction into conceptually disconnected quantitative and qualitative research approaches often involves alignment to singular disciplinary and ideological perspectives and little interchange. Thus, although during the past 30 years there has been no shortage of inquiry, it is possible that we are at a pivotal moment in the development of studies of physicians and patients with realistic prospects for reconciliation and integration. Approaches that deal with *practices* of talk and social interaction, which account for the meaningful character of social conduct in the medical encounter as an organized *verstehende* domain in its own right, also can provide the essential building blocks for generalizations about the causal significance of this meaningful social conduct and its relation to health outcomes.

References

Anspach R (1993) Deciding who lives: fateful choices in the intensive-care nursery. University of California Press, Berkeley

Atkinson P (1995) Medical talk and medical work. Sage, London

Atkinson P (1999) Medical discourse, evidentiality and the construction of professional responsibility. In: Sarangi S, Roberts C (eds) Talk, work and institutional order: discourse in medical, mediation and management settings. Mouton DeGruyter, Berlin, pp 75–107

Bales RF (1950) Interaction process analysis: a method for the study of small groups. Addison-Wesley, Reading, MA

Balint M (1957) The doctor, his patient and the illness. Pittman, London

Bloor M (1976) Bishop Berkeley and the adeno-tonsillectomy enigma: an exploration of variation in the social construction of medical diagnosis. Sociology 10:43–61

Bloor M (1997) Selected writings in medical sociological research. Ashgate, Aldershot, England

Boyd E (1998) Bureaucratic authority in the "company of equals": The interactional management of medical peer review. Am Sociol Rev 63(2):200–224

Boyd E, Heritage J (2006) Taking the patient's medical history: questioning during comprehensive history taking. In: Heritage J, Maynard D (eds) Communication in medical care: interactions between primary care physicians and patients. Cambridge University Press, Cambridge, England

Brown JB, Stewart M, Ryan BL (2003) Outcomes of patient-provider interaction. In: Thompson T, Dorsey A, Miller K, Parrott R (eds) Handbook of Health Communication. Lawrence Erlbaum, Mahwah, NJ

Brown P (1995) Naming and framing: the social construction of diagnosis and illness. J Health Soc Behav 35(Extra Issue):34–52

Brown P, Levinson S (1987) Politeness: some universals in language usage. Cambridge University Press, Cambridge

Byrne PS, Long BEL (1976) Doctors talking to patients: a study of the verbal behaviours of doctors in the consultation. HMSO, London

Carroll JG (1995) Evaluation of medical interviewing: concepts and principles. In: Lipkin M, Putnam S, Lazare A (eds) The medical interview: clinical care, education, and research. Springer-Verlag, New York, pp 451–459

Charon R, Greene MJ, Adelamn RD (1994) Multi-dimensional interaction analysis: a collaborative approach to the study of medical discourse. Soc Sci Med 39(7):955–965

Clair JM, Allman RM (eds) (1993) Sociomedical perspectives on patient care. University of Kentucky Press, Lexington, KY

Clayman S, Gill V (2004) Conversation analysis. In: Byman A, Hardy M (eds) Handbook of data analysis. Sage, Beverly Hill, CA, pp 589–606

Cohen-Cole SA (1991) The medical interview: the three function approach. Mosby Year Book, St. Louis

Cohen-Cole SA, Bird J (1991) Function 3: education, negotiation, and motivation. In: Cohen-Cole SA (ed) The medical interview: the three function approach. Mosby Year Book, St. Louis MO

Conrad P, Schneider JW (1992) Deviance and medicalization. Temple University Press, Philadelphia

Davis F (1963) Passage through crisis: polio victims and their families. Bobbs-Merrill, Indianapolis

Drew P, Sorjonen M-L (1997) Institutional discourse. In: Dijk TV (ed) Discourse studies: a multidisciplinaryintroduction. Sage, London, pp 92–118

Drummond K, Hopper R (1993) Backchannels revisited: acknowledgment tokens and speakership incipiency. Res Lang Soc Interact 26:157–177

Emanuel EJ, Emanuel LL (1992) Four models of the physician–patient relationship. J Am Med Assoc 267:2221–2226

Emerson J (1970) Behavior in private places: sustaining definitions of reality in gynecological examinations. In: Drietzel HP (ed) Recent sociology no. 2: patterns of communicative behavior. Macmillan Company, London, pp 73–97

Ende J, Kazis L, Ash A, Moskowitz MA (1989) Measuring patients' desire for autonomy: decision making and information seeking preferences among medical patients. J Gen Intern Med 4:23–30

Engel GL (1977) The need for a new medical model: a challenge for biomedicine. Science 196:129–136

Epstein RM, Franks P, Fiscella K, Shields CG, Meldrum SC, Kravitz RL et al (2005) Measuring patient-centred communication in patient-physician consultations: theoretical and practical issues. Soc Sci Med 61:1516–1528

Fisher S (1984) Doctor–patient communication: a social and micro-political performance. Soc Health Illn 6:1–27

Fisher S, Todd A (eds) (1986) Discourse and institutional authority: medicine, education and law. Ablex, Norwood, NJ

Fisher S, Todd A (eds) (1993) The social organization of doctor–patient communication. Ablex, Norwood NJ

Foucault, M. (1975). The birth of the clinic: an archeology of medical perception (A.M. Sheridan Smith, Trans.). Random House, New York.

Fox RC (1989) The sociology of medicine: a participant observer's view. Prentice Hall, Englewood Cliffs, NJ

Frankel R (1983) The laying on of hands: aspects of the organisation of gaze, touch and talk in the medical encounter. In: Fisher S, Todd AD (eds) The social organization of doctor–patient communication. Center for Applied Linguistics, Washington DC, pp 19–54

Frankel R (1984) From sentence to sequence: understanding the medical encounter through microinteractional analysis. Discourse Process 7:135–170

Frankel RM, Quill TE, McDaniel SH (2003) The biopsychosocial approach: past, present, future. University of Rochester Press, Rochester, NY

Freidson E (1970) Profession of medicine: a study of the sociology of applied knowledge. University of Chicago Press, Chicago

Freidson E (1985) The reorganization of the medical profession. Med Care Rev 42(Spring):11–35

Freidson E (1988) Afterword 1988. In: Friedson E (ed) Profession of medicine: a study of the sociology of applied knowledge. University of Chicago Press, Chicago

Frosch D, Kaplan R (1999) Shared decision making in clinical medicine: past research and future directions. AmJ Prev Med 17(4):285–294

Garfinkel H (1967) Studies in ethnomethodology. Prentice-Hall, Englewood Cliffs, N.J

Gill VT (1998) Doing attributions in medical interaction: patients' explanations for illness and doctors' responses. Soc Psychol Q 61:342–360

Gill VT (2005) Patient "demand" for medical interventions: exerting pressure for an offer in a primary care clinic visit. Res Lang Soc Interact 38:451–479

Gill VT, Maynard DW (2006) Explaining illness: patients' proposals and physicians' responses. In: Heritage J, Maynard D (eds) Communication in medical care: interaction between primary care physicians and patients. Cambridge University Press, Cambridge

Goffman E (1955) On face work. Psychiatry 18:213–231

Goffman E (1983) The interaction order. Am Soc Rev 48:1–17

Goodwin C, Heritage J (1990) Conversation analysis. Annu Rev Anthropol 19:283–307

Gray B (1991) The profit motive and patient care. Harvard University Press, Cambridge MA

Greenfield S, Kaplan SH, Ware JE, Yano E, Frank HJL (1988) Patients' participation in medical care: effects of blood sugar control and quality of life in diabetes. J Gen Intern Med 3:448–457

Greenfield SH, Kaplan S, Ware JE (1985) Expanding patient involvement in care: effects on patient outcomes. Ann Intern Med 102:520–528

Guthrie A (1997) On the systematic deployment of okay and mmhmm in academic advising sessions. Pragmatics 7(3):397–415

Halkowski T (2006) Realizing the illness: patients' narratives of symptom discovery. In: Heritage J, Maynard D (eds) Communication in medical care: interactions between primary care physicians and patients. Cambridge University Press, Cambridge

Hall JA, Irish JT, Roter DL, Ehrlich CM, Miller LH (1994a) Gender in medical encounters: an analysis of physician and patient communication in a primary care setting. Health Psychol 13(5):384–392

Hall JA, Irish JT, Roter DL, Ehrlich CM, Miller LH (1994b) Satisfaction, gender and communication in medical visits. Medical Care 32(12):1216–1231

Heath C (1982) The display of recipiency: an instance of sequential relationship between speech and body movement. Semiotica 42:147–161

Heath C (1986) Body movement and speech in medical interaction. Cambridge University Press, Cambridge

Heath C (1992) Diagnosis and assessment in the medical consultation. In: Drew P, Heritage J (eds) Talk at work: interaction in institutional settings. Cambridge University Press, Cambridge, pp 235–267

Heritage J (2005) Conversation analysis and institutional talk. In: Sanders R, Fitch K (eds) Handbook of language and social interaction. Erlbaum, Mahwah NJ

Heritage J, Boyd E, Kleinman L (2001) Subverting criteria: the role of precedent in decisions to finance surgery. Sociol Health Illn 23:701–728

Heritage J, Maynard D (eds) (2006) Communication in medical care: interactions between primary care physicians and patients. Cambridge University Press, Cambridge

Heritage J, Raymond G (2005) The terms of agreement: indexing epistemic authority and subordination in talk-in-interaction. Soc Psychol Q 68:15–38

Heritage J, Robinson J (2006a) Accounting for the visit: patients' reasons for seeking medical care. In: Heritage J, Maynard D (eds) Communication in medical care: interactions between primary care physicians and patients. Cambridge University Press, Cambridge

Heritage J, Robinson J (2006b) The structure of patients' presenting concerns 1: physicians' opening questions. Health Commun 19:89–102

Heritage J, Robinson JD, Elliott MN, Beckett M, Wilkes M (2007) Reducing patients' unmet concerns in primary care: the difference one word can make. J Gen Intern Med 22:1429–1433

Heritage J, Sefi S (1992) Dilemmas of advice: aspects of the delivery and reception of advice in interactions between health visitors and first time mothers. In: Drew P, Heritage J (eds) Talk at work. Cambridge University Press, Cambridge, pp 359–417

Heritage J, Stivers T (1999) Online commentary in acute medical visits: a method of shaping patient expectations. Soc Sci Med 49(11):1501–1517

Heritage J, Elliott M, Stivers T, Richardson A, Mangione-Smith R (2010) Reducing inappropriate antibiotics prescribing: the role of online commentary on physical examination findings. *Patient Educ Couns*.

Hutchby I, Wooffitt R (1998) Conversation analysis. Blackwell, Malden MA

Inui T, Carter WB (1985) Problems and prospects for health service research on provider-patient communication. Med Care 23(5):521–538

Inui TS, Carter WB, Kukull WA, Haigh VH (1982) Outcome based doctor–patient interaction analysis: 1. Comparison of technique. Medical Care 20:535–549

Jefferson G (1980) On "trouble-premonitory" response to inquiry. Sociol Inq 50:153–185

Jefferson G (1988) On the sequential organization of troubles-talk in ordinary conversation. Soc Probl 35(4):418–441

Kaplan S, Greenfield SH, Ware JE (1989) Assessing the effects of physician–patient interactions on the outcomes of chronic disease. Med Care 27:S11–S127

Katz J (1983) A theory of qualitative methodology: the social system of analytic fieldwork. In: Emerson RM (ed) Contemporary field research. Little Brown, Boston MA

Kleinman LC, Boyd E, Heritage J (1997) Adherence to prescribed explicit criteria during utilization review: an analysis of communication between attending and reviewing physicians. J Am Med Assoc 278:497–501

Kollock P, Blumstein P, Schwartz P (1985) Sex and power in interaction: conversational privileges and duties. Am Sociol Rev 50:24–46

Korsch BM, Negrete VF (1972) Doctor–patient communication. Sci Am 227:66–74

Koschmann T, Lebaron CD, Goodwin C (2005) Formulating objects in the operating room. Paper presented at the International Institute on Ethnomethodology and Conversation Analysis Conference, Bentley College, Boston MA, August 2005.

Kravitz RL, Epstein RM, Feldman MD, Franz CE, Azari R, Milkes MS et al (2005) Influence of patients' requests for direct-to-consumer advertized antidepressants: a randomized controlled trial. JAMA 293(16): 1995–2001

Lazare A, Putnam S, Lipkin M (1995) Three functions of the medical interview. In: Lipkin M, Putnam S, Lazare A (eds) The medical interview: clinical care, education, and research. Springer-Verlag, New York, pp 3–19

Light D (2000) The medical profession and organizational change: from professional dominance to countervailing power. In: Bird C, Conrad P, Fremont AM (eds) Handbook of medical sociology. Prentice Hall, Upper Saddle River NJ, pp 201–216

Lutfey K (2004) Assessment, objectivity, and interaction: the case of patient compliance with treatment regimens. Soc Psychol Q 67:343–368

Lutfey K (2005) On practices of "good doctoring": reconsidering the relationship between provider roles and patient adherence. Sociol Health Illn 27:421–447

Mangione-Smith R, McGlynn E, Elliot M, Krogstad P, Brook R (1999) The relationship between perceived parental expectations and pediatrician antimicrobial prescribing behavior. Pediatrics 103:711–718

Mangione-Smith R, Stivers T, Elliott M, McDonald L, Heritage J (2003) Online commentary during the physical examination: a communication tool for avoiding inappropriate prescribing? Social Science and Medicine 56:313–320

Maynard DW (1991a) Interaction and institutional asymmetry in clinical discourse. Am J Sociol 97(2):448–495

Maynard DW (1991b) The perspective display series and the delivery and receipt of diagnostic news. In: Boden D, Zimmerman DH (eds) Talk and social structure. University of California Press, Berkeley, pp 164–192

Maynard DW (1992) On clinicians co-implicating recipients' perspective in the delivery of diagnostic news. In: Drew P, Heritage J (eds) Talk at work: social interaction in institutional settings. Cambridge University Press, Cambridge, pp 331–358

Maynard DW (1996) On "realization" in everyday life: the forecasting of bad news as a social relation. Am Sociol Rev 60(1):109–132

Maynard DW (2003) Bad news, good news: conversational order in everyday talk and clinical settings. University of Chicago Press, Chicago

Maynard DW (2004) On predicating a diagnosis as an attribute of a person. Discourse Stud 6:53–76

Maynard DW, Clayman S (1991) The diversity of ethnomethodology. Annu Rev Sociol 17:385–418

Maynard DW, Frankel RM (2006) On diagnostic rationality: bad news, good news, and the symptom residue. In: Heritage J, Maynard D (eds) Communication in medical care: interaction between primary care physicians and patients. Cambridge University Press, Cambridge

Maynard DW, Heritage J (2005) Conversation analysis, doctor–patient interaction, and medical communication. Med Educ 39:428–435

Maynard DW, Hudak PL. (2008) "Small talk, high stakes: interactional disattentiveness in the context of prosocial doctor–patient interaction." Lang Soc. 37:661–688.

Maynard DW, Zimmerman D (1984) Topical talk, ritual and the social organization of relationships. Soc Psychol Q 47:301–316

McKinlay JB (1999) The end of the golden age of medicine. N Engl Res Inst Network, Summer 1:3

McWhinney I (1989) The need for a transformed clinical method. In: Stewart M, Roter D (eds) Communicating with medical patients. Sage, Newbury Park

Mead N, Bower P (2000) Patient centredness: a conceptual framework and review of the empirical literature. Soc Sci Med 51:1087–1110

Miller G, Holstein JA (1993) Reconsidering social constructionism. Aldine DeGruyter, Hawthorne NY

Mishler E (1984) The discourse of medicine: dialectics of medical interviews. Ablex, Norwood NJ

Mishler EG (1986) Research interviewing: context and narrative. Harvard University Press, Cambridge, MA

Mondada L (2003) Working with video: how surgeons produce video records of their actions. Vis Stud 18:58–73

Parsons T (1951) The social system. Free Press, New York

Pendleton D (1983) Doctor–patient communication: a review. In: Pendleton D, Hasler J (eds) Doctor–patient communication. Academic, New York, pp 5–53

Peräkylä A (1995) AIDS counselling: institutional interaction and clinical practice. Cambridge University Press, Cambridge

Peräkylä A (1998) Authority and accountability: the delivery of diagnosis in primary health care. Soc Psychol Q 61:301–320

Peräkylä A (2002) Agency and authority: extended responses to diagnostic statements in primary care encounters. Res Lang Soc Interact 35(2):219–247

Peräkylä A (2006) Communicating and responding to diagnosis. In: Heritage J, Maynard D (eds) Practicing medicine: structure and process in primary care consultations. Cambridge University Press, Cambridge

Pescosolido B, McLeod J, Alegría M (2000) Confronting the second social contract: the place of medical sociology in research and policy for the twenty-first century. In: Bird C, Conrad P, Fremont AM (eds) Handbook of medical sociology. Prentice Hall, Upper Saddle River, NJ

Potter S, McKinlay JB (2005) From a relationship to encounter: an examination of longitudinal and lateral dimensions in the doctor–patient relationship. Soc Sci Med 61:465–479

Robinson J (2006) Soliciting patients' presenting concerns. In: Heritage J, Maynard DW (eds) Communication in medical care: interaction between physicians and patients. Cambridge University Press, Cambridge

Robinson J, Heritage J (2005) The structure of patients' presenting concerns: the completion relevance of current symptoms. Soc Sci Med 61:481–493

Robinson J, Stivers T (2001) Achieving activity transitions in primary-care consultations: From history taking to physical examination. Hum Commun Res 27(2):253–298

Robinson JD (2003) An Interactional Structure of Medical Activities During Acute Visits and its Implications for Patients' Participation. Health Commun 15(1):27–59

Robinson JD, Heritage J (2006) Physicians' opening questions and patients' satisfaction. Patient Educ Couns 60:279–285

Rodwin M (1993) Medicine, money and morals: physicians' conflicts of interest. Oxford University Press, New York

Roter D (1977) Patient participation in the patient-provider interaction: The effects of patient question asking on the quality of interaction, satisfaction and compliance. Health Educ Monogr 5:281–315

Roter D, Frankel R (1992) Quantitative and qualitative approaches to the evaluation of the medical dialogue. Soc Sci Med 34(10):1097–1103

Roter D, Hall J (1992) Doctors talking with patients/patients talking with doctors: improving communication in medical visits. Auburn House, Westport Conn

Roter D, Larson S (2001) The relationship between residents' and attending physicians' communication during primary care visits: an illustrative use of the roter interaction analysis system. Health Commun 13(1):33–48

Roter D, Larson S (2002) The roter interaction analysis system (RIAS): utility and flexibility for analysis of medical interactions. Patient Educ Couns 42:243–251

Roter D, McNeilis KS (2003) The nature of the therapeutic relationship and the assessment of its discourse in routine medical visits. In: Thompson T, Dorsey A, Miller K, Parrott R (eds) Handbook of health communication. Lawrence Erlbaum, Mahwah NJ, pp 121–140

Roter D, Stewart M, Putnam S, Lipkin M, Stiles W, Inui TS (1997) Communication patterns of primary care physicians. J Am Med Assoc 227(4):350–356

Roter DL, Hall JA, Katz NR (1988) Physician–patient communication: a descriptive summary of the literature. Patient Educ Couns 12:99–109

Sacks H, Schegloff EA, Jefferson G (1974) A simplest systematics for the organization of turn-taking for conversation. Language 50:696–735

Schegloff EA (1993) Reflections on quantification in the study of conversation. Res Lang Soc Interact 26:99–128

Schegloff EA, Jefferson G, Sacks H (1977) The preference for self-correction in the organization of repair in conversation. Language 53:361–382

Shorter E (1985) Bedside manners: the troubled history of doctors and patients. Simon and Schuster, New York

Silverman D (1987) Communication and medical practice. Sage, London

Silverman D (1997) Discourses of counselling: HIV counselling as social interaction. Sage, London

Spector M, Kitsuse J (1977) Constructing social problems. Cummings, Menlo Park

Starr P (1982) The social transformation of american medicine. Basic Books, New York

Stewart M (1995) Effective physician–patient communication and health outcomes: a review. Can Med Assoc J 152:1423–1433

Stewart M (2003) Evidence for the patient-centered clinical method as a means of implementing the biopsychosocial approach. In: Frankel RM, Quill TE, McDaniel SH (eds) The biopsychosocial approach: past, present, future. University of Rochester Press, Rochester NY, pp 123–132

Stiles WB (1989) Evaluating medical interview process components: null correlations with outcomes may be misleading. Med Care 27(2):212–220

Stivers T (2002a) Participating in decisions about treatment: overt parent pressure for antibiotic medication in pediatric encounters. Soc Sci Med 54:1111–1130

Stivers T (2002b) "Symptoms only" and "candidate diagnoses": presenting the problem in pediatric encounters. Health Commun 14:299–338

Stivers T (2005a) Non-antibiotic treatment recommendations: delivery formats and implications for parent resistance. Soc Sci Med 60:949–964

Stivers T (2005b) Parent resistance to physicians' treatment recommendations: one resource for initiating a negotiation of the treatment decision. Health Commun 18(1):41–74

Stivers T (2006) Treatment decisions: negotiations between doctors and patients in acute care encounters. In: Heritage J, Maynard D (eds) Communication in medical care: interactions between primary care physicians and patients. Cambridge University Press, Cambridge

Stivers T (2007) Practicing patienthood: determinants of children's responses to physicians' questions in routine medical encounters. Unpublished manuscript. Max Planck Institute of Psycholinguistics, Nijmegen, The Netherlands

Stivers T, Majid A (2007) Questioning children: interactional evidence of implicit bias in medical interviews. Soc Psychol Q 70:424–441

Stivers T, Mangione-Smith R, Elliot M, McDonald L, Heritage J (2003) What leads physicians to believe that parents expect antibiotics? A study of parent communication behaviors and physicians' perceptions. J Fam Pract 52:140–148

Strong P (1979) The ceremonial order of the clinic. Routledge, London

Szasz PS, Hollender MH (1956) A contribution to the philosophy of medicine: the basic model of the doctor–patient relationship. Arch Inter Med 97:585–592

Tates K, Elbers E, Meeuwesen L, Bensing J (2002) Doctor–parent–child relationships: a "pas de trois". Patient Educ Counsel 48:5–14

ten Have P (1999) Doing conversation analysis. Sage Publications, London

Thompson T (ed) (2001) Coding patient-provider interaction. A special issue of health communication 13(1). Erlbaum, Mahwah, NJ

Todd AD (1989) Intimate adversaries: cultural conflict between doctors and women patients. University of Pennsylvania Press, Philadelphia

Tuckett D, Boulton M, Olson C, Williams A (1985) Meetings between experts: an approach to sharing ideas in medical consultations. Tavistock, London

Tuckett D, Williams A (1984) Approaches to the measurement of explanation and information-giving in medical consultations: a review of empirical studies. Soc Sci Med 7:571–580

Waitzkin H (1985) Information giving in medical care. J Health Soc Behav 26:81–101

Waitzkin H (1990) On studying the discourse of medical encounters: a critique of quantitative and qualitative methods and a proposal for reasonable compromise. Med Care 28(6):473–488

Waitzkin H (1991) The politics of medical encounters. Yale University Press, New Haven CT

Waitzkin H (2000) Changing patient–physician relationships in the changing health-policy environment. In: Bird C, Conrad P, Fremont AM (eds) Handbook of medical sociology. Prentice Hall, Upper Saddle River NJ, pp 271–283

Waitzkin H (2001) At the front lines of medicine. Rowman and Littlefield, Lanham MD

Wasserman RC, Inui T (1983) Systematic analysis of clinician-patient interactions: a critique of recent approaches with suggestions for future research. Med Care 21(3):279–293

Weber M (1947) The theory of social and economic organization. (Translated by Henderson AM and Talcott Parsons). The Free Press: NY.

West C (1984) Routine complications: troubles with talk between doctors and patients. Indiana University Press, Bloomington IN

West C, Frankel R (1991) Miscommunication in medicine. In: Coupland N, Giles H, Wiemann JM (eds) Miscommunication and problematic talk. Sage, Newbury Park CA, pp 166–194

Williams GC, Frankel RM, Campbell TC, Deci EL (2000) Research on relationship-centered care and healthcare outcomes from the rochester biopsychosocial program: a self-determinatioin theory integration. Fam Syst Health 18:79–90

Zimmerman DH (1988) On conversation: the conversation analytic perspective. In: Anderson JA (ed) Communication Yearbook II. Sage, Newbury Park, CA, pp 406–432

Zimmerman DH (1993) Acknowledgment tokens and speakership incipiency revisited. Res Lang Soc Interact 26(2):179–194

Zola IK (1964) Illness behavior of the working class: implications and recommendations. In: Shostak AB, Gomberg W (eds) Blue-collar world. Prentice Hall, Englewood Cliffs NJ, pp 350–361

Zola IK (1973) Pathways to the doctor: from person to patient. Soc Sci Med 7:677–689

Chapter 18
Enter Health Information Technology: Expanding Theories of the Doctor–Patient Relationship for the Twenty-First Century Health Care Delivery System

Eric R. Wright

Abstract Since the publication of the Institute of Medicine's landmark report *To Err is Human* (1999), health care industry leaders and policymakers have emphasized the central importance of improving the quality of care and reducing the number of medical errors. More recently, various health information technologies (HIT) have been identified by many as essential quality improvement tools. Indeed, over the past two decades, HIT has expanded dramatically. While originally viewed as a hospital-based resource, HIT is increasingly entering the exam rooms of both primary care and specialty providers. The enthusiasm for HIT is undeniable, yet the impact of the expanded use of HIT on the care delivery process, especially the impact on the doctor–patient relationship, is still unclear. Available research highlights an emerging paradox. On the one hand, the strength and quality of the doctor–patient relationship have been shown to have important implications for understanding both the quality and outcome of care provided. At the same time, a growing body of literature suggests that physicians' utilization of HIT during consultations may be changing the nature of their relationships with patients. This chapter reviews the literature on the expansion of HIT in primary care settings and explores the sociological implications of this emerging trend for the social dynamics of doctor–patient interaction.

Introduction

In 1999, the Institute of Medicine published To *Err Is Human*. This report found that 98,000 people per year die due to medical errors. The report also cited the importance of health information technology (HIT) – including computers, personal data assistants (PDAs), decision support software, and electronic medical records (EMRs) – as a core component of infrastructure of the health care system to improve quality. President George W. Bush (2004), in his 2004 State of the Union Address, proclaimed that HIT – particularly the use of EMRs and HIT systems that included electronic billing – is a critical investment that would improve efficiency and help to slow the rising cost of health care. Initially seen as resources reserved for academic medical centers and research hospitals, the diffusion of various forms of HIT has increased exponentially over the past 3 decades.

E.R. Wright (✉)
Center for Health Policy, Indiana University School of Medicine, Department of Public Health, IUPUI,
410 W. Tenth Street, HS 3119, Indianapolis, IN 46202, USA
e-mail: ewright@iupui.edu

At the same time, a long history of research on doctor–patient interaction has concluded that high quality communication is essential for delivering high-quality care (Booker 2005; Ong et al. 1995; Shaw et al. 2007). When patients and doctors trust each other, they are more likely to engage in collaborative decision making, which increases both physician and patient satisfaction and improves outcomes (Epstein et al. 2004; Guadagnoli and Ward 1998). In recent years, however, as computers have entered more and more consultation rooms, providers and researchers have begun to ask: What impact do computers have on the nature and quality of the relationship between doctors and their patients? In this chapter, I offer a brief overview of the expansion and diffusion of HIT in primary care settings and explore the sociological implications of this emerging trend for the social dynamics of doctor–patient interaction.

Diffusion of Health Information Technology Within the Health Care System

HIT is becoming increasingly common in health care delivery settings (Robert Wood Johnson Foundation 2006). HIT has emerged as an umbrella term to refer to an enormously diverse set of information and communication technologies, including automated medical order systems, e-prescribing, electronic health record (EHR) management systems maintained by providers, personal health record (PHR) systems that patients manage, email communication with patients and among providers, electronic transfer of medical and/or billing information, and electronic medical resource and diagnostic/assessment support software. While most people conceptualize HIT as a particular piece of hardware or software (e.g., a computer, electronic physician desk reference), the U.S. Department of Health and Human Services defines it as the array of information and communication technological tools that "allows the comprehensive management of medical information and its secure exchange between health care consumers and providers" (U.S. Department of Health & Human Services 2008).

The earliest form of HIT dates back to the mid 1960s with the advent of multifunction, hospital-based information systems developed for major tertiary care centers in California, Massachusetts, Utah, and North Carolina (Staggers et al. 2001). Since the 1960s, the use of health IT has steadily increased; however, the most dramatic increase in the use of health IT began in the early 1990s (American Hospital Association 2007; Bates and Gawande 2003; Connors 2001; Division of Information Technology and Research 2007). From its inception, the use of HIT was driven by a desire to reduce medical errors and improve efficiency (Robert Wood Johnson Foundation 2006). Indeed, developers and more recent advocates maintain that moving from a largely paper driven record system to an automated one will reduce the amount of paper, facilitate more accurate and timely exchange of critical health information, cut down on medical errors, improve billing practices, and ultimately reduce health care costs (Association of American Medical Colleges 2004; Institute of Medicine 2001).

While HIT covers a wide range of discrete and increasingly sophisticated technologies, most providers and patients interface with these comprehensives systems through the management and use of EHRs and more elaborate health information systems to support provider and patient decision making, typically via a desktop or bedside computer, or handheld computer devices such as PDA's that are connected to the internet and/or large secure networks (Al Ubaydli 2004; American Hospital Association 2007). Because my central interest in this paper is on exploring the sociological implications of HIT for the physician–patient relationship, I do not explore in great depth the technological aspects of HIT in the broad sense, but rather focus on the ways that providers and patients utilize and experience HIT (e.g., interacting with computers/internet, the information gleaned from an EHR).

Before turning to the sociological implications, I briefly describe the nature and extent that HIT is being used by health care providers as they go about their work with patients.

The most fundamental building block of any HIT system is the EHR. Most experts agree that a well-designed EHR has the potential to revolutionize health care and possibly reduce health care costs (Institute of Medicine 2001; Powell 2004). Health informaticians and policymakers suggest that EHRs should be a comprehensive repository of patient data (including patients' past, present, and prospective health-related information) in digital form, stored and exchanged securely, and accessible by multiple, authorized users (Institute of Medicine 2001; Robert Wood Johnson Foundation 2006). The experts further agree that the primary objective of EHRs is to support continuing, efficient, and quality integrated health care (Schloeffel 2004). While EHRs first came into use with the advent of computers in the 1960s, the current use of EHRs was encouraged by the Institute of Medicine in 1991 when it recognized EHRs as an essential part of health care (Rubin et al. 2006).

Unfortunately, the data available to assess the extent to which health care providers are using HIT in their daily work are surprisingly limited. There have been surveys conducted of providers, physician practices, and hospitals, and all indications are that the number of providers across all types of clinical settings that utilize HIT in providing clinical care is increasing. In 2006, the Robert Wood Johnson Foundation convened an Expert Consensus Panel to evaluate the state of HIT use in the USA. Their report synthesized data from multiple surveys and estimated that nationally, approximately 24% of physicians' offices were using EHRs. Not surprisingly, they found that practice setting matters, with 39% of physicians in large offices and only 16% of physicians in solo practices reporting use of EHR systems. In a survey of 847 ambulatory care clinics in Massachusetts, Simon et al. (2008) also found that primary care-only practices and mixed practices were significantly more likely to report using EHRs than special care practices (23 and 25% versus 14% respectively). In another recent study, DesRoches and colleagues (2008) found that only 17% of doctors surveyed have EHRs. More importantly, they also found that only four percent of the physicians had "fully functional" EHRs, while 13% had only "basic" EHRs, which lacked two critical functional components: computerized physician order-entry and clinical decision support software. The prospects for adoption of EHRs by providers appear to be strong. In Simon et al.'s (2008) survey, they asked practices that did not currently have an EHR system about their plans to implement one in the near future and found that "13% plan to implement one within the next 12 months, 24% within the next two years, [and] 11% within the next 3–5 years."

The potential for improving both the quality and efficiency of health care delivery has led payers and policymakers to call for the wider diffusion and integration of HIT throughout the health care system (Bush 2004; Institute of Medicine 1999). Both the federal and state governments in the USA and the National Health Service in the UK have recently announced extensive initiatives to increase the use of HIT as part of routine ambulatory care (Bush 2004; Dixon et al. 2007; Powell 2004). Based on its review of the HIT evidence base, the Department of Health and Human Services' Agency for Healthcare Research and Quality (AHRQ) concluded, "HIT has the potential to enable a dramatic transformation in the delivery of health care, making it safer, more effective, and more efficient" (Shekelle et al. 2006).

According to AHRQ and other researchers, HIT has positively affected the quality, efficiency, and cost of medical care (Shekelle et al. 2006). The three major benefits of HIT on the quality of health care include an increased adherence to guideline-based care, enhanced surveillance and monitoring, and a reduction in medication errors (Asch et al. 2004; Chaudhry et al. 2006; Garg et al. 2005; Harrison and Palacio 2006; Jain et al. 2005; Kucher et al. 2005). The major efficiency benefit of HIT has been to decrease utilization of care, primarily of laboratory and radiology testing. While the impact of HIT on costs has proven difficult to measure, AHRQ and other independent researchers have concluded that based on available data, implementation of EHR systems predicted substantial costs savings with the benefits of implementation outweighing the initial investment costs in the long run (Shekelle et al. 2006; Wang et al. 2003). Although the reviews completed by AHRQ have demonstrated the efficacy of HIT for improving healthcare quality, efficiency, and reducing costs, the authors agree that the effectiveness of these technologies in the practice setting, where physicians deliver most health care, remains less clear. Thus, some experts warn of potentially negative consequences resulting from HIT such as shifting ambulatory care to telephone contacts (Garrido et al. 2005) or they point to the failure of HIT to improve adherence to treatment plans for patients with heart disease and hypertension (Murray et al. 2004; Tierney et al. 2003).

Many barriers exist that prevent physicians from using EHRs (Robert Wood Johnson Foundation 2006; Rothschild et al. 2006). Some barriers are related to the EHR software itself, which is often developed for large hospitals and not small, private practices. Early EHR systems were designed to record clinical and billing data on hospital-based acute care services rather than the kinds of data needed by primary care providers to monitor patients over the long-term, especially those with chronic care needs where frequent follow-up is needed. Other barriers include the location of one's practice, with urban centers being more likely than rural areas to have some form of EHR system. The cost of an EHR system can also be an obstacle to implementation (Robert Wood Johnson Foundation 2006; Rothschild et al. 2006; Shekelle et al. 2006; Simon et al. 2008). An EHR system for a small practice might require an initial investment of $15,000. In addition to the capital cost, a significant amount of time would be required to get the system operational and to train the staff in its use. During the transition to an EHR system, physicians may have to see fewer patients, which could lead to a temporary loss of income. For the physician in private practice, the implementation of an EHR system can be a daunting task (DesRoches et al. 2008; Rothschild et al. 2006).

Most often providers gain access to HIT systems using internet-connected computers on desktops or at the bedside. Handheld computer devices or PDAs have become increasingly popular, as they often provide access to some functional components of clinical HIT systems in a small, handheld, easily portable device. Because of their portability, PDAs have proven useful for storing data to which physicians may need regular access, such as pharmaceutical reference guides (Garritty and Emam 2006). Generally, physicians use PDAs mainly as reference guides to look up drug information, obtain lists of recommended drugs for specific conditions, check for drug interactions, determine if pregnant women can take certain medications, and access medical textbooks online. Some PDAs also perform medical calculations. Recently, many physicians have begun using PDAs to write e-prescriptions. When used in this fashion, the physician can enter the prescription into the PDA, transmit it directly to the pharmacy, and, if available, record it in the patient's EHR (Al Ubaydli 2004). In a recent survey of PDA-using -physicians, 39% reported using the pharmaceutical reference software on their handheld devices in more than 50% of their patient encounters. A significant majority of these physicians also admitted that the software prevented either adverse drug interactions or other medical errors three or more times in the four weeks prior to the survey (Rothschild et al. 2006). Similarly, Dee et al. (2005) reported that 87% of physicians they surveyed reported using a PDA during doctor–patient consultations. Of all the physicians surveyed, 32% said they were occasional PDA users. Of the occasional users, 54% stated they had changed a patient's treatment plan based entirely on information acquired from their PDA. Due to their affordability, ease of use, and ever-increasing capabilities, it is estimated that by 2011, 70% of medical doctors will be relying on PDAs to help them complete their patient care activities (Pizzi 2007).

HIT is no longer just for providers, either. The number of consumers who use the internet to access basic health information has increased exponentially in recent years (Tu and Cohen 2008). More recently, private corporations and health insurance providers have begun to market PHRs as a parallel to EHR systems (Aetna Intelihealth Inc. 2008; Gustafson et al. 1997; Hassol et al. 2004; MyPHR.com 2008; Pizzi 2006). These systems are designed to allow patients to construct, usually via the internet, a permanent and easily portable record of pertinent medical information, ranging from basic demographic information, medical history, and allergies. In some cases, these systems are deeply integrated with EHR systems, and both patients and providers can input and access information as needed (Hartley 2007; Hassol et al. 2004). Alternatively, patients can maintain control over the record and share it only with providers and payers as needed to support their own clinical care, often by simply informing their providers or by the swipe of a PHR card (MyPHR.com 2008; Pizzi 2006). As patient-centered PHRs represent one of the newest features of HIT, these systems have not yet been widely adopted by consumers, and little research has examined their impact on clinical care.

While the specific type may vary, HIT is clearly quickly becoming a more common feature of clinical care settings. More importantly, HIT is dramatically changing the nature of medical work (Aydin 1989; Heath et al. 2003; Stoeckle 1988) and, as a result, changing the way providers and patients interact. The question of how HIT is affecting the doctor–patient relationship has received surprisingly little attention in medical sociology. In the remainder of this paper, I explore some of the sociological implications of this emerging trend and highlight potential directions for future medical sociology research.

HIT and the Sociological Study of Doctor–Patient Interaction

Both sociological and health services research reminds us that health care delivery is, at its core, about the interactions that occur between patients and their health care providers, usually in the privacy of the provider's office (Heritage and Maynard 2006a; Hohmann 1999). As described above, the role of the computer in health care delivery is changing rapidly from being primarily a tool for information management and processing to one in which HIT actually influences, to varying degrees, the patient–provider relationship. In more extreme cases, the HIT equipment may even serve as a proxy by embodying providers, as in the case of telemedicine, or even more dramatically as automated health data collectors (eHealth Magazine 2008). Prior research on the effects of HIT on the patient–provider relationship has highlighted a number of potential concerns for the quality of provider–patient relationships; however, the extant research has been conducted nearly exclusively by communications, health informatics, and health services researchers. As a relatively new area, this research is largely atheoretical and, more importantly, neglects the structure and socially dynamic nature of patient–provider relationships.

Here, I assert that HIT is rapidly becoming an increasingly influential and powerful *social* actor in health care settings. In this regard, I believe that medical sociologists have an important role to play in the advancement of research on patient and provider experiences with HIT. Consistent with classical theoretical concerns, sociological research on the patient–provider relationship could help understand how different types of HIT impact interpersonal dynamics in clinical settings. The increasing sophistication of HIT also raises new theoretical questions regarding the social dynamics of clinical information processing and how they affect or mediate the outcomes of care. Moreover, I argue that the expansion of HIT poses even broader challenges for the status and definition of the profession of medicine. In the following sections, I explore these domains in more depth and highlight health services research that emphasizes the social significance of HIT, and discuss the potential value thinking sociology has for the study of HIT across these three areas.

HIT and Patient–Provider Rapport

Health services and health informatics researchers have become increasingly interested in the effects of HIT on the nature and quality of the interpersonal relationships of providers and patients. Underscoring the potentially dramatic social impact of HIT, some have gone as far as to argue that

EHRs can be seen as a separate entity or even a third party to exam room conversations, with both the patients and doctors projecting their perceptions on it (Margalit et al. 2006; Schloeffel 2004). Guided primarily by an interpersonal communications framework, researchers have tended to focus on process analyses of clinical interactions in which HIT is utilized. Reminiscent of classical interaction process analyses (Bales 1950) and informed by more recent strategies for coding clinical interaction (Roter and Larson 2002), researchers have constructed objective measures of provider–computer interaction as well as computer-mediated provider–patient interaction behavior.

Verbal and nonverbal behaviors such as empathy and support, posture, gesture, and tone of voice have been related to many important outcomes of care such as patient satisfaction and adherence to treatment. In an observational study of computer-using physicians, Frankel et al. (2005) found that physicians were able to maintain communication with patients during computer use in several ways. Physicians often sustained verbal contact with the patient by talking with him or her while typing on the keyboard or reading the screen. Physicians kept visual contact with patients by making eye contact intermittently with them during computer use. Physicians also adopted some level of postural closeness to patients during computer use by positioning their head or torso toward the patient rather than having their back toward the patient. Computers adversely affected the quality of the communication between physicians and patients when physicians demonstrated poor skills in organizing a patient's visit or poor data gathering skills. Rouf et al. (2007) came to a similar conclusion when interviewing patients of computer-using physicians at a medical school. Patients seeing the less experienced residents, compared to those seeing faculty, were more likely to agree that the computer adversely affected the amount of time the physician spent talking to, looking at, and examining them, overall decreasing the amount of interpersonal contact they received. Therefore, the effective use of computers depends on a clinician's baseline skills that are amplified with the introduction of HIT, either positively or negatively, in their effects on clinician–patient communication (Frankel et al. 2005). Still other researchers have found that well designed electronic patient records do not disturb the clinician–patient relationship, particularly when one gives careful consideration to the positioning of computers in exam rooms and the way it affects both patient and physician nonverbal behavior (Christensen and Grimsmo 2008; Margalit et al. 2006). While these process-oriented studies suggest the important impact HIT can have on the quality of provider–patient interaction, they generally conceptualize the medical encounter in very traditional ways, emphasizing rapport or patients' willingness to disclose information to providers so that they can make appropriate clinical decisions (Emanuel and Emanuel 1992).

Sociological work on the physician–patient interaction over the past several decades, however, emphasizes that the development of clinical rapport is a much more dynamic process that is heavily influenced by the social contexts of medical encounters (Heritage and Maynard 2006b). Classical discourse analyses of physician–patient interaction have highlighted the highly structured nature of the medical interview, the sharp differences in the interactional objectives of physicians and patients, and the power dynamics that tend to subordinate patients' needs to the diagnostic work of the physician (Mishler 1984; Waitzkin 1991; West and Frankel 1991). More recently, Heritage and Maynard (2006a) suggest that conversation analysts have augmented and deepened our understanding by focusing on the sequencing of action (Goffman 1983; Sacks et al. 1974; Schegloff et al. 1977), the substantive focus of clinical interaction (Jefferson 1988; Maynard 2003), and the social construction and negotiation of meaning (Heritage and Raymond 2005; Maynard and Frankel 2006; Maynard and Heritage 2005).

With the exception of the role technology plays in the construction of meaning, such as in discussions of medical information (Maynard 2003), sociologists have paid surprisingly little attention to the impact of technology on provider–patient interaction. The case of HIT, however, is important for understanding the development of clinical rapport because it, as evidenced above, affects the behavior and interactional processes occurring between patients and their providers. Perhaps even more important for the future, HIT is sociologically significant because it changes the social context of the medical encounter. These technologies – by their very nature – connect participants to society beyond the immediate medical setting and may have an effect on the rapport between providers and patients and the extent that patients may be willing to trust their health care providers.

While few studies have evaluated specifically the issue of trust between physicians and patients when HIT is utilized, research has suggested that patient involvement and participation in medical decision-making creates a more trusting doctor–patient relationship (Guadagnoli and Ward 1998; Roter 1977). If patients have established a trusting relationship with the doctor, technology seems to be seen as a means of communicating their concerns to the doctor in a more comprehensive way by stimulating personal language. E-mediated communication (contacting doctors via computers) can strengthen patients' trust in the doctor despite other trust-reducing trends in health care such as growing health care costs, malpractice crisis, and medical commercialism (Ventres et al. 2005). Studies revealed that patients were mostly uninformed as to how the EHR was used in their medical care (Als 1997; Schloeffel 2004; Ventres et al. 2006). Although patients' fears and doubts were common, they generally remained unexpressed to their physicians. Doctors, in turn, did not often explain the role of the computer to their patients. Reported barriers to using EHR by physicians included loss of eye contact with patients and falling behind schedule (Linder et al. 2006; Makoul et al. 2001; Margalit et al. 2006). Possible loss of confidentiality poses a challenge to doctors' technical and communication skills and remains the key concern in patients trusting the use of HIT (Linder et al. 2006).

Closely related to the issue of trust is the growing concern regarding the confidentiality of personal health information (DeCew 2000; U.S. Department of Health & Human Services 2008). Indeed, the main concerns undermining patients' trust in HIT were security and confidentiality issues (Chin 2003; Ornstein and Bearden 1994; Ridsdale and Hudd 1994), including accessibility by the government or insurers, and a possibility of technical failure. As society has become more dependent on computer technology and the amount of data transferred via the internet has increased, the general public has become ever more interested in accessing health information via the internet, and concern about the security and confidentiality of personal information has intensified because of highly publicized cases of data theft or mismanagement (Tu and Cohen 2008). Most recently, new ethical questions have emerged regarding the control and ownership of individuals' personal health information. Generally, EHR systems are owned and operated by health care facilities, while PHRs typically controlled and managed questions. How these systems connect (or not) is likely to become a more salient policy question with the push to integrate HIT systems.

Nevertheless, the exchange of health information holds great promise for reducing the cost of health care by reducing repetitive tests and timely sharing of critical medical information (Institute of Medicine 1999, 2001; Shekelle et al. 2006). The push to exchange health information among providers will also contribute to dramatic changes in the perception of the social context of medical interaction. This is not surprising as part of the promise of HIT is that providers can reduce costs through centralized billing and sharing critical information to coordinate care across providers (Institute of Medicine 1999; Shekelle et al. 2006), and the federal and state governments have already taken major steps to create regional health information exchanges (Dixon et al. 2007). These systems could prove invaluable for providing medical care in emergency situations (e.g., an emergency physician could potentially access an unconscious patient's medical records to help guide treatment decision making) or for controlling over- or inappropriate utilization (e.g., patients who seek unnecessary treatment or drugs from multiple providers).

Presently, health information does not flow easily within the system – at least not among providers – without intentional efforts to share patient information because of HIPAA and professional standards calling for strict confidentiality (Dixon et al. 2007). As health information becomes more freely accessible within the health care system, how this information is shared (or not shared) among providers and with patients will likely contribute to a redefinition of the social context of provider–patient interaction and change both patient and provider behavior. The expanded sharing of information among providers could also contribute to a structural deterioration in the movement toward patient-centered care, as medical knowledge regarding individual patients will extend beyond the immediate information shared by the patient and shift the balance of power even more toward the physicians and other providers involved in a patient's care. Thus, on many levels, HIT technology within medical settings has the potential for redefining the social context, and sociologists could contribute by moving beyond simple process studies to understanding how HIT influences patient and providers perceptions of the social context of the medical encounter.

The Social Dynamics of Health Information Processing

The impact of HIT on the social context of the medical encounter also affects the social dynamics of how patient information is collected, managed, and used. Indeed, a central premise guiding the dissemination of HIT is that it will improve provider performance, and there is a growing body of research demonstrating many tangible performance-related benefits including offering real-time access to information and clinical resources, improving adherence to preventive care guidelines, reducing inpatient medication errors, and improving familiarity with patients (Asch et al. 2004; Garg et al. 2005; Harrison and Palacio 2006; Hsu et al. 2005; Jain et al. 2005; Kucher et al. 2005). Among the many application areas of HIT, much attention is often given to the use of EHRs, predominantly used in examination rooms. Currently, less than 1 in 5 practices in the USA use EHRs in the exam room; however, their use is expected to spread widely in the coming years (Robert Wood Johnson Foundation 2006; Versel 2005). When using EHRs in an exam setting, the activities most commonly completed by physicians are correcting or updating the patient's medication list and writing at least part of the visit note. Other functions frequently performed with EHRs include reviewing a patient's allergy, family, social, and immunization history. Clinical information management and decision support tools available within an EHR system help to make patient data readily accessible and to improve the collection of clinical information, empowering providers in their work (Shekelle et al. 2006). Not surprisingly, research has also documented when the use of HIT is less likely to lead to improved effectiveness, specifically in situations where the workload is particularly high, when clinicians have not had adequate training, and when unique clinical situations do not match well with the structure of the HIT in use (Linder et al. 2006). Nevertheless, the consensus in this research appears to be that HIT can improve outcomes and the quality of care (Asch et al. 2004; DesRoches et al. 2008; Garg et al. 2005; Jain et al. 2005; Kucher et al. 2005; Liu et al. 2007; Osheroff et al. 2007; Rothschild et al. 2006; Rubin et al. 2006; Shekelle et al. 2006).

A number of studies have reported high levels of satisfaction with HIT among both physicians and patients, particularly with regard to the ease of storing and accessing information contained within EHR's (Harrison and Palacio 2006; Ornstein and Bearden 1994; Shekelle et al. 2006). According to Ventres et al. (2006), accessibility of the EHR gave both physicians and patients a sense of seamless communication because of the shared belief that the convenient availability of computers enables adding patient information to the medical record in real time. Besides having real time access to charts, other sources of patient satisfaction include participation in the decision-making process and in the explanation of diagnoses and treatment. Studies showed that patient satisfaction with the physician's use of the latest medical technology increased after computer introduction because of a better chance to participate in the decision-making process during a visit and a more active role of physicians in clarifying information (Hsu et al. 2005; Makoul et al. 2001; Margalit et al. 2006). It is noted that spatial arrangement of HIT devices is important since a computer screen more accessible to patients allows them to view their own record and/or participate in the consultation (Makoul et al. 2001; McGrath et al. 2007).

Traditionally, as noted above, clinical medicine has viewed the purpose of the medical interview as an information retrieval process intended for treatment decision-making (Heritage and Maynard 2006a, b; Ong et al. 1995). Theoretical conceptualizations of this physician–patient relationship often are designed to highlight differences in strategies physicians use to elicit essential and valid information from patients (Inui and Carter 1985; Roter, et al. 1988; Roter and Hall 2006). More recently, attention has focused on how HIT affects this process, and one ethnographic study (Ventres et al. 2005) identified three emerging practice styles: informational (where the principal focus of attention is on gathering data as prompted by the screen), interpersonal (where the physician focuses their nonverbal body language and on patients), and managerial (where the physician alternates his/her attention between patients and computers in defined intervals).

From a sociological perspective, Ventres et al.'s (2005) study is especially interesting because it highlights the emerging social and symbolic salience of HIT in the provider–patient interaction. At the simplest level, the physical presence of HIT is demanding that patients and providers negotiate new norms of interaction in medical settings. Several recent studies have documented some potential challenges in the use of HIT from the patient's perspective. Specifically, some patients report concerns that using HIT is shifting the physician's attention away from face-to-face engagement, and toward the computer screen. Research seems to support this view, as patients report that time spent navigating the computer system, searching for information, and documenting the visit are reducing the time available to address patients' needs and psychosocial concerns (Christensen and Grimsmo 2008; Hsu et al. 2005; Warshawsky et al. 1994). HIT proponents, however, counter that such adverse effects are likely temporary and due mainly to physicians having to adapt to using a computer and learning new skills (Hsu et al. 2005). Nevertheless, it is clear that the verbal and nonverbal communication skills of doctors may play a key role in increasing or decreasing patient satisfaction with HIT-enhanced visits (Ventres et al. 2005), which may explain the mixed results of many studies. While some studies observed an increase in communication (Andreassen et al. 2006) and some no change in satisfaction with time available and expressing psychosocial concerns (Christensen and Grimsmo 2008; Hsu et al. 2005; Legler and Oates 1993; Ridsdale and Hudd 1994; Solomon and Dechter 1995), most report decreased communication between patients and physicians as a result of incorporating HIT into medical practice (Makoul et al. 2001; Margalit et al. 2006).

There will likely be other ways that HIT may change the social dynamics of health information collection. Indeed, while most believe that the accuracy of health care will improve with HIT, some studies suggest that the social context of how health information is collected and disseminated may also be a source of error (Ash et al. 2004; Grondahl 2005, 2008). There may also be other changes to how information is collected. For example, some health policy leaders have questioned how involved physicians should be in the collection of patient's health information. Why couldn't a nurse, nurse practitioner, physician assistant, or lay health advisor work with individual patients to enter critical health information which then is accessed by the physician to plan treatment? Reorganizing the collection of personal health information in this way could reduce health care costs by utilizing the advanced skills of physicians more efficiently (Roob 2006). Telemedicine and remote diagnostic testing and information processing, in many ways, represent a precursor to this model, and there is some evidence that patients increasingly are using email and other forms of e-mediated communication with their doctors (Andreassen et al. 2006).

At the same time, primary care providers have increasingly relied on simple screening tools to help identify important health needs that may be difficult to address directly in face-to-face interaction, such as alcohol and drug use or sexual behavior (Cloud 2001; Dennis and Newman 1996). While many of these are still administered by paper and pencil, it isn't hard to imagine a future with paperless emergency departments (EDs) or clinics where patients may be asked to complete these questionnaires on a computer or other remote data collection tool so that results added immediately to the patients EHR for the physician to utilize in treatment planning. As noted above, health insurance and health informatics companies are launching web-based PHRs for patients to enter and manage their own health records and share them with their treatment providers. While the broader trend toward the McDonaldization of society (Ritzer 1993) and "self-service" has not, as yet, been fully realized in the health care system, trends in other sectors certainly suggest that the public could be comfortable with adopting this mode of operation – at some level – within our health care system.

In many ways, the organization and effectiveness of HIT depend on highly structured data that are collected, managed, and utilized in systematic ways. Indeed, HIT proponents such as the Institute of Medicine (1999) and others (Chaudhry et al. 2006; Robert Wood Johnson Foundation 2006; Shekelle et al. 2006) argue that if we could reduce the variability in both what and how health care is delivered, we would improve both treatment outcomes and population health. Practically, this has meant that there is an increased emphasis on collecting discrete measures of health status (e.g., symptom checklists, fields for clinical values, discrete categorical information [e.g., age, race, gender, family history]) that can be used for diagnostic and treatment planning purposes by clinicians working directly or remotely with patients or by automated clinical decision support systems (Osheroff et al. 2007).

Not surprisingly, the highly structured nature of HIT data processing is having a significant impact on the social dynamics within the medical encounter. In many ways, the medical interview is being restructured and standardized to conform with HIT to facilitate the collection and management of health information within EHRs. That is, the medical encounter is evolving into a semi-structured research interview that deemphasizes personal narratives over discrete answers to questions about diagnostically-relevant information. Waitzkin (1991) critically observed that physicians' emphasis on diagnostic decision-making often resulted in physicians overlooking the broader social context of patients' complaints and/or the imposition of subtle forms of social control, tendencies that could be exacerbated by a greater reliance on EHRs and HIT. Indeed, both providers and patients often report feeling dissatisfied with the decreased appeal of personal narratives in favor of the new more structured ways of conducting medical encounters (Liu et al. 2007; Makoul et al. 2001). From a provider's perspective, EHR notes are concise and easy to ready, but they lack the depth and intricacy of more traditional narrated notes. Physicians express concerns of the greater reliance on templates and quick-text features that produce more analogous-looking notes but may also promote the practice of "cookbook medicine" (Harding 1994; Steinberg 2006). Most EHR templates do not address patients' emotional issues and have significant limitations when it comes to providing information necessary to help manage the complexities of patients with multiple or chronic complaints (Chin 2003; Schloeffel 2004). Some physicians also report frustration with the apparent shift in the administrative workload from health secretaries to physicians as they are required to enter information that was once entered by support staff (Christensen and Grimsmo 2008). Increasingly, doctors are being burdened with filling in forms, scheduling patients, updating patient contact information, and preparing referral letters.

HIT and the Deprofessionalization of Medicine

The sociological implications of the increasingly structured medical encounter extend beyond these more practical considerations. HIT, and in particular computerized decision support systems (DSS), have the potential to hasten the "deprofessionalization" of medicine (Ritzer and Walczak 1988). Traditionally, sociologists have focused on the many ways that government and industry regulation, as well as health-related consumer movements, have challenged medical authority (Hafferty and Light 1995; Light 1989). Nevertheless, HIT also appears to be making it easier for both regulators and consumers to take control over medical care away from physicians and other health care providers.

Clearly, medical knowledge is vast and continues to grow at a rapid pace. However, much of physicians' authority is based on their command of a well-defined and controlled body of scientific knowledge (Freidson 1970; Starr 1982). Initially, HIT and decision support software were designed to assist providers not just to document health care encounters and patients but also to make more accurate diagnoses, reduce medical errors, and even choose the most clinically efficacious and economically efficient treatment plans (Chaudhry et al. 2006; Institute of Medicine 2001; Shekelle et al. 2006; Staggers et al. 2001). Data from these support systems are used to support a wide range of administrative and business functions within health care facilities, ranging from documenting the array of services provided, human resource planning, and billing. In addition to establishing the importance of patient confidentiality of EMRs, another objective of the U.S. Congress (1996) was to promote the standardization of computer records to facilitate more efficient billing and reporting information critical for monitoring and evaluating the health care system. The Centers for Medicare and Medicaid Services (CMS) is increasingly reliant on these types of services information for monitoring the cost and quality of care and is investigating initiatives to monetarily reward providers based on the quality of their performance using clinical and billing data supplied to them electronically (Centers for Medicare and Medicaid Services 2005). Private insurance companies have also used information collected through various HIT to examine patterns of utilization and outcomes in the populations they insure. Most importantly, payers – both public and private – use HIT and the type of data it generates to regulate physician behavior, something that physicians are complaining about more frequently as payers work to control costs more aggressively (Centers for Medicare and Medicaid Services 2005; Rosenthal 1993; Starr 2002; The Medical Society of the State of New York 2008).

The threat of HIT to physician authority extends even deeper to the level of the medical encounter. Computers and PDAs are becoming standard reference tools for new and more senior physicians to access critical diagnostic and pharmaceutical information both in and outside the exam room, and similar tools are usually available within hospital and clinic settings via desktop and bedside computers (Carroll et al. 2002; Lottridge et al. 2006; Rothschild et al. 2006). These tools, however, have the potential to change the nature of the critical thinking required by physicians to deliver basic health care. Often described by critics as "cookbook medicine," the growing perception that some providers – whether voluntarily or involuntarily – are following assessment and treatment protocols generated by software algorithms may convey an impression – rightly or wrongly – that the profession of medicine is no longer in control of the practice of their craft (Harding 1994; Steinberg 2006). Studies of patient responses to this type of HIT in the consultation room suggest that some patients view these tools as a potentially valuable check on their physicians' knowledge (Rouf et al. 2007; Winkelman et al. 2005). Still other consumers may view the computers and PDA's as crutches for the physicians and that the computer/PDA is the real decision-making authority. Interestingly, in one study of physicians' attitudes about using PDA's in medical consultation interviews, physicians were divided about whether it was a good or bad idea to use them in front of the patient because it might give patients an impression that the physician is not competent (Lottridge et al. 2006).

As HIT systems develop, though, the impact of HIT may be even more significant. Presently, with the exception of services that require "preauthorization" from payers, decisions about coverage are typically determined after the medical encounter. Truly integrated EMRs will likely alter medical decision making even more directly at the point of care. Physicians will be able to determine which procedures, tests, or treatments are covered or not covered under a particular patient's health plan, increasingly the likelihood that patients will view their providers as not being in control of their care. Thus, while DSS and related HIT may facilitate improvements in clinical care, it also has the potential to undermine the interpersonal authority that physicians have enjoyed because of their professional dominance over the body of medical knowledge and health care.

At the level of the consumer, the Internet is already changing the way consumers interact with their health care providers, and HIT has the potential to expand consumers' access to more and increasingly sophisticated health information. Consumers are already seeking information about their own health on the Internet (Tu and Cohen 2008), and despite disclaimers that the information provided is only for educational purposes and that "only a physician can diagnose," many patients are now entering the provider–patient relationship with more information and, in some cases, even a preconceived understanding of their health problem or preliminary self-diagnosis (Ahmad et al. 2006; Grady 2008; Gustafson et al. 1997). In an effort to encourage people to use their services or products, some companies have even posted symptom checklists or screeners online to allow potential patients to "educate" themselves about the severity of their health problems and even to refer them to places where they can get health care, most often the web-site sponsor's product or service. "Ask a Nurse" and similar "hotlines," once a popular initiative sponsored by many hospital systems, also appear to be migrating to the web. More objective sources of information are also becoming more readily available for consumers. Policymakers and health industry leaders have launched initiatives to improve the "transparency" of information about health care providers (Colmers 2007). Specifically, they are working to make data regarding the cost, quality, and outcomes of health care services public (usually via the internet) to facilitate "comparison shopping." More recently, consumer advocacy groups, such as "Angie's List" (www.angieslist.com), have begun collating and disseminating consumers' reports on health care providers, typically physicians (McManis 2008; Murphy 2007). Online networks and support groups of people facing similar health challenges also have emerged as important sources of information and have encouraged patients to take more control of their health care (Cotten 2001; van Uden-Kraan et al. 2008).

Unfortunately, there is very little systematic research on how consumers are accessing information via publicly available HIT or how health care providers are responding to consumers who do. Much of what we know is based on small and anecdotal studies. Some applaud this development, citing the improvements in health literacy (Ahmad et al. 2006; Hardey 2001; Norman and Skinner 2006; Tyson 2000). Consumers who have a better understanding of their health conditions can be more effective communicators with their health care providers (Norman and Skinner 2006; Patel et al. 2002). At the same time, providers – especially physicians – report frustrations with patients who "second guess" them and ask "too many questions" (Ahmad et al. 2006; Hardey 2001).

Clearly the demand for publicly available HIT is great; a simple internet search will yield hundreds of web-resources on even the most obscure health conditions. All indications are that this market will continue to expand and that health informatics companies will develop more sophisticated internet resources for consumers. While the publicly available HIT will probably lag behind the development of professional HIT, developers will likely build on ideas and resources designed for decision support systems as they search for new professional and lay consumers for HIT products. Many of these web resources include explicit endorsements from physicians, nurses, or health care organizations; however, many do not. Regardless, there are many unanswered questions regarding consumers and publicly available HIT. Which consumers are accessing this type of information? How do consumers make sense of the information they acquire? How, if at all, does this information affect their health and utilization behavior? How does this type of information affect their attitudes toward and interactions with their health care providers? Perhaps most important for medical sociology, to what extent and in what ways does the expanding market of publicly available HIT undermine medical authority in the minds of consumers and other professional constituencies?

Conclusion

Whether simply sitting on a desktop or mounted on a wall, the entry of computers into medical offices is yielding significant changes in the provider–patient relationship. Given the growing public and industry policymakers' push for integrated health information systems, expanding consumers demand for online health information products, and the extraordinary potential for economic profit, it seems clear that the diffusion and utilization of HIT will probably only accelerate and expand exponentially in the decades to come. Yet, our understanding of the social impact of HIT is clearly not keeping up with its uptake. In this chapter, I tried to highlight why HIT represents an important theoretical concern for sociologists interested in physician/provider–patient interaction. Specifically, I argued that HIT is becoming an increasingly important social force in medical settings by reshaping the interpersonal dynamics of provider–patient interaction, changing the social dynamics of the collection and management of health information critical for medical work, and challenging medical authority. Research on HIT has been limited by an insider's perspective that has ignored the importance of the social context of the medical encounter. In this regard, medical sociologists can contribute to this important and ongoing public policy debate by helping consumers, providers, and health care system leaders better understand the many ways that HIT is reshaping medical work and the interactions patients have with their health care providers.

Acknowledgements The author would like to thank Harold Kooreman, Brian Dixon, Ainur Aiypkhanova, and Oluyemi Aladejebi for their research assistance.

References

Aetna Intelihealth Inc (2008) "InteliHealth." Retrieved 10/16/2008 (http://www.intelihealth.com/IH/intIH/WSIHW000/408/408.html).
Ahmad F, Hudak P, Bercovitz K, Hollenberg E, Levinson W (2006) Are physicians ready for patients with internet-based health information? J Med Internet Res 8:e22
Als AB (1997) The desk-top computer as a magic box: patterns of behaviour connected with the desk-top computer; GPs' and patients' perceptions. Fam Pract 14:17–23
AlUbaydli M (2004) Handheld computers. Br Med J 328:1181–1184
American Hospital Association (2007) Continued progress: hospital use of information technology
Andreassen HK, Trondsen M, Kummervold PE, Gammon D, Hjortdahl P (2006) Patients who use e-mediated communication with their doctor: new constructions of trust in patient-doctor relationship. Qual Health Res 16:238–247
Asch SM, McGlynn EA, Hogan MM, Hayward RA, Shekelle P, Rubenstein L, Keesey J, Adams J, Kerr EA (2004) Comparison of quality of care for patients in the veterans health administration and patients in a national sample. Ann Intern Med 141:938–945
Ash JS, Berg M, Coiera E (2004) Some unintended consequences of information technology in health care: The nature of patient care information system-related errors. J Am Med Inform Assoc 11:104–112
Association of American Medical Colleges (2004) Learning from others: a literature review and how-to guide from the health professions partnership initiative. The Robert Wood Johnson Foundation and the W.K. Kellogg Foundation, Washington, DC
Aydin CE (1989) Occupational adaptation to computerized medical information systems. J Health Soc Behav 30:163–179
Bales RF (1950) Interaction process analysis: a method for the study of small groups. Addison-Wesley, Reading, MA
Bates DW, Gawande AA (2003) Improving safety with information technology. N Engl J Med 348:2526–2534
Booker R (2005) Effective communication with the patient. Eur Respir Rev 14:93–96
Bush GW (2004) Executive order: incentives for the use of health information technology and establishing the position of eth national health information technology coordinator. Retrieved August 25, 2008 (http://www.whitehouse.gov/news/releases/2004/04/20040427-4.html)
Carroll AE, Saluja S, Tarczy-Hornoch P (2002) The implementation of a personal digital assistant (PDA) based patient record and charting system: Lessons learned. In: American Medical Informatics Association Annual Symposium
Centers for Medicare and Medicaid Services (2005) Medicare pay for performance (P4P) initiatives. Retrieved 10/16/2008 (http://www.cms.hhs.gov/apps/media/press/release.asp?counter=1343)
Chaudhry B, Wang J, Shinyi Wu, Maglione M, Mojica W, Roth E, Morton SC, Shekelle PG (2006) Systematic review: impact of health information technology on quality, efficiency, and costs of medical care. Ann Intern Med 144(10):742–752

Chin JJ (2003) The use of information technology in medicine: defining its role and limitations. [comment]. Singapore Med J 44:149–51

Christensen T, Grimsmo A (2008) Instant availability of patient records, but diminished availability of patient information: a multi-method study of GP's use of electronic patient records. BMC Med Inform Decis Mak 8:12

Cloud R (2001) Internet screening and interventions for problem drinking: results from the www.carebetter.com pilot study. Alcohol Treat Q 19:23–44

Colmers JM (2007) Public reporting and transparency. The commonwealth fund: commission on a high performance health system

U.S. Congress (1996) Health insurance portability and accountability act of 1996.

Connors HR (2001) Technology: telehealth on the rise. J Prof Nurs 17:73

Cotten SR (2001) Implications of internet technology for medical sociology in the new millennium. Sociol Spectr 21:319–340

DeCew JW (2000) The priority of privacy for medical information. Soc Philos Policy 17:213–234

Dee CR, Teolis M, Todd AD (2005) Physicians' use of personal digital assistants in clinical decision making. J Med Libr Assoc 93:480–6

Dennis A, Newman W (1996) Supporting doctor–patient interaction: using a surrogate application as a basis for evaluation. In: Conference on human factors in computing systems. ACM, Vancouver, BC, Canada

DesRoches CM, Campbell EG, Rao SR, Donelan K, Ferris TG, Jha RK, Levy DE, Rosenbaum S, Shields AE, Blumenthal D (2008) Electronic health records in ambulatory care – a national survey of physicians. N Engl J Med 359:50–60

Division of Information Technology and Research (2007) Electronic health record overview. Retrieved 09/03/2008 (http://www.ehrweb.org/ehrweb/ehroverview/pages/ehroverview.htm)

Dixon BE, Wright DE, Quantz SD, Wright ER (2007) Health information exchange may cut costs and reduce medical errors, but raise challenges. Indiana University, Indianapolis, IN

eHealth Magazine (2008) Hospital robot expands doctors' reach. Retrieved September 16, 2008 (http://www.ehealthonline.org/news/news-details.asp?newsid=15359)

Emanuel EJ, Emanuel LL (1992) Four models of the physician-patient relationship. J Am Med Assoc 267:2221–2226

Epstein RM, Alper BS, Quill TE (2004) Communicating evidence for participatory decision making. J Am Med Assoc 291:2359–2366

Frankel R, Altschuler A, George S, Kinsman J, Jimison H, Robertson NR, Hsu J (2005) Effects of exam-room computing on clinician-patient communication. J Gen Intern Mede 20:677–682

Freidson E (1970) Profession of medicine: a study of the sociology of applied knowledge. Dodd, Mead, New York, NY

Garg AX, Neill KJ, Adhikari Heather McDonald, Patricia Rosas-Arellano M, Devereaux PJ, Beyene J, Sam J, Brian Haynes R (2005) Effects of computerized clinical decision support systems on practitioner performance and patient outcomes: a systematic review. J Am Med Assoc 293:1223–1238

Garrido T, Jamieson L, Zhou Y, Wiesenthal A, Liang L (2005) Effect of electronic health records in ambulatory care: retrospective, serial, cross sectional study. BMJ (Clinical Research Ed) 330:581–581

Garritty C, El Emam K (2006) Who's using PDAs? Estimate of PDA use by healthcare providers: a systematic review of surveys. J Med Internet Res 8:e7

Goffman E (1983) The interaction order. Am Sociol Rev 48:1–17

Grady D (2008) Self-diagnosis by internet? Tricky business. In International Herald Tribune

Grondahl HH (2005) The machine made me do it!: an exploration of ascribing agency and responsibility to decision support systems. Master's Thesis, Department of Religion and Culture, Centre for Applied Ethics, Linköping University, Linköping, Sweden

Grondahl HH (2008) Are agency and responsibility still solely ascribable to humans? The case of medical decision support systems. In: Duquenoy P, George C, Kimppa K (eds) Ethical, legal, and social issues in medical informatics. Medical Information Science Reference, Hershey, NY

Guadagnoli E, Ward P (1998) Patient participation in decision-making. Soc Sci Med 47:329–339

Gustafson DH, Gustafson RC, Wackerbarth S (1997) CHESS: health information and decision support for patients and families. Generations 21:56

Hafferty FW, Light DW (1995) Professional dynamics and the changing nature of medical work. J Health Soc Behav (Extra Issue):132–153

Hardey M (2001) Doctor in the house: the internet as a source of lay health knowledge and the challenge to expertise. Sociol Health Illn 21:820–835

Harding J (1994) Cookbook medicine – advisability and efficacy of practice guidelines. Physician Exec Retrieved 10/16/2008 (http://findarticles.com/p/articles/mi_m0843/is_/ai_15786956)

Harrison JP, Palacio C (2006) The role of clinical information systems in health care quality improvement. Health Care Manag 25:206–212

Hartley CP (2007) Hey doc, can you update my PHR? Retrieved 10/16/2008 (http://www.fortherecordmag.com/archives/ftr_02192007p6.shtml)

Hassol A, Walker JM, Kidder D, Rokita K, Young D, Pierdon S, Deitz D, Kuck S, Ortiz E (2004) Patient experiences and attitudes about access to a patient electronic health care record and linked web messaging. J Am Med Inform Assoc 11:505–513

Heath C, Luff P, Svensson MS (2003) Technology and medical practice. Sociol Health Illn 25:75–96

Heritage J, Maynard DW (2006a) Communication in medical care: interaction between primary care physicians and patients. Cambridge University Press, Cambridge

Heritage J, Maynard DW (2006b) Problems and prospects in the study of physician-patient interaction: 30 years of research. Annu Rev Sociol 32:351–74

Heritage J, Raymond G (2005) The terms of agreement: indexing epistemic authority and subordination in talk-in-interaction. Soc Psychol Q 68:15–38

Hohmann AA (1999) A contextual model for clinical mental health effectiveness research. Ment Health Serv Res 1:83–91

Hsu J, Huang J, Fung V, Robertson N, Jimison H, Frankel R (2005) Health information technology and physician-patient interactions: impact of computers on communication during outpatient primary care visits. J Am Med Inform Assoc 12:474–480

Institute of Medicine (1999) To err is human: building a safer health system. National Academy Press, Washington, DC

Institute of Medicine (2001) Crossing the quality chasm: a new health system for the 21st century. National Academy Press, Washington, DC

Inui TS, Carter WB (1985) Problems and prospects for health services research on provider-patient communication. Med Care 23(5):521–538

Jain A, Ashish Atreja C, Harris M, Lehmann M, Burns J, Young J (2005) Responding to the rofecoxib withdrawal crisis: a new model for notifying patients at risk and their health care providers. Ann Intern Med 142:182–186

Jefferson G (1988) On the sequential organization of troubles-talk in ordinary conversation. Soc Probl 35:418–441

Kucher N, Koo S, Quiroz R, Cooper JM, Paterno MD, Soukonnikov B, Goldhaber SZ (2005) Electronic alerts to prevent venous thromboembolism among hospitalized patients. N Engl J Med 352:969–977

Legler JD, Oates R (1993) Patients' reactions to physician use of a computerized medical record system during clinical encounters. J Fam Pract 37:241–244

Light DW (1989) Social control and the American health care system. In: Freeman H, Levine S (eds) Handbook of medical sociology. Prentice Hall, Englewood Cliffs NJ, pp 456–474

Linder JA, Schnipper JL, Tsurikova R, Melnikas AJ, Volk LA, Middleton B (2006) Barriers to electronic health record use during patient visits. AMIA Annu Symp Proc 2006:499–503

Liu X, Sawada Y, Takizawa T, Sato H, Sato M, Sakamoto H, Utsugi T, Sato K, Sumino H, Okamura S, Sakamaki T (2007) Doctor–patient communication: a comparison between telemedicine consultation and face-to-face consultation. Intern Med 46:227–232

Lottridge D, Chignell M, Straus S (2006) Social impacts of handheld computer information retrieval during physician-patient communication. In: 20th International Symposium on Human Factors in Telecommunication. Sophia-Antipolis, France

Makoul G, Curry RH, Tang PC (2001) The use of electronic medical records: communication patterns in outpatient encounters. J Am Med Inform Assoc 8:610–615

Margalit RS, Roter D, Dunevant MA, Larson S, Reis S (2006) Electronic medical record use and physician-patient communication: An observational study of Israeli primary care encounters. Patient Educ Couns 61:134–141

Maynard DW (2003) Bad news, good news: conversational order in everyday talk and clinical settings. University of Chicago Press, Chicago, IL

Maynard DW, Frankel RM (2006) On diagnostic rationality: bad news, good news, and the symptom residue. In: Heritage J, Maynard DW (eds) Communication in medical care: interactions between primary care physicians and patients. Cambridge University Press, Cambridge

Maynard DW, Heritage J (2005) Conversation analysis, doctor–patient interaction and medical communication. Med Educ 39:428–435

McGrath JM, Arar NH, Pugh JA (2007) The influence of electronic medical record usage on nonverbal communication in the medical interview. Health Inform J 13:105–18

McManis S (2008) A checkup on web-side manners: patient-generated doctor reviews abound, but are they accurate? Retrieved 10/16/2008 (http://company.angieslist.com/Visitor/News/PressDetail.aspx?i=1189)

Mishler EG (1984) The discourse of medicine: dialectics of medical interviews. Ablex, Norwood, NJ

Murphy T (2007) Angie's to-do list: doctors. Retrieved 10/16/2008 (http://www.angieslist.com/AngiesList/Visitor/PressDetail.aspx?i=818)

Murray M, Harris L, Overhage JM, Zhou X-H, Eckert G, Smith F, Buchanan NN, Wolinsky F, McDonald C, Tierney W (2004) Failure of computerized treatment suggestions to improve health outcomes of outpatients with uncomplicated hypertension: results of a randomized controlled trial. Pharmacotherapy 24:324–337

MyPHR.com. (2008) Your personal health information: a guided tour. Retrieved 10/16/2008 (http://www.myphr.com/resources/tour.asp)

Norman CD, Skinner HA (2006) e-Health literacy: essential skills for consumer health in a networked world. J Med Internet Res 8:e9

Ong LML, de Haes JCJM, Hoos AM, Lammes FB (1995) Doctor–patient communication: a review of the literature. Soc Sci Med 40:903–918

Ornstein S, Bearden A (1994) Patient perspectives on computer-based medical records. J Fam Pract 38:606–610

Osheroff J, Teich J, Middleton B, Steen E, Wright A, Detmer D (2007) A roadmap for national action on clinical decision support. J Am Med Inform Assoc 14:141–145

Patel V, Arocha J, Kushniruk A (2002) Patients' and physicians' understanding of health and biomedical concepts: relationship to the design of EMR systems. J Biomed Inform 35:8–16

Pizzi R (2006) Insurance industry reps reveal PHR plan. Retrieved 10/16/2008 (http://www.healthcareitnews.com/story.cms?id=6052)

Pizzi R (2007) Smartphones gain appeal with more docs. Retrieved 09/03/2008 (http://www.healthcareitnews.com/story.cms?id=8176&page=2)

Powell JC (2004) NHS national programme for information technology: changes must involve clinicians and show the value to patient care. BMJ 328:1200

Ridsdale L, Hudd S (1994) Computers in the consultation: the patient's view. Br J Gen Pract 44:367–369

Ritzer G (1993) The McDonaldization of society. Pine Forge Press, Los Angeles, CA

Ritzer G, Walczak D (1988) Rationalization and the deprofessionalization of physicians. Soc Forces 67:1–22

Robert Wood Johnson Foundation (2006) Health information technology in the United States: the information base for progress

Roob M (2006) Health care affordability and quality for hoosiers. Indiana Family and Social Services Administration, Indianapolis, IN

Rosenthal E (1993) Insurers second-guess doctors, provoking debate over savings. In: The New York Times. New York, NY

Roter DL (1977) Patient participation in the patient-provider interaction: the effects of patient question asking on the quality of interaction, satisfaction and compliance. Health Educ Monogr 5:281–315

Roter DL, Hall JA (2006) Doctors talking with patients/patients talking with doctors: improving communication in medical visits, 2nd edn. Praeger, New York, NY

Roter DL, Larson S (2002) The roter interaction analysis system (RIAS): Utility and flexibility for analysis of medical interactions. Patient Educ Couns 42:243–251

Roter DL, Hall JA, Katz NR (1988) Physician-patient communication: a descriptive summary of the literature. Patient Educ Couns 12(2):99–109

Rothschild J, Fang E, Liu V, Litvak I, Yoon C, Bates D (2006) Use and perceived benefits of handheld computer-based clinical references. J Am Med Inform Assoc 13:619–626

Rouf E, Whittle J, Na L, Schwartz MD (2007) Computers in the exam room: differences in physician-patient interaction may be due to physician experience. J Gen Intern Med 22:43–48

Rubin M, Bateman K, Donnelly S, Stoddard G, Stevenson K, Gardner R, Samore M (2006) Use of a personal digital assistant for managing antibiotic prescribing for outpatient respiratory tract infections in rural communities. J Am Med Inform Assoc 13:627–634

Sacks H, Schegloff EA, Jefferson G (1974) A simplest systematics for the organization of turn-taking for conversation. Language 50:696–735

Schegloff EA, Jefferson G, Sacks H (1977) The preference for self-correction in the organization of repair in conversation. Language 53:361–382

Schloeffel P (2004) Current EHR developments: an Australian and international perspective – Part 1. Health care and informatics review Online TM, September 2004

Shaw B, Han JY, Hawkins R, Stewart J, McTavish F, Gustafson D (2007) Doctor–patient relationship as motivation and outcome: examining uses of an interactive cancer communication system. Int J Med Inform 76:274–282

Shekelle P, Morton S, Keeler E (2006) Costs and benefits of health information technology. Evid Rep Technol Assess:1–71

Simon S, McCarthy M, Kaushal R, Jenter C, Volk L, Poon E, Yee K, Orav J, Williams D, Bates D (2008) Electronic health records: which practices have them, and how are clinicians using them? J Eval Clin Pract 14:43–47

Solomon GL, Dechter M (1995) Are patients pleased with computer use in the examination room? J Fam Pract 41:241–4

Staggers N, Thompson CB, Snyder-Halpern R (2001) History and trends in clinical information systems in the United States. J Nurs Scholarsh 33:75–81

Starr P (1982) The social transformation of American medicine. Basic Books, New York, NY
Starr P (2002) Health care reform and the new economy. Health Aff 19:23–32
Steinberg KE (2006) Cookbook medicine: recipe for disaster? J Am Med Dir Assoc 7:470–472
Stoeckle JD (1988) Reflections on modern doctoring. Milbank Q 66:76–91
The Medical Society of the State of New York (2008) Survey reveals that doctors feel pressured by health insurers to alter treatment of patients. Retrieved 10/16/2008 (http://www.medicalnewstoday.com/printerfriendlynews.php?newsid=120875)
Tierney W, Overhage M, Murray M, Harris L, Zhou X-H, Eckert G, Smith F, Nienaber N, McDonald C, Wolinsky F (2003) Effects of computerized guidelines for managing heart disease in primary care. J Gen Intern Med 18:967–976
Tu Ha T, Cohen G (2008) Tracking report 20: striking jump in consumers seeking health care information. Center for Studying Health System Change, Washington, DC
Tyson TR (2000) The internet: tomorrow's portal to non-traditional health care services. New developments in informatics and ambulatory care. J Ambul Care Manage 23:1–7
U.S. Department of Health & Human Services (2008) Health information technology home. Retrieved 10/16/2008 (http://www.hhs.gov/healthit)
van Uden-Kraan CF, Drossaert CH, Taal E, Seydel ER, van de Laar MA (2008) Participation in online patient support groups endorses patients' empowerment. Patient Educ Couns 74:61–69
Ventres W, Kooienga S, Marlin R, Vuckovic N, Stewart V (2005) Clinician style and examination room computers: a video ethnography. Fam Med 37:276–281
Ventres W, Kooienga S, Vuckovic N, Marlin R, Nygren P, Stewart V (2006) Physicians, patients, and the electronic health record: an ethnographic analysis. Ann Fam Med 4:124–31
Versel N (2005) One in five group practices now use EHRs. Health IT World, Health IT World News Newsletter 2. 1-25-2005
Waitzkin H (1991) The politics of medical encounters. Yale University Press, New Haven CT
Wang S, Middleton B, Prosser L, Bardon C, Spurr C, Carchidi P, Kittler A, Goldszer R, Fairchild D, Sussman A, Kuperman G, Bates D (2003) A cost-benefit analysis of electronic medical records in primary care. Am J Med 114:397–403
Warshawsky S, Pliskin J, Urkin J, Cohen N, Sharon A, Binztok M, Margolis C (1994) Physician use of a computerized medical record system during the patient encounter: a descriptive study. Comput Meth Programs Biomed 43:269–273
West C, Frankel R (1991) Miscommunication in medicine. In: Coupland N, Giles H, Wiemann JM (eds) Misscommunication and problematic talk. Sage, Newbury Park, CA, pp 166–194
Winkelman W, Leonard K, Rossos P (2005) Patient-perceived usefulness of online electronic medical records: employing grounded theory in the development of information and communication technologies for use by patients living with chronic illness. J Am Med Inform Assoc 12:306–314

Part V
Connecting Personal & Cultural Systems

Chapter 19
Culture, Race/Ethnicity and Disparities: Fleshing Out the Socio-Cultural Framework for Health Services Disparities

Margarita Alegría, Bernice A. Pescosolido, Sandra Williams, and Glorisa Canino

Introduction

There is little question that the issue of "health disparities" has been given a central place across medicine and contemporary society of late (e.g., Institute of Medicine 2002). From research, to policy and even to the popular press, the unmasking of the disparities in health and health care for individuals who belong to certain race and ethnic groups has been a prominent theme (van Ryn and Fu 2003). While the attention to these matters is welcome by sociologists and other social scientists, the existence of inequality in health, illness, and healing is hardly a revelation. From the earliest times in our history, the focus on the differential in infant mortality; the incidence and prevalence of disease; and access to, treatment in, and the outcomes of care for those at the lower ends of the stratification hierarchy in any society have been the mainstay of both the sociological and public health enterprises. From Marx, to Durkheim, to Weber in sociology, and from Virchow to Snow to the Roemers outside of sociology, the understanding that stratification plays itself out, in part, in morbidity and mortality statistics represented a principal theme of theory, empirical investigation and the design of interventions (Pescosolido and Kronenfeld 1995).

Recaptured by the notion of "fundamental causes" (Link and Phelan 1995) and Lutfey and Freese (also in this volume), the focus on social class is now accompanied by concerns about how race and ethnic differences structure the life chances of individuals (Kumanyika 1993). In fact, given the recent, pioneering work by David Williams and his colleagues, we now have a distressingly clear picture of the way that African Americans are disadvantaged in American society (see, e.g., Williams 2005; Williams and Jackson 2005; Wilson and Williams 2004). The focus on Latino or Hispanic Americans and that of Asian-Americans is, for the most part, more recent; yet, the bulk of the message is similar (Alegría et al. 2008). Race and ethnicity do play a role in health and health care.

Mirroring the larger terrain of medical sociology in recent decades, our attention to documenting these race and ethnic differences in morbidity and mortality has been greater than just trying to unpack the social mechanisms that underlie them. Equally sparse is our general focus on the organizational response to health problems, whether that is the lay response to the onset of health problems, the focus on the interaction between the community and treatment systems, the nature of the profession (Hafferty and Castellani 2010), or the operations of the health care system itself (see Caronna 2010; Mechanic 2004). Given this differential distribution of effort, this chapter concentrates on developing the under-

M. Alegría (✉)
Cambridge Health Alliance and Harvard Medical School, 120 Beacon St., 4th Floor, Somerville, MA 02143, USA
e-mail: malegria@charesearch.org

standing of the forces and structures that create the disparities in health care that cumulate across the illness career to shape disparities in chronic health and mortality. That is, we do not contend that health disparities are rooted, first and foremost, in the problems associated with access to or treatment in the formal medical and mental health systems. Nor do we claim that health care, as a mediating factor in understanding health gradients, will eliminate health disparities. However, we argue that, whatever the issues, disparities are compounded in the nature of the health care system available to individuals, their ability to access it, the suitability of the treatments and providers that are available in medicine, and the way care is provided to individuals from different social strata.

In sum, this chapter is designed to fill a gap – the lack of an overall framework to guide the investigation of the structures, processes, and mechanisms that underlie health care disparities and hinder the development of interventions to redress problems. The Socio-Cultural Framework for Health Service Disparities (SCF-HSD) has been introduced elsewhere and to different audiences (e.g., Alegría et al. 2009). However, the limitations of these venues, in either length or focus, have prevented an in-depth exploration of the specific propositions and hypotheses that can be drawn from such a frame. Here, we take the opportunity to review the basic sociological, social science, and public health roots of the framework. We introduce the SCF-HSD by level (societal, organizational and individual), describing first the dual structures (community and treatment system) that come together to produce six mechanisms central to the development and maintenance of health disparities. This approach allows us to flesh out the kinds of research questions, propositions, and hypotheses that, we believe, would improve our knowledge of the health and health care differential among race and ethnic groups in America, and in doing so, provide a better empirical base to develop treatment, educational, and policy interventions to close the gaps.

The Sociological and Social Science Roots of a Framework to Understand Health Service Disparities

In our initial development of the SCF-HSD (Alegría et al. 2009), we began by defining the scope of the problem and the nature of cultural difference on two critical issues.

First, on the nature of health care or health service disparities, the definition we employ differs. Above, we acknowledged the Institute of Medicine's Report and its definition – "racial and ethnic differences in the quality of healthcare that are not due to clinical needs, preferences and appropriateness of intervention" (pg. 2–4). However, 1 year later, the U.S. Department of Health and Human Services (2003) expanded this definition in terms of time and groups. Disparities now included differences in access associated with race, ethnicity, income, education, and place of residence. While this was an improvement, the definition of health services disparities that we proposed was even broader. We defined disparities as *racial and ethnic differences in access, health care quality or health care outcomes that are not due to clinical needs or the appropriateness of treatment.*

As such, the most radical modification lies in the exclusion of preferences as a potential *allowable* explanation for disparities. We do not suggest that the focus on preferences translates into the absence of service use because of ignorance, lack of education, low health literacy, or parochialism, as was suggested by theories of the mid-twentieth century (Parsons 1951; Suchman 1965). Rather, we believe that patient preferences are shaped by the same social structures and dynamics that create disparities along other points in the illness career. Differences in the endorsement of the health care system may result, in part, from the options that people have and from the community repository of "stories" about providers, practices, and facilities (Olafsdottir and Pescosolido 2009).

Second, and following directly from this, we proposed that it is equally critical to shift the focus in theory and empirical research away from categorical "boxes" or socio-demographic variables that try to capture an increasingly diverse patchwork of race and ethnic affiliations in the U.S. to a view that targets culture as a whole. At each level of society, embedded structures and processes shape the attitudes, beliefs, values, and cultural scripts that both clients and providers use in everyday life. Understanding if and how these are shaped either by membership in select race and ethnic groups or by how others respond to these categories requires a view that conceptualizes culture as a veil, filter, or screen that overlays each process and structural level. As Tilly (2002) points out, categories *do* matter, but they matter because society has bundled together cultural understandings of the practices, routines, and relationships of people who are separated out and labeled. This bundling facilitates inequality and its reproduction through organizations and institutions over time. Unpacking this bundle regarding health and health care for members of race and ethnic groups by looking to new insights on culture speaks directly to the roots of health disparities.

Putting Disparities in the Context of Social Science Knowledge. Three sets of research are directly or indirectly tied to elaborating the basic building blocks of health service disparities – contemporary empirical work on illness careers and its inevitable connection to the larger focus on life course models, research on inequality and cumulative disadvantage in occupational careers or incomes, and recent sociological and anthropological developments on the nature and role of culture. Certainly, the first set brings in the dynamic nature of the lay response to the onset of health problems, while the second suggests that health is not the only societal arena in which disparities continue to plague certain race and ethnic groups. The third set provides conceptual tools to rethink the nature of race and ethnic difference and how they play out in life styles and life chances.

We realize that these research literatures, like our efforts here, have drawn from one another over time and are often intertwined. For example, scientific careers work through a process of cumulative advantage (the "Matthew Effect," Merton 1957). Not surprisingly, cumulative (dis)advantage is seen as a mechanism that underlies many forms of inequality (DiPrete and Eirich 2006). For our purposes, tracing the unique lines that build to the SCF-HSD's complicated dynamic, multilevel approach provides a more solid foundation for asking how they may come together in health care outcomes for underrepresented minority individuals.

Our initial foundation – that disparities cumulate over the course of an illness career shaped by whole cultural systems – synthesizes insights from these established lines of research to produce three assumptions underlying the SCF-HSD described below.

The Life Course and Illness Careers. The life course perspective sees any experience in individuals' lives embedded in a larger social process and cannot be understood outside of it. By fiat, then, to understand the kinds of problems that individuals face at any one point in dealing with the health care system requires a dynamic approach that sees later experiences influenced by earlier ones (Elder 1992; Elder and Caspi 1990). Lives are "socially organized in biological and historical time" (Elder 1998:9), where these large contexts are seen as central to understanding experiences and outcomes.

In fact, this approach was influential in the development of the other recent research lines we consider in this section. For example, while the illness career approach had roots in early, qualitative studies of illness and illness behavior (Clausen and Yarrow 1955; Zola 1973), it reemerged as a central theme when life course research became more prominent and as medical sociologists faced a disappointing, inconsistent body of research on service utilization. New models, particularly the Network-Episode Model (Pescosolido 1991, 2006), reframed the decision to seek care as part of larger process of coping with the onset of illness. The dynamic approach suggested examining patterns and pathways rather than, for example, the single experience of visiting a doctor (see also McLeod and Fettes 2007; Pavalko et al. 2007). Key entrances and exits (e.g., the sick role, patient role, and disabled role) were reframed as linked across the career to produce a more complex but better understanding of service use, adherence, and outcomes. These exits and entrances are connected to health through the routine and normative expectations surrounding events in the life course (e.g., see the case of mental health and the ordering of marriage and giving birth;

Jackson 2004). And, they are shaped by the content and structure of interactions in social networks.

In sum, the SCF-HSD maintains that larger social context raises opportunities and places limits on access, quality, and outcomes of health care that exist for racial and ethnic groups in American society. Our approach is multilevel, focusing on how social structure includes national and local policy, organizational, and informal domains for both the treatment system and the community system. According to the Network-Episode Model (Pescosolido 1991, 2006; Pescosolido and Boyer 1999), the illness career becomes the critical point at which the influences of the larger community and the health care system meet to shape the lives of persons facing illness. The result may be attempts from both sides to construct and reconstruct the meaning of illness, treatment, and outcomes for individuals. These efforts may reinforce one another, overwhelm one or the other system, or set up a clash of cultures (Pescosolido et al. 1995).

Considerations of the life course perspective and, more specifically, the illness career leads to our first foundational assumption:

> *Building Block 1*: Cross-Pressures at the interface of community and treatment systems create the engines of disparities that individuals may face in their illness careers.

Cumulative Disadvantage in Scientific Careers and Societal Inequality. While the notion of careers, including but not restricted to occupational careers, was introduced early in sociology (Merton 1957), the more recent study of scientific careers has taken an explicit life course approach, conceptualizing careers "as a series of linked events occurring over time within specific contexts" (Long and Fox 1995: 53–54). In the study of the scientific careers of women, for example, the basic idea is that scientists who have early success in terms of job placement or publication will have an easier time in acquiring resources to continue, even expand, their productivity or reputation (Long 1987). While researchers argue about details (e.g. will early advantage be maintained or will inequality increase over time), there has been a broad acceptance of explanations that conceptualize time-ordered processes that benefit or penalize individuals.

From this research, three points translate easily to and set an additional building block for understanding disparities in health care outcomes. *First*, the observed inequality in careers "demands explanations of the processes generating the inequality" (Long and Fox 1995: 53) rather than simply the continued documentation of differences and untested hypotheses about the underlying mechanisms. *Second*, "successive filtering" (Zuckerman and Cole 1975) represents an important phenomenon; that is, each career stage erodes participation and positive outcomes, little by little. *Third*, "cumulative disadvantage," the process by which initial disadvantages, however they occurred, are reinforced and magnified across the career, may be especially important for understanding sex and race differences (Long and Fox 1995).

More generally, the idea of cumulative dis/advantage has been applied across numerous areas of social science, "wherever we have searched for a general mechanism of inequality across any temporal process" (DiPrete and Eirich 2006: 271). At base, an initial favorable or unfavorable position sets in motion a process that produces further gains or losses, respectively. This is due, in part, to the role of organization in reproducing inequality (or in Tilly's 1999 terms, producing "durable inequality" based on categorical assignments; also Tilly 2000). According to Allison et al. (1982), the notion of cumulative disadvantage is powerful in explanation, intuitively plausible, and appealing to both supporters and critics of stratification. This leads to our second building block:

> *Building Block 2*: Health service disparities represent a social process of inequalities that cumulate across a dynamic illness career.

Race and Ethnic Differences in Cultural Perspective. In our view, cultural processes not only refer to ethnicity/race as a particular set of values, norms, and beliefs but also include the circumstances and experiences leading to a group's social, economic, and political status in the social structure (Guarnaccia and Rodriguez 1996). Our rejection of a simplistic view of culture or cultural differences based solely on categorical assignment reflects current thinking in sociology and anthropology. Cultural processes are now routinely conceptualized as a fundamental thread running through communities, health systems, providers, and clients (Rogler 1996) and their interactions with each other.

Socio-demographic categories are now seen as poor proxies for culture (Pescosolido 1992). Rather, the emphasis is on understanding the "cultural toolboxes" that individuals, organizations, and systems have at their disposal (Swidler 2001) and the direct (exploitation) and indirect (e.g. opportunity hoarding; Tilly 2000) social processes that reinforce categorical cultural differences. Thus, cognitive worldviews embedded in culture structure human action by creating available cultural repertoires based, in part, in historical experience including barriers to resources (DiMaggio 1997; DiMaggio and Powell 1991; Strauss and Quinn 1997; Swidler 2001: 220ff). Such cultural repertoires are resident not only in individuals but also in communities and treatment systems.

We acknowledge the difficulty in conceptualizing and measuring culture, race, ethnicity, and social factors influencing help-seeking and health care outcomes. Our specific challenge, with regard to health disparities, targets how to translate a general consensus on the importance of culture into research ideas and approaches that expose the meaning and impact of culture in ethnic groups, treatment organizations, and institutional systems (Bernal et al. 2003). This leads to our final assumption:

Building Block 3: Culture is omnipresent and enacted.

The SCF-HSD: Outlining and Specifying the Frame

From our building blocks, we conceptualize health service disparities as arising from a dynamic illness career that links the community and treatment system experiences and routines that race and ethnic groups have at each stage of dealing with health and illness problems. Inequities are not located in one unique part of the career; rather, a set of inequities, sometimes seen as minor by themselves, cumulate to a career of disadvantage and often gross disparities. In sum, our underlying assumptions focus on the dynamic nature of disadvantage; the active, guiding role of culture; and the multiple layers of social structures that come into play in response to illness.

Each point of interaction between the two major systems – community and treatment – represents a key site of understanding and potential for change. Each domain is conceptualized to operate at three levels – the societal level (macro; larger policy or environmental contexts), the organizational level (meso; formal organizations or lay sectors), and the individual level (micro; provider or patient). In the section below, we reorient our approach to the SCF-HSD by considering the structural elements at each level, first introducing the mechanisms at work. We tailor our discussion here to the case of mental health and substance abuse problems (Alegría et al. 2009). The utility of the framework can be more easily illustrated through a particular case (Pescosolido 1992). This facilitates the explication of the general theoretical framework since the primary and secondary level hypotheses are stated in very general terms.

When Health Care Systems and Community Systems Meet: Mechanisms Producing Disparities

Dual Systems in Operation – Health Care and Community

Perhaps not surprisingly, the IOM's *Unequal Treatment* (Institute of Medicine 2002) focuses on three arenas, each operating at different levels, within the healthcare system: (1) federal, state, and

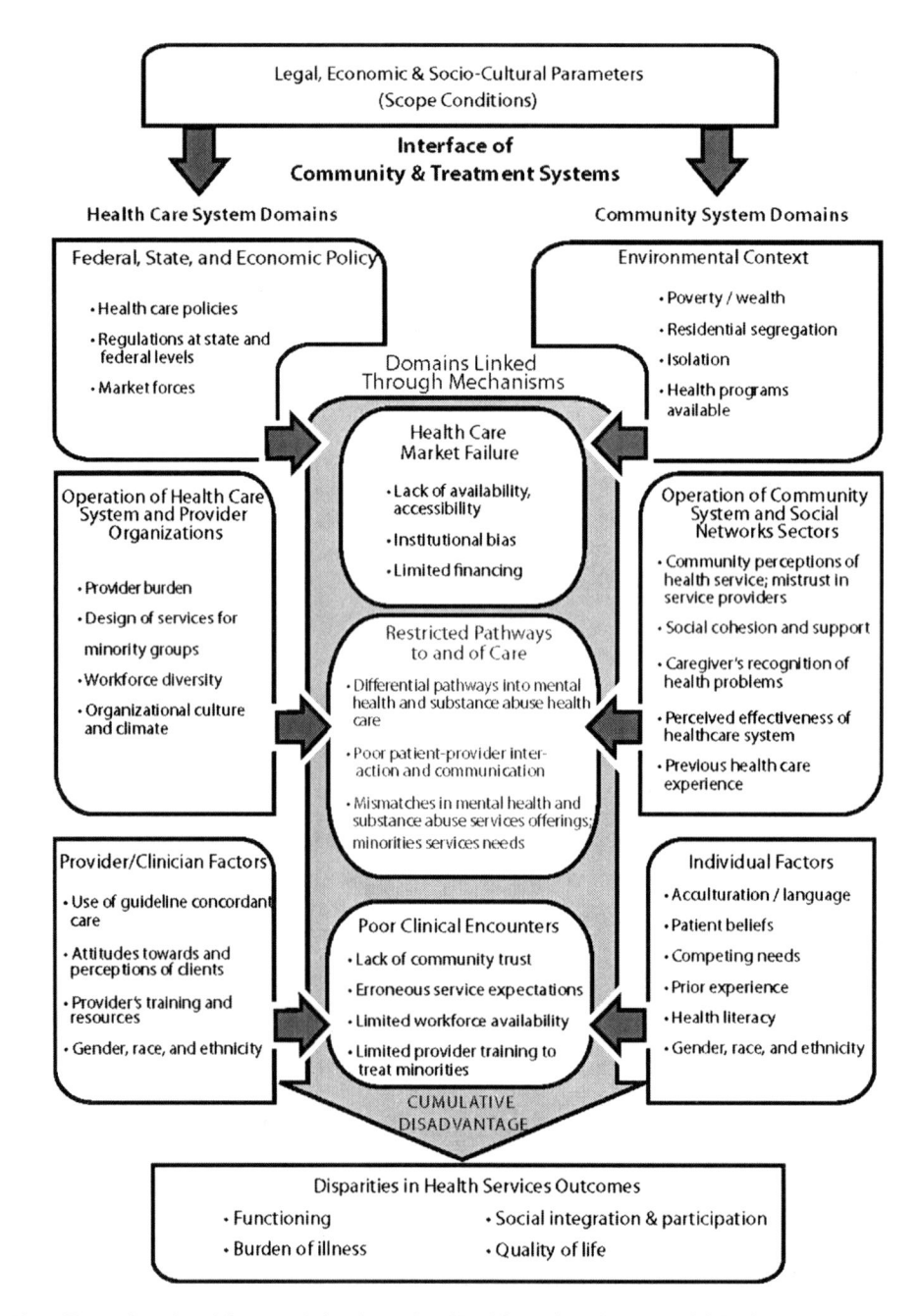

Fig. 19.1 The socio-cultural framework for the study of health service disparities (SCF-HSD)

economic health care policies and regulations at the state and federal levels; (2) the operation of the health care system and provider organizations; and (3) provider/clinician-level factors (Fig. 19.1, left-hand side). However, the SCF-HSD adds a parallel community concern along the same three levels; social forces may differentially impact access to services or quality in services. Community, family, friends, and individuals shape ethno-cultural individuals' referral, entry, and retention in mental health or substance abuse services. These three additional domains or levels are drawn from utilization, "take-up" or help-seeking models: (1) the environmental context, specifically social and economic forces affecting ethno-cultural populations; (2) the operation of the community and social networks system, including family, friends, and the lay sector; and (3) patient-level factors (Fig. 19.1, right-hand side).

Below, we discuss each level, looking to how the domain interactions may operate to impact services disparities. We provide concrete examples; however, the levels are heuristic, to an extent because the essential cross-cutting nature of effects creates overlap both in our descriptions and in individuals' experiences. While we train our focus on mental health and substance abuse, we sometimes bring in other concepts and findings to help identify more general, potential leverage points to reduce disparities.

The Macro-Level: Federal State and Economic Policy and Environmental Context

Health care policies and regulations at the state and federal level shape systems in health care domains. Specific policies on health care as well as other economic policies and regulations create a set of market forces. As a result of legal cases against the health care industry, many admissions and treatment polices that indirectly limited service delivery for persons of color no longer exist (Rosenbaum 2002). Lack of access due to uninsurance serves as a potential mechanism promoting services disparities. Hargraves and Hadley (2003) argue that expanding insurance coverage for minorities would significantly reduce access disparities. Furthermore, a sizeable share of disparities in usual sources of care could be reduced if Hispanics and African Americans were insured at levels comparable to those of Whites (Lillie-Blanton and Hoffman 2005).

Insurance coverage is significant for children's access to health care, with the state of the child's residence influencing restrictions on eligibility for government health programs and the likelihood of receiving health care, even after controlling for ethnic and racial differences in the population of children and the level of need (Shone et al. 2005). Health care polices such as SCHIP play a crucial role in reducing access barriers that create health services disparities among minority youth.

The rising costs of health service delivery prior to the mid-1980s contributed to an increase in the number of uninsured individuals. Much of this was due to employers' decisions to stop offering insurance to employees and employees choosing not to purchase employer health insurance (Kaiser Family Foundation 2008). State and federal regulations aimed toward cost control also contributed to the increase in the number of uninsured. For example, individuals were excluded from Medicaid as states responded to increased costs by enacting more stringent eligibility criteria (Bodenheimer 2005). These consequences of market failure contributed to disparities in health services delivery for ethno-cultural populations since minorities are overrepresented among the under- and uninsured (U.S. Bureau of the Census 2002). When states raise eligibility thresholds for Medicaid, individuals who depend on public insurance are affected. Although federal legislation mandates the criteria for the federal poverty line (FPL), states are given flexibility to set their own poverty line criteria as long as eligibility does not exceed 185% of the poverty line (Perry et al. 2001). Since ethnic minorities tend to be overrepresented among the poor (U.S. Bureau of the Census 2002), the flexibility of states to set their own eligibility criteria may have implications for minorities' access to and quality of care. In fact, Shone et al. (2005) found that preexisting racial/ethnic disparities in access, unmet need, and usual sources of care between White, Hispanic, and African American youth were virtually eliminated during the first year of enrollment in SCHIP in New York State. Further, the 2003 AHRQ *National Healthcare Disparities* Report indicates that improvements in access to care among White, Black, Hispanic, and the poor coincided with the implementation of SCHIP.

If states with higher minority proportions of populations are less generous in their health care coverage for poor populations, a disproportionate number of individuals may remain uninsured.

Despite their detrimental impact, policies have been met with very little resistance as they tend to affect vulnerable populations who lack social power (i.e. low income earners, immigrants, and children). These groups have limited political and organizational power to protest and advocate against such policies. Further, because certain medical providers and institutions tend to serve a disproportionate share of the poor and under- or uninsured, disproportionate burdens may have been placed on those organizations and individuals who do serve underrepresented minorities. In addition, the number of providers accepting new Medicaid patients has been reduced over the past 10 years (Cunningham and Hadley 2008). Just over 20% of physicians surveyed were no longer accepting new Medicaid patients in 2004–2005, which is five times the rate for private insurance. In addition, the majority (84%) of physicians surveyed alluded to low Medicaid payment rates as the primary reason for not taking Medicaid patients. Low Medicaid capitation payments (Alegría et al. 2002) and limited provider networks for Medicaid health maintenance organizations (HMOs) enrolling minority beneficiaries (Tai-Seale et al. 2001) may also restrict the group of available providers.

The disproportionably low geographic supply of providers, particularly multilingual service providers in communities with ethnic and racial minorities as compared to nonminority communities (Derose and Baker 2000) may influence availability of physicians, consequently impacting service disparities. Communities with high proportions of African-American and Latino residents were four times as likely as non-Latino Whites to have a shortage of physicians regardless of community income (Putsch and Pololi 2005). The end result may be insufficient health plan competition that thwarts the power of governments to push the health care system, consequently producing a failure of the market to provide more and better quality care to ethnic and racial minorities.

The Macro-Level: Communities

Link and Phelan (2000, 2005) among others have argued that the greatest impact in reducing health differentials might be achieved by changing the social conditions for those in lower social positions. For example, housing policies play a particularly vital role in affecting disparities in mental health and substance abuse. Public housing units are primarily occupied by vulnerable populations and overwhelmingly by minorities (Alegría et al. 2003). Supportive housing policies can directly reduce housing cost burden and ambient hazards and indirectly increase access to community resources or to safer conditions.

However, the larger geographical area in which ethnic minorities live helps to create a social context that, in itself, fosters a lack of connection with treatment systems and the dominant culture. Geographical segregation continues, perhaps even at greater levels than would be expected for many minority populations. Even among Hispanics who have generally been more successful in living in integrated communities than African Americans, Puerto Ricans stand out as having been significantly less able to break through residential segregation barriers (Massey and Denton 1998). The implications of this are profound, from the lack of geographically available employment (Wilson 1990, 1997) that, in itself, creates lower levels of insurance coverage. In turn, the viability of health care facilities, even public hospitals, in areas of concentrated minority and poverty populations remains in question. Social and geographical contexts are often intertwined and overlapping for ethno-cultural populations. Similarly, public reaction and social policies are often intertwined, also influencing service access and, likely, health outcomes directly or indirectly. According to Keogan (2002), illegal immigrants in the Los Angeles (LA) and New York (NY) metropolitan areas during the 1990s experienced very different climates. Those in LA were considered threats to job security and burdens to taxpayers, facilitating the passing of anti-immigrant legislation such as Proposition 187 that denied education, welfare, and all but emergency medical services to immigrants and their children. In contrast, the period of economic stability in New York in the 1990s saw public attention focused on immigrants as victims, particularly in the face of a maritime tragedy involving illegal Chinese immigrants. In LA, then, illegal Mexican immigrants were unable to obtain medical care or utilize other social services, whereas the Chinese immigrants in NY were offered refugee status as permanent lawful residents with limited access to health and social resources.

Differences in problem recognition of mental health issues in the community, differential referral by the social network, and higher barriers to care serve as potential precipitating factors to disparities. For example, as Stiffman and her colleagues (Stiffman et al. 2000; Stiffman et al. 2004) theorized and documented for adolescents with mental health and substance abuse problems, an individual's first service contact may not be with a specialty professional, but rather with a formal or informal "gateway provider" (e.g., a social worker, general practitioner, teacher) who has a powerful role in determining whether and what type of health services should be included in a referral. Factors that may influence gateway providers' perceptions of an individual's need for mental health or substance abuse treatment include the providers' familiarity with and links to health services resources, the providers' perceptions of the clients' willingness to accept mental health services, and any organizational boundaries that may limit the gateway providers' time or fiscal resources (Stiffman et al. 2001). For example, while adult minorities are more likely to seek mental health care in primary care clinics (Williams et al. 1999), this may not be optimal. As Tai-Seale et al. (2007) reported, individuals who seek mental health treatment in the primary sector will receive only 2 min on average of mental health treatment for depression during a 15–16 min primary care visit.

Other pathways may result in disparities with both short and long term effects. For example, Latino and African-American children are overrepresented in the juvenile social service sectors. They receive fewer therapeutic services compared with "clinically comparable" white children (Garland et al. 2001). Further, independent of clinical factors, individuals in ethno-cultural populations have higher rates of involuntary psychiatric hospitalization. Afro-Caribbean adults (McGovern and Cope 1991) are much more likely to have higher rates of involuntary commitment and, like many other minorities, are referred to less psychotherapy or talk therapy than Whites. Minorities are also more likely to encounter higher rates of police involvement and involuntary detainment in psychiatric settings or other institutional settings (Massoglia 2008; Pescosolido et al. 1998; Rogers and Pilgrim 2003). Such pathways may translate into disparities in service delivery through misdiagnosis or delays in diagnosis.

In sum, the larger parameters of a society shape the health care system. In turn, the nature of these policies often interacts with community context to facilitate or disadvantage ethnic and racial minorities in the health care system. Specifically, we suggest:

Proposition 1. The failure of healthcare markets, institutional bias, and limited financing leads to decreased access to and utilization of mental health and substance abuse services.

Proposition 2. Differential community networks shape pathways into services that lead to differential experiences in service, delayed utilization, no service, or inadequate service.

The Meso-Level: Operation of the Health Care System and Provider Organizations

As a result of the parameters described above, health care systems face differential costs and opportunities associated with treating individuals from ethnic and racial minority populations. As noted, reimbursement by the state or the federal government holds a central role in shaping provider burden, service design, workforce diversity, and organizational climate of health care organizations. In 2000, the Department of Health and Human Services published guidelines for Cultural and Linguistically Appropriate Services (U.S. Department of Health & Human Services 2000). These guidelines urged providers to have trained interpreters on staff when servicing non-English speakers and to provide critical health information or medical forms that have been linguistically and culturally adapted. Lack of compliance with guidelines such as CLAS produces less diverse workforces, which leads to greater disparities in mental health and substance use services for racial and ethnic minority groups.

Managed care penetration has had significant effects on the composition of Medicaid caseloads and on reducing (Balsa et al. 2007; Daley 2005) or increasing disparities in care (Rylko-Bauer and Farmer 2002; Schneider et al. 2002). After the adoption of managed behavioral health care plans among those enrolled in Medicaid, higher managed care penetration was associated with an increase among Black children with chronic conditions going without care, but with parallel decreases among Latino children and poor teens (Currie and Fahr 2004). Health care packages may offer poor mental health and substance abuse treatments as a way to limit access to costly services that are prevalent for ethnic and racial minorities (Cao and McGuire 2003; Wells et al. 2001).

While the research on the patient–provider match by race/ethnicity or gender is somewhat mixed, there is little question that the influence of shared expectations and poor patient–provider interaction is not. While limited research does suggest that patient–provider matching improves retention of clients and intervention outcomes (Kurasaki et al. 2000), it is not clear if it reduces service disparities (Antshel 2002; Beutler et al. 1994). Similarly, physicians' race concordance with patients appears to be associated with use and quality of care only for preventive services (Saha et al. 1999). Uncertainty may also enter the clinical encounter for individuals from ethnic populations when a provider faces clinical symptoms, signs, or tests due to atypical symptom presentation, to a lack of information about the efficacy of a therapeutic intervention (Bloche 2001) resulting from underrepresentation of minorities in clinical trials (Rogers 2004).

Once in treatment, more individuals from ethno-cultural populations report feeling devalued and dismissed (14.1% of African-Americans, 19.4% of Latinos, and 20.2% of Asians) than non-Latino Whites (94%; Blow et al. 2004; Littlewood and Lipsedge 1981; McGovern and Cope 1991). Further, they express beliefs that attribute this unfair treatment to race or language spoken (Blanchard and Lurie 2004). In one study alone, language barriers between provider and patient accounted for a $38 increase in charges for testing, and increased length of stay in the emergency room (Hampers et al. 1999). Patients who reported being treated with disrespect were less likely to go for routine physical exams within the last year, to have received state-of-the-art care for a chronic condition, and to have followed their doctor's advice (Blanchard and Lurie 2004). However, recent efforts to integrate cultural and linguistic competence requirements in the health care system have been met with concern and resistance (Flores et al. 2003), since health systems may be required to cover additional costs and recruit scarce bilingual staff.

In sum, disparities resulting from mechanisms in this domain include discordance in the understanding that patients and providers have regarding cause of disease and effectiveness of treatments, significantly lower reports of physician participatory decision-making styles by minority patients as compared to nonminority patients, and lower rates of receiving preventative and necessary medical care (Cooper-Patrick et al. 1999; Roter and Hall 1992). Each of these likely plays a role in shaping treatment outcomes. Perceptions of poor provider behavior and lack of ancillary resources impede effective communication and medical errors, as well as the development of treatment partnerships (Cooper-Patrick et al. 1999; Mull 1993). However, the critical link to disparities lies not only in what happens in the clinical encounter but also in how it extends back into the community.

The Meso Level: The Informal Community System – Family/Friend/Lay Network Sectors

While the line between the environmental context and the proximate "community" in which individuals live their lives is sometimes subtle, the difference is important. While the larger social context can shape lower levels of social organization, the community is often seen as representing the "small worlds" of individuals (Fischer 1982). That is, the actual nature of social ties those individuals have inside and outside a geographic area constitutes their "community of meaning" and the largest source of health care resources, including information and influence (Wellman and Potter 1999). With regard to health and health care, the neighborhood and local social networks are seen as key.

Community systems can differ dramatically in ways that can facilitate the use of services and offer protection against health problems. The overall level of community social cohesion, or network interconnectedness, may play a role in health disparities by influencing factors that have been shown to affect services outcomes. For example, organized and cohesive communities have been more likely to ensure that state budget cuts do not affect their community and, in turn, increased access to health care is maintained (Sampson and Raudenbush 1997). However, in neighborhoods where aggression and violence are common, community ties may not be stable or cohesive; and as a result, the recognition of mental health and substance abuse problems may occupy a lower level priority (Cauce et al. 2002).

Three types of service mismatch to the community's needs (van Ryn and Fu 2003) may fuel service disparities. First, where practice guidelines exist, they often do not include common manifestations of symptoms among ethno-cultural populations. Symptom presentation does vary across racial and ethnic groups and differs from what most clinicians are trained to expect, particularly between the endorsement of psychotic symptoms and the diagnosis of psychotic disorders (Olfson et al. 2002; Vega and Lewis-Fernandez 2008). Misdiagnosis can occur in the form of underdiagnosing when genuine manifestations of mental illness are misinterpreted (Lopez 1989). Second, clients may respond to the therapy situation in ways consistent with their cultural socialization regarding options that are available and/or desirable for therapist and client roles. Thirdly, clinicians may stereotype patients' requests, especially when they are ambiguous or unfamiliar (Kunda and Sherman-Williams 1993), or when the decisions are more discretionary. Under such conditions of uncertainty, clinicians may inadvertently incorporate a prior or what is the "expected" condition (Balsa and McGuire 2003). Individual data may be disregarded and, consequently, a mismatch of services to needs results.

In sum, like other mechanisms we have described, this mismatch of services to needs can result in the accumulation of disparities in use, retention, adherence, and outcome, for individuals themselves and for those whom they advise on health and health care. In the absence of cultural and contextual information that supplants stereotypes, the probability of misdiagnoses and inappropriate treatment formulations are elevated (Alarcon et al. 2002; Fabrega 1990; Kirmayer and Young 1999; Lopez 1989). In turn, this boomerangs into greater disease burden and differential health outcomes. For example, both African American and Latino injection drug users report that drug treatment programs are difficult to access and poorly designed to meet their needs (Walton et al. 2001; Wells et al. 2001), potentially playing a role in the documented greater disease burden. In fact, African Americans report longer addiction problems and a greater likelihood to relapse, despite the fact that African Americans tend to start drug use later and have a lower lifetime prevalence rate compared to whites (Buka 2002). Formally, then, we suggest:

Proposition 3. Poor patient–provider interaction leads to miscommunication, clinical uncertainty, low therapeutic alliance, stereotyping, clinical errors, and poor outcomes.

Proposition 4. Mismatches between mental health and substance use service offerings and minorities' services needs and living circumstances lead to drop out, low "adherence," and poor outcomes.

The Micro-Level: Provider–Client Interactions

Although the implementation of evidence-based guidelines in medicine has improved treatment for disadvantaged groups (Rogers 2004), the treatment of minorities by health care providers frequently does not adhere to evidence-based standards of care (Alegría et al. 2008; Flores 2000; Young et al. 2001). Whether the deviation from evidence-based treatments (EBT) is greater among providers who serve primarily ethnic and racial minorities, or whether providers are less likely to provide EBTs to their minority clients whatever the case be, this issue has rarely been investigated. Greater mistrust of pharmacological treatments in depression treatment for African Americans appears to exacerbate unmet need.

The uncertainty and stereotyping discussed above continue to have ramifications, which appear to be at the center of many of these problems, especially when the provider has incomplete information about the efficacy of a therapeutic intervention (Bloche 2001). In part, these problems result from the underrepresentation of minorities in clinical trials that establish efficacy or effectiveness of EBTs (Miranda et al. 2005).

Categorizations such as race, age, sex, and socioeconomic status are overgeneralized (Abreu 1999; Balsa and McGuire 2003). Providers tend to see African-American patients, assigning them less complicated (and less effective) diabetes regimens (Lutfey and Freese 2005), as less educated than non-Latino white patients. Psychiatrists characterized African-American patients, who were indistinguishable from white patients in sociodemographics and clinical data (except for race) as "less articulate, competent, introspective, self-critical, sophisticated about mental health centers, and psychologically minded" and consequently less able to profit from psychotherapy (Van Ryn and Burke 2000).

For Afro-Caribbeans, experiences of mistreatment and social exclusion by health professionals reverberated on future utilization and on community sentiments toward the mental health system (McLean et al. 2003). Community mistrust of health care providers translates into a decreased likelihood of using health care or of supporting the use of psychoactive medication (Croghan et al. 2003; LaVeist et al. 2000; McLeod et al. 2004). Even for children, African American families report fearing that taking their children to treatment for mental health issues would result in institutionalization and, as a result, avoid treatment (Takeuchi et al. 1993). Thus, repeated negative contacts are compounded by a lack of trust in key gateway providers such as teachers to produce community-held beliefs that produce health services disparities for ethno-cultural populations (LaVeist et al. 2000).

However, there appears to be a paradox here. Analyses of African-Americans and Latinos in the USA indicate that they hold *higher* expectations for medical care than non-Hispanic Whites (Schnittker et al. 2005). While there may be some differences by specialty (e.g. greater concern regarding mental health as opposed to physical health issues), the idea that the cultural context in ethno-cultural communities is not supportive of the potential of health care needs to be reconsidered.

The Micro-Level: Individual Level Factors Excluding Need or Clinical Appropriateness

While all of the factors mentioned above target structural and interactive factors, individuals do bring unique profiles in terms of their "readiness," knowledge, beliefs, cognitive, and psychological tendencies (Pescosolido 2006). Perhaps among the most stable, documented influence is education, a variable directly linked to economic welfare, healthy lifestyles, full-time employment, and health.

Greater educational attainment has been shown to positively impact mental health by increasing one's resources to cope with adversity or increasing a sense of control over one's destiny (Chartier et al. 2001). Conversely, not only are lower levels of educational attainment a strong predictor of poor mental health and substance abuse outcomes for children, but the effect also remains significant for mid-age and older cohorts. Education's effect on services use and even cultural support for mental health services, however, is more mixed (Croghan et al. 2003; Pescosolido and Boyer 1999; Pescosolido et al. 2008).

While not coterminous with educational attainment, health literacy, a more specific form of knowledge, includes individuals' basic literacy skills and the degree to which those skills can be applied in order to access health services and obtain or process health information in treatment (Gazmararian et al. 2005; Safeer and Keenan 2005). Low literacy skills create barriers to successful navigation and functioning within the US health care system. They increase the inability to register for health insurance, the difficulty in interpreting coverage benefits and rules, and the avoidance or delay in accessing health services requiring forms to be filled out in physician offices (Dewalt et al. 2004; Gazmararian et al. 2005; Pawlak 2005; Safeer and Keenan 2005). According to The Commonwealth Fund 2001 Health Care Quality Survey, 33% of Latinos, 27% of Asian Americans and 23% of African Americans (compared to 16% of Whites) reported that their doctor did not listen to everything they said, or that they did not fully understand their doctor, but did not ask questions during their visit (Collins et al. 2002). Misunderstanding treatment directives likely leads to poor adherence to medications, itself a disparity in services delivery. All totaled, individuals with low literacy skills are 1.3–3 times more likely to experience adverse health outcomes than individuals with high literacy levels (Dewalt et al. 2004).

In the lay cultural sphere, individuals' general beliefs can add to the production of health services disparities for ethno-cultural populations. For example, fatalism, the belief that fate controls one's destiny, continues to be more common among Latinos, African Americans and Asians than non-Latino Whites, even when controlling for SES and education (Green et al. 2004). And, fatalistic individuals tend to delay seeking health care (Nelson et al. 2002). In addition, the catalog of possible options to respond to mental health and addiction issues varies for different ethnic groups in the U.S. Whites and African-Americans, for example, endorse the use of general and mental health specialists at the same rates, African-Americans are significantly less likely to suggest (Pescosolido and Boyer 1999). Finally, ethnic and racial minority individuals who come from disadvantaged backgrounds come to treatment with complex social needs that cumulate into greater disparities. In a recent study, 25% of patients in Los Angeles County who delayed using care reported that competing necessities such as food, shelter, or clothing had higher priority (Diamant et al. 2004), or were unable to leave work or take time off from work because of lack of benefits (Perez and Fortuna 2005). In sum, what individuals bring to the conceptualization of health problems and treatment options and to the clinical encounter matters. To the extent that individuals present unique or more complicated problems and hold different views, pathways to care are longer, more complex and convoluted from the medical system's perspective. Taken together with the limits at the macro and meso levels, these individual profiles can result in health, health care, and treatment disparities.

On the treatment side, a disproportionately low supply of providers, particularly multilingual service providers in geographical communities with ethnic and racial minorities, not seen in nonminority communities, can impact services disparities (Derose and Baker 2000). This can be caused or compounded by the way that health care organizations staff services. Physicians from ethno-cultural backgrounds represent only 9% of all US physicians in the USA (Association of American Medical Colleges 2000), and most US health care providers tend to be monolingual English speakers (Fiscella and Franks 2001). The likelihood of encountering a "match" in terms of either background or culturally competent training is predictably low. And, of course, for Medicaid beneficiaries, particularly those with limited English language skills, the chances are further diminished as competition draws physicians to a more lucrative and less difficult caseload of privately insured patients (Tai-Seale et al. 2001). Not surprisingly, then, communities with high proportions of Black and Latino residents are four times as likely as non-Latino Whites to confront a physician shortage regardless of community income (Putsch and Pololi 2005). Similarly, health care services available through the Indian Health Services vary widely across tribes, even as the IHS partially offsets the lack of insurance for some American Indian and Alaska Natives (AIANs). AIANs were more than two times as likely to be uninsured than non-Latino Whites (Zuckerman et al. 2004) and face limited provider networks for Medicaid health maintenance organizations (HMOs) enrolling minority beneficiaries (Tai-Seale et al. 2001). Following on this, we suggest two propositions:

> *Proposition 5.* Lack of community trust and erroneous expectations of services lead to disengagement and poor collaboration in healthcare services systems.
>
> *Proposition 6.* Limited workforce availability and training of service providers to treat ethnic and racial minority populations lead to reliance on informal or poorly trained providers and stress the capacity of well-trained providers.

We end with propositions because the development of testable hypotheses require a unique and tailored understanding of the particular health problems and specifically targeted beliefs. For example, while concerns about obesity or colorectal cancer turn researchers' attention to cultural issues surrounding food and invasive community screening procedures, concerns about mental health and substance abuse do not. They raise cultural issues about health and health care, but different ones. Issues about stigma of mental illness, the efficacy of mental health care, and more negative views of particular treatment options [e.g., psychiatric medication (Schnittker et al. 2005)] require that we consider both generalized cultural issues and specific ones, locating where and whether each may play a role in how patients and providers respond to the onset of health problems or even to the willingness to engage in health behavior. Too often, this narrowing down and customizing is left out, leaving researchers and policymakers with more global challenges to confront in understanding and changing communities and health care systems. From our perspective, this has been part of the reason why multilevel frameworks have been underutilized – the reliance on standardized batteries about what Hispanics are like or what African Americans thinks rob us of the very insights that can come from initial, exploratory, or rich ethnographic work (see Pescosolido (2006) on more issues on this point).

Discussion and Conclusion

By drawing together research documenting glaring discrepancies in patterns of health service use and outcomes for racial and ethnic groups considered to be underrepresented minorities in the U.S. (e.g. augmented age-adjusted mortality), a series of reports signaled a shift in medical science's attention to social inequalities outside and inside their purview (Institute of Medicine 2002; National Center for Health Statistics 2004). Despite a perennial concern with social inequality in health and health care among certain disciplines and organizations, this recent effort marks a concerted health policy shift in medicine and medical science to confront systematic and pressing differences facing certain groups projected to make up nearly a third of the US population by the year 2020.

At present, we are just beginning to develop systematic theoretical models that reflect the complex structures and mechanisms to guide empirical research necessary to get underneath inequities and provide a foundation for the science-to-services translation called for by NIH and other policy-making bodies [see Warnecke et al. (2008) as a recent example; see Hohmann and Shear (2002); National Advisory Mental Health Council Workgroup on Clinical Treatment and Services Research (1997) on the calls]. The SCF-HSD was designed to help close that gap. It represents only a start, requiring the development of specific hypotheses, complex and innovative research designs, multi-level and/or longitudinal data, and well-considered analytical choices (Alegría et al. 2009).

The point of the SCF-HSD is a deceptively simple one: Disparities arise when disadvantages in the health care system interact with those in the community system. Simple, in that when considered in light of the literature, it seems obvious. Individuals "bring" ideas, beliefs, and behaviors to the treatment system, whether as patients or providers, rather than just their problems and expertise, respectively. Deceptive, in that this is rarely done. Research tends to be bifurcated as epidemiology or services research, as patient or provider focused, and as individual or macro focused. Among the key challenges that remain in the constantly touted call for transdisciplinary and translational research agendas is how to do these effectively. As we suggest above, this will require moving outside of the standard approaches to research design, methods, and analytic techniques. While it will not be easy to convince those who hold resources necessary to do such research that complex community-based designs are necessary at this stage of understanding disparities, consideration of the SCF-HSD requires, at minimum, an understating of these processes in context, whether across levels or within them.

The SCF-HSD is intended to help conceptualize and carry out the next stages of research directed at understanding and eliminating ethnic and racial disparities. Yet, it is also designed to go beyond basic research. A consideration of complexity and context may have utility in training health and social agency personnel. Finally, the SCF-HSD aims to supply services planners and policy makers with working propositions, initially, and a science-base, eventually, on how to intervene and eliminate services disparities (Alegría et al. 2009). At each level or domain, the SCF-HSD suggests basic mechanisms that produce disparities for ethno-cultural populations and suggests points of intervention that can be directed to the health care system, existent policies, clinical training, and community programs.

Research that addresses the complexity of the multiple levels and two major domains that produce health and health care disparities continues to evolve, producing more tailored and effective efforts to eliminate disparities. Our goal here has been to draw the foundational elements that suggest one approach to help stimulate the research and policy thinking that can foster change for health care systems and communities.

Acknowledgements The writing of this chapter was supported by NIH Research Grant # 1P50 MHO 73469 and U01 MH 06220-06A2, both funded by the National Institute of Mental Health, as well as Grant #P60 MD0 02261, funded by the National Center for Minority Health and Health Disparities. In addition, support as provided from the College of Arts and Sciences, Indiana University, to the Indiana Consortium for Mental Health Services Research.

References

Abreu J (1999) Consciout and nonconsciout African American stereotypes: impact on first impression and diagnostic ratings by therapists. J Consult Clin Psychol 67:387–393

Alarcon DR, Bell CC, Laurence Kirmayer J, Lin K-M, Ustun B, Katherine Wisner L (2002) Beyond the funhouse mirrors. In: First BM, Regier DA (eds) A research agenda for DSM-V. American Psychiatric Association, Washington, DC, pp 219–281

Alegría M, Canino G, Rios R, Vera M, Calderon J, Rusch D, Ortega AN (2002) Inequalities of use in specialty mental health services among Latinos, African Americans, and non-Latino Whites. Psychiatr Serv 53:1547–1555

Alegría M, Chatterji P, Wells KB, Cao Z, Chen Chih-nan, Takeuchi D, Jackson J, Meng Xiao-Li (2008) Disparity in access to and quality of depression treatment among racial and ethnic minorities in the US. Psychiatr Serv 59:1264–1272

Alegría M, Perez DJ, Williams S (2003) The role of public policies in reducing disparities in mental health status for people of color. Health Aff 22:51–64

Alegría M, Pescosolido BA, Canino G (2009) A socio-cultural framework for health services disparities: illustrating the case of mental health and substance abuse. In: Sadock BJ, Sadock VA, Ruiz A (eds) Comprehensive textbook of psychiatry. Wolters Kluwer Health, Lippincott Williams & Wilkins, Baltimore, MD, pp 4370–4379

Allison PD, Scott Long J, Krauze TK (1982) Cumulative advantage and inequality in science. Am Sociol Rev 47:615–625

Antshel KM (2002) Integrating culture as a means of improving treatment adherence in the Latino population. Psychol Health Med 7:435–449
Association of American Medical Colleges (2000) Minority graduates of U.S. medical schools: trends, 1950–1998. Association of American Medical Colleges, Washington DC
Balsa A, Cao Z, McGuire TE (2007) Does managed health care reduce unfair differences in health care use between minorities and Whites? J Health Econ 26:101–121
Balsa A, McGuire TE (2003) Prejudice, clinical uncertainty and stereotypes as sources of health disparities. J Health Econ 22(1):89–116
Bernal G, Trimble JE, Burlew AK, Leong F (2003) Handbook of racial and ethnic minority psychology. In: Leong FTL (ed) Racial and ethnic minority psychology series. Sage Publications, Thousand Oaks
Beutler LE, Machado PPO, Neufeldt SA (1994) Therapist variables. In: Bergin AE, Garfield SL (eds) Handbook of psychotherapy and behavior change. Wiley, New York, pp 229–269
Blanchard J, Lurie N (2004) R-E-S-P-E-C-T: patient reports of disrespect in the health care setting and its impact on care. J Fam Pract 53:721–730
Bloche MG (2001) Race and discretion in American medicine. Yale J Health Policy Law Ethics 1:95–131
Blow F, Zeber J, McCarthy J, Valenstein M, Gillon L, Raymond Bingham C (2004) Ethnicity and diagnosis patterns in veterans with psychoses. Soc Psychiatry Psychiatr Epidemiol 39:841–851
Bodenheimer T (2005) High and rising health care costs, part 1: seeking an explanation. Ann Intern Med 142:847–854
Buka SL (2002) Disparities in health status and substance use: ethnicity and socioeconomic factors. Public Health Rep 117:S118–S125
Cao Z, McGuire TE (2003) Service-level selection by HMOs medicare in medicare. J Health Econ 22:915–931
Caronna CA (2010) Clash of logics, crisis of trust: entering the era of public for-profit health care? Forthcoming In: Pescosolido BA, McLeod JD, Martin JK, Rogers A (eds) The handbook of the sociology of health, illness, and healing: blueprint for the 21st century. Springer, New York.
Cauce AM, Domenech-Rodriguez M, Paradise M, Cochran B, Shea J, Srebnik D, Baydar N (2002) Cultural and contextual influences in mental health help seeking: a focus on ethnic minority youth. J Counsel Clin Psychol 70:44–55
Chartier MJ, Walker JR, Stein MB (2001) Social phobia and potential childhood risk factors in a community sample. Psychol Med 31:307–315
Clausen JA, Yarrow MR (1955) Pathways to the mental hospital. J Soc Issues 11:25–32
Collins KS, Hughes DL, Doty MM, Ives B, Edwards J, Tenney K (2002) Diverse communities, common concerns: assessing health care quality for minority Americans. In: Findings from The Commonwealth Fund 2001, Health Care Quality Survey. The Commonwealth Fund, New York, NY
Cooper-Patrick L, Gallo L, Gonzales JJ, Vu H, Powe NR, Nelson C, Ford D (1999) Race, gender, and partnership in the patient-physician relationship. J Am Med Assoc 282:583–589
Croghan TW, Tomlin M, Pescosolido BA, Martin JK, Lubell KM, Swindle R (2003) Americans' knowledge and attitudes towards and their willingness to use psychiatric medications. J Nerv Ment Dis 191:166–174
Cunningham PJ, Hadley J (2008) Effects of changes in incomes and practice circumstances on physicians' decisions to treat charity and medicaid patients. Millibank Q 86:91–123, Center for Studying Health System Change
Currie J, Fahr J (2004) Hospitals, managed care, and the charity caseload in California. J Health Econ 23:421–442
Daley M (2005) Race, managed care, and the quality of substance abuse treatment. Adm Policy Ment Health 32:457–476
Derose KP, Baker DW (2000) Limited english proficiency and latinos' use of physician services. Med Care Res Rev 57:76–91
Dewalt D, Berkman N, Sheridan S, Lohr KN, Pignone M (2004) Literacy and health outcomes: a systematic review of the literature. J Gen Intern Med 19:1228–1239
Diamant AL, Hays RD, Morales LS, Ford W, Calmes D, Asch S, Duan N, Fielder E, Kim S, Fielding J, Sumner G, Shapiro MF, Hayes-Bautista D, Gelberg L (2004) Delays and unmet need for health care among adult primary care patients in a restructured urban public health system. Am J Public Health 94:783–789
DiMaggio PJ (1997) Culture and cognition. Annu Rev Sociol 23:263–287
DiMaggio P, Powell W (1991) Introduction. In: Powell W, DiMaggio P (eds) The new institutionalism in organizational analysis. University of Chicago Press, Chicago
DiPrete TA, Eirich GM (2006) Cumulative advantage as a mechanism for inequality: a review of theoretical and empirical developments. Annu Rev Sociol 32:271–297
Elder GH Jr (1992) The Life Course. In: Borgatta E, Borgatta M (eds) The encyclopedia of sociology, vol 3. MacMillan, New York, pp 1120–1130
Elder GH Jr (1998) Children of the great depression. Westview Press, New York
Elder GH Jr, Caspi A (1990) Studying lives in a changing society: sociological and personological explorations. In: Rabin AI, Zucker RA, Emmons RA, Frank S (eds) Studying persons and lives. Springer, New York, pp 201–247
Fabrega H Jr (1990) Hispanic mental health research: a case for cultural psychiatry. Hisp J Behav Sci 12:339–365

Fiscella K, Franks P (2001) Impact of patient socioeconomic status on physician profiles: a comparison of census-derived and individual measures. Med Care 39:8–14
Fischer CS (1982) To dwell among friends. University of California Press, Berkeley, CA
Flores G (2000) Culture and the patient–physician relationship: achieving cultural competency in health care. J Pediatr 136:14–23
Flores G, Laws MB, Mayo SJ, Zuckerman B, Abreu M, Medina L, Hardt EJ (2003) Errors in medical interpretation and their potential clinical consequences in pediatric encounters. Pediatrics 111:6–14
Garland AF, Hough RL, Yeh McCabe M, Wood P, Aarons G (2001) Prevalence of psychiatric disorders for youth in public sectors of care. J Am Acad Child Adolesc Psychiatry 40:409–418
Gazmararian JA, Curran JW, Parker RM, Bernhardt JM, DeBuono BA (2005) Public health literacy in America: an ethical imperative. Am J Prev Med 28:317–322
Green BL, Lewis RK, Wang MQ, Person S, Rivers B (2004) Powerlessness, destiny, and control: the influence on health behaviors of African Americans. J Commun Health 29:15–27
Guarnaccia PJ, Rodriguez O (1996) Concepts of culture and their role in the development of culturally-competent mental health services. Hisp J Behav Sci 18:419–443
Hafferty FW, Castellani B (2010) Two cultures – two ships: the rise of a professionalism movement within modern medicine nad medical sociology's disappearance from the professionalism debate. Forthcoming In: Pescosolido BA, McLeod JD, Martin JK, Rogers A (eds) The handbook of the sociology of health, illness, and healing: blueprint for the 21st century. Springer, New York.
Hampers L, Cha S, Gutglass D, Binns H, Krug S (1999) Language barriers and resource utilization in a pediatric emergency department. Pediatrics 103:1253–1256
Hargraves JL, Hadley J (2003) The contribution of insurance coverage and community resources to reducing racial/ethnic disparities in access to care. Health Serv Res 38:809–829
Hohmann AA, Katherine Shear M (2002) Community-based intervention research: coping with the "noise" of real life in study design. Am J Psychiatr 159:201–207
Institute of Medicine (2002) In: Smedley BD, Stith AY, Nelson A (eds) Unequal treatment: confronting racial and ethnic disparities in health care. The National Academies Press, Washington, DC
Jackson PB (2004) Role sequencing: does order matter for mental health? J Health Soc Behav 45:132–154
Kaiser Family Foundation (2008) Employee health benefits: 2008 annual survey. Health research & educational trust, 2008 summary of findings.
Keogan K (2002) A sense of place: the politics of immigration and the symbolic construction of identity in southern California and the new york metropolitan area. Sociol Forum 17:223–253
Kirmayer LJ, Young A (1999) Culture and context in the evolutionary concept of mental disorder. J Abnorm Psychol 108:446–452
Kumanyika SK (1993) Diet and nutrition as influences on the morbidity/mortality gap. Ann Epidemiol 3:154–158
Kunda Z, Sherman-Williams B (1993) Stereotypes and the construal of individuating information. Pers Soc Psychol Bull 19:90–99
Kurasaki K, Sue S, Chun C, Gee K (2000) Ethnic minority intervention and treatment research. In: Aponte J, Boston JW (eds) Psychological intervention and cultural diversity. Allyn and Bacon, MA, pp 2324–2349
LaVeist TA, Diala C, Jarrett NC (2000) Social status and perceived discrimination: who experiences discrimination in the health care system, how, and why. In: Hogue C, Hargraves M, Scott-Collins K (eds) Minority health in America. Johns Hopkins University Press, Baltimore, MD, pp 194–208
Lillie-Blanton M, Hoffman C (2005) The role of health insurance coverage in reducing racial/ethnic disparities in health care. Health Aff 24:398–408
Link BG, Phelan JC (1995) Social conditions as fundamental causes of disease. J Health Soc Behav 35:80–94, Extra issue
Link BG, Phelan JC (2000) Evaluating the fundamental cause explanation for social disparities in health. In: Bird CE, Conrad P, Fremont AM (eds) Handbook of medical sociology. Prentice-Hall, Inc, Upper Saddle River, NJ, pp 33–46
Link BG, Phelan JC (2005) Fundamental sources of health inequalities. In: Mechanic D, Rogut L, Colby D (eds) Policy challenges in modern health care. Rutgers University Press, New Brunswick, NJ, pp 71–84
Littlewood R, Lipsedge M (1981) Acute psychotic reactions in caribbean-born patients. Psychol Med 11:303–318
Long JS (1987) Problems and prospects for research on sex differences in the scientific career. In: Dix LS (ed) Women: their underrepresentation and career differentials in science and engineering. National Academy Press, Washington DC, pp 163–169
Long JS, Fox MF (1995) Scientific careers: ascription and achievement. Annu Rev Sociol 21:45–71
Lopez SR (1989) Patient variable biases in clinical judgment: conceptual overview and methodological considerations. Psychol Bull 106:184–203
Lutfey KE, Freese J (2005) Toward some fundamentals of fundamental causality: socioeconomic status and health in the routine clinic visit for diabetes. Am J Sociol 110:1326–1372

Massey DS, Denton N (1998) American apartheid: segregation and the making of the underclass. Harvard University Press, Cambridge, MA
Massoglia M (2008) Incarceration as exposure: the prison, infectious disease, and other stress-related illnesses. J Health Soc Behav 49:56–71
McGovern D, Cope R (1991) Second generation Afro-Caribbeans and young Whites with a first admission diagnosis of schizophrenia. Soc Psychiatry Psychiatr Epidemiol 26:95–99
McLean C, Campbell C, Cornish F (2003) African-Caribbean interactions with mental health services in the U.K.: experiences and expectations of exclusion as (re)productive of health inequalities. Soc Sci Med 56:657–669
McLeod JD, Fettes DL (2007) Trajectories of failure: the educational careers of children with mental health problems. Am J Sociol 113:655–656
McLeod JD, Pescosolido BA, Takeuchi DT, White TF (2004) Public attitudes toward the use of psychiatric medications for children. J Health Soc Behav 45:53–67
Mechanic D (2004) The rise and fall of managed care. J Health Soc Behav 45:76–86, Extra issue
Merton RK (1957) Social theory and social structure. Free Press, Glencoe, IL
Miranda J, Bernal G, Lau A, Kohn L, Hwang WC, Lafromboise T (2005) State of the science on psychosocial interventions for ethnic minorities. Annu Rev Clin Psychol 1:113–142
Mull J (1993) Cross-cultural communication in the physician's office. West J Med 159:609–613
National Advisory Mental Health Council Workgroup on Clinical Treatment and Services Research (1997) Bridging science and service. National Institutes of Health/National Institute of Mental Health, Bethesda, MD
National Center for Health Statistics (2004) Health, United States, 2004. National Center for Health Statistics Hyattsville, MD
Nelson K, Geiger AM, Mangione CM (2002) Effect of health beliefs on delays in care for abnormal cervical cytology in a multi-ethnic population. J Gen Inter Med 17:709–716
Olafsdottir S, Pescosolido BA (2009) Drawing the line: the cultural cartography of utilization recommendations for mental health problems. J Health Soc Behav 50(2):228–244
Olfson M, Lewis-Fernandez R, Weissman MM, Feder A, Gameroff M, Pilowsky D (2002) Psychotic symptoms in an urban general medicine practice. Am J Psychiatry 159:1412–1419
Parsons T (1951) The social system: the major exposition of the author's conceptual scheme for the analysis of the dynamics of the social system. Free Press, New York, NY
Pavalko EK, Harding CM, Pescosolido BA (2007) Mental illness careers in an era of change. Soc Probl 54:504–522
Pawlak R (2005) Economic considerations of health literacy. Nurs Econ 23:173–180
Perez MC, Fortuna L (2005) Psychosocial stressors, psychiatric diagnoses and utilization of mental health services among undocumented immigrant Latinos. J Immigr Refug Serv 3:107–123
Perry M, Kannel S, Riley T, Pernice C (2001) What parents say: why eligible children lose SCHIP. National Academy for State Health Policy, Portland, ME
Pescosolido BA (1991) Illness careers and network ties: a conceptual model of utilization and compliance. In: Albrecht GL, Levy JA (eds) Advances in medical sociology. JAI Press, CT, pp 161–184
Pescosolido BA (1992) Beyond rational choice: the social dynamics of how people seek help. Am J Sociol 97:1096–1138
Pescosolido BA (2006) Of pride and prejudice: the role of sociology and social networks in integrating the health sciences. J Health Soc Behav 47:189–208
Pescosolido BA, Boyer CA (1999) How do people come to use mental health services? Current knowledge and changing perspectives. In: Horwitz AV, Scheid TL (eds) A handbook for the study of mental health: social contexts, theories, and systems. Cambridge University Press, New York, pp 392–411
Pescosolido BA, Brooks-Gardner C, Lubell KM (1998) How people get into mental health services: stories of choice, coercion and 'muddling through' from 'first-timers'. Soc Sci Med 46:275–286
Pescosolido BA, Kronenfeld J (1995) "Health, illness, and healing in an uncertain era: Challenges from and for medical sociology." Journal of Health and Social Behavior 35:5–33
Pescosolido BA, Jensen P et al (2008) Public knowledge and assessment of child mental health problems: findings from the national stigma study–children. J Am Acad Child Adolesc Psychiatry 47:339–349
Pescosolido BA, Wright ER, Sullivan WP (1995) Communities of care: a theoretical perspective on care management models in mental health. In: Greenwich GA (ed) Advances in medical sociology, vol 6. JAI Press, CT, pp 37–80
Putsch R, Pololi L (2005) Distributive justice in American healthcare: institutions, power, and the equitable care of patients. Am J Manag Care 10:SP45–SP53
Rogers A, Pilgrim D (2003) Mental health and inequality. Palgrave MacMillan, New York
Rogers WA (2004) Evidence-based medicine and justice: a framewrok for looking at the impact of EBM upon vulnerable or disadvantaged groups. J Med Ethics 30:141–145
Rogler HL (1996) Research on mental health services for Hispanics: targets of convergence. Cult Divers Ment Health 2:145–156

Rosenbaum PR (2002) Observational studies. Springer-Verlag, New York, NY

Roter D, Hall J (1992) Doctors talking with patients/patients talking with doctors: improving communication in medical visits. Praeger/Greenwood, London

Rylko-Bauer B, Farmer P (2002) Managed care or managed inequality? A call for critiques of market-based medicine. Med Anthropol Q 16:476–502

Safeer RS, Keenan J (2005) Health literacy: the gap between physicians and patients. Am Fam Physician 72:463–468

Saha S, Komaromy M, Koepsell TD, Bindman AB (1999) Patient-physician racial concordance and the perceived quality and use of health care. Arch Inter Med 159:997–1004

Sampson RJ, Raudenbush SW (1997) Neighborhoods and violent crime: a multilevel study of collective efficacy. Science 277:918–924

Schneider E, Zaslavsky AM, Epstein A (2002) Racial disparities in the quality of care for enrollees in medicare managed care. J Am Med Assoc 287:1288–1294

Schnittker J, Pescosolido BA, Croghan TW (2005) Are African Americans really less willing to use health care? Soc Probl 52:255–271

Shone L, Dick A, Klein J, Zwanziger J, Szilagyi P (2005) Reduction in racial and ethnic disparities after enrollment in the state children's health insurance program. Pediatrics 115:e679–e705

Stiffman AR, Hadley-Ives E, Dore P, Polgar MF, Horvath VE, Striley C, Elze D (2000) Youths' access to mental health services: the role of providers' training, resource connectivity, and assessment of need. Ment Health Serv Res 2:141–154

Stiffman AR, Pescosolido BA, Cabassa LJ (2004) Building a model to understand youth service access: the gateway provider model. Ment Health Serv Res 6:189–198

Stiffman AR, Striley C, Horvath V, Hadley-Ives E, Polgar M, Elze D, Pescarino R (2001) Organizational context and provider perception as determinants of mental health service use. J Behav Serv Res 28:188–204

Strauss C, Quinn N (1997) A cognitive theory of cultural meaning. Cambridge University Press, Cambridge

Suchman EA (1965) Social patterns of illness and medical care. J Health Hum Behav 6:2–16

Swidler A (2001) Talk of love: how culture matters. University of Chicago Press, Chicago, IL

Tai-Seale M, Freund D, LoSasso A (2001) Racial disparities in service use among medicaid beneficiaries after mandatory enrollment in managed care: a difference in differences approach. Inquiry 38:49–59

Tai-Seale M, McGuire T, Colenda C, Rosen D, Cook M (2007) Two-minute mental health care for elderly patients: inside primary care visits. J Am Geriatr Soc 55:1903–1911

Takeuchi DT, Bui Khanh-Van T, Kim L (1993) The referral of minority adolescents to community mental health centers. J Health Soc Behav 34:153–164

Tilly C (1999) Durable Inequality. In: Moen P, Dempster-McClain D, Walker H (eds) A nation divided: diversity, inequality, and community in American society. Cornell University Press, Ithaca, NY, pp 15–33

Tilly C (2000) Chain migration and opportunity hoarding. In: Dacyl JW, Westin C (eds) Governance of cultural diversity. Centre for research in international migration and ethnic relations, Stockholm

Tilly C (2002) Event catalogs as theories. Sociol Theory 20(2):248–254

U.S. Bureau of the Census (2002) Statistical abstract of the united states. U.S. Government Printing Office, Washington, DC

U.S. Department of Health & Human Services (2000) National standards on culturally and linguistically appropriate services (CLAS). Office of Minority Health, Rockville, MD

U.S. Department of Health and Human Services (2003) National healthcare disparities report. Agency for Healthcare Research and Quality, Rockville, MD

Van Ryn M, Burke J (2000) The effect of patient race and socio-economic status on physicians' perceptions of patients. Soc Sci Med 50:813–828

van Ryn M, Fu S (2003) Paved with good intentions: do public health and human service providers contribute to racial/ethnic disparities in health? Am J Public Health 93:248–255

Vega WA, Lewis-Fernandez R (2008) Ethnicity and variability of psychotic symptoms. Curr Psychiatry Rep 10:223–228

Walton MA, Blow FC, Booth BM (2001) Diversity in relapse prevention needs: gender and race comparisons among substance abuse treatment patients. Am J Drug Alcohol Abuse 27:225–240

Warnecke RB, Oh A, Breen N, Gehlert S, Paskett E, Tucker KL et al (2008) Approaching health disparities from a population perspective: the National Institutes of Health Centers for Population Health and Health Disparities. Am J Public Health 98:1608–1615

Wellman B, Potter S (1999) The elements of personal communities. In: Boulder BW (ed) Networks in the global village: life in contemporary communities. Westview Press, CO, pp 49–82

Wells K, Klap R, Koike A, Sherbourne C (2001) Ethnic disparities in unmet need for alcoholism, drug abuse, and mental health care. Am J Psychiatry 158:2027–2032

Williams DR, Jackson PB (2005) Social sources of racial disparities in health. Health Affairs 24(2):325–334

Williams D (2005) Patterns and Causes of Disparities in Health. In: Policy Challenges in Modern Health Care. New Brunswick, NJ: Rutgers University Press. pp 115–134

Williams JW Jr, Rost K, Dietrich AJ, Ciotti MC, Zyzanski SJ, Cornell J (1999) Primary care physicians' approach to depressive disorders: effects of physician specialty and practice structure. Arch Fam Med 8:58–67

Wilson WJ (1990) The truly disadvantaged: the inner-city, the underclass, and public policy. University of Chicago Press, Chicago

Wilson WJ (1997) When work disappears: the world of the new urban poor. Vintage, New York

Wilson CM, Williams DR (2004) Mental Health of African Americans. In: Praeger Handbook of Black American Health: Policies nad Issues Behind Disparities in Health, Vol. 1. I.L. Livingston, Ed. Westport, CT: Praeger Publishers. pp 369–382

Young A, Klap R, Sherbourne CD, Wells KB (2001) The quality of care for depressive and anxiety disorders in the United States. Arch Gen Psychiatry 58:55–61

Zola IK (1973) Pathways to the doctor – from person to patient. Soc Sci Med 7:677–689

Zuckerman H, Cole JR (1975) Women in American science. Minerva 13:82–102

Zuckerman S, Haley JM, Roubideaux Y, Lillie-Blanton M (2004) Access, use, and insurance coverage among American Indians/Alaska Natives and Whites: what role does the Indian health service play? Am J Public Health 94:53–59

Chapter 20
Health Disparities and the Black Middle Class: Overview, Empirical Findings, and Research Agenda

Pamela Braboy Jackson and Jason Cummings

Health disparities may follow along a series of "…events signified by a difference in (1) environment, (2) access to, utilization of, and quality of care, (3) health status, or (4) a particular health outcome that deserves scrutiny" (Carter-Pokras and Baquet 2002: 427). This chapter focuses on three types of health disparities assessed by evaluating the gap in health status or a given health outcome. First, we describe Black–White differences across health and refer to these patterns as general health disparities. Second, we present some research demonstrating the standard SES-health gradient where those at the top of the economic hierarchy are in much better health than those at the bottom of the economic hierarchy. We focus specifically on the health of African Americans since our ultimate goal is to better understand differences within this population. Third, we emphasize a more recent disparity highlighted by some health scholars – that of a paradox among the Black middle class. These inequalities are surprising (and hence referred to as paradoxical) because the patterns are counter-intuitive to the SES-health gradient.

Overview

General Health Disparities

Recent research has drawn attention to growing racial disparities in health (Jackson 2005; Williams and Jackson 2005). Over the past three decades, the Black–White gap in both life expectancy and all cause mortality has shown a marked trend toward increasing disparities. In fact, the overall death rate of Blacks today still lags behind the death rate of Whites from nearly 30 years ago. According to Levine et al. (2001), there is an excess of approximately 100,000 Black deaths in USA compared to other racial groups. African Americans have higher death rates for most major chronic diseases, including heart disease, cancer, diabetes, and cirrhosis/liver disease (NCHS 2007).

Unlike the growing and convincing body of work on racial disparities in physical health, a mixed set of findings continue to be reported across studies on mental health. Prevalence studies using DSM (Diagnostic and Statistical Manual of Mental Disorders) criteria show that Blacks have lower lifetime rates of having any mental disorder when compared to their non-Hispanic White counterparts (Breslau et al. 2005; Kessler et al. 1994). It would appear, however, that while Blacks have

---

P.B. Jackson (✉)
Department of Sociology, Indiana University, Ballantine 744, Bloomington, IN 47405, USA
e-mail: pjackson@indiana.edu

lower rates of major depressive disorder (Riolo et al. 2005), they have higher rates of dysthymia (Somervell et al. 1989) than non-Hispanic Whites. In terms of hedonic well-being (Keyes et al. 2002), African Americans report lower assessments than Whites on life satisfaction and general happiness measures (Thomas and Holmes 1992). In sum, the literature suggests that general health disparities exist in favor of non-Hispanic Whites when compared to Blacks on biological measures of disease and self-reports of hedonic well-being. Evidence of Black–White disparities in mental disorder depends on the outcome of interest.

SES-Health Gradient

One of the most robust findings in the health literature is the positive association between SES and physical health across populations (Crimmins and Saito 2001; Marmot et al. 1997; Preston and Elo 1995). The US health data reveal a consistent education-health gradient among African Americans across a wide range of outcomes including infant mortality, low birth weight, limitations of physical activity, and rates of homicide (Pamuk et al. 1998). High death rates from heart disease are also associated with income declines (Pamuk et al. 1998). Community-level data confirm many of these patterns by showing that overall perceptions of health are conditioned by SES among African Americans (Drevenstedt 1998). Research on hypertension, however, has yielded mixed findings with some scholars reporting an inverse association with SES (measured by education and occupation; Keil et al. 1977), a positive association with SES (measured as education; Williams 2003), and no association with SES (measured as education; Vargas et al. 2000). We focus on composite self-reports of medical conditions as well as general assessments of physical health. We are comfortable using these indicators of physical health, especially since self-assessed health is a consistent predictor of mortality (Idler and Benyamini 1997).

In terms of mental health, Kessler and Neighbors (1986) conclude that Blacks in high-income categories report fewer symptoms of depression than those in low-income categories. More recent evidence from the National Study of American Life (NSAL) finds no association between SES (education or income) and rates of lifetime major depressive disorder among African Americans and Caribbean Blacks (Williams et al. 2007), but SES (education and income) is associated with a higher prevalence of reporting any lifetime substance abuse disorder among African Americans (Broman et al. 2007). In other research, Forman (2003) shows that Blacks in higher level occupations report lower levels of psychological distress than their working class counterparts. Thomas and Holmes (1992) find that Blacks in higher SES categories report greater life satisfaction than those in lower SES categories. In fact, the widest Black–White disparity in mental health has been found among those in the lowest (Kessler and Neighbors 1986) as well as at the highest (Cockerham 1990) SES levels. Supportive evidence is provided by Ellison (1990) who finds that African Americans with high levels of education and income report higher levels of life *happiness* than their lower class peers and that those with high incomes report higher life *satisfaction* than their counterparts with lower income (also see Musick 2000). Thus, albeit scant, research provides a somewhat predictable SES-mental health gradient within the Black population.

We assess mental health in terms of diagnostic-type assessments, scores on a symptom checklist, and quality of life measures (or hedonic well-being). Many scholars show the importance of distinguishing distress from disorder (Williams et al. 1992), and others have convincingly argued that indicators of quality of life are distinct from psychiatric diagnoses (Schuessler and Freshnock 1978; Schuessler 1982). More revealing are the arguments suggesting that African Americans may experience better psychiatric health while simultaneously experiencing lower life satisfaction (Thomas and Holmes 1992). We investigate this possibility in this study.

The Health Paradox

Despite evidence of a somewhat predictable SES-health gradient among African Americans, another pattern is emerging in the health literature. This particular disparity suggests that the social position of African Americans does not translate into the life chances one would expect from having higher SES when compared to non-Hispanic Whites of lower SES standing. It would appear that a wide range of health problems are not conditioned by SES in the expected ways, for at least some members of the middle class. The most frequently-cited examples suggesting a health paradox facing the Black middle class are (1) Black women who are college graduates have a higher infant mortality rate than White women who did not complete high school; (2) the highest SES group of Black women have equivalent or higher rates of hypertension, overweight, and low-birth weight than the lowest SES group of White women (Pamuk et al. 1998); (3) Black female college graduates report substantially lower perceived health scores than the health scores reported by White women with a high school diploma (Cummings and Jackson 2008); and (4) the homicide rate of Black men in the highest education category exceeds that of White men in the lowest education group (Pamuk et al. 1998). As suggested by this potpourri of health outcomes, Black–White differences in health range from internal (e.g. chronic health conditions) to external (e.g. homicide) factors – both of which can ultimately result in premature death.

Figure 20.1 illustrates this paradox using the case of infant mortality, the most widely used indicator of national health. As shown here, an African American infant is almost twice as likely to die before his/her first birthday compared to a non-Hispanic White infant (general disparities). Those with higher education report lower infant death rates (SES-health gradient). More striking is the Black middle class health paradox where we find a higher infant death rate among Black women with a college degree or more (~11.4) when compared to non-Hispanic White women who have less than a high school education (~9.9). The health paradox holds if middle-class Blacks report worse health than non-Hispanic Whites in lower class positions *or* there are no differences between these two groups.

We believe that racism remains a fundamental cause of health disparities (Williams 1997) and elucidate this position below by expounding on two critical starting points: Who is Black and who is the Black Middle Class? We argue that the challenges faced by those attempting to adopt the categories "Black" and "middle class" make it difficult to assess overall health disparities between certain groups. Nonetheless, we present empirical analyses using information in the NSAL to examine whether disparities are evident among all "Blacks" and consistent across measures of SES and a wide range of health outcomes.

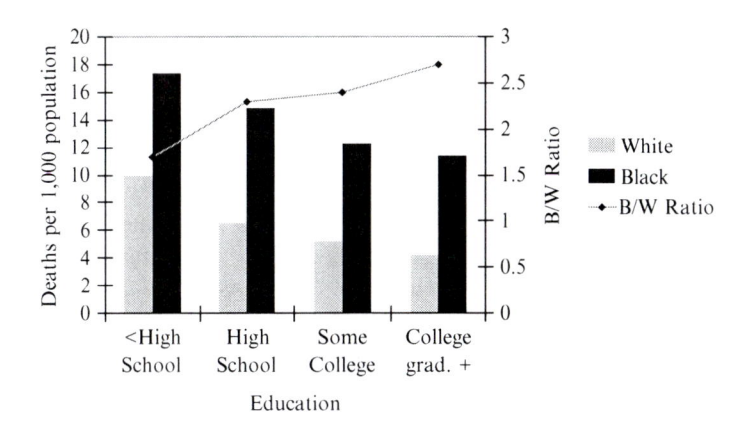

Fig. 20.1 A visual example of the health paradox: infant death rates by mother's education, 1995 (Pamuk et al. 1998)

Our ultimate goal is to offer a parsimonious explanation of certain health disparities reported among the Black middle class. This discussion relies heavily on research focusing on hyper-segregation and its unequivocal relationship to social networks. If our logic is correct, public policy efforts to reduce health disparities will have to consider the role of these social contextual factors as part of a broader set of social processes reflecting responses to negative racial attitudes in American society.

Who Is Black in the USA?

The topic of Black identity in America has a long and varied history (see Kennedy 2004). We do not wish to engage in this debate, but to simply describe those individuals who fall within this category utilized in much health research, especially statistics generated by the US Census Bureau. The US federal government's Office of Management and Budget (OMB) provides guidelines for categorizing race and ethnicity. According to Statistical Directive No. 15, federal agencies are required to provide statistics for four racial groups (American Indian and Alaskan Native, Asian or Pacific Islander, African American, and White) and one ethnic group (Hispanic). A revision to these guidelines was provided by the OMB in 1997, altering these categories by placing Asians in a separate group and creating a new category for Native Hawaiians and other Pacific Islanders (Grieco and Cassidy 2001).

According to general consensus, the category of Black includes any person with known African Black ancestry (Bahr et al. 1979: 27–28; Williamson 1980). This definition is reflected in the "one drop rule," which states that a single drop of "black blood" results in a person being designated as black. Others have referred to this rule as the "one black ancestor rule," the "traceable amount rule," or the "hypodescent rule" (Davis 1991; Rockquemore and Brunsma 2002). There is ample evidence that racial definitions shift over time and vary across social contexts. For example, in USA, the terms mulatto, Colored, Negro, Black and African American have all come to refer to people with any known black African ancestry (Blank et al. 2004, Table 2-1). On the contrary, in Latin America and the Caribbean, any degree of non-African ancestry means that a person is not black (Winn 1992).

The US Census continues to define a Black or African American as someone "…having origins in any of the Black racial groups of Africa. It includes people who indicate their race as 'Black, African American, or Negro' or provide written entries such as African American, Afro-Americans, Kenyan, Nigerian, or Haitian" (U.S. Census Bureau 2000).[1] The measurement of race remains an important concern because of the growing diversity of the US Black population – mostly due to immigration from Africa and the Caribbean.

The number of Black African immigrants to the USA began to grow dramatically in the 1970s (Gordon 1998). There were approximately one million African immigrants in the USA in 2002 compared to just 364,000 in 1990 (Grieco 2004), and more than 50% of the current immigrants from Africa settled in the USA between 1990 and 2000 (U.S. Census Bureau 2000). Due to the selectiveness of the migrant pool, almost a fourth of these legal immigrants are well-educated, professional, technical, and skilled workers (Champion 1994; U.S. Department of State 2002).

The Caribbean has always been the primary source of the USA's largest Black immigrant group with Afro-Caribbeans representing approximately 4% of the total US Black population (Logan and Deane 2003). Many of the Caribbean immigrants who entered the USA in the early part of the

---

[1] The number of individuals who identify as Black may be decreasing as more Blacks adopt a biracial or immigrant identity (Korgen 1998; Rockquemore and Brunsma 2002; Waters 1996, 1999).

twentieth century were well-educated professional workers (James 2002; Martinez 2003) as were many Afro-Caribbeans from English-speaking states who entered the USA in the twenty-first century (Kalmijn 1996). Haitian immigrants represent an exception to this pattern since many current immigrants are less skilled than individuals in previous generations (Fouron 1983; Jacobson 2003). In fact, immigrants from Haiti have levels of SES very similar to those of African Americans. The influx of African and Caribbean foreign-born in the USA has important implications for this chapter on health disparities primarily because these immigrant groups increase the variation in socioeconomic status (SES) within the Black population (Read and Emerson 2005; Williams et al. 2007).

In this chapter, Blacks are African Americans who self-identify as Black but who do not report Caribbean ancestry. Caribbean Blacks also self-identify as Black but affirm some form of Caribbean descent (referred to as Afro-Caribbeans). Different ethnic groups were considered more closely within the Caribbean Black sample: adults from Spanish-speaking Caribbean countries, English-speaking Caribbean countries, Haitians, and other Caribbeans. When possible, the health profile of these groups is compared to non-Hispanic White adults who were part of the NSAL. Later, we provide evidence suggesting that African Americans and Afro-Caribbeans present health profiles that are sufficiently different to challenge the practice of combining these heterogeneous groups into a single census category.

Who Are the Black Middle Class?

The definition and composition of the Black middle class has also changed over time. As early as 1899, W.E.B. DuBois (1899) characterized this group as "Families of undoubted respectability, earning sufficient income to live well; not engaged in menial service of any kind…" (310). Much of DuBois' work draws attention to the top ten percent of Black adults who attain high levels of education (Battle and Wright 2002). This image of the Black middle class resonates with Drake and Cayton (1945) and Frazier (1957) who sought to describe the lives of the growing professional class of Black workers in the USA. Frazier (1957) refers to the professional class as Black bourgeoisie and defines this group along occupational and economic lines. He also includes a discussion of a set of values (e.g. morality, piety, thrift) and behaviors (membership in certain organizations) that seem prevalent among the middle class (also see Rose 1997).

There has since been little consensus in the choice of criteria for defining the Black middle class (see Kronus 1971 for a discussion of this issue; Battle and Wright 2002). Most measures, however, are grounded in a general body of work on class analysis (Giddens 1973; Kohn 1977; Marshall et al. 1996; Treiman 1977; Wright 1979) that takes as its starting point a certain level of occupational prestige for defining class position (see Gatewood 2000). For example, in his well-cited work proclaiming the declining significance of race for determining the life chances of African Americans, Wilson (1978) defined the Black middle class simply as those who occupy white-collar jobs. Although he includes some nonprofessional occupations in this category, he argues that access to the jobs included in his category of middle class requires a certain level of educational attainment and therefore should be considered within this class position. Many scholars follow suit and simply adopt this particular single indicator of class position using the same job categories (e.g. see Hwang et al. 1998), further restricting the type of jobs included among white-collar workers (Landry 1987; Lareau 2002), or adopting individual measures of social class (see Durant and Sparrow 1997; Hochschild 1995).

Oliver and Shapiro (1995) identify the Black middle class along traditional lines of stratification but include consideration for wealth accumulation (defined primarily by home ownership). Interestingly, among Black adults living in the "middle class" neighborhood of Groveland in Chicago, Pattillo-McCoy (1999) describes mowing your lawn, getting married, going to church, and voting as evidence of middle class status. More recently, Lacy (2007) argues that personal income is a key determinant of middle class status among a group of Black suburbanites living outside of Washington, DC. She believes that single adults comprise a growing contingent of the Black middle class who work in professional jobs (also see Marsh et al. 2007) but who may live in quite distinct residential spaces where some neighborhoods border on impoverished areas within a city (e.g. Groveland) and others are located in isolated suburbs (see Appendix A for more conceptualizations of the Black middle class).

In general, though, the percentage of adults who fall within the middle class varies based on the dimension of stratification that is adopted. We demonstrate this point using a 5% sample of individual records in the Integrated Public Use Microdata Series (IPUMS), for the year 2000 (Ruggles et al. 1995). As few as 15% but as many as 59% of Black adults are members of the middle class, depending upon the dimension of stratification adopted by the investigator (see Appendix A for more detailed statistics). Here, we report on disparities in health using traditional measures of social class position. We adopt Oliver and Shapiro's (1995) definition of middle class status given their specificity on these multiple class dimensions (adjusting income for 2002 dollars; the time frame when the NSAL was being conducted). What is important is the overall theoretical position that middle class status should afford individuals a health advantage.

Can We Explain the Health Paradox of the Black Middle Class?

We offer two possible explanations for the health paradox of the Black middle class. First, the heterogeneity of the category Black may explain some of the anomalies currently reported in the health literature. An initial comparison across racial/ethnic groups should give an indication of potential variation in health outcomes. There is ample evidence that African Americans differ from some Afro-Caribbeans on health indicators such as infant mortality (Singh and Yu 1996), adult mortality (Hummer et al. 1999; Singh and Miller 2004), and psychiatric disorders (Williams et al. 2007).[2] We extend this list of health outcomes in our initial assessment across groups to include self-assessed physical and mental health. If significant differences are found between African Americans and Afro-Caribbeans, then it is possible that the aggregation of the Black population is obscuring the health profile of the Black middle class.

Second, the different ways in which middle class status is assessed may reveal why there are inconsistent reports of a health disadvantage among some members of the Black middle class. Perhaps education, for example, is a more sensitive indicator of mental health differences within a racial/ethnic group, whereas income and/or occupation may reveal a consistent SES-physical health gradient. In this case, there may very well be a real paradox faced by the middle class, which does not necessarily translate into patterns across SES measures. Once social class position is isolated within racial/ethnic groups and across dimensions of health, there may be some suggestive evidence that certain anomalies should be further investigated. Williams (2004) argues that traditional indicators of SES are not equivalent across groups. Instead, these indicators may represent different forms of capital among and within racial/ethnic groups. We investigate this possibility.

---

[2] In another series of studies of overall birth weight, African-born Black women experienced lower rates of very low birth weight compared to African American women (Williams and Collins 1995), and Black Caribbean (75% from Jamaica, Haiti, Belize) women immigrants gave birth to heavier infants than African-American women (Pallotto et al. 2000).

Where Do We Stand? Investigating the Paradox

We utilize data from the National Study/Survey of American Life (NSAL), a survey of 6,082 adults in the US households begun in February 2001 and completed in June 2003 by the University of Michigan (see Heeringa et al. 2004; Jackson et al. 2004). This project was part of the National Institute of Mental Health Collaborative Psychiatric Epidemiology Surveys Initiative and was approved by the human subjects committee of the University of Michigan. The NSAL is the first known study to include a household probability sample of African Americans ($n=3,570$; 58%), Afro-Caribbeans ($n=1,621$; 26%), and non-Hispanic Whites ($n=891$; 16%) aged 18 years and older. Most (86%) of the interviews were completed face-to-face and conducted in English using a computer-assisted personal interview that lasted approximately 2 h and 20 min. The remaining interviews were conducted by telephone. The Caribbean sample included persons from English-, French-, Spanish-, and Dutch-speaking Caribbean countries. The overall response rate was 72.3%: 70.7% for African Americans, 77.7% for Caribbean Blacks, and 72.3% for Whites. The NSAL is unique in its comprehensive assessment of health problems. We retain the sample of adults aged 25- to 64-years-old in order to speak to some of the patterns described above that have been found in the US Census data. Additionally, this age restriction captures both prime working years and excludes younger individuals who have yet to finish their education (see Appendix B for operationalizations).

We explore design-adjusted prevalence rates for each race/ethnic and SES subgroup. The percentages in each table represent weighted means/proportions. When possible (based on sample size), we conduct difference in means test across groups to determine the extent to which the distributions are statistically significant. Significant differences within racial/ethnic groups are discussed in the results section of the paper. Given the vast number of across-group comparisons, several of these patterns are simply noted as superscripts in the designated tables ($p \leq 0.05$).

General Health Disparities: Are Blacks in Worse Health than Non-Hispanic Whites?

The simple answer is no. As shown in Table 20.1, there are no significant differences in reports of medical conditions between Blacks (African Americans and Black Caribbeans) and non-Hispanic Whites. However, while African Americans report equivalent perceptions of physical health as non-Hispanic Whites (see Cummings and Jackson 2008; Schnittker 2007 for similar results), Afro-Caribbeans report better perceptions of their physical health than non-Hispanic Whites (especially those from English-speaking countries). Again, perceived physical health is the indicator that is most closely tied to actual mortality among adults, even more so than reports of physical conditions (Idler and Benyamini 1997); thus we strongly emphasize these differences within the Black population as they are compared to reports by non-Hispanic Whites.

Turning our attention to mental health, we find a lower prevalence of lifetime mood disorder among Blacks (African Americans and Afro-Caribbeans) compared to non-Hispanic Whites – a finding consistent with other prevalence studies (Kessler et al. 1994). A mixed picture emerges when considering subjective assessments of mental health. African American and Afro-Caribbeans report fewer symptoms of non-specific distress (see Farmer and Ferraro 1997; Williams 2000) and better perceived mental health, but they are not as happy with their lives as non-Hispanic Whites (see Hughes and Thomas 1998). There are few significant differences between racial/ethnic groups in their reports of life satisfaction (see Herzog et al. 1982 for similar findings), with the exception of Blacks from Spanish-speaking countries reporting significantly lower levels of life satisfaction than non-Hispanic Whites.

Table 20.1 Descriptive statistics of health profile by race/ethnicity: National Study of American Life (NSAL)

	Race/ethnicity						
	Black						
	African American	Afro-Caribbean					Non-Hispanic White
Health profile		All	Haitian	E-S	S-S	F/D-S	
Physical health							
# Chronic health problems	1.21[a,b]	1.10	0.79	0.96	0.90	1.39	1.20
# Acute health problems	0.76	0.78	0.75	0.66	0.96	0.83	0.79
Perceived physical health	3.41[a,c,d]	3.70[e]	3.62	3.90[f]	3.46	3.64	3.45
Mental health							
Diagnostic (lifetime)							
Mood disorder	0.13[a,g]	0.14[e]	0.13	0.09[f]	0.19	0.18	0.24
Anxiety disorder	0.20[h]	0.18	0.08	0.15	0.31	0.18	
Substance use disorder	0.13[a,b,c]	0.09	0.02	0.06	0.19	0.13	
Any disorder	0.33[a,c,h]	0.26	0.19	0.20	0.41	0.29	
Symptom checklist							
Non-specific distress	5.79[a,b,c]	5.26[e]	5.07[i]	4.22[f]	6.41[j]	5.92	7.88
Quality-of-life							
Perceived mental health	3.82[a,c,g]	3.98[c]	3.90	4.19[f]	3.94	3.80	3.67
Life satisfaction	3.17	3.15	3.13	3.17	3.05[j]	3.19	3.25
Happiness	3.12[g]	3.10[e]	3.02	3.13	3.15	3.10	3.20
N	2,668	1,227	225	527	134	323	647

E-S English-speaking, *S-S* Spanish-speaking, *F/D-S* French/Dutch-speaking countries of origin

$p<0.05$

[a] African American versus E-S Caribbean
[b] African American versus S-S Caribbean
[c] African American versus Afro-Caribbean
[d] African American versus F/D-S Caribbean
[e] Afro-Caribbean versus non-Hispanic White
[f] E-S Caribbean versus non-Hispanic White
[g] African American versus non-Hispanic White
[h] African American versus Haitian
[i] Haitian versus non-Hispanic White
[j] S-S Caribbean versus non-Hispanic White
[k] F/D-S Caribbean versus non-Hispanic White

Do All Blacks Present the Same Health Profile?

The not so simple answer is no. African Americans report lower levels of perceived physical health than the combined group of Afro-Caribbeans (especially those from English- and French/Dutch-speaking countries). African Americans also report a higher prevalence of mood disorder than Afro-Caribbeans from English-speaking countries; and they report a higher prevalence of lifetime substance use disorder (and having any disorder; Williams et al. 2007) than the combined group of Afro-Caribbeans [these differences seem to be confined to adults with Haitian and English-speaking heritage; see also Broman et al. (2008)].

Symptoms of non-specific distress among African Americans seem to fall between those reported by adults from the English-speaking Caribbean (who have lower scores) and those from Spanish-speaking Caribbean countries (who have higher scores). The quality of life measures also suggest important differences within the category of "Black" such that African Americans report lower evaluations of their mental health when compared to all Afro-Caribbeans (with those from English-speaking countries having the highest perceptions of their mental health). No differences are found between Blacks in reports of life satisfaction and happiness.

In essence, this general assessment across racial/ethnic groups demonstrates that (1) African Americans have a distinct-enough health profile from Afro-Caribbeans to distinguish the groups in future health research (especially Afro-Caribbeans from English-speaking countries), (2) there is consistency in the mental health profile of African Americans compared to non-Hispanic Whites using diagnostic categories and symptom checklists, and (3) quality of life measures continue to yield contradictory findings when comparing African Americans to non-Hispanic Whites. Perhaps a more coherent theme can be found in the distribution of mental health problems if we consider SES further within the category of "Black." Here our focus turns to whether the Black middle class are more (or less) likely to report different areas of problematic health. Again, social class is measured using the indicators of education, household income, and occupation.

SES-Health Gradient and the Health Paradox: Education?

African Americans

As shown in Table 20.2, there is a clear education – physical health gradient for African Americans. That is, the most health problems (chronic and acute) are reported by those with the least amount of education. Not surprisingly, positive perceptions of physical health are highest among the middle class. More importantly, the African American middle class (those with a college degree) report better physical health than the non-Hispanic White lower class (those with less than a high school education), offering no support for a physical health paradox.

There are no significant differences across educational groups in terms of the prevalence of lifetime mood disorder. There is a lower prevalence of anxiety, substance use or any disorder among the African American middle class compared to their counterparts with less education. This pattern is consistent with symptoms of NSD as well, with the middle class reporting fewer distress symptoms than the lower class. These patterns indicate a typical SES-mental health gradient among African Americans.

In terms of a mental health paradox, the Black middle class evaluate their quality of life better than non-Hispanic Whites in the lower class. There is partial support for a mental health paradox since we would expect middle class African Americans to say they are happier with their lives than non-Hispanic Whites who are part of the lower class. Here, we find no significant differences in reports of life happiness.

Table 20.2 Descriptive statistics of health profile by race/ethnicity and education (those with some college and more representing the middle class): National Study of American Life (NSAL)

Race/ethnicity and education	N	Health profile				Mental health						Quality of life		
		Physical health				Diagnostic assessments (lifetime)				Symptoms			
		# Chronic health problems	# Acute health problems	Perceived physical health	Mood (%)	Anxiety (%)	Substance (%)	Any (%)	NSD	PMH	LS	Happy
African American												
<High school	582	1.61[a]	0.98[a,h]	3.10[a,b,c]	0.14[a,b,d]	0.29[a,b]	0.24[a,b,c,f]	0.46[a,b,c]	7.80[b,c]	3.51[a,b]	3.20	3.11
HS graduate	1,024	1.11[b,d,e]	0.72[f]	3.42[e,d]	0.11[c]	0.16	0.11[a,b,d,e,f]	0.28[a,b]	5.97[b,c]	3.83[f]	3.16[c]	3.10
Some college	657	1.12[a,b,d]	0.72[a,h]	3.49[a,b,c]	0.13[a,c]	0.18[a]	0.11[a]	0.31[a]	4.90[a,c]	3.94[b,c]	3.13	3.16[a,d]
>College	405	1.05	0.59	3.66	0.15	0.19[a,d]	0.05[e]	0.32[b]	4.17[c]	3.99[b,c]	3.25	3.14
Afro-Caribbean												
<High school	206	2.01	0.98	3.40[g]	0.10	0.21	0.09	0.24	7.45	3.66	3.14	2.96
HS graduate	349	0.68[g]	0.74	3.57[g]	0.13[g]	0.18	0.03	0.22	5.76[g]	3.86	3.14[g]	3.02
Some college	331	1.06	0.79	3.84[g]	0.11[g]	0.18	0.12	0.25	4.14[g]	4.09[g]	3.11	3.08[g]
>College	341	0.99	0.70	3.73	0.19	0.16	0.14	0.32	4.36[g]	4.21	3.23	3.30
Haiti												
<High school	45	0.46[h]	0.48[h]	3.68[h]	0.03[h]	0.02	0.00	0.04	7.01[h]	3.91[h]	3.15	3.13
HS graduate	62	0.69[h]	0.58	3.50	0.08[h]	0.14	0.00	0.15	5.11	4.01	3.26	3.00
Some college	59	0.44[h]	0.40[h]	3.98[h]	0.01[h]	0.05	0.03	0.09	4.06[h]	3.96	3.09	2.87[h]
>College	59	1.27	1.23	3.41	0.30	0.10	0.04	0.35	4.98[h]	3.77	3.04	3.11
English												
<High school	96	1.49	0.54	4.09[i]	0.03[i]	0.08	0.01	0.11	3.69[i]	4.35[i]	3.37	3.14
HS graduate	154	0.70[i]	0.67	3.70	0.08[i]	0.14	0.03	0.18	4.75[i]	3.94	3.11	3.03
Some college	137	0.86[i]	0.77	4.06[i]	0.11[i]	0.19	0.13	0.26	4.12[i]	4.23[i]	3.12	3.16
>College	140	0.95	0.60	3.75	0.11[i]	0.16	0.04	0.20	4.09[i]	4.35[i]	3.17[i]	3.21

Spanish										
<High school	18	2.29	1.51	2.36	0.39	0.46	0.05	0.46	11.03	3.10	2.85	2.61
HS graduate	43	1.02	1.38[b]	3.21	0.17	0.21	0.04	0.24	6.80	3.42[j]	2.99	3.00[j]
Some college	44	0.93	0.89[b]	3.43	0.12[j]	0.30	0.19	0.40	4.64[j]	3.64	3.06	3.00
>College	29	0.41	0.58	3.94	0.17	0.33	0.32	0.49	5.52	4.60	3.14	3.44
French/Dutch										
<High School	38	3.18	1.65	2.34	0.02	0.41	0.37	0.45	14.53	2.71	2.80	2.76
HS graduate	84	0.55[k]	0.62	4.19[k]	0.20	0.20	0.03	0.24	6.29	3.84	3.14	2.96
Some college	89	1.80[k]	0.98	3.48	0.17	0.16	0.10	0.23	4.04[k]	3.99[k]	3.13	3.04
>College	112	1.23	0.64	3.72	0.22	0.08	0.14	0.30	3.70[k]	4.04	3.40	3.37
Non-Hispanic Whites										
<High school	87	1.95	0.91	2.70	0.20				11.23	3.31	3.00	3.10
HS graduate	209	1.13	0.78	3.38	0.25				7.41	3.70	3.29	3.21
Some college	155	1.26	0.92	3.49	0.29				8.27	3.65	3.16	3.16
>College	196	0.94	0.68	3.74	0.21				6.92	3.80	3.36	3.28

E-S English-speaking, *F/D-S* French/Dutch-speaking countries of origin

$p < 0.05$

[a] African American versus Haitian
[b] African American versus E-S Caribbean
[c] African American versus non-Hispanic White
[d] African American versus F/D-S Caribbean
[e] African American versus Afro-Caribbean
[g] Afro-Caribbean versus non-Hispanic White
[f] African American versus S-S Caribbean
[h] Haitian versus non-Hispanic White
[i] E-S Caribbean versus non-Hispanic White
[j] S-S Caribbean versus non-Hispanic White
[k] F/D-S Caribbean versus non-Hispanic White

Afro-Caribbeans

We find a mixed set of results for the SES-health gradient among the sample of Afro-Caribbean adults. Members of the middle class report fewer physical health problems and better perceived physical health than their lower class peers – a pattern similar to that reported above for African Americans. However, the prevalence of substance use disorder is actually higher among members of the Afro-Caribbean middle class (specifically those from Spanish-speaking countries). Overall, Afro-Caribbeans who occupy middle class positions report better mental health (as indicated by NSD, perceived mental health, life satisfaction, and happiness) than their lower class peers.

More importantly, the Afro-Caribbean middle class report better health outcomes than non-Hispanic White adults with less than a high school education across most of the health measures. There is a single exception with the prevalence of mood disorder (although there is much variation within the Black Caribbean groups) where we find no differences between these groups. In other words, we find very little support for the health paradox (across physical and mental health measures) when college educated Afro-Caribbeans are compared to non-Hispanic Whites with less than a high school education.

SES-Health Gradient and the Health Paradox: Income?

African Americans

Table 20.3 reveals the most consistent set of SES-health patterns when using household income as the indicator of social class position. African Americans who earn between $40,000 and $80,000 annually in household income (the middle class) report fewer chronic and acute physical health problems than their peers who earn less than $40,000 (the lower class). Those in the middle range income category also report better perceived health than those in the lower income category. At no point are the African American middle class (measured by income) at a perceived physical health disadvantage when compared to non-Hispanic Whites of lower class standing.

When we look at the mental health profile of the Black middle class, we also see that the African American middle-income group report better mental health (across all of the measures) than those with less income. We find no evidence of a mental health paradox when comparing the African American middle class to non-Hispanic Whites of lower class standing.

Afro-Caribbeans

Afro-Caribbeans of middle class standing report fewer acute health problems than those in the lower class. Among Afro-Caribbeans of middle-class standing, there is a trend toward better mental health when compared to the lower class. However, there is a significant U-shaped relationship between household income and anxiety and substance use disorder (and subsequently any disorder). That is, Afro-Caribbeans at the high end of the household income continuum have a higher prevalence of substance use disorder than the lower and middle class.

We find little evidence that Afro-Caribbean adults who earn a middle-class income report poorer health outcomes than the non-Hispanic White adults who earn less money. We should

Table 20.3 Descriptive statistics of health profile by race-ethnicity and household income (with those earning $40,000–$80,000 representing the middle class)

Race/ethnicity HH income	N	Health profile					Mental health						Quality of life		
		Physical health				Diagnostic assessments (lifetime)				Symptoms				
		# Chronic health problems	# Acute health problems	Perceived physical health		Mood (%)	Anxiety (%)	Substance (%)	Any (%)	NSD	PMH	LS	Happy
African American													
≤$39,999	1,795	1.35[a,b]	0.88[a,c]	3.28[a,b,d,e]		0.14[a,f]	0.23[a,c]	0.16[a,d]	0.38[a,d]	6.62[a,b,f]	3.70[b,f]	3.11[e]	3.06[d]
$40,000–$80,000	708	0.97	0.54	3.59[b]		0.12[f]	0.15[d]	0.07[b,d]	0.25[b]	4.73[b,f]	3.99[b,f]	3.25	3.21
≥$80,001	165	1.08	0.64[c]	3.64[b,c,d]		0.10[f]	0.15	0.10[b,c,d]	0.28[b,c]	3.77[c,f]	4.05	3.37	3.28
Afro-Caribbean													
≤$39,999	678	1.12[g]	0.96	3.64[g]		0.14[g]	0.23	0.09	0.28	6.42[g]	3.81[g]	3.01	2.96
$40,000–$80,000	393	1.01	0.70	3.63		0.15	0.10	0.04	0.22	4.37[g]	4.07[g]	3.25	3.15
≥$80,001	156	1.23	0.41	4.09[g]		0.10	0.20	0.21	0.30	3.58[g]	4.32	3.42	3.45
Haiti													
≤$39,999	153	0.49[h]	0.51[h]	3.69[h]		0.04[h]	0.05	0.00	0.09	5.01[h]	3.91[h]	3.10	2.87
$40,000–$80,000	57	1.21	1.05	3.48		0.24	0.09	0.04	0.30	5.30	3.82	3.13	3.23
≥$80,001	15	0.56	0.64	3.93		0.12	0.24	0.00	0.24	3.94	4.28	3.24	2.94
English													
≤$39,999	274	0.87[i]	0.80	4.09[i]		0.10[i]	0.18	0.09	0.24	4.98[i]	4.10[i]	3.00	3.00
$40,000–$80,000	176	0.81	0.56	3.70[i]		0.09[i]	0.12	0.03	0.16	3.59[i]	4.27[i]	3.31	3.23
≥$80,001	77	1.60	0.43	4.06[i]		0.03[i]	0.11	0.05	0.13	3.03[i]	4.34[i]	3.45	3.29
Spanish													
≤$39,999	76	1.34	1.69[j]	3.04[d]		0.25	0.34	0.09	0.37	7.98	3.36	2.96	2.93
$40,000–$80,000	42	0.79	0.65	3.26		0.21	0.08	0.04	0.28	5.68	4.10	3.12	3.06
≥$80,001	16	0.26	0.18	4.66		0.02	0.72	0.68	0.74	4.92	4.71	3.08	3.72

(continued)

Table 20.3 (continued)

Race/ethnicity HH income	N	Health profile					Mental health						Quality of life		
		Physical health			Perceived physical health	Diagnostic assessments (lifetime)				Symptoms				
		# Chronic health problems	# Acute health problems			Mood (%)	Anxiety (%)	Substance (%)	Any (%)	NSD	PMH	LS	Happy
French/Dutch													
≤$39,999	166	1.52	1.05	3.64[k]		0.18	0.27	0.16	0.34	7.94[k]	3.55	2.90	2.89
$40,000–$80,000	109	1.21	0.76	3.52		0.17	0.11	0.04	0.24	4.65	3.94	3.10	3.10[k]
≥$80,001	48	1.37[k]	0.47	3.84		0.19	0.06	0.19	0.26	3.48	4.13	3.55	3.55
Non-Hispanic Whites													
≤$39,999	304	1.54	0.97	3.20		0.29				9.42	3.48	3.07	3.06
$40,000–$80,000	249	1.00	0.71	3.59		0.20				7.19	3.80	3.33	3.27
≥$80,001	94	0.86	0.58	3.65		0.22				5.75	3.82	3.49	3.40

E-S English-speaking, *F/D-S* French/Dutch-speaking countries of origin
$p < 0.05$
[a]African American versus Haitian
[b]African American versus E-S Caribbean
[c]African American versus S-S Caribbean
[d]African American versus Afro-Caribbean
[e]African American versus F/D-S Caribbean
[f]African American versus non-Hispanic White
[g]Afro-Caribbean versus non-Hispanic White
[h]Haitian versus non-Hispanic White
[i]E-S Caribbean versus non-Hispanic White
[j]S-S Caribbean versus non-Hispanic White
[k]F/D-S Caribbean versus non-Hispanic White

note, however, that there are less dramatic differences between the Afro-Caribbean middle class (those from English-speaking countries) and lower class non-Hispanic Whites on the number of chronic health problems, suggesting to some, then, that a paradox exists at some level (although minimal).

SES-Health Gradient and the Health Paradox: Occupation?

African Americans

As shown in Table 20.4, there are very few instances where members of the African American middle class (as defined by occupation) are disadvantaged in their physical or mental health when compared to African Americans who do not occupy White collar positions. More specifically, we find significant differences in reports of chronic health problems, perceived physical health, substance use disorder, nonspecific distress, and perceived mental health. Thus, the African American middle class report better health outcomes across the range of measures considered in this study.

There is little evidence that non-Hispanic Whites who occupy nonprofessional jobs report better health outcomes than African American professional workers – thus providing no support here for the health paradox. The exception again appears to be in reports of quality of life where middle class African Americans report *no difference* in life quality when compared to non-Hispanic Whites of lower class standing.

Afro-Caribbeans

As a group, there are no significant within-group differences in reports of physical health or mental disorder among Afro-Caribbeans. However, White collar workers report higher levels of life satisfaction than their peers who do not hold these types of professional jobs. In other words, there is no clear SES-health gradient in operation among this group of Afro-Caribbeans across the wide range of health outcomes (see Williams et al. 2007 for a similar set of findings). There is some suggestive evidence that Afro-Caribbeans who occupy middle class jobs report better physical health than lower class non-Hispanic Whites.

In some instances, there are few differences between Afro-Caribbeans and non-Hispanic Whites, especially when evaluating the quality of their lives. This finding is similar to those reported above for African Americans where we can conclude that partial support is provided for the health paradox since we would expect significant differences between middle-class Afro-Caribbeans and non-Hispanic Whites who occupy lower class positions.

SUMMARY: Health Disparities in sum, the different measures of SES yield a consistent pattern of better physical and mental health among the African American middle class compared to their lower class peers (African American and non-Hispanic White) with household income demonstrating a more robust set of findings for physical and mental health across the different racial/ethnic groups than education or occupation. Among Afro-Caribbeans, however, Haitians are distinct in their health profile in two important ways (1) unlike other Afro-Caribbeans, household income is not associated with any measure of health and (2) like African Americans, occupation is associated with the same set (although a lower number) of health outcomes.

Partial (although limited) support is found for the middle class health paradox in terms of finding few differences between middle class "Blacks" and non-Hispanic Whites (on quality of life measures for education and occupation). There is no evidence that the Black middle class have a health

Table 20.4 Descriptive statistics of health variables by race/ethnicity and occupation (with *White Collar* workers representing the middle class): National Study of American Life (NSAL)

		Health profile				Mental health					Quality of life		
		Physical health				Diagnostic assessments (lifetime)				Symptoms			
Race/ethnicity and occupation	N	# Chronic health problems	# Acute health problems	Perceived physical health		Mood (%)	Anxiety (%)	Substance (%)	Any (%)	NSD	PMH	LS	Happy
African American													
Other	1,369	1.28[a,b,c,d]	0.80	3.31[a,c,d]		0.12[c,e,f]	0.21[b,c]	0.16[a,b,d]	0.35[a,c]	6.43[c,f]	3.78[c,e]	3.16	3.12[a,b]
White collar	1,071	1.12	0.70[h]	3.53[b,c]		0.14[b,f]	0.18[b,c]	0.09[b,c]	0.32[b,c]	4.92[b,c]	3.90[b,c,f]	3.17[f]	3.13
Afro-Caribbean													
Other	586	1.01[g]	0.79	3.65[g]		0.13[g]	0.17	0.06	0.23	5.63[g]	3.87	3.10	3.03
White collar	555	1.29	0.79	3.71		0.15[g]	0.17	0.09	0.27	4.93	4.01[g]	3.23	3.13
Haiti													
Other	138	0.66[h]	0.99	3.19		0.17	0.07	0.01	0.23	6.49[h]	3.54	2.97	2.93[h]
White collar	74	0.99	0.43[h]	4.17[h]		0.08[h]	0.11	0.03	0.14	3.24[h]	4.35[h]	3.32	3.15
English													
Other	259	0.90[i]	0.69	3.84[i]		0.07[i]	0.16	0.08	0.19	4.55[i]	4.12[i]	3.13	3.12
White collar	229	1.08	0.66	3.98[i]		0.11[i]	0.14	0.05	0.21	3.54[i]	4.26[i]	3.26	3.13
Spanish													
Other	57	1.63	1.33	3.07		0.27	0.39	0.10	0.43	7.73	3.32[j]	3.06	2.99
White collar	66	0.76	0.77	3.31		0.22	0.09	0.04	0.29	6.26	4.03	3.05[j]	2.99

	n											
French/Dutch												
Other	118	0.86[k]	0.63	3.83[k]	0.14	0.16	0.05	0.22	5.99[k]	3.94	3.08	3.03
White collar	183	1.78	0.97	3.53	0.19	0.19	0.18	0.33	6.05	3.67	3.26	3.13
Non-Hispanic Whites												
Other	212	1.40	0.82	3.23	0.24				9.42	3.68	3.16	3.16
White collar	354	1.08	0.79	3.60	0.25				7.18	3.66	3.32	3.23

$p < 0.05$; *E-S* English-speaking, *F/D-S* French/Dutch-speaking countries of origin

[a] African American versus Afro–Caribbean
[b] African American versus Haitian
[c] African American versus E-S Caribbean
[d] African American versus F/D-S Caribbean
[e] African American versus S-S Caribbean
[f] African American versus non-Hispanic White
[g] Afro-Caribbean versus non-Hispanic White
[h] Haitian versus non-Hispanic White
[i] E-S Caribbean versus non-Hispanic White
[j] S-S Caribbean versus non-Hispanic White
[k] F/D-S Caribbean versus non-Hispanic White

disadvantage to non-Hispanic Whites regardless of how SES is measured (this assessment includes African Americans and Afro-Caribbeans).

Discussion: Remaining Questions

What We Found

We examined health profiles utilizing information gathered in the National Study of American Life – the first national survey that included a group of African Americans and Afro-Caribbeans. We were able to take into account the ethnicity of "Black" people and explore variation across multiple dimensions of stratification and health outcomes. As such, we broaden research on health disparities including the generalizability of the health paradox of the Black middle class. We initially support existing research demonstrating some Black–White disparities in health, but there was much variation across health outcomes. There is strong evidence for the SES-health gradient for all ethnic/racial groups across most indicators of SES and a wide range of health outcomes. In terms of the health paradox, we find little evidence that the Black (African American or Afro-Caribbean) middle class are at a health disadvantage when compared to lower class non-Hispanic Whites.

What May Underlie These Findings

We offer two explanations for the paradox facing some members of the Black middle class. First, it is possible that the category of "Black" has been too-loosely applied such that foreign-born Blacks of African or Caribbean ancestry (an ever-changing immigrant population) significantly alter health profiles when included among the African American population. This thesis is well-developed by scholars who also argue the role played by ethnicity in explaining health disparities (Read and Emerson 2005). Given the wide variation we found in the subjective health profiles of African Americans and Afro-Caribbeans (combined group), this thesis is not without merit. In other words, some degree of overall health disparities may be an artifact of the ethnic and nativity heterogeneity within the "Black" race.

Second, race may not be generating these anomalies as much as the indicators of SES may be capturing an important middle class experience that is unique to some Blacks. *Perhaps the health paradox represents subtle variations within the middle class that manifest in only a certain class of diseases: diseases of adaptation.* The outcomes that surface as anomalies in the health literature have a common denominator of stress exposure (Collins et al. 1998; Geronimus et al. 2006). We have argued elsewhere that the Black middle class is especially sensitive to certain forms of stress (Cummings and Jackson 2008; Jackson and Stewart 2003). This position is supported by a growing body of empirical work showing that the Black middle class report more frequent episodes of racism in the form of perceived discrimination (Kessler et al. 1999) and perceptions of being treated unfairly in a variety of settings (Schulz et al. 2000) than their lower class peers. The perception of these personal assaults may lead to changes in physiological processes that adversely affect health. For example, perceived discrimination has been linked to high blood pressure (Harrell et al. 2003). The more proximate (or immediate) cause of such physiological changes might be measured in allostatic load. Allostatic load is conceptualized as an index of indicators of cumulative strain on multiple organs and tissues that accumulates through the wear and tear associated with acute shifts in physiologic activity in response to negative stimuli

(McEwen and Seeman 1999). Allostatic load is higher among nonpoor Black women compared to poor White women (Geronimus et al. 2006) and has been linked to hypertension (Seeman et al. 1997) and poor birth outcomes (Lu and Halfon 2003). In the final section, we draw special attention to the outcomes of infant mortality, hypertension, and homicide since these indicators are oft-used to draw attention to the health paradox (Williams 2001).

Next Steps: Taking the Best from Past Research to Build a Promising Future Research Agenda

A new line of research highlights the fact that the static conceptions of SES are underestimating an important part of the process of becoming a member of the Black middle class. James and colleagues (2006), for example, demonstrate that hypertension is lowest among Black men who grew up in middle class households and who now hold middle class status. Hypertension levels were four times higher among those who ascended to the middle class from initially lower class backgrounds. Similarly, Colen and colleagues (2006) find that upward mobility is unrelated to giving birth to a low-birth weight baby among Black women but is associated with improved health outcomes among White women. Thus, the upwardly mobile (rather than the stably middle class) may be generating the hypertension paradox. This line of thought requires a consideration of the way in which social mobility differentiates childhood and adulthood experiences, a position that has been argued in some work on infant birth weight (Colen et al. 2006) and more general health research (Hayward et al. 2000; Neighbors 1987). The future study of health disparities among the Black middle class should compare SES trajectories to non-Hispanic Whites who occupy lower class positions.

Typically, it is the combination of stress exposure and limited resources that produce poor health outcomes. Thus, we propose that a missing element to the puzzle of the health paradox of the Black middle class is a discussion of the lack of sufficient *network-generating capital* that one typically assumes underlies the structural position of middle class. This component of our theoretical model is what leads to a more parsimonious explanation of each of the life-threatening experiences aforementioned as evidence of a health paradox among the Black middle class: hypertension, infant mortality, and homicide. We elaborate on this thesis below, taking advantage of the intellectual strides that have been made across a broad range of sociological research.

Social Networks: The Elephant in the Paradox Room

Individuals typically attempt to manage stressful situations by evoking coping strategies or responses. Seeking out social support is, unequivocally, the most effective coping response involving the activation of the social network (Berkman and Glass 2000; Ross and Mirowsky 2002; Thoits 1995). Lin (2000) has argued that socioeconomic origins often result in inequality in the social capital of individual network members where social capital is defined as "...investment and use of embedded resources in social relations for expected returns" (p. 786). The basic process by which inequality in social networks is perpetuated is homophily or "...the tendency for individuals to interact and share sentiment with others with similar characteristics" (Lin 2000:787). To link Lin's (2000) social capital theory to the discussion of health disparities among the Black middle class, consider the following evidence and discussion. Colen and colleagues (2006) show that the presence of grandmothers in a household is associated with more positive pregnancy outcomes among African American women, and yet upwardly mobile Black women are less likely to reside in households that include a coresidential grandmother. As speculated by these authors "...If upward mobility decreases the likelihood that young Black women can fully participate in extended kin networks and thereby obtain important forms of social support, our findings suggest that the health of their newborns may suffer despite beneficial changes in social class status" (Colen et al. 2006:2037). We find this possibility quite intriguing, and its exploration would enrich the current body of research on social networks as well as health disparities research (see Smith and Christakis 2008 for a review).

Evidence that the social networks of the Black middle class may not be generating sufficient social capital can also be garnered from the literature on racial residential segregation. Pattillo-McCoy (1999) convincingly demonstrates that while upwardly mobile African Americans leave their low-income communities, they often maintain social relationships with poor and working class African Americans through various organizations such as social clubs and churches. Oliver (1988) provides a brilliant analysis of social networks among African Americans residing in three Los Angeles communities (predominantly Black lower class urban neighborhood, predominantly Black middle class urban neighborhood, and a multiracial suburb outside of Los Angeles). He finds that African Americans residing in the middle class urban neighborhood actually report more social ties and higher levels of support than their peers residing in the racially integrated suburb. More telling, however, is the fact that kin are the most likely, and co-workers the least likely, group to be represented in any network (regardless of where African Americans reside).

This pattern has since been replicated in a national study of Black Americans. Chatters and colleagues (1989) find, for example, that high-income Blacks have more individuals in their "helper networks" than their low-income counterparts, but kin are more prevalent in these networks than nonkin. The Black middle class are less likely to consider coworkers as viable sources of social support, and African Americans, overall, believe their neighbors make life more difficult for them (Taylor and Turner 2002). It is not surprising, then, that Blacks have smaller, more homogenous networks than Whites (Marsden 1988). Overall, African Americans have a higher number of informal ties with relatives, friends, and neighbors than Whites (Martineau 1977). Thus, while Oliver's (1988) study dispels the myth of social disorganization within Black communities; it provides suggestive evidence that the Black middle class seek social support from family members who are who reside outside of their immediate neighborhoods.

The majority of African American homeowners reside in cities rather than suburbs; therefore, it stands to reason that many members of the middle class who live in suburbs venture into the city after forming social contacts with other African Americans who reside in the city. Lacy (2007) shows that upper middle-class Black parents engage in active socialization techniques that will expose their children to "Black" spaces and places so that they can learn what it means to be Black. She finds that Blacks who live in the predominantly White suburb of Lakeview are more likely than other Blacks to "...attend a Black church, be an active member of a Black sorority, fraternity, or participate in Jack and Jill, an exclusive Black social organization" (p. 171). Even upper middle class Blacks, then, are deliberate in their interactions in Black spaces in order to retain ties with the Black community. In fact, she argues that "...all believe that racial identity is constructed primarily through social interaction in the Black world, and that Blacks who grow up outside the larger black community miss many important aspects of the experience, such as learning black slang, childhood games, and other formal and informal norms." Thus, the social networks of the upwardly mobile may very well include a higher percentage of individuals who are not reciprocating important knowledge (cultural capital gained through education), relationships (social capital generated through occupational position or place of residence), or finances (money capital generated by higher incomes) that may be associated with positive health behaviors (Portes 1998).

A similar case can be made for understanding excessive rates of homicide among Black middle class men. Research shows the physical vulnerability of the Black middle class given their geographical proximity to low-income neighborhoods (McNulty and Holloway 2000; Morenoff and Sampson 1997; Owens 1997) and the likelihood that they will frequent these neighborhoods to visit family and friends (Pattillo 1999). The neighborhood often serves as the backdrop for the exchange of social capital, which includes a sense of mutual trust and shared expectations (Sampson and Morenoff 1997). Some low-income Black neighborhoods (where there is high concentrated disadvantage) are characterized by the combined lack of social control (Krivo and Peterson 2000; Peterson and Krivo 1999) and a tolerance for criminal behavior (Kubrin and Weitzer 2003; Pattillo-McCoy 1999). The decision to underreport crime stems from the desire to maintain positive relationships with neighbors (Browning et al. 2004). This perspective is consistent with social disorganization and collective efficacy theory (Sampson and Morenoff 1997) as well as the growing body of research linking neighborhood characteristics to individual health (Kawachi and Berkman 2003).

More likely, however, are scenarios where the Black middle class are unable to escape from crime since most reside in neighborhoods that are as crime-prone as the poorest White neighborhood (Alba et al. 1994). In fact, in a study of Black and White families in Philadelphia, Massey and colleagues (1987) find that the probability of encountering someone who lives in your neighborhood who is on welfare is 22% for college-educated Blacks but a mere 8% for college-educated Whites. A similar pattern was found when considering contact with the unemployed, high-school dropouts, and blue-collar workers. Most urban neighborhoods, of course, are not characterized by high crime rates and serve as important sources of community engagement (Oliver 1988). Nonetheless, one of the key factors that link SES, social stressors (and their corresponding physiological reactions), and neighborhoods to the range of health outcomes heralded as paradox among the Black middle class is the structure of the social network. The implications of this social milieu are important for the upwardly mobile portions of the Black middle class. What we add to this discussion, however, is a consideration of the fact that the Black middle class may very well *live* in neighborhoods that are affluent and promote healthy behaviors but they *play* in neighborhoods that have concentrated disadvantage which often encourages violence. Thus, neighborhood conditions may influence health regardless of the social profile of individuals who visit those neighborhoods.

Although our alternative explanations for the discrepancy between the health paradox reported in the broader health literature and our findings of predictable SES-health relationships may be compelling, the real challenge faces those who embrace both explanations of the health paradox of the Black middle class. For those most convinced by the explanation that the paradox is real and therefore the category "Black" should be unpacked in future research, they may ask: what types of health patterns might we expect if the upward mobility experience for African Americans is quite different than that of Afro-Caribbeans? Is there evidence that the social networks of certain Caribbean groups function in a different manner than those of African Americans or perhaps they offer different types (and levels) of capital (see Chap. 10 in this volume on the NEM framework)? For those focused on the meaning of SES, you may ask: what is the process by which upwardly mobile Blacks acquire, maintain, and utilize different types of social capital over the life course? What is the association between network-generating capital and health among the upwardly mobile? These are the questions we believe mark the new era of research on health disparities, especially as they pertain to the Black middle class.

Appendix A. The dimensions of stratification identified by a select group of scholars to define the black middle class

Scholar	Occupation	Income	Education	Home ownership	Place of residence	Other
DuBois (1899)	X and	X	and	X	and	Respectable; politically active
Drake and Cayton (1945)		X	and X		and	Political power
Frazier (1957)	X or	X			and	Moral values; Org. membership
Willie (1974)	X and/or	X	and/or X		and	Dual earner household
Wilson (1978)	X		X			
Oliver and Shapiro (1995)	X or	X	and/or X	X	and/or	Wealth
Durant and Sparrow (1997)		X	and X			
Pattillo-McCoy (1999)	X or	X	or X	X	and X	Voting
Willie and Reddick (2003)	X and/or	X	and/or X			
Lacy (2007)		X			and X	

Appendix B. Percentage of Black adults who qualify as members of the middle class based on select criteria linked to the dimensions of stratification

Scholar	Occupation Criteria	% MC	Income[a] Criteria	% MC	Education Criteria	% MC	Home ownership Criteria	% MC
Willie (1974)	b,c	39.9	Above Ntl. median[d]	35.0	SC	44.7		
Wilson (1978)	b,c,e	56.1						
Landry (1987)	b,c,f	48.6						52.5
Oliver and Shapiro (1995)	b,c	39.9	$33,664	52.9	College	14.6		52.5
Hochschild (1995)			Upper one-third of income for Blacks[g]	30.3	SC	44.7		
Durant and Sparrow (1997)			$16,608[h]	53.9	SC	44.7		
Pattillo-McCoy (1999)	b,c	39.9	Income-to-needs ratio 2 or more	58.5	College	14.6		52.5
Lareau (2002, 2003)	b	19.9						
Lacy (2007)			$30,000 and higher[h]	30.4				

[a]1999 Inflation adjusted values are presented for income in 1999 (Consumer Price Index)
[b]Professional/managerial
[c]Technical, sales, administrative
[d]$53,000
[e]Craftsmen, foremen
[f]Limited service jobs (police, firemen, and kindred workers)
[g]Upper one-third of income for $58,300
[h]Personal income
SC refers to Some College

Appendix C. Description of measures used from the National Study of American Life

Variable name	Description
Social characteristics	
Race/ethnicity	African-Americans; all Caribbeans (then subdivided into Haitians, English-speaking Caribbean Blacks, Spanish speaking Caribbean Blacks, French/Dutch speaking Caribbean Blacks), and non-Hispanic Whites
Social class	
Education	
Lower class	Less than high school, high school diploma, and some college = 1
Middle class	College degree and higher = 1
Income	
Lower class	<$39,999 = 1
Middle class	$40,000–$80,000 = 1
Upper class	$80,001 and higher = 1
Occupation	
Lower class	Other profession = 1
Middle class	Professional/managerial (white collar) = 1

(continued)

Appendix C (continued)

Variable name	Description
Physical health	
Chronic health problems	Have you ever been diagnosed by a physician or health professional with any of the following (1) arthritis, (2) ulcers, (3) cancer, (4) hypertension, (5) diabetes, (6) liver problems, (7) kidney problems, (8) stroke, (9) asthma, (10) chronic lung disease, (11) blood circulation, (12) sickle cell disease, (13) heart trouble, (14) glaucoma, (15) fertility problems, and (16) osteoporosis. These items were summed to form a chronic health index.
Acute health problems	Have you had any of these in the past 12 months (1) migraines/bad headaches, (2) hearing problems, (3) visual problems, (4) allergies or infections, and (5) back problems? These items were summed to form an acute health index.
Perceived physical health	How would you rate your overall physical health? Response categories were: 1 = excellent, 2 = very good, 3 = good, 4 = fair, and 5 = poor. Recoded such that high scores represent higher perceived health.
Mental health	
Diagnostic assessments (lifetime DSM-IV)[a]	
Mood	Lifetime rates of mood disorders (major depression, dysthymia, and bipolar)
Anxiety	Lifetime rates of anxiety disorders (panic disorder, agoraphobia, social phobia, generalized anxiety disorder, post-traumatic stress disorder)
Substance	Lifetime rates of substance use disorders (alcohol abuse, alcohol dependence, drug abuse, drug dependence)
Any disorder	Lifetime rates of any disorder (a combination of the DSM-IV disorder groups listed below)
Symptoms	
Non-specific	Non-specific distress (NSD) is a 30-day symptoms checklist consisting of ten items. "In the past 30 days, how often did you feel (1) you had crying spells; (2) restless; (3) depressed; (4) you could not get going; (5) you enjoyed life; (6) hopeful about the future; (7) everything you did was an effort; (8) you had trouble focusing; (9) happy; (10) people were unfriendly?" Response categories for both subscales were (1) most or all of the time; (2) occasionally; (3) some of the time; (4) rarely or never. All items were reverse coded and summed so that a high score represents high NSD (*alpha* = 0.76)
Quality of life	
Perceived mental health (PMH)	"How would you rate your overall mental health at the present time?" Responses included 1 = excellent; 2 = very good; 3 = good; and 4 = poor. Recoded such that high scores represent high perceived mental health
Life satisfaction (LS)	"In general, how satisfied are you with your life as a whole these days?" Responses ranged from 1 = very dissatisfied to 4 = very satisfied
Happiness	"Taking all things together, how would you say things are these days?" Responses ranged from 1 = very happy these days, to 4 = not happy at all these days. Recoded such that high scores represent much happiness

$n = 6,082$
[a] Assessed using the Composite International Diagnostic Interview (CIDI)

References

Alba RD, Logan JR, Bellair PE (1994) Living with crime: the implications of racial/ethnic differences in suburban location. Soc Forces 73:395–434

Bahr H, Chadwick BA, Stauss JH (1979) American ethnicity. D.C. Heath and Company, Massachusetts, pp 128–129

Battle J, Wright E (2002) W.E.B. Du Bois's talented tenth: a quantitative assessment. J Black Stud 32:654–672

Berkman LF, Glass T (2000) Social integration, social networks, social support, and health. In: Berkman LF, Kawachi I (eds) Social epidemiology. Oxford University Press, New York, pp 137–173

Blank RM, Dabady M, Citro CF (eds) (2004) Measuring racial discrimination. National Academies Press, Washington, DC

Breslau J, Kendler KS, Maxwell Su, Gaxiola-Aguilar S, Kessler RC (2005) Lifetime risk and persistence of psychiatric disorders across ethnic groups in the United States. Psychol Med 35:317–327

Broman CL, Neighbors HW, Delva J, Torres M, Jackson JS (2008) Prevalence of substance use disorders among African Americans and Caribbean Blacks in the national survey of American life. Am J Public Health 97:1–9

Browning CR, Feinberg SL, Dietz RD (2004) The paradox of social organization: networks, collective efficacy, and violent crime in urban neighborhoods. Soc Forces 83:503–534

Carter-Pokras O, Baquet C (2002) What is a 'health disparity'? Public Health Rep 117:426–433

Champion AG (1994) International migration and demographic change in the developed world. Urban Studies 31:653–678

Chatters LM, Taylor RJ, Neighbors HW (1989) Size of informal helper network mobilized during a serious personal problem among Black Americans. J Marriage Fam 51:667–676

Cockerham WC (1990) A test of the relationship between race, socioeconomic status, and psychological distress. Soc Sci Med 31:1321–1331

Colen CG, Geronimus AT, Bound J, James S (2006) Maternal upward socioeconomic mobility and Black–White disparities in infant birth weight. Am J Public Health 96:2032–2039

Collins JW Jr, David RJ, Symons R, Handler A, Wall S, Andes S (1998) African-American mothers' perception of their residential environment, stressful life events, and very low birth weight. Epidemiology 9:286–289

Crimmins EM, Saito Y (2001) Trends in healthy life expectancy in the United States, 1970–1990: gender, racial, and educational differences. J Soc Sci Med 52:1629–1641

Cummings JL, Jackson PB (2008) Race, gender, and SES disparities in self-assessed health, 1974–2004. Res Aging 30:137–167

Davis JF (1991) Who is Black? State University of Pennsylvania, University Park, PA

Drake SC, Cayton HR (1945) Black metropolis: a study of Negro life in a northern city. Harper & Rowman, New York

Drevenstedt GL (1998) Race and ethnic differences in the effects of religious attendance on subjective health. Rev Relig Res 39:245–263

DuBois WEB (1899) The philadelphia negro. University of Pennsylvania Press, Philadelphia, PA

Durant TJ, Sparrow KH (1997) Race and class consciousness among lower- and middle-class Blacks race and class consciousness among lower- and middle-class Blacks. J Black Stud 27:334–351

Ellison CG (1990) Family ties, friendship, and subjective well-being among Black Americans. Journal of Marriage and the Family 52:298–310

Farmer MM, Ferraro KF (1997) Distress and perceived health: mechanisms of health decline. J Health Soc Behav 38:298–311

Forman T (2003) The social psychological costs of racial segmentation in the workplace: a study of African Americans' well being. J Health Soc Behav 44:332–352

Fouron G (1983) The Black dilemma in the US: the Haitian experience. J Caribb Stud 3:242–265

Frazier EF (1957) Black bourgeoisie: the rise of a new middle class. Free, New York

Gatewood WB (2000) Aristocrats of color: the Black elite, 1880–1920. University of Arkansas Press, Fayetteville

Geronimus AT, Hicken M, Keene D, Bound J (2006) Weathering' and age patterns of allostatic load scores among Blacks and Whites in the United States. Am J Public Health 96:826–833

Giddens A (1973) The class structure of the advanced societies. Hutchinson University Library, London

Gordon A (1998) The new diaspora – African immigration to the United States. J Third World Stud 15:79–103

Grieco E (2004) U.S. in focus: the african foreign born in the United States. Migration Policy Institute, Washington, DC

Grieco EM, Cassidy RC (2001) Overview of race and Hispanic origin: census 2000 brief. U.S. Census Bureau, Washington, DC

Harrell JP, Hall S, Talliaferro J (2003) Physiological responses to racism and discrimination: an assessment of the evidence. Am J Public Health 93:243–248

Hayward MD, Miles TP, Crimmins EM, Yang Yu (2000) The significance of socioeconomic status in explaining the racial gap in chronic health conditions. Am Sociol Rev 65:910–930

Heeringa SG, Wagner J, Torres M, Duan N, Adams T, Berglund P (2004) Sample designs and sampling methods for the collaborative psychiatric epidemiology studies (CPES). Int J Methods Psychiatr Res 13:221–240

Herzog AR, Rodgers WL, Woodworth J (1982) Subjective well-being among different age groups. The University of Michigan, Institute for Social Research, Survey Research Center, Ann Arbor, MI

Hochschild J (1995) Facing up to the American dream: race, class, and the soul of the nation. Princeton University Press, Princeton, NJ

Hughes M, Thomas M (1998) Race, class, and quality of life in America. 1972–1996. Am Sociol Rev 63:785–795

Hummer RA, Rogers RG, Nam CB, LeClere FB (1999) Race/ethnicity, nativity, and U.S. adult mortality. Soc Sci Q 80:136–153

Hwang SS, Fitzpatrick KM, Helm D (1998) Class differences in racial attitudes: a divided Black America? Sociol Perspect 41:367–380

Idler EL, Benyamini Y (1997) Self-rated health and mortality: a review of twenty-seven community studies. J Health Soc Behav 38:21–37

Jackson JS, Torres M, Caldwell CH, Neighbors HW, Nesse RM, Taylor RJ, Trierweiler SJ, Williams DR (2004) The national survey of American life: a study of racial, ethnic, and cultural influences on mental disorders and mental health. Int J Methods Psychiatr Res 13:196–207

Jackson PB (2005) Health inequalities among minority populations. J Gerontol 60B(Special issue II):63–67

Jackson PB, Stewart Q (2003) A research agenda for the Black middle class: work stress, survival strategies, and mental health. J Health Soc Behav 44:442–455

Jacobson E (2003) An introduction to haitian culture for rehabilitation service providers. Center for International Rehabilitation Research Information and Exchange (CIRRIE). University of Buffalo, State University of New York, New York. http://cirrie.buffalo.edu/monographs/haiti.pdf

James S, Van Hoewyk J, Belli RF, Strogatz DS, Williams DR (2006) Life-course socioeconomic position and risk for hypertension in African American men: the pitt county study. Am J Public Health 96:812–817

James W (2002) Explaining Afro-Caribbean social mobility in the United States: beyond the Sowell thesis. Comp Stud Soc Hist 44:218–262

Kalmijn M (1996) The socioeconomic assimilation of Caribbean American Blacks. Soc Forces 74:911–930

Kawachi I, Berkman LF (eds) (2003) Neighborhoods and health. Oxford University Press, New York, NY

Keil JE, Tyroler HA, Sandifer SH et al (1977) Hypertension: effects of social class and racial admixture. The results of a cohort study in the Black population of Charleston, South Carolina. Am J Public Health 67:6234–6639

Kennedy R (2004) Finding a proper name to call Black Americans. Journal of Blacks in Higher Education 46:72–83

Kessler RC, Neighbors H (1986) A new perspective on the relationships among race, social class, and psychological distress. J Health Soc Behav 27:107–115

Kessler RC, Katherine A, McGonagle SZ, Nelson CB, Hughes M, Eshleman S, Wittchen H-U, Kendler KS (1994) Lifetime and 12-month prevalence of DSM- III-R psychiatric disorders in the United States. Arch Gen Psychiatry 51:8–19

Kessler RC, Mickelson KD, Williams DR (1999) The prevalence, distribution, and mental health correlates of perceived discrimination in the United States. J Health Soc Behav 40:208–30

Keyes C, Shmotkin D, Ryff CD (2002) Optimizing well-being: the empirical encounter of two traditions. J Pers Soc Psychol 82:1007–1022

Kohn M (1977) Class and conformity: a study in values, with a reassessment. University of Chicago Press, Chicago

Korgen K (1998) From Black to biracial. Praeger, Westport, CT

Krivo LJ, Peterson RD (2000) The structural context of homicide: accounting for racial differences in process. Am Sociol Rev 65:547–559

Kronus S (1971) The Black middle class. Merrill, Columbus, OH

Kubrin C, Weitzer R (2003) Retaliatory homicide: concentrated disadvantage and neighborhood culture. Soc Probl 50:157–180

Lacy KR (2007) Blue-chip Black: race, class, and status in the new Black middle class. The University of California Press, Berkeley

Landry B (1987) The new Black middle class. University of California Press, Berkeley

Lareau A (2002) Invisible inequality: social class and child rearing in Black families and White families. Am Sociol Rev 67:747–776

Levine R, Foster JE, Fullilove RE, Fullilove MT, Briggs NC, Hull PC, Hennekens CH (2001) Black–White inequalities in mortality and life expectancy, 1933–1999: implications for healthy people 2010. Public Health Rep 116:474–483

Lin N (2000) Inequality in social capital. Contemp Sociol 29:785–795

Logan JR, Deane G (2003) Black diversity of metropolitan America. University at Albany Lewis Mumford Center for Comparative Urban and Regional Research, Albany, NY

Lu MC, Halfon N (2003) Racial and ethnic disparities in birth outcomes: a life-course perspective. Mater Child Health J 7:13–30

Marmot MG, Ryff CD, Bumpass LL, Shipley MJ, Marks NF (1997) Social inequalities in health: next questions and converging evidence. Soc Sci Med 44:901–910

Marsden PV (1988) Homogeneity in confiding networks. Soc Networks 10:57–76

Marsh K, Darity WA Jr, Cohen P, Casper L, Salters D (2007) The emerging Black middle class: single and living alone. Soc Forces 86:735–762

Marshall G, Roberts S, Burgoyne C (1996) Social class and underclass in Britain and the United States. Br J Sociol 47:22–44

Martinez R Jr (2003) Moving beyond Black and White violence: African American, Haitian and Latino homicides in Miami. In: Hawkins DF (ed) Interpersonal violence: the ethnicity, race and class nexus. Cambridge University Press, New York City, pp 22–43

Martineau WH (1977) Informal social ties among urban Black Americans: some new data and a review of the problem. J Black Stud 8:83–104
Massey D, Condran GA, Denton NA (1987) The effect of residential segregation on Black social and economic well-being. Soc Forces 66:29–57
McEwen BS, Seeman T (1999) Protective and damaging effects of mediators of stress: elaborating and testing the concepts of allostasis and allostatic load. Annu NY Acad Sci 896:30–47
McNulty TL, Holloway SR (2000) Race, crime, and public housing in Atlanta: testing a conditional effect hypothesis. Soc Forces 79:707–729
Morenoff J, Sampson RJ (1997) Violent crime and the spatial dynamics of neighborhood transition – Chicago, 1970–1990. Soc Forces 76:31–64
Musick MA (2000) Theodicy and life satisfaction among Black and White Americans. Sociol Relig 61:267–287
National Center for Health Statistics (NCHS) (2007) Health, United States with chartbook on trends in the health of Americans. U.S. Government Printing Office, Hyattsville, Maryland
Neighbors HW (1987) Improving the mental health of Black Americans: lessons from the community mental health movement. Milbank Q 65:348–380
Oliver ML (1988) The urban Black community as network: toward a social network perspective. Sociol Q 29:623–645
Oliver ML, Shapiro T (1995) Black wealth, White wealth: a new perspective on racial inequality. Routledge, New York
Owens ML (1997) Renewal in a working-class black neighborhood. J Urban Aff 19:183–205
Pallotto EK, Collins JW Jr, David RJ (2000) Enigma of maternal race and infant birth weight: a population-based study of US-born Black and Caribbean-born black women. Am J Epidemiol 151:1080–1085
Pamuk E, Makuc D, Heck K, Reuban C (1998) Socioeconomic status and health chartbook. National Center for Health Statistics, Health, United States, Hyattsville, MD
Pattillo-McCoy M (1999) *Black picket fences: privilege and peril among the Black middle class.* University of Chicago Press, Chicago
Peterson R, Krivo L (1999) Racial segregation, the concentration of disadvantage, and Black and White homicide victimization. Sociol Forum 14:465–493
Portes A (1998) Social capital: its origins and applications in modern sociology. Ann Rev Sociol 22:1–24
Preston S, Elo IT (1995) Are educational differentials in adult mortality increasing in the United States. J Aging Health 74:476–496
Read JG, Emerson MO (2005) Racial context, Black immigration and the U.S. Black/White health disparity. Soc Forces 84:181–199
Riolo S, Nguyen TA, Greden JF, King CA (2005) Prevalence of depression by race/ethnicity: findings from the national health and nutrition examination survey III. Am J Public Health 95:998–1000
Rockquemore KA, Brunsma DL (2002) Beyond Black: biracial identity in America. Sage Publications, Newbury Park, CA
Rose F (1997) Toward a class-cultural theory of social movements: reinterpreting new social movements. Sociol Forum 12:461–494
Ross CE, Mirowsky J (2002) Family relationships, social support and subjective life expectancy. J Health Social Behav 43:469–489
Ruggles S, David Hacker J, Sobek M (1995) Overview of the integrated public use microdata series. Hist Methods 28:33–39
Sampson RJ, Morenoff JD (1997) Ecological perspectives on the neighborhood context of urban poverty: past and present. In: Brooks-Gunn J, Duncan GJ, Aber JL (eds) Neighborhood poverty. Russell Sage Foundation, New York, NY, pp 1–22
Schnittker J (2007) Working more and feeling better: women's health, employment and family life, 1974–2004. Am Sociol Rev 72:221–238
Schuessler RF (1982) Measuring social life feelings. Jossey-Bass, San Francisco.
Schuessler RF, Freshnock L (1978) Measuring attitudes toward self and others in society: state of the art. Social Forces 56:1228–1244
Schulz A, Williams D, Israel B, Becker A, Parker E, James SA, Jackson J (2000) Unfair treatment, neighborhood effects, and mental health in the detroit metropolitan area. J Health Social Behav 41:314–332
Seeman TE, Singer BH, Rowe JW, Horwitz RI, McEwen BS (1997) Price of adaptation – allostatic load and its health consequences. Arch Intern Med 157:2259–2268
Singh GK, Miller BA (2004) Health, life expectancy, and mortality patterns among immigrant populations in the United States. Can J Public Health 95:114–121
Singh GK, Yu SM (1996) Adverse pregnancy outcomes: differences between U.S. and foreign-born women in major U.S. racial and ethnic groups. Am J Public Health 86:837–843
Somervell PD, Leaf PJ, Weissman MM, Blazer DG, Bruce ML (1989) The prevalence of major depression Black and White adults in five United States communities. Am J Epidemiol 130:725–735
Smith KP, Christakis NA (2008) Social networks and health. Ann Rev Sociol 34:405–429

Taylor J, Turner RJ (2002) Perceived discrimination, social stress, and depression in the transition to adulthood: racial contrasts. Soc Psychol Q 65:213–225

Thoits PA (1995) Stress, coping and social support processes: where are we? What next? J Health Social Behav 35:53–79, Extra Issue

Thomas ME, Holmes BJ (1992) Determinants of satisfaction for Blacks and Whites. Sociol Q 33:459–472

Treiman DJ (1977) Occupational prestige in comparative perspective. Academic, New York

Census Bureau US (2000) Statistical abstract of the United States: 2000. U.S. Government Printing Office, Washington, DC

U.S. Department of State (2002) 1990 and 1992 statistical yearbook of the immigration and naturalization service. U.S. Department of Justice, 1991, and 1993, Washington, DC

Vargas CM, Ingram DD, Gillum RF (2000) Incidence of hypertension and educational attainment the NHANES I epidemiologic follow-up study. Am J Epidemiol 152:272–278

Waters MC (1996) Ethnic and racial groups in the USA: conflict and cooperation. In: Rupensinghe K, Tishkov V (eds) Ethnicity and power in the contemporary world. United Nations, Tokyo, pp 236–262

Waters MC (1999) Black identities: West Indian immigrant dreams and American realities. Russell Sage Foundation, New York, NY

Williams DR (1997) Race and health: basic questions, emerging directions. Ann Epidemiol 7:322–333

Williams DR (2000) Race and health in Kansas: data, issues, directions. In: Tarlov AR, St Peter RF (eds) The society and population health reader. New, New York, pp 236–258

Williams DR (2001) Racial variations in adult health status: patterns, paradoxes, and prospects. In: Smelser NJ, Wilson WJ, Mitchell F (eds) America becoming: racial trends and their consequences, vol II. National Academy Press, Washington, DC, pp 371–410

Williams DR (2003) The health of men: structured inequalities and opportunities. Am J Public Health 93:724–731

Williams DR (2004) Health and the quality of life among African Americans. In: Daniels LA (ed) The state of Black America. National Urban League, New York, NY, pp 115–138

Williams DR, Collins C (1995) U.S. socioeconomic and racial differences in health. Annu Rev Sociol 21:349–386

Williams DR, Jackson PB (2005) Social sources of health disparities. Health Aff 24:325–334

Williams DR, Gonzalez HM, Neighbors H et al (2007) Prevalence and distribution of major depressive disorder in African Americans, Caribbean Blacks, and Non-Hispanic Whites: results from the national survey of American life. Arch Gen Psychiatry 64:305–315

Williams, DR, Takeuchi, D, Adair, R (1992) Socioeconomic status and psychiatric disorder among Blacks and Whites. Social Forces 71:179–194

Williamson J (1980) New people: miscegenation and mulattoes in the United States. Free, New York

Willie CV (1974) The Black family and social class. Journal of Orthopsychiatry 44:50–60

Wilson WJ (1978) The declining significance of race: Blacks and changing American institutions. University of Chicago Press, Chicago

Winn P (1992) Americas: the changing face of Latin America and the Caribbean. Pantheon, New York

Wright EO (1979) Class structure and income determination. Academic, New York

Chapter 21
Gender and Health Revisited

Jen'nan Ghazal Read and Bridget K. Gorman

Introduction

During the last 4 decades, we have seen a tremendous expansion in what we know about the health profiles of men and women. In the broadest terms, women enjoy an advantage over men when it comes to life expectancy and mortality but are disadvantaged when it comes to morbidity or illness. Put differently, women can expect to live longer than men, but their lives are more likely to be lived in poor health (Allendale and Hunt 2000). This general finding has garnered much attention, debate, and scrutiny in recent years, with the result being renewed interest in determining the exact size and scope of gendered health disparities as well as identifying the mechanisms that contribute to differences between men and women. Several key questions guide contemporary research, including but not limited to: Are women uniformly sicker than men across the range of mental and physical health outcomes? Does this vary by age and position in the life course? Is it the same for men and women in different racial/ethnic groups? How do biology, social structural position, behavioral, and lifestyle factors combine to differentially shape the mental and physical health of men and women?

In this chapter, we examine these questions with an eye towards the future: Given what we know about gender differences in health and what we know from other realms in the social and health sciences, where do we need to focus our attention in the coming years? To address this overarching question, we begin by documenting contemporary patterns in men's and women's mental and physical health and examining the extent to which the gender gap in US health has widened or narrowed over the past few decades. We then review the major sociological theories that have been used to explain these patterns. Our goal is not to replicate other excellent assessments of these theories (see Bird and Rieker 2008; Rieker and Bird 2000; Verbrugge 1985), but rather to focus on other existing theories, concepts, and perspectives in mainstream sociology that can be better used to understand gendered patterns in disease and death. In taking this approach, our overarching goal is to provide an agenda for future research.

Gender Differences in Health

Health status is a complex term that encompasses many dimensions of physical and mental well being. In this section of the chapter, we focus on three broad dimensions of health status that differentiate men's and women's lives in most nations of the world: mortality, physical health, and

J.G. Read (✉)
Department of Sociology, Duke University, 101 Trent Hall, Durham, NC 27708, USA
e-mail: jennan.read@duke.edu

mental health.[1] We pay particular attention to how gender intersects with other social status characteristics, namely race/ethnicity and socioeconomic status, to stratify the lives of adult Americans.

Mortality

Of all dimensions of health status, mortality is the most straightforward with respect to gender differences in health: women outlive men regardless of when life expectancy is measured (at birth or in later life), although the size of the female advantage shrinks with age. In 2004, life expectancy at birth was 80.4 years for women compared to 75.2 for men, a difference of 5.2 years and the smallest gap in more than 50 years (Table 21.1). The gap peaked in 1975 at 7.8 years and has been steadily declining ever since. However, if we move beyond birth, we see that the gender gap in mortality declines with age. For example, if men live to the age of 65, and especially 75, their life expectancies approach (but do not match) that of women of the same age. The gender gap shrinks with age because men are more likely to die at younger ages from a variety of causes such as heart disease, cirrhosis of the liver, homicide, and suicide. We will discuss this gender pattern in more detail in the next section on physical health.

Gender differences in mortality are more complicated when race/ethnicity and socioeconomic status are brought into the picture (Rogers et al. 2000). Overall, women fare better than men in their same racial/ethnic group, but black females have lower life expectancies than white females, roughly the same as white males at 76 years, and black males have the lowest life expectancies of any group at 69.5 years. Further, the gender gap in life expectancy is smaller for whites than for blacks (5.1 and 6.8 years, respectively), and whites as a group have a 5.2 year advantage over blacks as a group. With respect to socioeconomic status, persons of higher social class standing (whether measured by education, occupation, or income) outlive those of lower standing, but even here, this varies by gender and race with men benefiting more than women and whites more than blacks from socioeconomic success. For example, Fig. 21.1 shows that death rates are generally lower for women than men, but more highly educated men (who have at least a high school diploma) have lower death rates than women in lower educational attainment brackets. Similarly, black women benefit much less from their educational achievements than do white women. Figure 21.2 presents infant mortality rates and shows that black women have the highest rates by far (13.5), while white, Hispanic and Asian women have much lower rates (5.7, 5.6, and 4.8, respectively). Infant mortality rates drop for women in the highest educational attainment bracket, but the racial gap persists even among highly educated women with black women's rates nearly three times that of white women's (11.3 compared to 4.3). Moreover, the gap between white and black women actually widens with educational attainment.

Turning now to the leading causes of death, the top two causes are the same for men and women of all racial/ethnic groups (heart disease and cancer), but for men, the third leading cause is unintentional injuries followed by stroke, and for women, it is stroke followed by chronic lower respiratory disease. Suicide and liver disease rank in the top ten causes of death for men but not for women, and Alzheimer's ranks sixth for women but falls outside the top ten for men, in part reflecting the fact that women live to older ages where the onset of Alzheimer's disease is most prevalent. Again, race/ethnicity complicates the picture, and its impact is most evident for three causes of death: homicide, HIV, and Alzheimer's disease. For men as a group, neither homicide nor HIV is one of the top ten leading causes of death, but when examining cause of death by race, homicide is the fifth

---

[1] We will address the link between mental and physical health in the last section of the chapter, where we discuss an agenda for future research.

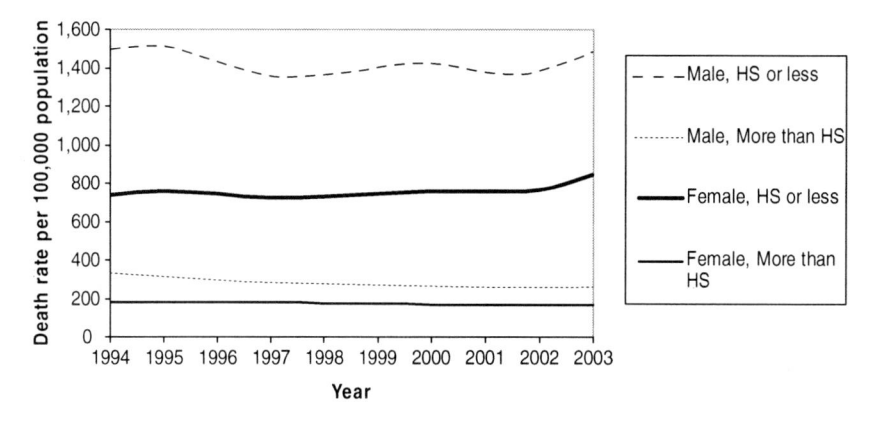

Fig. 21.1 Age-adjusted death rate by sex and education, 1994–2003. *Based on data from 43–47 states and the District of Columbia. National Center for Health Statistics (2006) Health, United States, 2006 with Chartbook on trends in the health of Americans. Hyattsville, MD

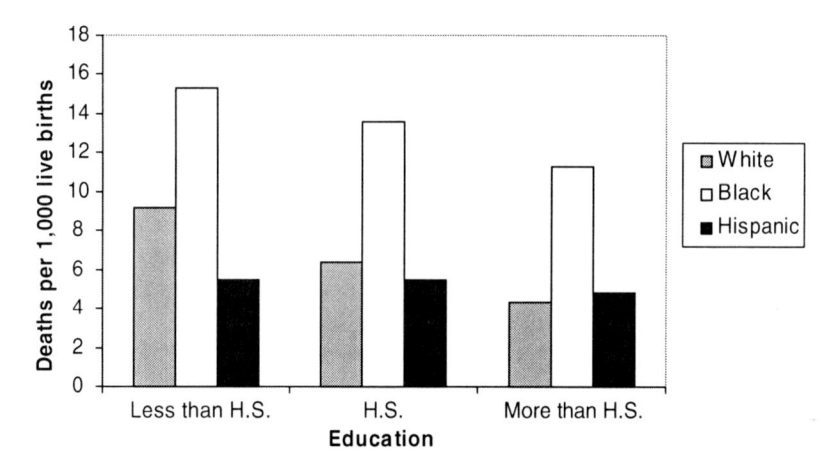

Fig. 21.2 Infant mortality rate by race and education, 2003. *Persons of Hispanic origin may be of any race. National Center for Health Statistics (2006) Health, United States, 2006 with Chartbook on trends in the health of Americans. Hyattsville, MD

leading cause for both Hispanic and Black males and HIV is sixth for Black males and tenth for Hispanic males. Neither of the two causes is in the top ten for White males. Among women, Alzheimer's as a leading cause of death is only prevalent in White women. These patterns clearly show that any discussion of the US mortality rates must consider the influence of social status categories, such as gender, race/ethnicity, and socioeconomic position.

Physical Health

Until recently, there was a general consensus that women had poorer health than men across the spectrum of physical health outcomes despite having lower mortality rates. This came to be known as the "morbidity paradox" (Verbrugge 1985) and waves of research were conducted to explain why women reported worse health than men but lived longer (for a review, see Macintyre et al. 1996). The tides have changed over the past decade, however, as newer scholarship began challenging this overgeneralized line of thinking on two grounds. The first underscored the multidimensionality of health and called for greater attention to gender differences across the full range of health outcomes, and the second highlighted the importance of age in defining men's and women's health status (for reviews, see Gorman and Read 2006; Macintyre et al. 1996; Williams 2003). Several systematic examinations of multiple health outcomes at different stages of the life cycle found that the paradox of women's poorer health but longer life expectancy was not really so paradoxical when one considers that men experience more life-threatening illnesses – such as heart disease – that result in death at younger ages, while women experience less serious, chronic illnesses – such as arthritis – that result in longer years spent in poor health (Gorman and Read 2006; Verbrugge 1989).

That being said, the physical health status of men and women certainly differs, but the difference is likely much smaller and more easily explained than commonly believed. In this section of the chapter we focus on the major physical health conditions that afflict men and women (e.g., heart disease and cancer) as well as the conditions on which men and women drastically differ, namely chronic, nonfatal problems such as physical disability. Our overview is not exhaustive, as the dimensions of physical health are potentially endless, ranging from global self-assessments of health status, to life-threatening conditions such as heart disease and cancer, to nonfatal chronic conditions such as ulcers and functional limitations.

We begin with self-rated health because it is frequently cited as evidence for the "morbidity paradox" (i.e., women's poorer health relative to men). Self-rated health is more broad and inclusive than more specific measures of health or impairment and captures something about an individual's health status that is above and beyond more objective measures of health, such as the presence of a chronic health condition, such as heart disease or cancer (Idler and Benyamini 1997). Men generally report better self-rated health than women, but the size of the gap decreases considerably with age. For example, Verbrugge (1985) first pointed out that men's advantage over women was much smaller among persons aged 65 and above; Ross and Bird (1994) found that younger women reported significantly worse health than men, but that the gap closed with age; and Marks (1996) showed that women aged 53 had better self-reported health than men. Data from Britain reveal a similar pattern. Macintyre et al. (1996) found significant differences in self-rated health only among 18-year olds, with no differences among older age cohorts, and Arber and Cooper (1999) found almost no difference in self-rated health among persons aged 60 and above. What might explain these patterns? One plausible explanation is that gender differences in self-rated health are more of a social construction than a health disparity – men's apparent advantage may be an artifact of gender role socialization whereby ideals of masculinity result in men being less likely to think that they are sick, less likely to seek medical advice and treatment (where they would be told that they are sick), and thus less likely to report that they are in poor health. The gender gap closes with age because the poorer social circumstances and higher stressors experienced by women (lower wages, more unpaid work) make them feel worse than men when younger, while men's higher status and the attendant expectations of masculine robustness incline them to report better health at younger ages (Ross and Bird 1994). As men age, several changes may affect how they view their health: (1) the adverse affects of their health behaviors (e.g., smoking and heavy drinking) take years to develop and begin to catch up to them, making them feel less healthy, (2) they are more likely to be married to spouses who encourage them to seek regular medical care where doctors tell them that they are less healthy, and (3) the inevitable physical decline that accompanies aging detracts from the robustness they felt at younger ages (Rosenfield 1999).

Disability, or functional limitations, is a more objective measure of physical health status that disproportionately hinders women's daily lives more than men's. Regardless of how disability is defined, research has consistently documented higher rates of disability among women than men

(Lubitz et al. 2003; Merrill et al. 1997; Newman and Brach 2001). This holds across the life course, with younger and older women reporting higher rates of disability than their male counterparts (Marks 1996; Merrill et al. 1997). Moreover, the size of women's disadvantage increases with age. For example, Newman and Brach (2001) report that the gender gap in functional limitations rises with age, climbing to a 15-point differential among persons aged 85 and above: 65.6% of women report at least one functional limitation, compared to 50.0% of men. More recently, we examined gender differences in health across the major US racial/ethnic groups and found that disability was the one outcome that consistently disadvantaged women, regardless of their racial/ethnic group, socioeconomic status, and age (Read and Gorman 2006). Like others before us, we argued that research and public policy must continue to address women's greater burden of poorer health on such a critical outcome that affects daily life (Arber and Cooper 1999; Lubitz et al. 2003).

While women fare worse than men with respect to disability, and to a lesser extent self-rated health, the story is quite different for chronic health conditions. Here we find that both men and women experience more chronic health conditions as they age, but they differ substantially in the type of problems they develop (Guralnik et al. 1989). Men suffer from more life-threatening conditions (e.g., heart disease, emphysema) that develop with age and shorten their life expectancy, while women suffer from more acute conditions (e.g., upper respiratory infections), nonfatal chronic conditions (e.g., arthritis, thyroid conditions), and more disabling conditions (e.g., functional limitations). In sum, women tend to suffer from conditions that cause them to feel poorly, while men tend to suffer from conditions that develop in later life and are often fatal, which partially explains gender differences in mortality and life expectancy.

Again, race/ethnicity further complicates these already complex gender patterns in physical health. In a recent national study, we assessed gender differences in multiple measures of physical health status across five major US racial and ethnic populations and found that gender patterns in health vary considerably by racial/ethnic group, comparison category (within vs. between groups), and health status measure (Read and Gorman 2006). We found that some racial/ethnic groups (e.g., Mexican Americans) have better health profiles than the majority white population, regardless of gender, while other groups (e.g., black women) are doubly disadvantaged by their gender and racial group membership. These findings resonate with similar research in the UK (Cooper 2002) and underscore the need for more research on the gender-race-ethnicity nexus.

Mental Health

As is the case for physical health, differences in men's and women's mental health depend in large part on how mental health is defined and measured. According to the World Health Organization (2001), mental health is a multidimensional concept that refers to more than just the lack of mental disorders and includes a person's subjective well-being, perceived self-efficacy, autonomy, competence, intergenerational dependence, and self-actualization of one's intellectual and emotional potential. A complete classification of mental disorders is beyond the scope of this chapter, but among the most severe in terms of gender differences in health are depressive disorders and substance use disorders (Rieker and Bird 2005).

Of all mental health outcomes, gender differences in depression have been the most documented, with recent studies reporting that women are about twice as likely as men to be depressed (Keyes and Goodman 2006). This oft-replicated finding has led to the general conclusion that women as a group have poorer mental health than men. However, this assumption neglects the key fact that men and women express psychological distress through different routes (Horwitz et al.

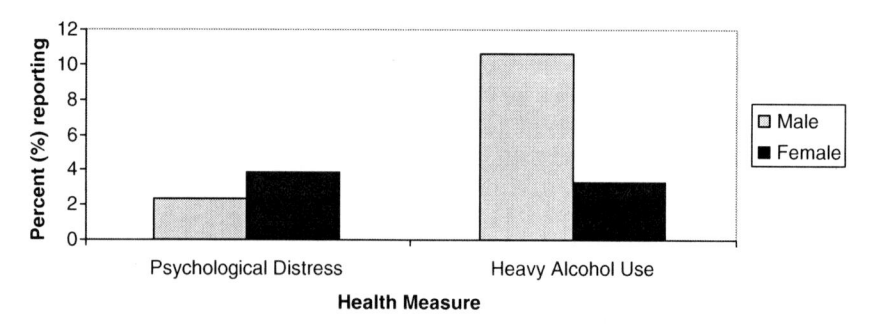

[Bar chart showing Percent (%) reporting for Male and Female across two Health Measures: Psychological Distress (Male ~2.3%, Female ~3.8%) and Heavy Alcohol Use (Male ~10.5%, Female ~3.2%).]

Fig. 21.3 Rates of heavy alcohol use and psychological distress among US adults, 18 and over by Sex, 2002–2004. *Serious psychological distress is measured by a six-question scale that asks respondents how often they experience each of six symptoms of psychological distress. National Center for Health Statistics (2006) Health, United States, 2006 with Chartbook on trends in the health of Americans. Hyattsville, MD

1996; Rieker and Bird 2000; Üstün 2000). Because of gender norms and role socialization, women are more likely to internalize stress and express their problems through conditions such as anxiety and depression, while men are more likely to externalize their feelings through behaviors such as heavy drinking and drug use (Horwitz and Davies 1994). More specifically, Rosenfield (1999) states that women internalize and men externalize their problems because of social beliefs about masculinity and femininity that are shaped through childhood socialization (whereby emotional displays are accepted and aggression is prohibited for girls, while boys are given more independence and allowed more risk-taking behavior) and social practices in adulthood (whereby women are more responsible for caretaking and emotional labor, and men are more responsible for economic support). These practices shape central dimensions of the self in women and men, and mental health problems reflect these gendered divisions. As Fig. 21.3 illustrates, women are much more likely to report psychological distress than men, while men are more than twice as likely to report heavy alcohol use.

These findings have led some scholars to argue that the common belief that women suffer from more emotional disturbance than men is more of a social construction than a reality and that feelings of distress (depression) should be distinguished from behaviors of distress (substance abuse) (see Umberson and Williams 1999). Indeed, several studies find no gender difference in the prevalence of psychological distress when measures common to men and women are jointly considered. For example, Kessler and Zhao (1999) analyzed data from the National Comorbidity Study and concluded that rates of mood and anxiety disorders are higher among women, rates of addictive disorders and antisocial personality disorder are higher among men, and if these disorders are combined, there is no sex difference in the overall prevalence of mental health problems.

However, most research on gender differences in mental health have focused on understanding the poorer health of women, particularly their higher rates of depression (Rieker and Bird 2000). In turn, the emphasis on depression has shaped the research literature around the discussion of how social conditions worsen the mental health of women vis-à-vis men, without a commensurate level of attention toward understanding the higher rate of problematic behaviors among men, such as heavy drinking (Horwitz and Davies 1994). As a result, it is likely that health professionals and laypersons underestimate the degree to which mental health problems exist among men, which in turn means that subsequent policies – both in the public and private sector – that are informed by these studies will likely be less efficacious for men than women.

Explanations for Gender Differences in Health

Leading explanations for gender differences in physical and mental health can be classified broadly into four categories: biological, behavioral, psychosocial, and social structural. We will briefly summarize biological explanations for the gender gap, and then discuss the latter three in more detail.

The oldest explanation for gender differences in health focused on biological differences between the sexes, namely physiological and genetic differences in the production of hormones. For example, research has found that estrogen reduces circulatory levels of harmful cholesterol and thereby reduces women's chances of heart disease; for men, the opposite occurs: testosterone increases low-density lipoprotein and thus increases their chances of heart disease (Newman and Brach 2001). Men also tend to have weaker immune systems than women because testosterone causes immunosuppression (Owens 2002). However, biological explanations alone cannot explain the persistent, but often changing nature of gendered health inequities across time and space, leading many to place more weight on the behavioral and social structural bases of gendered health inequalities.

Sociologists often frame the discussion of how social factors actually work to influence men's and women's health around two general hypotheses. The first is the *differential exposure hypothesis* that suggests that men and women have different levels of exposure to the conditions that foster good health. The second is the *differential vulnerability hypothesis* that indicates that not only are men and women differentially exposed to conditions that promote health, but they also react differently to these conditions (for good reviews see Denton et al. 2004; Rieker and Bird 2000). Evidence exists in support of both perspectives, and we frame our discussion of behavioral, psychosocial, and social structural explanations for the gender gap around these themes of differential exposure and differential vulnerability.

Behavioral explanations highlight differences in men's and women's lifestyle activities that either damage or protect their health. With few exceptions, men are exposed to more behavior that is harmful to their health, which is why adjusting for behavioral measures tends to narrow the gender gap in mortality. Most discussed are cigarettes and alcohol, given their legal status and high use among the teenage and adult populations. Men drink more frequently and more heavily than women, especially during young adulthood (Johnson et al. 1998; NCHS 2006). Smoking rates are also higher among men (23.9% of men and 18.1% of women in 2005), although the gender gap in smoking has closed among teenagers (CDC 2006), indicating that the contribution of smoking to gender differences in measures of morbidity and mortality will decline with time (see discussion by Gorman and Read 2007). In addition, while men (at least for now) participate in higher rates of smoking and heavy drinking, it also appears that men are more vulnerable to the effects of alcohol and cigarettes, as both influence the health status of men more than women (Denton et al. 2004; Denton and Walters 1999).

The gender pattern is somewhat mixed when we look at diet, exercise, and body mass index (BMI). Men engage in slightly higher levels of regular exercise (NCHS 2006), and they appear to benefit more from exercise when compared to women (Denton et al. 2004). However, they eat a less healthy diet than women (CDC 2007), and rates of overweight are higher for men – although obesity levels are slightly higher among women (NCHS 2006). However, across a wide array of risky behaviors (including illegal drug use, drunk driving, lack of seatbelt, and helmet use), men participate at higher levels than women (e.g., Everett et al. 2001; SAMHSA 2006). As such, it is not surprising that they experience more unintentional injuries than women, which has important consequences for daily functioning and mortality. For example, while 14.7% of premature mortality among women is due to unintentional injury, this accounts for 21.2% of premature deaths among men (CDC 2005).

Violence also plays an important role in shaping the health profiles of men and women, but the types of violence they experience tend to differ. For example, studies have shown that women experience much higher rates of sexual and intimate partner violence than men; 78% of victims of sexual assault and rape are women (Tjaden and Theonnes 2000), and intimate partner violence makes up 20% of all nonfatal violence against women, but only 3% of nonfatal violence against men (Rennison 2003). Men, however, experience more types of fatal violence. For example, rates of premature mortality due to suicide and homicide are more than twice as high among men when compared to women (CDC 2005). Lastly, with respect to behavioral patterns, adult women report more preventive health care visits than men, especially among persons aged 18–44 (when women are more than twice as likely to see a doctor), mostly because of medical care associated with reproduction. However, this gender gap closes with age; among persons aged 65 and older, the frequency of seeing a doctor is the same for men and women (NCHS 2006).

Psychosocial explanations focus on differences in men's and women's exposure and reaction to stressors and social support networks that in turn affect their health. These factors contribute in important ways to gender differences in health status but are less studied than behavioral or economic explanations. In terms of exposure, women report lower self-esteem and personal control than men, and women are more likely to experience stressful life events and chronic stressors in their social roles that, in turn, increase their likelihood of depression and poor physical health (Denton et al. 2004; Forthofer et al. 2001; Nazroo et al. 1998; Thoits 1995). In terms of vulnerability, it also appears that men and women are susceptible to different types of chronic stressors (Denton et al. 2004; McDonough and Walters 2001) and that men and women respond differently to stress (Aneshensel et al. 1991; Rieker and Bird 2000). On the other hand, women have stronger support networks than men that appear to enhance their well-being (Denton et al. 2004; Shye et al. 1995), and some studies suggest that women benefit more from social support than men (Denton et al. 2004; Denton and Walters 1999; Forthofer et al. 2001; Umberson et al. 1996). However, the evidence on this point is not conclusive (see Elliott 2001; Neff and Karney 2005; Shye et al. 1995). Part of the inconsistency likely results from higher involvement of women in the health needs and behaviors of family, friends, and other members of their social network. Thus, while this results in deeper social networks for women, this also results in substantial costs to their health – costs that men do not incur (Shye et al. 1995).

Of all explanations for gender differences in health, sociologists have lent the most weight to social structural disparities between men and women since contemporary research regularly acknowledges that inequities in men's and women's well-being are rooted in their different social structural locations in society and the attendant resources, roles, and opportunities associated with those locations (Blau et al. 2006; Graham 2000). More specifically, men and women occupy different social positions that mediate their exposure to risks that are harmful to health, their participation in health damaging behaviors, and perhaps most importantly, their access to goods and resources that promote well-being (Bird and Rieker 1999).

It is well-established that women occupy less privileged socioeconomic positions in society, which increases their exposure to hardship and stress and limits their access to the resources needed to prevent and cure disease (Phelan et al. 2004; Ross and Bird 1994; Walters et al. 2002). In the United States, women are more likely than men to work part-time, participate in unwaged labor, and receive unequal wages, all of which contributes to their lower socioeconomic position and drives down their health. Evidence also exists that women benefit more than men from full-time employment, making their weaker attachment to the labor market all the more detrimental to their health (Denton et al. 2004).

While socioeconomic status affects women's health directly through access to resources, it has a large, indirect influence on health through psychosocial factors and social roles (Denton et al. 2004; McDonough and Walters 2001). Lower socioeconomic position is associated with lower levels of perceived control and self-esteem, both of which are associated with greater levels of depression and poorer self-rated health (Denton et al. 2004; Rieker and Bird 2000). Depression further contributes to poorer physical health through decreased immune system and heightened blood pressure (see discussion by Ross and Bird 1994), and studies consistently report higher levels of depression among women (Kessler 2006). Socioeconomic status also helps explain the well-established positive relationship between marital status and health, operating through increased social support and decreased risky behavior for men and increased financial well-being for women (Lillard and Waite 1995). Married women typically have greater economic resources than their unmarried peers, which translates into greater access to health care, lower levels of stress, and better overall health (Meyer and Pavalko 1996).

In keeping with the chapter's goal of bringing in race/ethnicity to the analysis of gender, we must underscore the fact that the utility of these explanations is not uniform across racial and ethnic groups. Taking socioeconomic explanations as an example, research clearly shows that Whites benefit from their advantaged social and economic standing, and the depressed socioeconomic status of blacks is an important culprit behind their across-the-board poorer health status (Hayward et al. 2000). Mexican Americans, on the other hand, have more favorable health outcomes than would be expected given their high-risk socioeconomic profile (Palloni and Arias 2004; Singh and Siahpush 2002). Moreover, socioeconomic status is a much more powerful explanation for health differentials between racial/ethnic groups (e.g., whites relative to blacks) than for gender differences within racial/ethnic groups (Cooper 2002; Read and Gorman 2006). This pattern may reflect the fact that there are greater socioeconomic disparities between racial/ethnic populations than among men and women in the same racial/ethnic group. The point is that the utility of socioeconomic explanations for gender differences in health varies across racial/ethnic groups.

Looking to the Future: Prospects and Challenges for Understanding and Reducing Gendered Health Disparities

To this point, we have drawn from a vast literature in medical sociology to provide an overview of what is known about differences in US men's and women's health. We now shift our lens outward beyond medical sociology to ask what we can glean from other mainstream arenas that will move forward our thinking on gendered health inequalities. As we said at the beginning of the chapter, this list is potentially endless and by no means are we discounting the significance and potential contribution of other areas not discussed here. Rather, we have chosen to focus on three areas that have great potential to influence the nature of gender differences in health in the near future and have both theoretical and policy implications: (1) immigration (given the rapid and sustained growth of the foreign-born population), (2) life course perspective (given the aging of the population), and (3) the link between mental and physical health (given the increasing recognition of their interconnectedness).

Gender, Immigration, and Health

Over 33 million immigrants live in the USA today, totaling 11.5% of the US population and making the foreign-born population of considerable interest to health researchers, public health officials, and policymakers. Women make up one-half of the foreign-born population, and their immigration rates have outpaced men's in every decade since the 1960s (US Bureau of the Census, 1999, 2004), yet surprisingly little is known about how gender interacts with immigration to influence health. This is a crucial question because migration processes differ drastically for men and women, and therefore the theories and concepts historically used to explain immigrant health (e.g., selectivity, return migration, etc.) may be less useful for understanding the health profiles and trajectories of immigrant women. Furthermore, the explanations typically used to account for gender differences in US health (e.g., socioeconomic status) may be less relevant for understanding differences between immigrant men and women who share similar socioeconomic positions (Read and Gorman 2006).

The implications from existing research are that bringing gender into the picture may alter what we currently know about immigrant health patterns, and concurrently, that gendered immigrant health patterns may change how we think about gender differences in US health. How might gender matter for immigrant health? First, it appears that US migrants are a physically robust population. Several studies document that while the health profile of the foreign-born population is as good (and sometimes better) than the native-born US population, this advantage declines with duration in the USA (Antecol and Bedard 2006; Cho and Hummer 2001; Singh and Siahpush 2002). This pattern is often referred to as the "epidemiological paradox", since the health of new migrants is surprising, given the relatively limited socioeconomic resources of many groups of immigrants upon initial migration (Waters 1999). Indeed, this pattern runs counter to a great deal of research documenting poor health outcomes among lower socioeconomic groups in the USA (House and Williams 2000), and past studies frequently find that adjusting for socioeconomic status does not explain the relationship between immigrant characteristics and measures of physical health (e.g., Angel et al. 2001; Cho et al. 2004).

To account for this pattern, two complementary explanations are often applied. First, immigrants are healthier than their counterparts who did not migrate – appearing to represent a selective snapshot of residents from their country-of-origin (Jasso et al. 2004, Landale et al. 2000). Second, immigrants living in the USA benefit from cultural ties and norms that emphasize healthier behaviors and strong family support networks (see discussion by Jasso et al. 2004; Vega and Amaro 1994). Studies also indicate, however, that immigrant health deteriorates with increasing time spent in the USA, even when socioeconomic status rises (Jasso et al. 2002). Existing research suggests two conclusions: First, selection cannot completely account for the healthy immigrant effect, and researchers should also consider the role of acculturation (often measured by duration of residence in the USA, language use, and citizenship). Second, it suggests that over time, changes in other health-related factors (e.g., declining social support) may override the health gains associated with increased economic well-being.

While we have learned a lot about immigrant health in recent decades, gender has been largely missing from discussions of immigrant health patterns, which is somewhat surprising given the large and growing literature on gendered migration and incorporation patterns which indicates that gender might matter a great deal (Hondagneu-Sotelo 1994). Most work to date has focused on the Mexican case (from which the largest number of legal and unauthorized migrants come), and so our discussion draws mainly from this work. First, the decision to migrate is often based on very different factors for men and women (e.g., to find employment for men, vs. family reunification for women), and recent research has shown that even though more women are migrating from Mexico than in the past, explanations for male migration do not apply to women (Donato et al. 2006). If the decision for women to migrate is more of a family decision, based on gendered interactions and roles, then women may be less selective on health than their male counterparts – a factor which may contribute to the sicker profile of Mexican American women when compared to Mexican American men (Read and Gorman 2006). On the other hand, the relative costs of migration might be higher for women than men because of fewer and weaker network ties, often limited to kinship ties, suggesting that they may select more on health than their male counterparts (Curran and Saguy 2001; Kanaiaupuni 2000). Further, female migrants may be more positively selected with respect to education (and health) because the relative returns are potentially higher for them than for men (Kanaiaupuni 2000). This is turn implies that health advantages among Mexican women in the USA, at least initially, should exceed those of men, all else equal.

Second, cultural norms surrounding gender are very different in Mexico than in the USA and involve sharper divisions between men and women with women occupying relatively more inferior and subordinate positions both in the family and workforce. As a result, Mexican women tend to benefit from migration more than men, at least at the beginning, because they are offered a wider range of opportunities in the US context (Hondagneu-Sotelo 1994). At the same time, patriarchal cultural norms in Mexico result in women participating in less health-damaging behaviors than men in Mexico (see discussion by Lopez-Gonzalez et al. 2005). On arrival in the USA, immigrant women smoke and drink less than immigrant men, but with increasing acculturation, the health behavior of women becomes less positive, while the behavior of men changes little with acculturation (Lopez-Gonzalez et al. 2005).

These studies indicate that both migration and acculturation processes are gendered and suggest competing possibilities for both the initial and long-term health of immigrant men and women. At the onset, immigrant women may be less healthy than immigrant men due to weaker selectivity factors at work, or they may be healthier than men because the costs associated with migration may be higher for women. In the long term, the health profiles of both immigrant men and women may deteriorate, but at a faster pace for women than men, or they may deteriorate at different rates depending on the health outcome in question (faster for nonacute conditions for women but slower for fatal chronic conditions). These are empirical questions that need to be the center of future research on gender and health, as immigrants will continue to shape the demographic composition and health profile of the US population.

Gender and Health over the Life Course

The US population is aging rapidly. In 2000, one out of eight Americans was aged 65 and older; by 2030, this will grow to one out of five (Himes 2002), and the implications for the health profile of the United States is enormous. What is also clear is that the health status of elderly women will be particularly important, since the higher mortality rate of men has given the elderly population in the USA a decidedly female face. In 2000, there were three women for every two men aged 65 and older; by age 85, there were five women for every two men (Himes 2002). And, while this gender gap is closing due to faster improvements in male mortality in the last several years, elderly women will continue to outnumber elderly men for decades to come.

For measures of morbidity, the gender gap appears to vary by condition and age. For example, while women report worse self-rated health (physical and mental) in the younger adult ages, this gap closes with age; for measures of disability, however, women report higher rates than men, and the size of the gap increases with age (e.g., Cleary et al. 2004; Gorman and Read 2006). However, for life-threatening medical conditions, the gender gap is quite small in the early adult years and increases with age (Gorman and Read 2006).

While these types of cross-sectional studies of the gender-health gap are informative, an increasing number of researchers are applying a life course perspective to explore how health unfolds as people age. Known life course principles include (a) the significance of historical context; (b) the understanding that prior life course experiences shape subsequent life course experiences; and (c) the understanding that the life path of any individual is linked with the life courses of family, friends, and coworkers (see review by Moen 2001). This is an important concept because a person's health status at any one point in time is the cumulative result of a host of factors, either health-promoting or health-damaging, leading up to that point – and it appears that the life course trajectories of men and women differ, and these differences have important, long-term implications for health.

In particular, men's and women's different structural locations and life paths can result in cumulating advantage for men, but cumulating disadvantage for women (Moen and Spencer 2006; Moen and Chermack 2005; Moen 2001). For example, research on the long-term effects of conditions during childhood has begun to document how this cumulating disadvantage for women begins at an early age, in stark contrast to the experience of men. In general, a growing number of life course studies document how health unfolds from birth to death, with convincing evidence that the social and health conditions experienced in early life (e.g., parental socioeconomic status, family size, birth weight, childhood infectious disease) are strongly tied to adult disease and mortality (Kuh and Ben-Shlomo 1997). Most importantly, early and later life biological and social risk factors combine to influence adult health, forming "chains of risk" (both advantageous and disadvantageous), whereby "…certain experiences in early life increase the likelihood of future events which in turn lead to a change in the risk of adult disease" (Kuh and Ben-Shlomo 1997:7). While very few studies to date have examined the implications of childhood conditions for gender disparities in health, evidence is growing that childhood socioeconomic status has different implications for the health of adult men and women. For example, using data from the Health and Retirement Survey, Hamil-Luker and O'Rand (2007) show that while measures of childhood SES (i.e., never living with a father while growing up, economic disadvantage) increase the risk of heart attack for adult women (even with adjustment for adult risk factors), childhood SES is unrelated to heart attack risk for adult men. Hamil-Luker and O'Rand (2007:153) conclude that adult women are more susceptible to the negative health effects of early disadvantage because of their poorer structural location in relation to men: "The circumstances of women's childhood may more firmly anchor them in future health trajectories because life-course exposures in the realms of education, family, and work further solidify latent differences expressed in early life. In contrast, men's childhood SES may more weakly affect adult health trajectories because their greater access to power, resources, prestige, and knowledge over the life course renders early exposures less important than proximal resources." We need more studies like this, across a diverse array of disease and disability outcomes, to assess whether the weaker tie between childhood and adult health for men is consistent, or whether it is condition-specific.

We have also seen a growing number of studies that examine the health implications of men's and women's differential paths through a variety of adult roles, including work, parenting, marriage, and care-giving. For example, a substantial gender divide remains in the time men and women spend participating in paid and unpaid work, although this is dependent upon marital and parenting status. The gap is smallest between single men and women without children and largest between married fathers and mothers, with women participating in paid work less and unpaid work more (Sayer et al. 2004). In addition, men typically experience a straight-line occupational career path that moves from education to employment to retirement, while the education and work path of women is more sporadic due to the demands of children, family, and their husband's careers (see review by Moen and Chermack 2005). The stronger connection between work and home life demands for women can create strains and overloads, and can decrease personal control, emotional well-being, and especially economic well-being. Indeed, women accumulate less wealth over the life course than men and are less likely to receive pension funds (Himes 2002). Because of this, the health and well-being of older women is tightly bound to the financial status of their husbands.

This is quite troubling given that three-quarters of men over the age of 65 are married, but only 44% of women are married, and among persons aged 85 and older (who are the fastest growing segment of the elderly population), only 13% of women are married, compared to over half of men (Himes 2002). The lower marriage rate of senior women contributes strongly to their increased likelihood of living alone, entering a nursing home, and depending on nonspouses for care – even though women are more likely to become caregivers themselves (Himes 2002; Moen 2001). Indeed, older men, because of higher marriage rates, expect that that their wives will provide personal care as they age, while only a minority of older women feel they can count on spousal help with personal care (Spitze and Ward 2000). The presence and care provided by wives is particularly important for men; widowhood is a more psychologically disturbing experience for men, and social isolation in late life is more harmful to men than women (Lee and DeMaris 2007; Moen 2001).

In the end, the implications of an aging population are far-reaching, not the least of which is how healthy the US population will be in the years to come. In an ideal world, we would see a compression of morbidity, whereby longer life is associated with better health. For example, recent decades have seen improvement in several forms of disability (e.g., functional limitations) with overall prevalence rates for elder disability declining in the USA, although trends for more severe type of disability are unclear (Population Reference Bureau 2007). While this may be possible for certain selective groups, evidence suggests that for many groups – including women – longer life means a frailer population, where the gains of increasing life expectancy are accompanied by more years lived in sickness, rather than health (Hayward and Heron 1999). As such, we need more studies that apply a life-course framework to identify how circumstances in childhood and adult life combine to influence risk and shape the nature of the aging process for men and women. The good news is that an increasing number of longitudinal data sources are available today, and as long as studies that have started in earlier phases of the life course continue to follow-up with respondents as they age (e.g., The National Longitudinal Study of Adolescent Health, where Wave IV is currently underway), we will be able to tease out the gendered nature of healthy aging with greater precision in the years that come.

Linking Mental and Physical Health

The idea that mental and physical health problems are intricately related is not new, nor does anyone dispute the fact that men and women often experience very different mental and physical health outcomes. What has been missing to date is a merging of these multiple and diverse strands of literature to provide a deeper understanding of how and under what conditions the link between mental and physical health varies for men and women over the life course. We do not purport that this will be an easy task to undertake because it requires the foundation of some common ground where biological, epidemiological, and sociological arguments can each contribute in unison, rather than as separate voices. In this section of the chapter, we offer what we believe is one promising avenue for the future that can achieve this pressing, albeit lofty, goal. Before turning to the future, we briefly describe how mental and physical health relate to each other and discuss the importance of bringing gender into analyses of the mental–physical health connection.

Looking first at the physical health consequences of poor mental health, there are numerous longitudinal studies that provide good evidence that mental health problems have dreadful consequences for physical health. Depression (a female-typical form of emotional upset) is the most frequently studied mental health outcome and is associated with poorer self-rated health (Han 2001), hypertension (Bosworth et al. 2003; Davidson et al. 2000; Jones et al. 1997; Meyer et al. 2004), functional decline (Roberson and Lichtenberg 2003), and especially heart disease (see review pieces by Carney and Freedland 2003; Frasure-Smith and Lesperance 2005; Rugulies 2002; and Schwartzman and Glaus 2000). Longitudinal studies of alcohol abuse (a male-typical form of emotional upset) also show a link with diminished physical health across a variety of dimensions, including elevated blood pressure (Keil et al. 1998), poorer self-rated health (Friedmann et al. 1999), and increased risk of cancer, kidney disease, cardiovascular disease, and digestive tract disorders (for a review, see Bagnardi et al. 2001).

Second, longitudinal studies have established that having a physical health problem increases the likelihood of depression over time (Fultz et al. 2005; Lanteri-Minet et al. 2005; Karasz and Ouellette 1995). For example, a study by Schnittker (2005) found that cancer, stroke, heart condition, chronic obstructed pulmonary disease, diabetes, high blood pressure, and arthritis all increase depressive symptoms in adults over 50, as did several forms of disability. Physical health problems are also accompanied by increased levels of stress, which in turn, have been linked to increased likelihood of alcohol abuse (for a review see Brady and Sonne 1999).

While these studies tell us much about the interconnectedness of mental and physical health, two substantial gaps in our understanding of these processes remain. First, few studies systematically examine how gender impacts the relationship between mental and physical health. For example, most studies that examine how depression affects morbidity and mortality do not explore gender differences, and among the few that do, the pattern is not clear (see review by Sevick et al. 2000). This makes it difficult to gauge whether the nature of the relationship between depression and physical health is equally applicable to men and women. Yet, we have some evidence that mental health problems can result in different physical health consequences for men and women. A study by Van Hout et al. (2004) found that having an anxiety disorder increased the risk of mortality for men, but not for women. Since anxiety disorders are typically viewed as a "female" problem, the authors speculate that women might be better able to cope with anxiety by accepting help from others; alternatively, unwillingness to report anxiety may mean that among men who do report it, the condition is more severe, and thus the physical health consequences more dire than for women. Turning to alcohol use/abuse, while alcohol use disorders are more prevalent in men, physicians are less likely to identify alcohol problems in women, even though women are more sensitive to the toxic effects of alcohol (see review by Brienza and Stein 2002).

The second gap in this literature is the lack of information regarding bidirectionality: To what extent is mental health a cause and/or effect of physical health problems, and how does this vary by gender? For example, longitudinal research has established that depression is associated with an increase in physical health problems, and that having a physical health problem is associated with an increase in depression. However, while it is clear that an assumption of unidirectional causality is not tenable, all studies that we have found assume and test this relationship in only one direction. Frasure-Smith and Lesperance (2005) do discuss the potential for reciprocity in the relationship between depression and coronary heart disease by evaluating past studies that have examined causality in either direction. While they conclude that there is greater evidence that depression increases the risk of heart disease than heart disease increasing the risk of depression, they do not explicitly test for bidirectionality in their paper. Pearlin et al. (2007) conclude that the separation of research into mental or physical health categories fails to acknowledge the intimate connection between mental and physical well being, noting that more inclusive research exploring how mental and physical health influence one another (simultaneously, and over time) is needed. Furthermore, it is unclear whether these processes operate the same for men and women and across a variety of measures of both physical and mental health.

As these studies show, the nature of the relationship between mental and physical health remains an unsettled issue, and therein lies the conundrum: We can identify and recognize these patterns and we can acknowledge the importance of the intersection between mental and physical health at the theoretical level, but how do we how to build it into our theories, frameworks, and empirical assessments? It is clear that mental and physical health are interconnected and influence one another over the adult life course. However, systematic examinations of the mental–physical health link over time are rare, and gender differences in these processes are often overlooked. So, at the start, we need researchers to take better advantage of existing longitudinal data sources to test for reciprocity between markers of mental and physical health as people age, and to explore whether the ties that bind mental and physical health together are different, or the same, for men and women across a range of health conditions. Looking further into the future, one promising avenue is to establish more systematic efforts to collect longitudinal data that contain both clinical assessments of mental and physical health and survey-based assessments of health that rely on respondent self-assessments of their own mental and physical well-being. Not only would we benefit from increased validity of health conditions by comparing self-reports of hypertensive status with physician-assessed measures of blood pressure, but we would also benefit in that the meaningfulness of illness to the individual could be better assessed.

Conclusion

We end this chapter as we began it, with the acknowledgement that we have gained tremendous knowledge over the last few decades on gender disparities in health and well-being, both physical and mental. Not only do we have a better sense of the biological and social circumstances that shape the health status of the adult population, but we also have better insight into how the gender-stratified nature of US society differentially helps (and hurts) men and women. Indeed, one of the biggest contributions of sociological studies of gender and health in recent years has been teasing out how differences in men's and women's biological make-up, lifestyle behaviors, psychosocial well-being, and socioeconomic standing shape gender differences in health.

That being said, we still have a long way to go in our quest for understanding the mechanisms that produce gendered health disparities. Our examination of these processes to date has relied too heavily on cross-sectional information, which artificially partitions health into discrete life phases, obscuring the reality that an individual's health profile unfolds across the totality of the life course. We have also created artificial divisions between mental and physical health, often overlooking the mind–body link that together shape the mental and physical well-being of individuals. And, we cannot ignore the fact that the demographic make-up of the US population is in constant flux, due largely to increasing life expectancy and the continual addition of migrants from a host of different sending nations. These changes necessitate continued study of how the gender–health relationship varies across racial/ethnic and immigrant groups as people age, and more in-depth analyses of the possible implications that these demographic shifts will have for other social conditions that in turn shape health, most notably socioeconomic status given that economic well-being is unevenly distributed across age, racial/ethnic, and immigrant groups.

We thank Georgiana Bostean for her valuable help with producing the figures for this chapter.

References

Allendale E, Hunt K (2000) Gender inequalities in health: research at the crossroads. In: Allendale E, Hunt K (eds) Gender inequalities in health. Open University Press, Buckingham, pp 1–35

Aneshensel CS, Rutter CM, Lachenbruch PA (1991) Social structure, stress, and mental health: competing conceptual and analytic models. Am Sociol Rev 56:166–178

Angel JL, Buckley CJ, Finch BK (2001) Nativity and self-assessed health among pre-retirement age hispanics and non-hispanic whites. Int Migr Rev 35:784–804

Antecol H, Bedard K (2006) Unhealthy assimilation: why do immigrants converge to American health status levels? Demography 43(2):337–360

Arber S, Cooper H (1999) Gender differences in health in later life: the new paradox? Soc Sci Med 48:61–76

Bagnardi V, Blangiardo M, La Vecchia C, Corrao G (2001) Alcohol consumption and the risk of cancer: a meta-analysis. Alcohol Res Health 25(1):263–270

Bird CE, Rieker PP (2008) Gender and health: the effects of constrained choices and social policies. Cambridge University Press, New York

Bird CE, Rieker PP (1999) Gender matters: an integrated model for understanding men's and women's health. Soc Sci Med 48:745–755

Blau FD, Brinton MC, Grusky DB (eds) (2006) The declining significance of gender? Russell Sage Foundation, New York

Brady KT, Sonne SC (1999) The role of stress in alcohol use, alcoholism treatment, and relapse. Alcohol Res Health 23:263–71

Brienza RS, Stein MD (2002) Alcohol use disorders in primary care: do gender-specific differences exist? J Gen Intern Med 17(5):387–397

Bosworth HB, Bartash RM, Olsen MK, Steffens DC (2003) The association of psychosocial factors and depression with hypertension among older adults. Int J Geriatr Psychiatry 18:1142–1148

Carney RM, Freedland KE (2003) Depression, mortality, and medical morbidity in patients with coronary heart disease. Biol Psychiatry 54:241–247

Centers for Disease Control and Prevention (2005) Web-based injury statistics query and reporting system (WISQARS) [online], National Center for Injury Prevention and Control. Retrieved: 27 June 2007. Available from URL: www.cdc.gov/ncipc/wisqars

Centers for Disease Control and Prevention (2006) Cigarette use among high school students: United States, 1991–2005. MMWR 55(26):724–726

Centers for Disease Control and Prevention (2007) Fruit and vegetable consumption among adults: United States, 2005. MMWR 56(10):213–217

Cho Y, Hummer RA (2001) Disability status differentials across fifteen asian and pacific islander groups and the effect of nativity and duration of residence in the US. Soc Biol 48(3–4):171–195

Cho Y, Parker Frisbie W, Hummer RA, Rogers RG (2004) Nativity, duration of residence, and the health of hispanic adults in the United States. Int Migr Rev 38(1):184–211

Cleary PD, Zaborski L, Ayanian J (2004) Sex differences in health over the course of midlife. In: Brim OG, Ryff CD, Kessler RC (eds) How healthy are we? A national study of well-being in midlife. University of Chicago Press, Chicago, IL, pp 37–63

Cooper H (2002) Investigating socio-economic explanations for gender and ethnic inequalities in health. Soc Sci Med 54:693–706

Curran S, Saguy A (2001) Migration and cultural change: a role for gender and social networks? J Int Womens Stud 2:54–77

Davidson K, Jonas BS, Dixon KE, Markovitz JH (2000) Do depression symptoms predict early hypertension incidence in young adults in the CARDIA study? Arch Intern Med 160:1495–1500

Denton M, Walters V (1999) Gender differences in structural and behavioral determinants of health: an analysis of the social production of health. Soc Sci Med 48:1221–1235

Denton M, Prus S, Walters V (2004) Gender differences in health: a Canadian study of the psychosocial, structural and behavioural determinants of health. Soc Sci Med 58:2585–2600

Donato KM, Gabaccia D, Holdaway J, Manalansan M, Pessar PR (2006) A glass half full? Gender in migration studies. Int Migr Rev 40:3–26

Elliott M (2001) Gender differences in causes of depression. Women Health 33(3–4):163–177

Everett SA, Shults R, Barrios L, Sacks J, Lowry R, Oeltmann J (2001) Trends and subgroup differences in transportation-related injury risk and safety behaviors among high school students, 1991–1997. J Adolesc Health 28:228–234

Forthofer MS, Janz N, Dodge J, Clark N (2001) Gender differences in the associations of self-esteem, stress and social support with functional health status among older adults with heart disease. J Women Aging 13(1):19–37

Frasure-Smith N, Lesperance F (2005) Depression and coronary heart disease: complex synergism of mind, body, and environment. Curr Dir Psychol Sci 14:39–43

Friedmann PD, Jin L, Karrison T, Nerney M, Hayley DC, Mulliken R, Walter J, Miller A, Chin M (1999) The effect of alcohol abuse on the health status of older adults seen in the Emergency Department. Am J Drug Alcohol Abuse 25(3):529–542

Fultz NH, Jenkins KR, Ostbye T, Taylor Jr Donald, Kabeto M, Langa K (2005) The impact of own and spouse's urinary incontinence on depressive symptoms. Soc Sci Med 60:2537–2548

Gorman BK, Read JG (2006) Gender disparities in adult health: an examination of three measures of morbidity. J Health Soc Behav 47:95–110

Gorman BK, Read JG (2007) Why men die younger than women. Geriatr Aging 10(3):179–181

Graham H (2000) Socio-economic change and inequalities in men and women's health in the UK. In: Annandale E, Hunt K (eds) Gender inequalities in health. Open University Press, Buckingham, pp 90–122

Guralnik JM, La Croix A, Everett D, Kovar MG (1989) Aging in the eighties: the prevalence of comorbidity and its association with disability. Advance data from vital and health statistics. No. 170. National Center for Health Statistics, Hyattsville, MD

Hamil-Luker J, O'Rand A (2007) Gender differences in the link between childhood socioeconomic conditions and heart attack risk in adulthood. J Health Soc Behav 44(1):137–158

Han B (2001) The impact of age, gender, and race on the relationship between depression and self-rated health in community-dwelling older adults: a longitudinal study. Home Health Care Serv Q 20(3):27–43

Hayward MD, Heron M (1999) Racial inequality in active life among adult Americans. Demography 36(1):77–91

Hayward MD, Miles T, Crimmins E, Yang Yu (2000) The significance of socioeconomic status in explaining the racial gap in chronic health conditions. Am Sociol Rev 65:910–930

Himes CL (2002) Elderly Americans. Population Bulletin 56(4). Washington, DC: Population Reference Bureau

Hondagneu-Sotelo P (1994) Regulating the unregulated? Domestic workers' social networks. Soc Probl 41:50–64

Horwitz AV, Davies L (1994) Are emotional distress and alcohol problems differential outcomes to stress? An exploratory test. Soc Sci Q 75(3):607–621

Horwitz AV, White HR, Howell-White S (1996) Becoming married and mental health: a longitudinal study of a cohort of young adults. J Marriage Fam 58:895–907

House JS, Williams DR (2000) Understanding and reducing socioeconomic and racial/ethnic disparities in health. In: Smedley BD, Syme SL (eds) Promoting health: intervention strategies from social and behavioral research. National Academies Press, Washington, DC, pp 81–124

Idler EL, Benyamini Y (1997) Self-rated health and mortality: a review of twenty-seven community studies. J Health Soc Behav 38:21–37

Jasso G, Mark RR, Smith JP (2002) The earnings of US immigrants: world skill prices, skill transferability and selectivity. Unpublished manuscript

Jasso G, Massey D, Rosenzweig M, Smith J (2004) Immigrant health: selectivity and acculturation. In: Anderson N, Bulatao R, Cohen B (eds) Critical perspectives on racial and ethnic differences in health in later life, panel on race, ethnicity, and health in later life, National Research Council. National Academies Press, Washington, DC, pp 227–266

Johnson FW, Gruenewald P, Treno A, Taff GA (1998) Drinking over the life course within gender and ethnic groups: a hyperparametric analysis. J Stud Alcohol 59(5):568–581

Jones BS, Franks P, Ingram DD (1997) Are symptoms of anxiety and depression risk factors for hypertension? longitudinal evidence from the national health and nutrition examination survey I epidemiological follow-up study. Arch Fam Med 6:43–49

Kanaiaupuni SM (2000) Reframing the migration question: an analysis of men, women, and gender in Mexico. Soc Forces 78:1311–1347

Karasz A, Ouellette SC (1995) Role strain and psychological well-being in women with systemic lupus erythematosus. Women Health 23:41–57

Keil U, Liese A, Filipiak B, Swales JD, Grobbee DE (1998) Alcohol, blood pressure, and hypertension. Novartis Found Symp 216:125–144

Kessler RC (2006) The epidemiology of depression among women. In: Keyes CLM, Goodman SH (eds) Women and depression. Cambridge University Press, New York, pp 22–40

Kessler RC, Zhao S (1999) Overview of descriptive epidemiology of mental disorders. In: Aneshensel CS, Phelan JC (eds) Handbook of the sociology of mental health. Kluwer, New York, pp 127–150

Keyes CLM, Goodman SH (eds) (2006) Women and depression: a handbook for the social, behavioral, and biomedical sciences. Cambridge University Press, New York

Kuh D, Ben-Shlomo Y (1997) Introduction: a life course approach to the aetiology of adult chronic disease. In: Kuh D, Ben-Shlomo Y (eds) A life course approach to chronic disease epidemiology: tracing the origins of ill-health from early to adult life. Oxford University Press, New York, pp 3–14

Lanteri-Minet M, Radat F, Chautard M-H, Lucas C (2005) Anxiety and depression associated with migraine: influence on migraine subjects' disability and quality of life, and acute migraine management. Pain 118:319–326

Landale NS, Oropesa RS, Gorman BK (2000) Migration and infant death: assimilation or selective migration among Puerto Ricans? Am Sociol Rev 65:888–909

Lee GR, DeMaris A (2007) Widowhood, gender, and depression: a longitudinal analysis. Res Aging 29(1):56–72

Lillard LA, Waite LJ (1995) Til death do us part: marital disruption and mortality. Am J Sociol 5:1131–1156

Lopez-Gonzalez L, Aravena V, Hummer R (2005) Immigrant acculturation, gender and health behavior: a research note. Soc Forces 84:581–593

Lubitz J, Cai L, Kramarow E, Lentzner H (2003) Health, life expectancy, and health care spending among the elderly. N Engl J Med 349(11):1048–55

Macintyre S, Hunt K, Sweeting H (1996) Gender differences in health: are things really as simple as they seem? Soc Sci Med 42:617–624

Marks NF (1996) Flying solo at midlife: gender, marital status, and psychological well-being. J Marriage Fam 58:917–932

McDonough P, Walters V (2001) Gender and health: reassessing patterns and explanations. Soc Sci Med 52:547–559

Merrill SS, Seeman TE, Kasl SV, Berkman LF (1997) Gender differences in the comparison of self-reported disability and performance measures. J Gerontol A Biol Sci Med Sci 52A(1):M19–26

Meyer MH, Pavalko EK (1996) Family, work, and access to health insurance among mature women. J Health Soc Behav 37:311–325

Meyer CM, Armenian HK, Eaton WW, Ford DE (2004) Incident hypertension associated with depression in the Baltimore epidemiologic catchment area follow-up study. J Affect Disord 83:127–133

Moen P (2001) The gendered life course. In: Binstock RH, George LK (eds) Handbook of aging and the social sciences, 5th edn. Academic, San Diego, CA, pp 179–196

Moen P, Chermack K (2005) Gender disparities in health: strategic selection, careers, and cycles of control. J Gerontol B 60B (special issue):99–108

Moen P, Spencer D (2006) Converging divergences in age, gender, health, and well-being: strategic selection in the third age. In: Binstock R, George L (eds) Handbook of aging and the social sciences, 6th edn. Academic, San Diego, CA, pp 127–144

National Center for Health Statistics (2006) Health, United States, 2006: With chartbook on trends in the health of Americans. Author, Hyattsville, Maryland

Nazroo JY, Edwards A, Brown G (1998) Gender differences in the prevalence of depression: artifact, alternative disorders, biology or roles? Sociol Health Illn 20(3):312–330

Neff LA, Karney B (2005) Gender differences in social support: a question of skill or responsiveness? J Pers Soc Psychol 88(1):79–90

Newman AB, Brach J (2001) Gender gap in longevity and disability in older persons. Epidemiol Rev 23(2):343–350

Owens IPF (2002) Sex differences in mortality rate. Science 297(5589):2008–2009

Palloni A, Arias E (2004) Paradox lost: explaining the hispanic adult mortality advantage. Demography 41:385–415

Pearlin L, Avison W, Fazio E (2007) Sociology, psychiatry, and the production of knowledge about mental illness and its treatment. In: Avison WR, McLeod JD, Pescosolido BA (eds) Mental health, social mirror. Springer, New York, pp 33–53

Phelan Jo C, Link B, Diez-Roux A, Kawachi I, Levin B (2004) "Fundamental Causes" of social inequalities in mortality: a test of the theory. J Health Soc Behav 45:265–285

Population Reference Bureau (2007) Trends in disability at older ages: today's research on health. Issue 7. Population Reference Bureau, Washington, DC

Read JG, Gorman BK (2006) Gender inequalities in US adult health: the interplay of race and ethnicity. Soc Sci Med 62:1045–1065

Rennison CM (2003) Intimate partner violence, 1993–2001. Bureau of Justice Statistics, US Department of Justice, Washington, DC, Publication No. NCJ197838

Rieker PP, Bird CE (2000) Sociological explanations of gender differences in mental and physical health. In: Bird C, Conrad P, Fremont A (eds) The handbook of medical sociology. Prentice Hall, Upper Saddle River, NJ, pp 98–113

Rieker PP, Bird CE (2005) Rethinking gender differences in health: why we need to integrate social and biological perspectives. J Gerontol B 60B (special issue II):40–47

Roberson T, Lichtenberg P (2003) Depression, social support, and functional abilities: longitudinal findings. Clin Gerontol 26(3/4):55–67

Rogers RG, Hummer R, Nam C (2000) Living and dying in the USA: behavioral, health, and social differentials of adult mortality. Academic, San Diego, CA

Rosenfield S (1999) Splitting the difference: gender, the self, and mental health. In: Aneshensel CS, Phelan JC (eds) Handbook of the sociology of mental health. Kluwer, New York, pp 209–224

Ross CE, Bird C (1994) Sex stratification and health lifestyle: consequences for men's and women's perceived health. J Health Soc Behav 35:161–178

Rugulies R (2002) Depression as a predictor for coronary heart disease: a review and meta-analysis. Am J Prev Med 23:51–61

Sayer LC, Cohen P, Casper L (2004) Women, men, and work. Russell Sage Foundation and the Population Reference Bureau, New York and Washington, DC

Schnittker J (2005) Chronic illness and depressive symptoms in late life. Soc Sci Med 60:13–23

Schwartzman JB, Glaus KD (2000) Depression and coronary heart disease in women: implications for clinical practice and research. Prof Psychol Res Pr 31(1):48–57

Sevick MA, Rolih C, Pahor M (2000) Gender differences in morbidity and mortality related to depression: a review of the literature. Aging Clin Exp Res 12(6):407–416

Shye D, Mullooly JP, Freeborn DK, Pope CR (1995) Gender differences in the relationship between social network support and mortality: a longitudinal study of an elderly cohort. Soc Sci Med 41:935–947

Singh GK, Siahpush M (2002) Ethnic-immigrant differentials in health behaviors, morbidity, and cause-specific mortality in the united states: an analysis of two national data bases. Hum Biol 74:83–109

Spitze G, Ward R (2000) Gender, marriage, and expectations for personal care. Res Aging 22(5):451–469

Substance Abuse and Mental Health Services Administration (2006) Results from the 2005 national survey on drug use and health: national findings. Office of Applied Studies, NSDUH Series H-30, DHHS Publication No. SMA 06-4194. Rockville, MD

Thoits PA (1995) Stress, coping, and social support processes: Where are we? What next? J Health Soc Behav 35 (extra issue):53–79

Tjaden, Patricia, Nancy Thoennes (2000) Full report of the prevalence, incidence, and consequences of violence against women: findings from the national violence against women survey. Washington, DC: National Institute of Justice. Publication No. NCJ183781

Umberson D, Chen M, House J, Hopkins K, Slaten E (1996) The effect of social relationships on psychological well-being: are men and women really so different? Am Sociol Rev 61:837–857

Umberson D, Williams K (1999) Family status and mental health. In: Aneshensel C, Phelan J (eds) Handbook of the sociology of mental health. Springer, New York, pp 225–253

Larsen L (2004) The foreign-born population in the United States: 2003. Current population reports

Gibson C, Lennon E (1999) Historical census statistics on the foreign-born population of the United States: 1850–1990. Population division working paper no. 29

Üstün TB (2000) Cross-national epidemiology of depression and gender. J Gend Specif Med 3(2):54–58

Hout V, Hein PJ Aartjan, Beekman TF, De Beurs E, Comijs H, Van Marwijk H, De Haan M, Van Tilburg W, Deeg DJH (2004) Anxiety and the risk of death in older men. Br J Psychiatry 185:399–404

Vega WA, Amaro H (1994) Latino outlook: good health, uncertain prognosis. Annu Rev Public Health 15:39–67

Verbrugge LM (1985) Gender and health: an update on hypotheses and evidence. J Health Soc Behav 26:156–182

Verbrugge LM (1989) The Twain Meet: empirical explanations of sex differences in health and mortality. J Health Soc Behav 30:282–304

Walters V, McDonough P, Strohschein L (2002) The influence of work, household structure, and social, personal and material resources on gender differences in health: an analysis of the 1994 Canadian national population health survey. Soc Sci Med 54:677–692

Waters MC (1999) Immigrant dreams and American realities: the causes and consequences of the ethnic labor market in American cities. Work and Occup 26(3):352–364

Williams K (2003) Has the future of marriage arrived? A contemporary examination of gender, marriage, and psychological well-being. J Health Soc Behav 44:470–487

World Health Organization (2001) The world health report. Mental health: new understanding, new hope. http://www.who.int/whr/2001/en/. Accessed 5 June 2007

Chapter 22
Hearsay Ethnography: A Method for Learning About Responses to Health Interventions

Susan Cotts Watkins, Ann Swidler, and Crystal Biruk

Introduction

How can we know how health interventions – the dissemination of health knowledge and the promotion of behavior change – are received by the people whom our interventions address? In this paper, we describe a practical methodology that contributes to the project of studying collective meaning making as it unfolds and changes. By fixing episodes of public discourse as texts, rather than directly interrogating respondents in interviews or focus groups, conversational journals convey a sense of spontaneous issues that comprise the dynamic world of publicly available, collectively constituted meanings. While several theoretical traditions, from the Durkheimian to the symbolic-interactionist, posit such a dynamic public realm, few methods capture its texture.

At one extreme of research on health behaviors is survey research, collecting systematic data from a large sample representative of a defined population. At the other extreme is classical ethnography – full immersion in a field site, learning a language, coming to understand practices and institutions that first appeared strange, and then returning with a career's worth of field notes (Geertz 1973; Lindenbaum and Lock 1993; Scheper-Hughes 1992; Clifford and Marcus 1986). We introduce here a new research technique: asking members of local communities in rural Malawi to be our ears and eyes, observing, listening, and writing what they overheard in field journals that tell us about conversations in social networks from which outsiders are necessarily excluded. Our "hearsay ethnography" – invented originally as much by accident as by design – offers unique advantages over both traditional ethnography and over interview-based research approaches.

We focus on conversational interactions in order to capture more effectively the way meaning is produced and reproduced in everyday life, what the people health promoters aim to influence say to each other rather than to an outsider with a clipboard or a tape recorder. These interactions are transformed by cultural insiders into texts of who said what to whom. In the Geertzian sense, then, these texts, or collections of publically available cultural meanings, can be "read" to understand the manner in which health knowledge and behavior change discourses are taken up and incorporated into local systems of meaning. However, our approach views local Malawians, likely to be well enmeshed in Geertz' "webs of meaning," as active consumers and critics of these texts themselves. It also acknowledges that although meanings may be publically accessible, they are differentially accessible to insiders and outsiders, and differentially transmitted depending on, for example,

S.C. Watkins (✉)
Department of Sociology, University of Pennsylvania, 3718 Locust Walk,
McNeil Bldg., Ste. 113, Philadelphia, PA 19104-6299, USA
e-mail: scwatkins@gmail.com

whether the forum is an everyday conversation or a formal interview. Through hearsay ethnography, we can thus access health knowledge as it actually circulates: how the pro's and con's of behavior change are evaluated and debated, whether public health programs become part of the discussion, and what become authoritative resolutions.

The material here was gathered as part of a study of responses to the AIDS epidemic in Malawi, a very poor, largely rural country in southern Africa that is among those most ravaged by the epidemic. It is no accident that a new research approach emerged in a study of AIDS – both the epidemic and responses to it are shaped by social and cultural patterns that may be difficult for Western researchers to comprehend (Parker 2001). Through many journals, collected from multiple journalists in a wide variety of situations, we witness cultural understandings evolving, tacking back and forth, sometimes folding back on themselves or breaking down in confusion – but over time, even in the course of a single discussion, collective definitions have shifted. This observation is in agreement with the insights put forward by anthropologists and sociologists of science, who point out that knowledge is always partial, plural, and provisional, but that at any given moment there is agreement about some things (Schutz 1964; Crick 1982; Lambek 1993; Schmaus 1994; Longino 2002). At least in our setting, rural Malawi, and about an important issue like AIDS, which is problematic, frightening, salient, and challenging, people are not passive. Collectively and publicly, they dwell on the problem they face, piece together practical knowledge, gossip and authoritative opinion, to try to bring clarity, to construct a conversational and situational universe, and to map potential ways forward.

We argue that hearsay ethnography has three methodological advantages (as well as several practical ones): First, it provides data more authentically representative of local understandings than all other methods, including ethnography, that require the presence of an outsider.[1] This is especially valuable in places where people do not construct themselves as having "opinions" of the sort that pollsters ask about, and where their deference to those they see as more educated, urban, or cosmopolitan (or as potential sources of help) or their occasional desire to pull the leg of gullible outsiders may distort research interactions. Second, because our texts are records of ordinary conversation – including joking around, conversations on intimate issues among friends, and incidents from women's group meetings to barroom brawls – conversational journals show how culture is actually mobilized in natural social contexts (Swidler 2001; Eliasoph and Lichterman 2003). Third, and most important, hearsay ethnography makes visible what is *social* about social experience, thought, and culture.[2] Our method captures not what individuals think, even if one could, in principle, have complete, accurate access to their subjectivities (Wuthnow 1987). Rather it captures dynamic public discourse – the living reality of talk and dramatic incidents from the thick and thin of life – and thus tells us what goes on in the relational space between people. The practical advantages – that it takes in a much wider variety of people, places, and settings than even the most energetic ethnographer could do; that it records public dramas as well as casual conversation; that it permits local meta-commentary on public discourses instead of just documenting them; that it puts meat on the bare-bones notion of social networks; that compared both to ethnography and surveys it is relatively "cheap"; that the journalists already have local language and cultural knowledge; – will be addressed below.

---

[1] We are not the first to recruit "insiders" as research collaborators to avoid the distortions that come from local participants' interactions with outsiders. Williams and Kornblum (1985) had high school students keep diaries of their everyday lives to capture the texture of their daily experience. These moving documents convey the interior sense of life as it is lived by youth in poor neighborhoods with great poignancy; they do not attempt to capture the flow of public discussion. Power (1994) and Elliott et al. (2002) provide examples of the use of "indigenous fieldworkers" – current or former members of "covert communities" such as commercial sex workers or injecting drug users – recruited as "temporary research staff."

[2] See (Noelle-Neumann 1993) who explores how survey questions can capture this public aspect of public opinion. Focus groups are also meant to capture this collective property of cultural meanings (Gamson 1992). Some ethnographers, such as (Eliasoph 1998), give explicit attention to the group contexts in which public discussion occurs.

The Ethnographic Journals

In 1997, Watkins and several colleagues began a research project, the Malawi Diffusion and Ideational Change project (MDICP),[3] on the role of social networks in influencing responses to the AIDS epidemic in rural Malawi. Because the focus was demographic, the primary data they planned to collect would come from multiple waves of a survey, supplemented by semi-structured interviews. After the first round of the survey in 1998, the researchers had a great deal of data about the composition and structure of the social networks in which rural Malawians talked about AIDS. They had not, however, learned much about the content of the social interactions – what people said to each other about AIDS or their strategies for avoiding infection and death – and semi-structured interviews conducted in 1999 were disappointing. Unable to locate an anthropology (or sociology) graduate student willing to hang out and just listen to what people actually said in their social networks, the researchers improvised.

The researchers adapted classical ethnography to new purposes. They asked several high school graduates living in or near their study sites to be participant observers as they went about their daily routines. If they overheard anything concerning AIDS, they were to make mental notes of what people said and did, and then write their recollections in commonplace school notebooks that evening or soon thereafter (some include the exact time the ethnographer started writing, time off for a bath and dinner, several more hours before bed, then breakfast and writing again). The ethnographers wrote their journals in English, a language learned in high school; the handwriting and repetitions suggest they often wrote rapidly. Their notebooks were given to a local intermediary who mailed them to the researchers.

This approach depends on hearsay evidence: we hear only secondhand, through the journalists' ears. Although the "journalists" are relatively well-educated,[4] in rural Malawi many such people cannot find jobs in the modern sector. Rather, they live in villages, side-by-side with those who have no schooling, and engage in the same tasks as others – small-scale trading, tending their maize fields, attending their church, going to neighbors' funerals, and so forth. It will become obvious below that in places where only the fortunate few have battery-run television, where there is modest access to the radio, and where many are unemployed or spend long hours doing sometimes dull tasks – weaving palm mats, sitting all day in the market hoping to sell something, taking the bus from one town to another, washing clothes at the well – sociable conversation is a major source of interest in life.

What public health interview or survey could discover the myriad themes – revealed in the excerpt below – that roil the issue of condom use? The excerpt is long, in order to illustrate how one topic segues into another and how one argument is answered with another. As with the other excerpts in this paper, we use pseudonyms when proper names are mentioned and for the journalist; the journal is dated in year, month, and day format. In this excerpt, the journalist is on a bus going to a meeting of her Smallholder Marketing Action Group along with three other members of the group; the rest of the speakers are strangers. The bus has a breakdown, irritating the passengers. After complaining to the conductor, they debate whether it is better to die in an accident or from AIDS.

---

[3] The MDICP has conducted four surveys in rural Malawi (1998, 2001, 2004, 2006). The initial sample consisted of approximately 1,500 ever-married women and their husbands; in 2004, a sample of approximately 1,500 adolescents (aged 15–24) was added. Semi-structured interviews with randomly selected subsamples of the initial sample were also conducted. More detail is available at www.malawi.pop.upenn.edu.

[4] Few who go to school in rural Malawi attend high school, although men are more likely to do so than women. Those who complete high school hope for social mobility and thus try to leave the rural area for a city. Many who are unsuccessful in finding urban employment, like our journalists, remain in their village.

Someone who sat at the back seat added saying that the death by the Bus accident is the same as the death because of AIDS. The AIDS is better off because there are some things which one can use to protect himself or herself from being infected to it while an accident have no any protection. Once the accident has occurred, a person can die at the same spot. People began talking, everyone was speaking on what he or she wanted. Some people were speaking that the accident's death is better than the AIDS death.....

Mrs. Hajiri was among the people who were saying that it is better to die of Accident than die of AIDS. She said that if one has died at the same spot that the accident has done, [one] do[es] not feel any pain. He/she just dies. If any pain is there, it is just for a short time, but if you have been infected to the AIDS, it takes a long time for you to die. …. Mr. Chabwera said … but as far as I know, there is no anything which one can use to protect himself/herself from death. If the day has come for you to die, then you cannot do otherwise there. You have to die and you die, Mr. Chabwera said. Though many people are cheating themselves [fooling themselves] to use condoms in order to prevent themselves from death which can come because of AIDS, they just waste their time. The death will still come through other way round. God is very clever and nobody can compete with him. God has not vice or Deputy. If you don't be faithful to your Spouse you will die of AIDS. If you don't want to abstain from sex, you will die of AIDS. If you shall receive the unsterilized injection, you shall die of AIDS. If you [are] found sick and receive blood from the hospital, you shall die of AIDS. Many ways which can make one to suffer from AIDS and one can use condoms always when having sex but long at last, you can find that he/she has AIDS: Why? He also added that though he never used the condoms but he heard many people complaining that the condoms have some problems. When men use them they just see that the sores have come out and those sores itch and after some time, they began [to be] painful. Condoms cause other disease in addition to the AIDS disease. Those sores is also a disease because it causes itching and one feels painful. Unfortunately, nobody knows its kind of treatment unless you go to the hospital to explain about that problem.

When Mr. Chabwera finished speaking, the Bus Conductor who put on [wore] the Khaki short trousers and a Green T-shirt answered that AIDS is the dangerous disease because the only common way of being infected is through sex yet our God knows that there is that AIDS dangerous disease which can kill his people. He is the same God who created people and AIDS too because there is nobody who can create anything apart from God the great. God has an aim with us and that is why he is just looking on what is happening. His many people are passing away every day and many of them are sick. But still he is doing nothing. He would like to punish us but since everyone likes life, that is why we are trying to use the condoms always for protection. Using a condom is not a bad thing because it is the only way which we can save our lives. Since there is no any treatment that one can receive and get recovered from AIDS, then it is better to use the condoms which can protect our lives for some days before death.

Edah also put her comments on what the conductor said. She said that there is no good death or the bad death in the world. Both deaths by making an accident or getting sick for a long time is also the bad death. Death is death and no better death is in the world. She continued by saying the difference between the death because of AIDS and the death through accident. If one is sick, his/her relative know that one day, they will cry for their relative if he/she has shown the signs, while the one who dies of an accident cannot show the signs of anything but he/she stays normal and maybe a happy life. After some minutes or hours, people just see that they have made an accident. About the use [of] the condoms, Edah said that it is the good idea to use the condoms because the AIDS disease is very dangerous and many people are passing away every day because of AIDS and it has no treatment. If all the people in the country are not using the condoms, all the people will die of AIDS at a short time because they lack the knowledge and the lack of money for daily life. Many women are not married therefore they want to depend on men as their husbands though they are not their husbands. She also said that the use of condoms are very good though they encourage people in doing sex unnecessary and no matter they are causing problems like the sores our father Mr. Chabwera has said. It is better to suffer from sores than die of AIDS. If you use the condom and have sores, you can go to the hospital to explain and you can be helped by the Doctors while if you just have sex without any protection like condoms and be infected to AIDS, just know that the hospital can help you but you cannot get recovered until you die. Therefore it is good to use the condoms [rather] than having sex plain.

She stopped there because we reached at the roadblock and nobody continued speaking. (Alice 021025)

The Journals and the Journalists: How Good Are the Data?

More than 700 journals have been written since 1999. The current collection of diaries covers hundreds of distinct conversations, some overheard or witnessed by the journalists, others relayed to them through gossip. Since there are frequently several people conversing, we overhear, at second hand, thousands of people. The journalists' close networks, the ones in which they routinely spend most time, are homophilous, as are close networks elsewhere (McPherson et al. 2001), but many of the conversations they overhear have a very diverse cast of characters. For example, the most prolific of the female journalists is on many committees in her community and sometimes attends regional or national meetings of these groups, and many women, but also men, come to her for advice; the two most active male journalists spend much of their time hanging out in a nearby trading center, at the bus depot or at a bar, where there may be friends of friends or strangers. The male journalists write primarily about men's conversations, the women about women's, reflecting the gendered interaction typical of the communities in which they live (Marshall 1970).

Twenty-two journalists (9 females, 13 males) have contributed to our corpus of texts, with three (two males, one female) contributing very frequently, thirteen frequently, and six only occasionally. The diarists wrote in English, a language learned in school, and used parentheses or carets (< >) to set off their explanatory comments or untranslatable expressions in the local language. We have retained locutions that reflect local adaptations of English. English is taught in Malawian public schools starting in Standard 5, equivalent to US fifth grade, and has become somewhat indigenized. For example, to be sexually promiscuous is to be "movious" and one who has multiple partners is said to be "moving around," an Anglicization of a Chichewa expression, *woyendayenda*, derived from the earlier association of multiple partners with migrant labor. The naturalness with which the journalists adapt English to Chichewa, chiYao, or chiTumbuka linguistic forms means that their English is somewhat closer to local languages than is the standard English in which a Canadian, British, or American ethnographer might translate local languages. We have retained most of the idiosyncrasies in grammar and spelling, although on occasion we insert obviously missing words in brackets for greater legibility and make minor grammatical changes in the interest of legibility.

The journalists were paid US$30 for an 80-page school notebook; a typical notebook is about 10–12 typed single-spaced pages. The amount was deliberately set high relative to incomes in rural Malawi, as an incentive to continue with the project. The incentives raise the possibility of fakery. The journalists had worked for the MDICP as interviewers and shown themselves the most reliable, honest, thorough, and intelligent. But of course there is no way to know with absolute certainty whether the journals are honest and accurate. We have evaluated the journals in the light of other information (e.g., from the survey and the semi-structured interviews). In addition, because some of the more notorious characters in the area, such as the prostitute Miss Baidon, appear in the journals of more than one journalist, and some actors appear in more than one journal, we can examine internal and cross-journalist consistency. Most convincing, however, are the internal qualities of the journals. Kaler (2003) notes recurring themes in the journals, but the relative absence of clichéd situations and characters. We (and other readers of the journals) are struck by their quality of verisimilitude. While only extended excerpts from many journals could make this point fully convincing, it is evident as one reads these journals that only a writer as gifted as Chekov could have manufactured such a variety of voices, situations, incidents, and viewpoints. In fact, the sheer diversity of stories, characters, and experiences of the AIDS epidemic in Malawi found in the journals challenges international authoritative accounts of familiar figures such as the "grandparent-led family," the "orphan," or the "destitute widow" that color the pages of documents and reports.

A related concern is whether the pay motivates the journalists to seek out situations in which AIDS is likely to be discussed. No doubt this happens. Initially, the journalists produced journals at the rate of one or two a month, but their productivity increased, first after the poor harvest of 2001 and then dramatically with the famine of 2002 when grain prices rose by approximately 500% (Malawi National Vulnerability Assessment Committee 2002). The male journalists may indeed have begun going to the nearby trading center more often than they otherwise might, playing *bawo* or drinking at the local bar in hopes of hearing something for a journal. The female journalists tend mainly to report conversations that occur during their daily tasks – washing clothes at the borehole or walking to tend their gardens – or walking to or from the very frequent funerals. When journalists have sought to "pad" their journals, however, they have done things like report at numbing length on a village AIDS committee's informational meeting or reproduce nearly verbatim a pastor's sermon. We have not discouraged such tactics, feeling that it is better not to censor what the journalists write. But this increased output does not directly undermine the value of the evidence they give about where and when discussions of AIDS take place. In fact, these robust accounts may help us to better understand the complicated context rife with multiple circulating ideas and claims into which AIDS dialog and debate enters.

Agency and Action

Neither of the two "gold standards," survey research nor ethnography, can adequately capture the drama, the joking, the contradictions, and disagreements of everyday talk (Billig 1987; Swidler 2001). Surveys that ask about the characteristics of those with whom the respondents talk provide information that permits analyses of network structure and inferences about the causal impact of variations in that structure (Kohler et al. 2002. But even supplementing short-response survey questionnaires with semi-structured interviews provides only a very partial glimpse of what transpires in social interaction. For example, the excerpt below comes from the MDICP semi-structured interviews on informal conversations conducted in 1999. Although the area in which this interview took place is the same as one of the areas in which the conversational journals were produced, notice the inhibited, laconic answers, and the repetition of standard safe-sex slogans:

Interviewer: And right now there is this disease of AIDS, what do the people say about this disease?
Respondent: Aaah, what people say is that you should be holding your heart without doing any sexual intercourse with other women. That's why they say on that AIDS. Only holding the heart, be sure of your wife only.
Interviewer: And where did you hear this?
Respondent: Also this I heard on the radio.
Interviewer: Okey. Did you ever hear from your friends?
Respondent: Yes, they do talk.
Interviewer: What are they saying?
Respondent: They were saying that we [i.e. husbands] should be holding our hearts from these women, just believe in your wife because if you keep on going with other women, you will catch AIDS. (M 6504)[5]

This is far from the complex conversations we showed earlier, with the variety of gossip, detailed narrative, and the varied moral and practical concerns in which the narrative of AIDS is framed.

Why the difference? As Wendy Griswold (Griswold 1987) has argued in a paper on methods for studying culture, cultural artifacts are produced by agents implementing their agendas in contexts that constrain what they can accomplish. In our case, those producing AIDS talk are evaluating and debating information, entertaining their friends, seeking advice, and assessing potential actions, in pursuit of their own agendas, both collective and personal. They do so in a variety of quotidian contexts that offer constraints and possibilities, both real and imagined.

---

[5]This excerpt is identified by the survey identification number of the respondent.

It is this sense of purposive agendas, social performance, and evolving collective production that differentiates hearsay ethnography from the pallid interview above. In the semi-structured interviews conducted as part of the MDICP, even though the interviewers had unusual latitude in the order and wording of the questions, the interview setting itself elicited condensed and sanitized generalizations rather than the vivid, sometimes ribald, back and forth of actual talk. Focus groups are not much better. Rather than pursuing agendas that are part and parcel of everyday life, participants follow the agenda imposed by the researcher. These difficulties are exacerbated in Africa. Focus groups are meant to stimulate natural discussion and debate. But transcripts of focus groups, including our own, show that natural talk rarely happens. Rather, moderators and participants follow the model of classroom instruction in Malawi, with the moderator asking questions and the participants answering one at a time, deferring to rather than joking with the moderator. In addition, the focus groups produce, as do the semi-structured interviews, responses that conform to current messages of AIDS prevention distributed through the prevention bureaucracy. Finally, in a time when many rural Malawians are feeling the effects of "research fatigue" or have grown tired of participating in multiple research projects, it is important that researchers adapt their previously mundane, tired methods to more effectively capture the meat of everyday life.

Classical ethnography permits an outsider to overhear everyday conversation, but it has several disadvantages when compared with the method of hearsay ethnography. One problem is that village talk is likely to take a different turn when the anthropologist joins the conversation. As Philip Salzman (1999:96) notes, ethnography "gives us a good idea of what people will say to anthropologists, what pronouncements it pleases them to make, which self-image they wish to present to us, [but] we have little way of knowing what people will actually do, how they will act in their encounters in the real world." Salzman may be too dismissive. A very good ethnographer, one who learns local slang and learns to relish eating grasshoppers, who observes and participates in at least some local settings, and who focuses on trying to retain and record the details of conversational exchanges would be able to capture some of the dynamics of everyday chatting. But it is significant that even in excellent ethnographies one almost never finds the back and forth of everyday talk. There is a further disadvantage of classical ethnography when compared with our journalists' conversational diaries, and that is simply the volume of material and the variety of situations on which our journalists report. An anthropologist might be in Malawi many months or years and hear relatively few spontaneous discussion of matters like the advantages and disadvantages of condoms or gossip about which neighbor is "moving with" which girlfriend. These topics might be less likely to come up in the anthropologist's presence, or, more likely, she or he might only rarely be in the contexts where such matters are discussed. Only multiple ethnographers of varying ages, gender, and lifestyle situations could have access to the varied contexts from which our journalists report.

A major advantage of hearsay ethnography is that it reveals the natural contexts in which people discuss the issues that interest the researcher. AIDS comes up at the borehole where women draw water, at the market, in buses and jitneys, on the village path, in bars and *bawo* parlors, and in homes as well as more formal public settings like churches and village meetings. These places of sociability are, of course, far different from the artificial settings of survey interviews or focus groups. And whereas interviewers are trained to seek a private place where the respondents' views cannot be overheard by others, in the day-to-day life of rural Malawians, they both announce their views publicly and overhear the opinions of others, perhaps in turn relaying what they hear to yet others. Indeed, the Western emphasis on informed consent and privacy is puzzling: people are used to solving problems together and cannot imagine why, for example, a son or daughter would be expected or permitted to chat with an interviewer out of their earshot. Our ethical concerns as well as our conventional methods limit what we can learn about how knowledge is made and evaluated locally. But more important than the physical location of conversations is that they are social activities that have a multiplicity of uses: scandalous stories provide entertainment; a chance meeting at the borehole offers an opportunity to seek advice for a deeply personal concern; gossip about other villagers, or those known to other villagers, provides narratives of moral instruction; and a chat at a funeral may turn into a philosophical discussion.

Diagnosing AIDS Without a Blood Test

To illustrate what we learn from the journals about how knowledge circulates and is put to use, we examine a frequent activity in rural Malawi: speculating on the HIV status of relatives, friends, and neighbors who are ill or who have died. In rural Malawi, it was difficult to get a blood test for HIV until 2005, when the government expanded access to voluntary counseling and testing (VCT) to district hospitals and some smaller rural health facilities. Before that expansion, sick patients in a hospital or at an STD clinic might be tested for HIV for the benefit of the health care personnel, but VCT was available only in freestanding clinics in the two major cities (a long and expensive bus trip for most rural Malawians) or in special projects. Even now, most Malawians have not been tested for HIV. Whether or not a relative, friend, or neighbor is sick from, or has died from, AIDS is, however, a topic of intense interest. Many conversations in the journals feature "social autopsies," where individuals discuss or debate the AIDS status of people around them, often apparently with a view toward learning lessons that might be helpful in their own efforts to prevent infection.

Usually, the participants begin by invoking a series of physical symptoms they have "seen with their own eyes." Speakers rarely debate the legitimacy of the constellation of the symptoms presented as evidence for infection with AIDS; rather, when they debate it is about whether they agree that an individual under discussion is infected. This usually involves moving away from an initial focus on visible, physical symptoms and moving toward discussions of the "movements" of that person or his/her moral fiber. The main physical symptom of infection is weight loss or becoming thinner. Thus, weight loss is given a certain primacy in the act of social diagnosis; in other words, it is usually present when people reflect publicly on a person's AIDS status. Variations on observations of weight loss include the notion of a "weak body" or "a body like a child's." Other times, people are sure that someone has AIDS because he/she is wealthy and eats a "well-balanced diet" but still loses weight. In addition, diagnoses of AIDS may be made based on the presence of other physical symptoms such as sores on the body and particularly on the face. An interesting physical symptom that recurs throughout the journals is change of the quality or coarseness of hair or hair loss. In the presence of weight loss, a person who has this kind of hair or change in hair type is likely to be viewed as HIV-positive. This symptom is interesting because it is not one of the symptoms that health prevention experts use to diagnose AIDS. However, its repetition in conversation indicates that it has become a legitimate sign of AIDS locally.

Because rural Malawians know that the symptoms of AIDS may be symptomatic of other illnesses, they often proceed to pool what the participants in the conversation know about the medical history of the person: did he have a sexually transmitted infection? Was she treated for TB? Most significant, did he or she have an illness that was treated at the hospital, only to fall ill again within days or weeks. The pooled local knowledge can be quite detailed, including who saw the person at the STD clinic or who paid for the trip to the hospital. Again, however, participants know that although those with TB or an STD are particularly likely to be HIV positive, some with TB or gonorrhea are not.

In addition, diagnoses of AIDS may be made based on the presence of other physical symptoms such as sores on the body, and particularly on the face, but especially when the physical symptoms are confirmed by elements of the moral biography.

> My friend Robert said that the man is extremely thin .... Beata said that the man is sick and that certainly he is dying, ... his coughing and sores are the signs of his dying. ... Robert said that the coughing started a long time ago and even his sores, but that not every person who suffers coughing and develops sores is dying. "Dying from what?", I asked. Beata said, "Dying of AIDS, I know the man's behavior very well". Robert said, "What kind of behavior?" Beata said that even though the man has two wives ... he goes with other extramarital partners, and that he had met him several times at night when he was going to his sexual partner at Nawangwa Village, and that the woman whom he is running with, her husband has died after a long illness, and people who know about the death of her husband are afraid to have an affair with her because ... her husband died of AIDS... (Simon 030918)

Following most discussions of the physical or bodily status of some individual, speakers usually move to speculate upon their sexual behaviors or movements. This social information is usually used to bolster the interpretations mobilized regarding the particular constellation of physical symptoms exhibited by an individual.

> On the 13th June 2003, I went to Vingula to attend a funeral at the village of my friend Qualida. The man who died, Mr. Tingo, was the older brother of her aunt, her mother's older sister. ... He worked in South Africa[6] but his sister Qualida did not know the type of job that he'd had.
>
> Mr. Tingo stayed there for about five years without coming home to see his parents and his wife. ... When his friends came back from South Africa to see their parents, they told his parents and relatives that he had got married in South Africa and also had other partners apart from his wife and that what he was doing was very bad. ....
>
> Now this fifth year, Mr. Tingo came back from South Africa because he was very ill. ...he was very thin, he could not walk or sit down by himself. At that time he was opening his bowels and he was also coughing very much. He was sometimes vomiting if he started to cough. ...he died in the third week after he arrived. (Alice 030618)

In another excerpt from a different journalist, the moral biography is decisive:

> A lady was walking on the other side of the road. One of the men greeted her, saying "God is great for keeping us alive so that we should meet again today," and the lady replied, "God is wonderful, and the time has not yet come for us to die."
>
> Then a man told his friend who sat with him, "That lady is found everywhere. I used to see her at Mzuzu, Salima, Mchinji, Kasungu, Zomba, Mangochi, Blantyre, everywhere she was going to these places with different men. Those days she was fat. She had to fight off the men. But now she is becoming sick, and I am sure that she has taken this HIV because her body talks." But his friend said that he was wrong to say that she had got this HIV because nowadays everyone has it.
>
> But his friend said, "... I say that the lady has got AIDS because of how she moved, I have seen her. If someone wishes to sleep with her he should know that he is making his grave." (Anna 050330)

On other occasions, AIDS is inferred from a person's appearance in combination with whatever is known of his or her past, even if that does not include knowledge of sexual behavior.

> Today, Monday, I was at the trading centre and saw a man, he wore shorts and a dirty ragged shirt. He was about 28 years of age and was very thin indeed and had sores all over his body. His legs were so thin ... I wished that he had hidden them ...with long trousers. ...I stood at Mr. Zex's Tomato Bench. I was not buying anything, but was just chatting with Mr. Zex who sells tomatoes, onions, cabbage, ground nuts, pepper, eggplants, rice and other sorts of vegetables. ...
>
> Then I asked, "Where was he living before?" Mr. Zex answered, "The man used to live in Thyolo district where he was working on the tea estates, he migrated there a long time ago, probably when he was young,

---

[6] Malawian men have long traveled to South Africa to work in the mines.

> ...and I heard that he had married there and when his spouse died he only stayed a short period of time and then came back here. He came here last year in December and when he arrived his body was not healthy and I believe it's the same disease which he is suffering from."
>
> I asked, "What do you think the man is suffering from?" He said, "I think I already said that the man is suffering from nothing apart from AIDS".
>
> Then I asked, "Where did he contract it?" Mr. Zex said that where he contracted this AIDS nobody knows but himself. ...He said that probably it was on the tea estates ...He said that on the Thyolo estates ...the trees are always high and leafy and what often happens is that a man and a woman go far away from their fellow laborers for sexual intercourse and in these estates a lot of fornication happens. I exclaimed, "Indeed?" (Simon 030224)

As we can see, in most cases informal diagnoses of AIDS rest on tacit knowledge, the now taken-for-granted association of HIV and AIDS with promiscuous sexual behavior and a corresponding set of physical symptoms. In some cases, however, people rely less on the tacit nature of the knowledge they share and attribute its legitimacy or authority to some source. Usually, these sources include: the radio, gossip, and stories. For example, when one of the journalists asks his wife how she came to know that a male secondary school student is suffering from what she calls, "an unknown disease," she responds by citing the social chain through which she became privy to the information. Though this social chain may amount to little more than gossip or rumor, it grounds the piece of knowledge (that the school boy is infected with AIDS) in embodied individuals who know or live near to the boy:

> My wife said she learnt from her mother, who is the best friend of Mrs. Nkolokosa and she has been going to visit him to see him when he was sick. She went on saying that the patient was nearly about to die because (the wife went on saying that) her mother said that she heard from her friend Mrs. Nkolokosa saying that a patient was to die because one day the patient called/summoned his Father. (Simon 030129)

In another case, a friend of the journalist asks a man how he came to know for sure that some members of a family died of AIDS. The excerpt highlighting this exchange is below. It is notable that Tingo legitimizes the knowledge by suggesting that it is something that is taken for granted or well known in Dausi village where he stays:

> Kili asked him from where he learned this information. Tingo said that he knows about this since the late [parents] were living in Dausi village and he also stays in Dausi village and the rumor is well known to many people within the village and outside the village and everyone knows that the man and his wife had died of AIDS in the way he was suffering together with his wife he said that anyone contracted AIDS is well noticed because of his or her health status becomes very unpleasant and he said that even you can see the way the young girl is looking. (Simon 030707)

The "Domestication" of Offical Aids Information

Malawians are very aware that they have been bombarded by official information about HIV and AIDS. Sometimes – as in the early years with condom messages – they remain skeptical, but they also often express the view that anyone who does not understand what AIDS is, how one contracts it, and how one could prevent it, is a fool, or as they often say, intentionally courted death.

People attribute knowledge they have about AIDS to sources like billboards, or the radio, and the MDICP project itself. Certainly, many reflect on their bombardment with AIDS messages and information. In a conversation among young men who speculate about their chances with a group of young women, one youth says, "but you guys we are receiving HIV/AIDS messages almost, every day through radios, newspapers, drama groups, political leaders, medical personnel, chiefs and the like even research teams like LET'S CHAT team yearly they come in Black T-shirts but you cannot take a lesson." (Daniel 050305) He cites this as one justification for the claim that anyone who does not know about AIDS or change his behavior is an idiot.

> Rafiyasi said that when one comes to suffer diseases like *chizonono, chindoko, mabomu* just know that it's likely the person has also AIDS, because even the radio also announces about this. (Simon 030206)

Also notable are the instances in which individuals compare one kind of knowledge to another or note possible discrepancies between two epistemologies for recognizing AIDS. For example, persons frequently use the phrase, "I am not a doctor" before making a claim about the serostatus of some individual. Below, a man acknowledges that because he is not a doctor, he may not be able to conclusively state that a man under question is infected, but he suggests that the knowledge he has regarding this matter is sufficient for him. He has heard the man refer to the large number of women he slept with "plain":

> And that he has AIDS, I believe he has indeed, even though I am not a doctor. But you heard yourself that even a Zasintha Bus can be filled by the ladies with whom he has slept plain [no condom] always. (Simon 020613)

Another example, in a discussion of a group of prostitutes:

> "What do you think is the purpose or reason why their body status has greatly and completely changed as you say?" Lawrence answered saying, "Nothing, apart from AIDS, definitely. Even though I am not a doctor that has examined them, but I absolutely believe that it's AIDS. They have this disease in their bodies because indeed they were the sex lovers and great prostitutes. They used to have several sexual partners and the partners were only the rich and not the poor." (Simon 020730)

In short, then, the kind of diagnosis we see in the journals is a social process. Part of the ability to make a diagnosis of AIDS rests on convincing those around you that the foundation for your diagnosis is a good one. In the series of excerpts presented here, we note a few ways in which speakers legitimatize or make their knowledge authoritative: attribution to sources such as radio, attribution to social chains or familiarity with local context, and a generalized tacit knowledge, or reference to facts or information that is so prevalent that it need not be elaborated upon. In this way, speakers are able to make diagnoses of individuals' serostatus without a blood test. Nonetheless, despite the absence of scientific evidence of infection, much of the speculation in the journals suggest that rural Malawians find their way of diagnosing those around them to be useful, generally correct and reliable regarding AIDS.

Aids in Malawi: Misconceptions that Matter

The international AIDS prevention community has identified several knowledge questions that it considers important that those at risk of HIV infection be able to answer correctly (WHO 2004:38). Those who claim that people need more correct information typically point to relatively high proportions of survey respondents who, when asked whether HIV can be transmitted by mosquitoes or by sharing plates, say Yes. The other indicators do not believe that condom use and fidelity can reduce HIV risk and that a healthy-looking person can still be infected. These are then considered "misconceptions" that need the attention of programs. The contrast between what respondents say on a survey and what they say to each other is illuminating: in the hundreds of social autopsies in our journals, it is extremely rare that mosquitoes or sharing plates are mentioned as a source of infection. Perhaps in their role as respondents, people think that it is theoretically possible that HIV can be transmitted by mosquitoes or sharing plates, but when they are in their natural settings and engaged in trying to figure out why a particular person they know has died of AIDS, these "misconceptions" are never used as an explanation. The social autopsies, as well as other types of conversations in the journals, do, however, expose fundamental misconceptions about the epidemiology of HIV, misconceptions that are not tracked by the WHO or used as Millennium Development Goals. In particular, rural Malawians vastly overestimate the transmission probabilities of HIV, and they drastically underestimate the time from infection with HIV to the appearance of the symptoms of AIDS. These misconceptions matter for local strategies of HIV prevention.

A critical misconception (partly created by the deluge of public health warnings) concerns how easily HIV is transmitted through sex. While the actual risk of infection from a single act of sexual intercourse is 1/1,000 or less (Gray, Wawer, Brookmeyer et al. 2001),[7] most Malawians have been led to believe that HIV is easily transmitted. In several MDICP surveys, respondents were asked how likely it was that one act of sexual intercourse with an HIV infected person would lead to infection for the other partner. Over 95% said the probability of transmission was either certain or highly likely. Since husbands and wives are expected to be having intercourse, it is not surprising that Malawians strongly believe that if a husband is infected then so must his wife be, and vice versa.

> She said, "Yes, indeed, people say that lying together is dying together. If he has HIV/AIDS, I have HIV/AIDS, but I know that we don't have it."
>
> And I asked, "How do you know? Did you go for a blood test?"
>
> She said, "I know myself and he told me one day that he doesn't have HIV/AIDS. He went for a blood test and found that he doesn't have it." (Simon 020319)

The belief that if one spouse is infected it is inevitable that the other is as well leads to considerable puzzlement when one dies, supposedly of AIDS, but the other survives.

> Miss Tinenenji said that she does not believe that her husband died of AIDS.
>
> During the time that Mr. Eliasi was ill, many people said that he had AIDS since he had several sexual partners. Women did not refuse Mr. Eliasi because he had money and when people said he was suffering from AIDS, she believed them. When his illness became serious, she took him to the hospital where VCT was done on him and the results were that he was HIV positive.
>
> The doctors at the hospital tried to save his life but failed. It is now almost seven years since Mr. Eliasi died but Miss Tinenenji does not show any signs that she has HIV. She said that if her husband was HIV positive she should be HIV positive as well because they slept together, having sex without ever using a condom (Alice 041124)

Kaler (2004) has written of the "fatalism" that, especially earlier in the epidemic, often entered conversations about AIDS. A terrible plague (*mlili* in Chichewa, the term for the Biblical plagues), AIDS was sometimes seen as inevitable: "AIDS is for people not for chickens," or as one man said, "Everyone will dies of AIDS because no one can resist sex either with a wife or other sexual partners" (Simon 030125). It turns out that actual fatalism is rare and becoming rarer, and people are actively trying to find ways to avoid infection with AIDS (Watkins 2004). On the other hand, their attempts to avoid infection are hampered by their belief in the perfect

---

[7] Following a study of monogamous, heterosexual discordant couples in Rakai, Uganda, Gray et al. (2001) estimate the overall probability of transmission per coital act was 0.0011. It is important to remember the transmission rate of HIV varies; some factors proposed to effect the variance in rate of transmission include: presence of sexually transmitted infections, male circumcision, and viral load of the HIV-positive individual. For example, a study of men who had acquired a sexually transmitted disease from a group of prostitutes with a prevalence of HIV infection of 85% found an overall cumulative HIV transmission rate of 0.03 Cameron et al. (1989). Still, the estimated rate from the Cameron et al. (1989) study is much lower than that estimated by respondents in the MDICP.

transmissibility of HIV. As one young man says when his friends urge him to break up with an unfaithful girlfriend:

> He went on speaking that since he had been sleeping with her for a long time and moreover plain sex, then there is no need that he can divorce her for if it is the matter of AIDS disease then he had already contracted it and how can he avoid AIDS and if she has it it means he had it.... (Simon 040130)

Malawians tend to assume that if one has had sex even once with someone who is already infected, then one is infected as well: "Lie together, die together." Thus, when a young man says, after his first sexual encounter with a young woman who he hopes will be his "real girlfriend," that "Indeed, friend, if Grace has AIDS, she has given it to me, I couldn't resist her attractions." (Simon July 8–10 2001) He is spontaneously offering a serious AIDS "misconception."

The second consequential misconception, seen frequently in the social autopsies, is a telescoping of the time between risky sexual behavior and the visible symptoms of AIDS. Hence, although people know and sometimes say spontaneously that a person can be infected with the AIDS virus and still look healthy, they often also attribute the illness to behavior that happened only a year or two before, or they insist that if someone really looks fat, she or he cannot be infected.

The central message of HIV prevention programs has been to practice the ABCs: abstinence before marriage, behave faithfully after, and, when that is not possible, use condoms consistently. The journals show that virtually all in rural Malawians know that these are effective measures of prevention. They also show, however, that for many the ABCs are considered unattainable or undesirable. They are unattainable because humans naturally want sex. They are undesirable because strictly following the ABCs would take away much of the pleasure of life. Thus, in conversations in their social networks, participants rework the strict ABCs into more flexible rules for sexual behavior, as well as discussing other strategies of prevention that are not on the international prevention agenda. Currently, local Malawian modifications of the ABCs are to reduce the number of partners, both premarital and extramarital, and to select these fewer partners with greater care by drawing on local knowledge of a prospective partner's medical history and sexual biography. The journals also expose local strategies of prevention that are not mentioned among the recommendations of the international prevention community. One of these is to divorce a spouse whose behavior threatens "to bring AIDS into the family"; a second is to turn to religion for support in resisting the temptations of multiple sexual partners.

Although these strategies of prevention are not perfect, when practiced by many they could reduce the incidence of new infections. It is surely better to avoid selecting a partner whose husband died of AIDS than to select a partner in ignorance of that local knowledge; similarly, a woman who is uninfected but worried because her husband is promiscuous might avoid infection by divorcing him. Yet these strategies, we believe, are likely to be more effective if rural Malawians have correct knowledge of the transmission probabilities of HIV and the duration from infection to symptoms. If joint testing were to become a routine precursor to initiating a sexual relationship, there might be no need to speculate about a potential partner's HIV status.[8] Since it is not, it would be better were the speculation grounded in what is scientifically known about the epidemiology of HIV. As it is, their misconceptions also put Malawians at risk as they try to navigate the epidemic (Watkins 2004) by deciding who might be a safe sexual partner and when to break off a relationship or divorce as a way to avoid infection (Reniers 2008). Additionally, a key current prevention approach, the promotion of VCT to learn one's status, is hindered by the misconception that "to lie together is to die together": in conversations about the advantages and disadvantages of VCT, a major reason given for not seeking testing is "There is no need, I know I must be infected." The apparent discordance

---

[8] The "window period" after a person is first infected, when viral load is very high but antibodies have not yet developed, makes even joint HIV testing less-than-perfect protection. See Epstein (2007).

between the kinds of misconceptions organizations like WHO are trying to address and those we found circulating in everyday conversation are clear, and we suggest that hearsay ethnography is one method by which researchers may be more likely to come across the actual motivations, ideas, and claims that affect AIDS-related behaviors in local Malawian settings.

Conclusions

As a method, conversational journals allow sociologists and health researchers access to spontaneous uses of health information by real people, on the ground, trying to harness their own understandings to protect themselves from a terrible disease. This method shows how health information can be integrated with local knowledge through local social processes and relations to become real in people's everyday decisions about their lives; and it can also reveal misunderstandings – often created by the international public health community itself – that can actually hinder local people's ability to take effective steps to avoid illness and death.

References

Billig M (1987) Arguing and thinking: a rhetorical approach to social psychology. Cambridge University Press, Cambridge, England

Cameron D, Simonsen J, D'Costa L, Ronald A, Maitha G, Gakinya M, Cheang M, Ndinya-Achola J, Piot P, Brunham R et al (1989) Female to male transmission of human immunodeficiency virus type 1: risk factors for seroconversion in men. Lancet 2:403–7

Clifford J, Marcus GE (eds) (1986) Writing culture: the poetics and politics of ethnography. University of California Press, Berkeley, CA

Crick MR (1982) Anthropology of knowledge. Annual Review of Anthropology 11:287–313

Eliasoph N (1998) Avoiding politics: how Americans produce apathy in everyday life. Cambridge University Press, Cambridge, England

Eliasoph N, Lichterman P (2003) Culture in interaction. American Journal of Sociology 108(4):735–794

Elliott E, Watson AJ, Harries U (2002) Harnessing expertise: involving peer interviewers in qualitative research with hard-to-reach populations. Health Expectations 5(2):172–178

Epstein H (2007) The invisible cure: Africa, the West, and the fight against AIDS. Farrar, Straus and Giroux, New York

Gamson WA (1992) Talking politics. Cambridge University Press, Cambridge, England

Geertz C (1973) The interpretation of cultures. Basic Books, New York

Gray RH, Wawer MJ, Brookmeyer R et al (2001) Probability of HIV-1 transmission per coital act in monogamous, heterosexual, HIV-discordant couples in Rakai, Uganda. The Lancet 357:1149–1153

Griswold W (1987) A methodological framework for the sociology of culture. Sociological Methodology 17:1–35

Kaler A (2003) My girlfriends could fill a Yanu-Yanu bus: rural Malawian men's claims about their own serostatus. Demographic Research Special Collection 1(11):349–372

Kaler A (2004) AIDS-talk in everyday life: the presence of HIV/AIDS in men's informal conversation in Southern Malawi. Social Science & Medicine 59:285–297

Kohler, Hans-Peter, Jere Behrman, Susan Cotts Watkins (2002) Social network influences and AIDS risk perceptions: tackling the causality problem. Paper presented at the annual meeting of the Population Association of America, Atlanta, GA, 9–11 May

Lambek M (1993) Knowledge and practice in Mayotte: local discourses of Islam, sorcery, and spirit possession. University of Toronto Press, Toronto

Lindenbaum S, Lock M (eds) (1993) Knowledge, power, and practice: the anthropology of medicine and everyday life. University of California Press, Berkeley, CA

Longino H (2002) The fate of knowledge. Princeton University Press, Princeton, NJ

Malawi National Vulnerability Assessment Committee (2002) Malawi: emergency food security assessment report. Malawi Vulnerability Assessment Committee and SADC FANR Vulnerability Assessment Committee, Lilongwe, Malawi

Marshall G (1970) In a world of women: field work in a Yoruba community. In: Goode P (ed) Women in the field. Aldine, Chicago, IL, pp 165–191

McPherson M, Smith-Lovin L, Cook J (2001) Birds of a feather: homophily in social networks. Annual Review of Sociology 27:415–444

Noelle-Neumann E (1993) The spiral of silence: public opinion – our social skin. University of Chicago Press, Chicago, IL

Parker R (2001) Sexuality, culture, and power in HIV/AIDS research. Annual Review of Anthropology 30:163–179

Power R (1994) Some methodological and practical implications of employing drug users as indigenous fieldworkers. In: Boulton M (ed) Challenge and innovation: methodological advances in social research on HIV/AIDS. Taylor & Francis, London, pp 97–111

Reniers G (2008) Marital strategies for regulating exposure to HIV. Demography 45(2):417–38

Scheper-Hughes N (1992) Death without weeping: the violence of everyday life in Brazil. University of California Press, Berkeley, CA

Schmaus W (1994) Durkheim's philosophy of science in the sociology of knowledge: creating an intellectual niche. Chicago University Press, Chicago, IL

Schutz A (1964) The well informed citizen: an essay on the social distribution of knowledge. In: Brodersen A (ed) Collected papers II: studies in social theory. Martinus, The Hague

Swidler A (2001) Talk of love: how culture matters. University of Chicago Press, Chicago, IL

Watkins SC (2004) Navigating the HIV/AIDS epidemic in rural Malawi. Population and Development Review 30(4):673–705

Williams TM, Kornblum W (1985) Growing up poor. Lexington Books, Lexington, MA

World Health Organization (2004) National AIDS programmes: a guide to indicators for monitoring and evaluating national HIV/AIDS prevention programmes for young people. World Health Organization, Geneva, Switzerland

Wuthnow R (1987) Meaning and moral order: explorations in cultural analysis. University of California Press, Berkeley,CA

Part VI
Connecting to Dynamics: The Health and Illness Career

Chapter 23
Life Course Approaches to Health, Illness and Healing

Eliza K. Pavalko and Andrea E. Willson

The life course perspective provides a theoretical framework, concepts, and analytical tools for examining how individual lives unfold in historical and institutional contexts. Nearly a half century ago, C. Wright Mills described the task and promise of the sociological imagination as the ability to "grasp history and biography and the relations between the two" (Mills 1959: 6). In the intervening decades since Mills' plea for the sociological imagination, life course scholars have illuminated both the challenge and promise of this endeavor, focusing on the importance of a dynamic view of individuals and their social contexts. The growth of a wide array of large, longitudinal data collections and the increasing availability of a wide range of statistical tools for longitudinal analysis have made attention to the dynamics of lives in context increasingly possible. In turn, interest in innovative methodologies and the availability of large, national data sets that focus on particular life stages, such as adolescence, midlife, or later life, have encouraged more scholars to incorporate elements of life course perspective in their research.

In many respects, scholars interested in health, illness, and healing are at the forefront of these endeavors as they increasingly frame research questions about health within the context of particular life stages, examine effects of early life events on later health outcomes, and explore dynamic pathways of health and health correlates across the life course. The rapid growth in attention to life course concepts in health research has moved from being a specialized perspective applied to a specific set of topics to a core framework that defines a wide range of research questions.[1]

While health scholars have embraced and enlightened many aspects of the life course perspective, there are other dimensions of this perspective that have remained underutilized in framing questions about health, illness, and healing. We contend that these neglected areas of the life course perspective can raise new questions and offer new insights into enduring questions about health, illness, and healing. In this chapter, we discuss two areas central to the life course perspective that have been underdeveloped in health research and explore some of the unique contributions that these dimensions of the life course perspective can bring to our understanding of health illness and healing. The first neglected area we will discuss is the life course perspective's emphasis on indi-

---

[1]For example, comparing the content of articles published in the *Journal of Health and Social Behavior* from 1986 to 2006, in 1986 none of the 28 articles published referred to the life course in the title or abstract and only four referred to life course concepts in either the title or the abstract. In contrast, 4 of the 28 articles published in 2006 mentioned the life course perspective explicitly in the title or abstract, and 11 (or nearly 40%) invoked key life course concepts such as timing, sequencing, life transitions, age/cohort analyses, or specific life stages.

E.K. Pavalko (✉)
Department of Sociology, Indiana University, Ballantine 744, Bloomington, IN 47405, USA
e-mail: epavalko@indiana.edu

vidual agency within constraints. The second neglected area is attention to intersections between historical and institutional change with life trajectories.

Before turning to these neglected areas of study, we first review key elements of the life course perspective, including attention to variation in North American and European approaches to the life course (Marshall and Mueller 2003). Next we review several emerging areas where attention to the life course perspective is already broadening our understanding of health and illness. We then turn to neglected areas and suggest the types of questions that might be raised when these elements of the life course perspective are taken seriously. We close with discussion of the challenges of taking these issues seriously and ways that health researchers might overcome these challenges.

Basic Principles of the Life Course Perspective

The life course perspective has been informed by a wide range of disciplines ranging from sociology and demography to history and human development. As scholars from these disparate perspectives have elaborated various life course themes, it has, at times, been difficult to clearly identify what is, or is not, within the domain of this perspective. In response to this growing interest in the life course, Glen Elder (Elder et al. 2003) has specified a systematic set of life course principles that are central to the study of social change and individual lives. Elder has developed these principles from his long and influential program of research on the life course. As noted by Marshall and Mueller (2003), Elder's approach reflects a North American approach to the life course. While there is substantial overlap, Western European approaches to the life course perspective tend to differ from those in North America, and these differences are instructive. We thus begin by discussing each of Elder's principles and then consider differences between North American and Western European uses of the life course perspective.

Principle #1: Human Development and Aging are Life-Long Processes

While individuals face unique challenges and opportunities at different points in the life course, one of the major contributions of the life course perspective has been to shift attention to connections and pathways across the life course. For health researchers, the recognition that biological, intellectual, and social developments are not just occurring in childhood and that experiences in later life are shaped by a life time of opportunities and constraints has generated a wide range of new questions about patterns and pathways across the life course, which life course patterns are most salient for health, and the mechanisms underlying the unfolding of those patterns.

Recent research documenting the connections between early and later life health (Blackwell et al. 2001; Hayward and Gorman 2004) and the impact of poverty or mental health problems on educational attainment and the transition to adulthood (Guo 1998; McLeod and Kaiser 2004) illustrates the importance of looking beyond temporally proximate influences to consider more distal processes. Likewise, questions about when advantage and disadvantage accumulate and when disparities are stable or decline across the life course offer new insights into the production of health disparities (DiPrete and Eirich 2006; Dupre 2007; Guo 1998; McLeod and Kaiser 2004; Willson et al. 2007).

Principle #2: The Antecedents and Consequences of Life Transitions, Events Vary According to Their Timing in a Person's Life

A natural extension of attention to dynamic processes is the recognition that the meaning of an event differs depending on when it falls within the life course. The timing of an event may be important because of where it falls relative to biological or psychological development, because it affects other age-graded roles (such as school completion, or retirement), or because of normative expectations about the correct time for events to occur. For example, the optimal age to become a parent in the USA falls roughly in the 20s (Mirowsky 2002). Those becoming parents earlier than this optimal age face interruptions in schooling and restricted investment in career development while those who become parents after this optimal age face greater risks of physical health problems. Norms about the correct timing for parenthood and other life events also exist to varying degrees across different racial/ethnic groups and persons may experience negative consequences if they violate these norms (Jackson 2004; Neugarten et al. 1965).

Principle #3: Lives are Lived Interdependently and Sociohistorical Influences are Expressed Through This Network of Shared Relationships

The life course perspective is not alone in its emphasis on the interdependence of each person's life with others, but it does offer unique insights into the dynamic interplay between the lives of significant others. For example, attention to the coupling of careers illustrates how career patterns and decisions such as retirement are often coordinated between spouses or partners and are often contingent on earlier work and family trajectories. Women's decisions about retirement are particularly likely to be shaped by the timing of the spouse's retirement as well as prior history of combining work and family (Han and Moen 1999; Henretta et al. 1993).

Health events clearly illustrate the interconnectedness of lives, the ways that an event in one person's life impacts others, and how these interconnections may play out over time. For example, when an individual has a serious health event they may need to leave the labor force or stop working for a period of time but the effects of that health event also spill over to the work decisions of other family members. Women, in particular, are likely to assume care of ill of disabled family members and are at increased risk of leaving the labor force and experiencing their own health decline when they do so (Dentinger and Clarkberg 2002; Pavalko and Artis 1997; Pavalko and Woodbury 2000). The effects of caregiving extend far beyond the period of time when care is provided, increasing the risk of poverty in later life (Kingson and O'Grady-LeShane 1993; Wakabayashi and Donato 2006), thus also increasing risk of future health problems.

Principle #4: The Life Course of Individuals is Embedded in and Shaped by the Historical Times and Places They Experience over Their Lifetime

Each birth cohort experiences historical events at a distinct point in their life course, thus creating unique experiences for each cohort that differ from those in other cohorts. This basic demographic fact provides a powerful engine of social change, because it means the same historical events will be experienced differently by different birth cohorts and that each cohort will experience a unique combination of events in their life time (Ryder 1965). Cohort differences will be particularly sharp when timing effects are strongest. For example, attitudes are malleable in late adolescence and young adulthood and then stabilize as individuals settle into work and family roles (Alwin et al. 1991; Alwin and McCammon 2003). This impressionable period in the life course can create unique cohort perspectives because each cohort encounters influential historical events at different points in their life course.

Given the rapid and widespread change in health care institutions, ranging from the current scaling back of national health insurance in Great Britain (Armstrong 1998), the rise of managed care (Scott et al. 2000; Wholey and Burns 2000), and the transformation of mental health care from institution to community (Grob 1994; Mechanic 1989), there are numerous ways that our understanding of health, illness, and healing may be better informed by attention to the ways that historical and institutional change. We will return to elaborate this issue later.

Principle #5: Individuals Construct Their Own Life Course Through the Choices and Actions They Take Within the Opportunities and Constraints of History and Social Circumstance

Given that the emphasis of many life course studies is on transitions and trajectories across individual lives, it is surprising that there is not greater attention to the choices, decisions and motivations behind these paths (but see Clausen 1993; Hagan 2001). However, an even greater challenge is simultaneously illuminating these choices and decisions and their boundedness within social structures, or what some refer to as agency within constraints. The life course perspective offers two avenues for incorporating agency within constraints into our understanding of health, illness, and healing. Instead of framing questions in terms of causation *or* selection, the life course perspective focuses our attention on the dynamic interplay of the two (George 2007). Second, attention to lives in historical and institutional contexts focuses our attention on variation, not only in outcomes but also in opportunities and constraints surrounding the choices individuals have available to them. We will further elaborate these potential contributions below.

Insights from European Approaches to the Life Course

Although the North American approach to the life course recognizes the importance of institutional structures in the life course, European models have tended to give more explicit attention to the role of institutions and structures in the life course (Leisering and Schumann 2003; Marshall and Mueller 2003). Marshall and Mueller (2003) argue that one reason for this difference may be the tendency for North American life course scholars to take a structural–functionalist approach defining structure by status positions and roles, while many European scholars invoke a more concrete and institutionally based concept of structure. The prominent role of the welfare state in many European nations and the dramatic change in state structures in countries such as Germany may also have contributed to the greater attention to the state and institutions in European life course research (Leisering and Schumann 2003). Regardless of the reasons for the difference, European theorizing and research on the life course provides numerous examples of the ways institutions regulate individual lives (e.g., Heinz and Marshall 2003; Leisering and Schumann 2003; Mayer and Schoepflin 1989; Schaeper and Falk 2003).

Medical institutions and the state play a key role in the regulation of health at all stages of the life course. In addition to defining who does or does not have access to care, institutions define what is or is not an illness (Conrad 1992), which problems have the highest priority for treatment and research, and how inequities that serve as fundamental causes of disease are tackled. Our understanding of these types of connections between institutions and individual health has been limited, but as we argue below, it is a critical area for future research for health scholars wishing to take the life course seriously. Before elaborating on this point below, we now review several areas of research where the life course is expanding our understanding of health, illness, and healing.

Emerging Life Course Contributions to Health, Illness, and Healing

In this section, we review examples of the current and emerging approaches to studying health from a life course perspective. Our review of this burgeoning field is by no means comprehensive or exhaustive, but it does reflect a core theme running through much of the current work in this area – attention to dynamic health processes across the life course. In particular, recent life course studies of health share a focus on the long-term processes that affect health over the life course and attention to changing circumstances over the life cycle. Much of this work seeks to understand the emergence of physical and mental health disparities, and as a result places a strong emphasis on the dynamic interplay of health with status characteristics such as socioeconomic status, gender, and race/ethnicity (McDonough and Berglund 2003).

Emerging research on health from a life course perspective is demanding methodologically and has been aided by recent statistical innovations and data collections. Research in this area is generally quantitative, data intensive, and technically sophisticated. The life course perspective's emphasis on long-term patterns, combined with the availability of longitudinal data sets that now cover substantial portions of the life course and advances in methodological techniques, has led to a proliferation of studies examining trajectories of dynamics such as individual change over time and important inter-individual differences in change over the life course. For example, growth curve models allow researchers to examine how factors such as the experience of long-term economic advantage or disadvantage, as well as individual characteristics such as race/ethnicity and gender, affect health and well-being. In one of the earliest examples of growth curve modeling in health research, Maddox and Clark (1992) examined age-related trajectories of functional impairment in a cohort of employed older adults just prior to retirement, finding variation in functional impairment and differences in both initial levels of impairment and subsequent trajectories of impairment. Patterns varied considerably by age, sex, economic status, and educational attainment, and their research pointed to the limitations in making broad generalizations about the degree and trajectories of impairment among older adults. In a recent examination of age growth trajectories in depression among older adults, Yang (2007) found that increases in depression with age were explained by life course events such as health decline, widowhood, economic hardship, and negative life events, demonstrating the importance of distinguishing between age and cohort effects in understanding depression. Yang's research advances the literature on age and depression through its focus on disentangling the confounding effects of age changes and cohort differences.

The life course perspective draws attention to cumulative processes that create variation in life trajectories such as health and economic status, and the majority of studies on health from a life course perspective in some way addresses this process. Cumulative advantage/disadvantage theory (CAD) explains a process through which early advantages and disadvantages become compounded over the life course, leading to greater intracohort inequality at the oldest ages (Dannefer 1987, 2003; Merton 1968; O'Rand and Hamil-Luker 2005). Within the CAD framework, inequality grows with age as the result of the accumulation of social and personal resources, human capital, and economic returns to education in the form of income and wealth (DiPrete and Eirich 2006; O'Rand 2001). In sum, in its most basic form, cumulative advantage suggests that early advantage continues to grow over time, conceptualized in terms of increasing returns to resources, such as education, and increases in intracohort inequality.

Used initially to explain variation in scientific careers and then later labor market inequalities by age (e.g., Dannefer 1987, 1988; Kerckhoff 1993; Merton 1968; O'Rand 1996), more recently researchers have begun using this theory to address the accumulating effects of socioeconomic and other resources over time on later life health. Although much of the literature can be characterized as motivated by CAD questions, studies take several different approaches. In a recent review of the CAD literature, DiPrete and Eirich (2006) identified a number of conceptual distinctions regarding cumulative advantage as a mechanism generating inequality across the life course. Although most studies address some combination of concepts, these distinctions can be identified in the health literature.

One strand of CAD research specifies a process whereby a prior state influences one's current state and has both direct and indirect long-term consequences (DiPrete and Eirich 2006). These studies link early life conditions to later life health and well-being, typically the relationship of early childhood diseases or hardships associated with low SES to mid- and later life outcomes. Numerous studies have demonstrated enduring effects of early life experiences on later life outcomes through both direct and indirect mechanisms that link childhood conditions to the health of adults, as well as direct effects of adult conditions. For example, Hayward and Gorman (2004) examine the effects of social conditions in early life on later life mortality and find that early disadvantage sets in motion are a series of "cascading socioeconomic and lifestyle events" that have negative long-term consequences for adult health. Using retrospective data on childhood economic hardship experienced by respondents now in old age, Kahn and Pearlin (2006) find that chronic economic strains have effects that are independent of current financial strain and income, and that the duration of strains is more important to well-being than their timing. And in their research on pathways between early environment and heart attack risk across the life course, O'Rand and Hamil-Luker (2005) find that early disadvantage leads to later disadvantage and an increasing difficulty managing and responding to new insults to health. These studies demonstrate that histories of hardship have enduring effects on well-being over time and the importance recognizing continuity and change in the dynamic relationship between social circumstances and health.

Other studies in this vein focus on the life course concept of *duration* to model the direct effects that long-term exposure to a particular status or state, such as the persistence and duration of poverty, may have on the rate of the accumulation process. The long-term processes examined in this conceptualization of CAD create extensive data requirements, and therefore relatively little empirical attention has been give to this area. One of the few examples is Kelley-Moore and Ferraro's (2004) analysis of the cumulative disadvantage of obesity across the life course from which they conclude that long-term obesity accelerates health decline. Their findings also point to the importance of considering compensatory mechanisms (in this case, exercise) in tempering the effects of early disadvantage. A second example is McDonough and Berglund's (2003) examination of the effect of poverty history on trajectories of health. From almost 30 years of longitudinal data, they observed that persistent poverty early in life predicted health disparities, but that cumulative exposure to poverty was not related to over-time change in health trajectories; initial differences in health remained constant over time (also see McDonough et al. 2005). Overall, our understanding of the cumulative effects of the duration of time spent in an advantaged or disadvantaged state as a mechanism generating health inequality across the life course is limited.

A second variation of cumulative advantage processes focuses on between-group inequality that results from the persisting direct effects of a status variable or as the result of variation across groups in rates of return to initial resources (DiPrete and Eirich 2006). Despite a growing body of research examining cumulative advantage as a mechanism generating life course inequality, little empirical attention has been given to whether cumulative advantage processes operate the same across groups over time (George 2005). Existing research has demonstrated that racial disparities in health result from a long-term and cumulative process of disadvantage that begins in early life (Hayward et al. 2000; Warner and Hayward 2006). Studies in this area attempt to disentangle complex relationships between race, socioeconomic status, and health, such as Kelley-Moore and Ferraro's (2004) research which finds that black–white trajectories of disability diverge until controlling for changes in social and health factors, which eliminates the racial gap in health. This is an area of research receiving increasing attention. For example, a special issue of *Research on Aging* is devoted to research on race, socioeconomic status, and health from a life course perspective, with a focus on age, cohort, and period.

A third line of research models cumulative advantage as a process that produces growing rates of return to socioeconomic status with age and examines the extent to which trajectories of health diverge and health inequality based on socioeconomic status increases over the life course. This cumulative process is typically specified through the estimation of growth curve models that include interaction terms between age and socioeconomic status, and a significant and positive interaction coefficient is interpreted as support for cumulative advantage. Studies of this type have produced the most inconclusive evidence. A key question still under debate is whether cumulative advantage implies a process that continues indefinitely, or whether it slows upon reaching a particular critical age. Some longitudinal studies find that the SES gap in health diverges throughout most of life and then converges in the oldest old, or in other words, that the health advantages of socioeconomic resources diminish upon reaching a critical age value, evidenced by converging trajectories in later life (Beckett 2000; Deaton and Paxson 1998; Herd 2006). This slowing of the cumulative advantage process is framed as the age-as-leveler hypothesis and is often presented in competition with cumulative advantage as a mechanism of change in levels of health, inequality across the life course. Other studies have found support for a process of status maintenance, whereby intracohort levels of inequality remain stable over the life course. For example, McDonough and Berglund (2003) observed that persistent poverty earlier in life predicted initial levels of health, but did not affect change in health as people age. In contrast, there also is evidence that the SES gap in health continues to grow into old age (Dupre 2007; Lynch 2003, 2006; Willson et al. 2007). For example, Lynch (2003) found that the relationship of education and health strengthens with age and is becoming stronger across cohorts. Importantly, Lynch demonstrates that without accounting for both age and cohort in the analysis, the patterns would not have been detected. Dupre's (2007) use of hazard models to predict the effect of education on disease onset suggests that, with age, less-educated persons experience increases in the incidence of disease at a higher rate than the well-educated. And Willson et al. (2007) find evidence of a slow process of accumulation of advantage and disadvantage that, over long periods of time, produces sizable disparities in health.

The inconsistent evidence produced by these studies stems from several factors. First, data sets cover different spans of time. In contrast to the research reviewed above, conclusions from early studies were based primarily on cross-sectional or longitudinal data covering very short periods of time (e.g., House et al. 1990, 1994; Miech and Shanahan 2000; Ross and Wu 1996). The inconsistent results produced by this body of research on cumulative advantage have been attributed in part to the confounding of the effects of age and cohort that occurs with the use of cross-sectional data. The issue of disentangling age, period, and cohort remains a challenge to life course research and is related to choice of methodology and model specification.

But perhaps most important is the debate around the impact of selective mortality and attrition, which has the potential to produce biased estimates, another potential source of conflicting results. The strong association between low SES and mortality at younger ages and across the life course leads to an increasingly nonrepresentative group of hardy survivors among the disadvantaged group. As a result, their health at older ages does not differ greatly from that of the advantaged group, producing health trajectories that begin to converge at older ages (Beckett 2000; Lauderdale 2001). The difficulty of assessing selective mortality has led to much discussion and concern but few empirical assessments regarding its influence. Studies that have incorporated corrections for selection bias into their analyses find evidence that selective attrition results in biased estimates (Ferraro and Kelley-Moore 2003; Willson et al. 2007). However, Beckett's (2000) lack of support for selective mortality as an explanation for converging health trajectories in later life has been the subject of debate (Lynch 2003; Noymer 2001). The disproportionate attrition of those with low SES contributes to the apparent convergence in health outcomes and affects conclusions regarding mechanisms of inequality across life course processes (Willson et al. 2007). Disentangling these methodological and conceptual issues will no doubt continue to generate innovative research with the potential to contribute to the conclusions we draw about inequality and age more generally.

Neglected Areas of the Life Course Perspective in Health, Illness, and Healing

While medical sociologists are increasingly using the life course perspective to ask new questions and gain new insights into health, illness, and healing, this focus on CAD processes draws primarily from the view of human development as a life-long, dynamic process that dominates much North American life course research. In the remainder of this chapter, we explore two additional ways that the life course perspective may offer new insights into health, illness, and healing. First, we discuss the role of individual agency in shaping the life course and discuss how life course concepts may contribute to our understanding of health. Second we turn to insights from both North American and European life course approaches that address the importance of historical and institutional change for shaping the life course and discuss how these might be applicable to questions of health, illness, and healing.

Agency Within Constraints: Applications to Health, Illness, and Healing

Social psychologists have recently called for greater attention to selection processes, and more broadly, to the importance of individual agency in understanding relationships between social structure and health (George 2007; McLeod and Lively 2007; Thoits 2006; Thoits and Hewitt 2001). The life course perspective's interest in agency within constraint is consistent with this call and offers several useful tools for this endeavor. As described by Peggy Thoits (2006), personal agency is "evidence that people make choices or decisions, acted intentionally or deliberately, formulated and followed plans of action, or set goals and pursued them (Bandura 2001)." Thoits (2006) also notes that not all selection processes reflect the same degree of agency, and she introduces the useful distinction between social selection and self-selection. While social selection processes reflect structural influences that define the opportunities available, self-selection reflects the choices and actions individuals take. We suspect that most selection processes do not fall neatly into one category or the other but rather fall somewhere on a continuum between the two. Nevertheless, when discussing agency and selection, Thoits' point that we are primarily interested in self-selection is an important one. There is growing evidence that attention to self-selection is important for understanding the health consequences of an event (Thoits 2006; Thoits and Hewitt 2001; Wheaton 1990).

Recent attention to agency and self-selection contrasts sharply to the traditional stress process model (Pearlin 1989, 1999), which frames much of the research examining the effect of social structures and inequalities on mental and physical health (Link 2003; Thoits 2006). In order to clarify the impact of social structures on health and well-being, causal effects of social structures on health have been separated from the influence of health and well-being on the roles and statuses people hold. The latter are isolated from the causal processes of interest and ruled out as either inconsequential or statistically controlled.

Attention to causal order is an important step, but by framing these processes solely in terms of "selection" and viewing them as nuisances to be controlled and ruled out, we have not given attention to ways that individuals actively construct their lives and enact the resources they have to avoid or deal with adversity, and how those decisions may interact with social structures. While we want to avoid "blaming the victim," we do not want to ignore the power individuals have and use in shaping their own lives but must also consider the role social processes play in shaping the extent of this power. The life course perspective embraces the role of agency in structuring the life course, while also recognizing that resources and constraints create wide variation in the degree of agency individuals hold. However, a concrete understanding of the ways that individual agency and social structures interact and relate to health and well-being remains in its infancy (Marshall and Mueller 2003).

One way that the life course can contribute to this broader interest in agency is through closer attention to the temporal unfolding of processes, including attention to trajectories and sequences of events. As noted by Linda George (2007), life course theorists rarely think in either or terms of causation and selection, focusing instead on the temporal unfolding of social processes and illness. "The pathways or trajectories often include lagged effects, reciprocal effects, and/or cyclical effects – temporal patterns that cannot be easily categorized as selection or causation effects" (George 2007: 191). The life course view of lives as cumulative and dynamic forces us to consider, not just where people are now and how that affects their health and well-being, but also where they have come from and how they got to this point.

Research investigating the effects of employment on health and well-being provides one example of both how research questions have typically been framed and how attention to this reciprocal, dynamic interplay can improve our understanding of health. A key interest in research on employment and health has been to identify the components of work, and more recently, work and family, promoting or endangering health. Just as work environments that require work with heavy machinery, fumes and other hazards place workers at greater risk of physical harm, and job stress also poses health risks. While a number of job stressors such as heavy demands and low control (Karasek and Theorell 1990) have been identified as risk factors for mental health problems and cardiovascular disease, researchers have increasingly recognized that health also selects persons into and out of the labor force and into and out of certain types of jobs, a process often referred to as the "healthy worker effect." The "healthy worker hypothesis" is often presented as an alternative to the primary theoretical interest in causal effects of work environments on health (Khlat et al. 2000; Klumb and Lampert 2004; Pavalko and Smith 1999; Ross and Mirowsky 1995; Waldron and Jacobs 1988).

Attending to health selection is an important first step, but it is limited because it frames selection and causation as competing, independent processes. There is growing evidence that these processes are not fully independent from one another but instead that the work–health relationship is reciprocal. In other words, health plays a role in whether and where people work, but health is also affected by those jobs (Link et al. 1993; Pavalko and Smith 1999). Rather than trying to isolate these independent influences, attention to the dynamic, reciprocal nature of these influences may improve our understanding of the work–health relationship. Job transitions and statuses are imbedded in a work history that includes an accumulation of work experiences and, in many cases, prior transitions. For example, a life course approach might raise the following questions: how do the job histories and cumulative work experiences of those who change jobs or leave the labor force because of health problems compare with those who have health crises but do not make job changes as well as with those who do not have health crises? Are those whose job histories include extensive work in high demand and low control jobs at greater risk of leaving the labor force because of health problems? Does longer duration or more recent work in a high demand and/or low control job put one at greater risk of a health-related job exit than more distant work experiences?

While each of the questions above focuses on the work career, they also offer a unique perspective on questions of causation and selection from that provided by traditional approaches. Rather than defining transitions out of the labor force because of poor health as independent of work structures and job decisions, they question whether these "selection" processes may themselves be influenced by previous work structures. By viewing work and work transitions as imbedded with a broader career, we thus gain greater tools for exploring the interdependence of work and health.

Historical and Organizational Change and Illness Careers

A second neglected contribution of the life course perspective in the study of health, illness, and healing is the focus on how lives unfold within organizational and historical contexts. While much of the growth in life course research has emphasized dynamics across individual lives, a recurrent theme has been the impact of historical context and change on life paths (Elder 1974/1999; Haraven 1982; Pavalko and Elder 1990). International research on the life course has emphasized the effects of the state or organizational structures on the life course (Heinz and Marshall 2003; Mayer and Schoepflin 1989; Titma et al. 2003; Zhao and Hou 1999).

The organization, financing, and delivery of health services have undergone dramatic change over the past half century, and these structural changes have consequences for individual health, access to care, doctor–patient relationships, and the power and autonomy of the healing professions. While scholars have documented and analyzed these organizational changes (e.g., Quadagno 2004; Scott et al. 2000; Wholey and Burns 2000) and an extensive body of research on health services has assessed how health service use and treatment effectiveness is altered by program changes, we lack a broad understanding of how the organization of health care shapes the illness experiences of those needing services (but see Pescosolido 1991, 1992, 2006; Rogers et al. 1999). The life course perspective's focus on historical and institutional change can provide valuable concepts and tools for addressing the intersection of health care organizations and illness experiences.

The illness career concept is particularly valuable for exploring the intersection of medical institutions and individual illness experiences. The initial development of the illness career concept stemmed from the early ethnographic studies of the Chicago School (Barley 1989; Goffman 1961; Hughes 1937). As defined by Hughes and others, the illness career was dual-sided. The illness career reflects, on one side, one's personal experience of the career and on the other side, institutional positions. While careers are experienced by individuals, those experiences only take shape as individuals move through positions and enact the roles associated with those positions (Barley 1989). Just as occupational careers take shape within occupations, illness careers take on form and meaning as an individual moves through formal and informal treatment systems (Clausen and Yarrow 1955; Pescosolido 1991, 1992, 2006). The dual-sided concept of illness career thus provides a potentially valuable tool for exploring how individual health is shaped by the organization of healing and health care.

The example of mental illness careers is illustrative of this dual-sided nature of the career. At the individual level, various life course concepts are useful for understanding patterns of treatment as people move into, out of, and through the mental health treatment system. For example, Fig. 23.1 highlights broad patterns of exit after a first hospitalization contrasting those who have a steady decline or improvement from those who have a more fluctuating course of care (Pavalko 1997). For purposes of illustration, we organize our example around the critical event of the first hospitalization, and focus on variation in paths after this key turning point. The bottom path indicates a pattern of recovery and independent living, while the top represents a course of steady disability requiring long-term residential care. While indicating very different outcomes, these two contrasting pathways reflect persons who remain relatively stable after initial treatment or hospitalization.

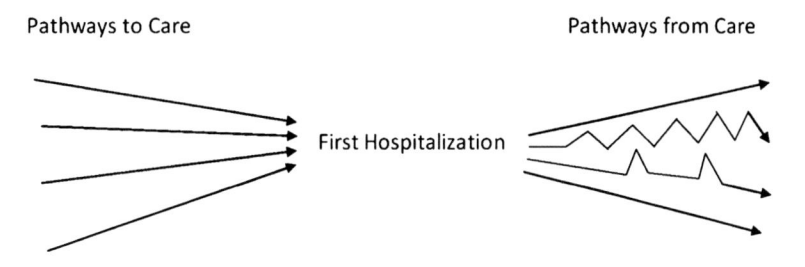

Fig. 23.1 Illustration of illness career patterns [source: Pavalko (1997)]

In contrast to these stable paths, the two middle paths represent fluctuating courses of care, for patients who either move back and forth between the hospital and the community (i.e., a revolving door model) or remain living independently in the community with only one or two short episodes of rehospitalization. The value added by focusing on the patterns of care, rather than just a snap shot of how people are doing at a single point in time, becomes more clear when we compare the bottom two lines on the right-hand side of the figure. If viewed at one point in time, persons following these two paths may look like they had similar levels of recovery, despite the fact that they reflect two very different courses of illness experience.

Beyond general patterns, the life course perspective offers a variety of additional concepts that may be useful for distinguishing different dynamic elements of the individual's movement through treatment and recovery. For example, turning points in the illness career, the sequence of movement between hospital, residential facilities, the criminal justice system, and independent living, and the pace of movement between any or all of these institutions all provide different types of information about the individual's treatment experience (Pavalko 1997).

However, mental illness careers do not just unfold across the individual's life course. They also take shape in a rapidly changing institutional context that in the USA included not only a move away from institutional care but also a complete transformation in the system of care as well as treatment philosophies. In the first half of the twentieth century, the mental hospital *was* the mental health system, but by the late twentieth century, a complex system of care including acute and long-term hospitals, day treatment, treatment teams, group homes, nursing homes and community mental health centers was in place to treat persons diagnosed with mental disorders (Pavalko et al. 2007). Because they unfold across both personal and historical time, illness careers thus reflect both individual and institutional dynamics.

In a recent study we took a first step toward following individual patients over time as they move into, out of and through the mental health system during a period of rapid institutional change to better understand how the organization of mental health care affects treatment experiences and outcomes (Pavalko et al. 2007). Sociologists have long questioned the extent to which treatment, or societal reaction to treatment, exacerbates or even creates mental disorder (Goffman 1961; Scheff 1966). In life course terms, this is a question of accumulation – whether there is an increasing intensity of illness or duration in treatment episodes as one accumulates more treatment experience, or what labeling theorists referred to as a downward spiral of care (Scheff 1966). Of even greater concern is whether this downward spiral is caused by the treatment rather than a natural progression of the illness but distinguishing these influences is difficult because they are so intertwined with one another. However, by assessing the extent of accumulation in the same patients before and after institutional reform we gain some leverage in addressing these questions. For example, we found that, prior to deinstitutionalization, there was strong evidence of accumulation, with length of prior hospitalization becoming an increasingly strong predictor of later hospitalizations, while illness characteristics a decreasing impact (Pavalko et al. 2007). However, after institutional reform the illness career was redirected, with prior hospitalizations no longer predicting risk of rehospitalization, but illness characteristics such as diagnosis and severity of the illness becoming more predictive of rehospitalization.

The transformation of the mental health system in the USA and other countries has been followed by equally important changes in the organization and financing of medical care, including the growth of managed care systems in the USA or the restructuring of the National Health Service in Great Britain. There is little question that these changes have altered how and when people seek medical care, their use of both formal and informal care, and their experiences of that care, but specific information on the experience of illness as people move into, out of, and through these various organizations of care remain largely unknown (but see Pescosolido 1996; Pescosolido and Rubin 2000). While the specific types of questions will vary depending on the substantive example, attention to individual illness careers as persons move through a changing health care system offers medical sociologists powerful tools for conceptualizing and measuring the intersection of health care institutions and health care consumers.

Conclusions

In the 1960s and 1970s, the emerging life course perspective challenged researchers from a variety of disciplines to study lives "the long way" encouraging attention to how lives take shape and change through childhood, adulthood, and old age, while also considering how historical context and social change shaped those lives (Elder et al. 2003; Marshall and Mueller 2003). While sociologists, particularly from the Chicago School, had long studied careers and longitudinal paths across lives (e.g., Goffman 1961; Hughes 1937; Thomas and Znaniecki 1918/1920), attention to dynamic processes was viewed as the domain of qualitative research. In contrast, the emerging multidisciplinary field of life course studies viewed the study of aging processes, life course transitions and trajectories as critical in both qualitative and quantitative research and in samples both large and small. The challenge of studying lives over time was great, particularly since most large-scale surveys at that time were cross-sectional and statistical tools for analyzing these data were designed to assess variation across, rather than within, cases.

The progress in data and methods available for the dynamic study of the life course in the span of just a few short decades has been remarkable. Beginning with the investment in the 1960s in national longitudinal studies such as the Panel Study of Income Dynamics and the National Longitudinal Surveys, we now have numerous longitudinal data collections focusing on specific birth cohorts, life stages, and substantive areas. The growth in statistical methodologies to analyze longitudinal data has been equally impressive, and as a result, life course researchers have ample tools available for the dynamic study of change within and across lives including identifying trajectories and detailed analysis of the timing of specific events.

Research focusing on health, illness, and healing has been central to many of these endeavors. Just as health research has been broadened by the life course perspective, studies of health and health professions have contributed to the empirical and conceptual bases of life course studies. The emerging interest in CAD reviewed in this chapter is just one of many examples of this synchrony between health and life course. While we have made significant progress in understanding health dynamics, the life course perspective has much more to offer to health researchers. We have highlighted a few critical but understudied areas in health research, particularly the dynamics of selection processes and the intersection of organizational change and illness experience, that we feel can be better understood with conceptual and methodological tools offered by the life course perspective.

Even with the wide array of tools available to life course researchers today, including advances in data collection and statistical techniques, the task of fully engaging the life course perspective presents several challenges. Data requirements for long-term longitudinal analysis are extensive. Despite major improvements in longitudinal data collection, researchers wishing to study paths across long periods of the life course are limited to available data collected during the time period of interest. In most cases, state-of-the-art measures and sampling procedures in place 30 or 40 years ago are out of date by today's standards, and one is restricted to the measures collected during that prior era (Elder et al. 1993). In other cases, longitudinal archives have updated or discontinued measures that are no longer in vogue, thus making it difficult to separate real change from measurement change in longitudinal designs. Thus, long-term longitudinal analyses are limited to the available data, but we contend that there is much that can be learned from longitudinal analyses of imperfect measures.

Advances in statistical techniques such as latent growth curve modeling, hierarchical linear modeling, latent class analysis, sequence analysis, and event history analysis all offer life course researchers powerful tools for temporal analysis of continuity and change. With this exciting array of tools, the greatest analytical challenge may be to retain life course theory and concepts as the driving force rather than having the newest methodology guiding research design.

However, probably the greatest challenge for life course researchers is presented by a core tension inherent in the life course perspective itself. Life course goals that emphasize understanding systematic patterns across lives and at the same time that attend to contextual variation create an inherent tension in life course research. For example, the process of identifying a manageable set of career paths in a particular domain, be it work, family, or health, requires that we obscure some of the complexity of people's lives. We might ignore key transitions or assume that those transitions mean the same thing for all persons following an identified trajectory. However, closer attention to the variation in the timing, meaning, or consequences stemming from a single transition risks losing sight of the broader trajectory in which that transition is imbedded. The strength of the life course perspective comes from the combination of these two dynamic elements, particularly when guided by a strong theoretical foundation, such as we have in research on health, illness, and healing.

References

Alwin DF, McCammon RJ (2003) Generations, cohorts and social change. In: Mortimer JT, Shanahan MJ (eds) Handbook of the life course. Kluwer Academic/Plenum, New York, pp 23–50

Alwin DF, Cohen R, Newcombe TM (1991) Political attitudes over the life-span: the Bennington women after fifty years. University of Wisconsin Press, Madison, WI

Armstrong D (1998) Decline of the hospital: reconstructing institutional dangers. Sociol Health Illn 20:445–457

Bandura A (2001) Social cognitive theory: an agentic perspective. Annu Rev Psychol 52:1–26

Barley SR (1989) Careers, identities, and institutions: the legacy of the Chicago school of sociology. In: Arthur MB, Hall DT, Lawrence BS (eds) Handbook of career theory. Cambridge University Press, Cambridge, MA, pp 41–65

Beckett M (2000) Converging health inequalities in later life – an artifact of mortality selection? J Health Soc Behav 41:106–119

Blackwell DL, Hayward MD, Crimmins E (2001) Does childhood health affect chronic morbidity in later life? Soc Sci Med 52:1269–1284

Clausen JA (1993) American lives: looking back at the children of the great depression. Free Press, New York

Clausen JA, Yarrow M (1955) Paths to the mental hospital. J Soc Issues 11:25–33

Conrad P (1992) Medicalization and social control. Annu Rev Sociol 18:209–232

Dannefer D (1987) Aging as intracohort differentiation: accentuation, the Matthew effect, and the life course. Sociol Forum 2:211–237

Dannefer D (1988) Differential gerontology and the stratified life course: cross fertilizing age and social science theory. Annu Rev Gerontol Geriatr 8:3–36

Dannefer D (2003) Cumulative advantage/disadvantage and the life course: cross-fertilizing age and social science theory. J Gerontol B Psychol Sci Soc Sci 58B:S327–S337

Deaton AS, Paxson CH (1998) Aging and inequality in income and health. Am Econ Rev 88:248–253

Dentinger E, Clarkberg ME (2002) Informal caregiving and retirement timing among men and women: gender and caregiving relationships in late midlife. J Fam Issues 23:857–879

DiPrete TA, Eirich GM (2006) Cumulative advantage as a mechanism for inequality: a review of theoretical and empirical developments. Annu Rev Sociol 32:271–297

Dupre ME (2007) Educational differences in age-related patterns of disease: reconsidering the cumulative disadvantage and age-as-leveler hypotheses. J Health Soc Behav 48:1–15

Elder GH Jr (1974/1999) Children of the great depression: social change in life experience. University of Chicago Press/Westview Press, Chicago

Elder GH Jr, Pavalko EK, Clipp EC (1993) Working with archival data: studying lives. Sage, Newbury Park, CA

Elder GH Jr, Kirkpatrick Johnson M, Crosnoe R (2003) The emergence and development of the life course. In: Mortimer JT, Shanahan MJ (eds) Handbook of the life course. Plenum, New York

Ferraro KF, Kelley-Moore JA (2003) Cumulative disadvantage and health: long-term consequences of obesity? Am Sociol Rev 68:707–729

George LK (2005) Socioeconomic status and health across the life course: progress and prospects. J Gerontol B Psychol Sci Soc Sci 60B:135–139

George LK (2007) Life course perspectives on social factors and mental illness. In: Avison WR, McLeod JD, Pescosolido BA (eds) Mental health, social mirror. Springer, New York, pp 191–218

Goffman E (1961) Asylums. Anchor Books, Garden City, NJ

Grob G (1994) The mad among us: a history of the care of America's mentally Ill. Harvard University Press, Cambridge, MA

Guo G (1998) The timing of the influences of cumulative poverty on children's ability and achievement. Soc Forces 77:257–288

Hagan J (2001) Northern passage: American Vietnam war resisters in Canada. Harvard University Press, Cambridge, MA

Han S-K, Moen P (1999) Clocking out: temporal patterning of retirement. Am J Sociol 105:191–236

Haraven T (1982) Family time and industrial time. Cambridge University Press, New York

Hayward MD, Gorman BK (2004) The long arm of childhood: the influence of early-life social conditions on men's mortality. Demography 41:87–107

Hayward MD, Crimmins EM, Miles TP, Yang Y (2000) The significance of socioeconomic status in explaining the racial gap in chronic health conditions. Am Sociol Rev 65:910–930

Heinz WR, Marshall VW (2003) Social dynamics of the life course: transitions, institutions, and interrelations. Aldine de Gruyter, New York

Henretta JC, O'Rand AM, Chan CG (1993) Joint role investments and synchronization of retirement: a sequential approach to couples' retirement timing. Soc Forces 71:981–1000

Herd P (2006) Do functional inequalities decrease in old age? Educational status and functional decline among the 1931–1941 birth cohort. Res Aging 28:375–392

House J, Kessler R, Herzog A, Mero R, Kinney A, Breslow M (1990) Age, socioeconomic status and health. Milbank Q 68:383–411

House J, Lepkowski J, Kinney A, Mero R, Kessler R, Herzog AR (1994) The social stratification of aging and health. J Health Soc Behav 35:213–234

Hughes EC (1937) Institutional office and the person. Am J Sociol 43:404–143

Jackson PB (2004) Role sequencing: does order matter for mental health? J Health Soc Behav 45:132–154

Kahn JR, Pearlin LI (2006) Financial strain over the life course and the health of older adults. J Health Soc Behav 47:17–31

Karasek RA, Theorell T (1990) Healthy work: stress, productivity, and the reconstruction of working life. Basic, New York

Kelley-Moore JA, Ferraro KF (2004) The black/white disability gap: persistent inequality in later life? J Gerontol B Psychol Sci Soc Sci 59B:S34–S43

Kerckhoff AC (1993) Diverging pathways: social structure and career deflections. Cambridge University Press, New York

Khlat M, Sermet C, Le Pape A (2000) Women's health in relation with their family and work roles: France in the early 1990s. Soc Sci Med 50:1807–1825

Kingson ER, O'Grady-LeShane R (1993) The effects of caregiving on women's social security benefits. Gerontologist 33:230–239

Klumb PL, Lampert T (2004) Women, work, and well-being 1950–2000: a review and methodological critique. Soc Sci Med 58:1007–1024

Lauderdale DS (2001) Education and survival: birth cohort, period, and age effects. Demography 38:551–561

Leisering L, Schumann KF (2003) How institutions shape the German life course. In: Heinz WR, Marshall VW (eds) Social dynamics of the life course: transitions, institutions, and interrelations. Aldine de Gruyter, New York

Link BG (2003) The production of understanding. J Health Soc Behav 44:457–469

Link BG, Lennon MC, Dohrenwend BP (1993) Socioeconomic status and depression: the role of occupations involving direction, control and planning. Am J Sociol 98:1351–1387

Lynch SM (2003) Cohort and life-course patterns in the relationship between education and health: a hierarchical approach. Demography 40:309–331

Lynch SM (2006) Explaining life course and cohort variation in the relationship between education and health: the role of income. J Health Soc Behav 47:324–338

Maddox G, Clark DO (1992) Trajectories of functional impairment in later life. J Health Soc Behav 33:114–125

Marshall VW, Mueller MM (2003) Theoretical roots of the life course perspective. In: Heinz WR, Marshall VW (eds) Social dynamics of the life course: transitions, institutions, and interrelations. Aldine de Gruyter, New York, pp 3–32

Mayer KU, Schoepflin U (1989) The state and the life course. Annu Rev Sociol 15:187–209

McDonough P, Berglund P (2003) Histories of poverty and self-rated health trajectories. J Health Soc Behav 44:198–214

McDonough P, Sacker A, Wiggins RD (2005) Time on my side? Life course trajectories of poverty and health. Soc Sci Med 61:1795–1808

McLeod JD, Kaiser K (2004) Childhood emotional and behavioral problems and educational attainment. Am Sociol Rev 69:636–658

McLeod JD, Lively KJ (2007) Social psychology and stress research. In: Avison WR, McLeod JD, Pescosolido BA (eds) Mental health, social mirror. Springer, New York, pp 275–306

Mechanic D (1989) Mental health and social policy, 3rd edn. Prentice Hall, Englewood Cliffs, NJ

Merton RK (1968) The Matthew effect in science. Science 159:56–63

Miech RA, Shanahan MJ (2000) Socioeconomic status and depression over the life course. J Health Soc Behav 41:162–176

Mills CW (1959) The sociological imagination. Oxford University Press, New York

Mirowsky J (2002) Parenthood and health: the pivotal and optimal age at first birth. Soc Forces 81:315–349

Neugarten BL, Moore JW, Lowe JC (1965) Age norms, age constraints, and adult socialization. Am J Sociol 70:710–717

Noymer A (2001) Mortality selection and sample selection: a comment on Beckett. J Health Soc Behav 42:326–327

O'Rand AM (1996) The precious and the precocious: understanding cumulative disadvantage and cumulative advantage over the life course. Gerontologist 36:230–238

O'Rand AM (2001) Stratification and the life course: the forms of life-course capital and their interrelationships. In: Binstock RH, George LK (eds) Handbook of aging and the social sciences. Academic, San Diego, CA, pp 197–210

O'Rand AM, Hamil-Luker J (2005) Processes of cumulative adversity: childhood disadvantage and increased risk of heart attack across the life course. J Gerontol B Psychol Sci Soc Sci 60B:117–124

Pavalko EK (1997) Beyond trajectories: multiple concepts for analyzing long-term process. In: Hardy MA (ed) Studying aging and social change: conceptual and methodological issues. Sage, Thousand Oaks, CA, pp 129–147

Pavalko EK, Artis JE (1997) Women's caregiving and paid work: causal relationships in late midlife. J Gerontol B Psychol Sci Soc Sci 52:S170–9

Pavalko EK, Elder GH Jr (1990) World War II and divorce: a life-course perspective. Am J Sociol 95:1214–1234

Pavalko EK, Smith B (1999) The rhythm of work: health effects of women's work dynamics. Soc Forces 77:1141–1162

Pavalko EK, Woodbury S (2000) Social roles as process: caregiving careers and women's health. J Health Soc Behav 41:91–105

Pavalko EK, Harding CM, Pescosolido BA (2007) Mental illness careers in an era of change. Soc Probl 54:504–522

Pearlin LI (1989) The sociological study of stress. J Health Soc Behav 30:241–256

Pearlin LI (1999) The stress process revisited: reflections on concepts and their interrelations. In: Aneshensel CS, Phelan JC (eds) Handbook of the sociology of mental health. Kluwer Academic/Plenum, New York, pp 395–415

Pescosolido BA (1991) Illness careers and network ties: a conceptual model of utilization and compliance. Adv Med Sociol 2:161–184

Pescosolido BA (1992) Beyond rational choice: the social dynamics of how people seek help. Am J Sociol 97:1096–1038

Pescosolido BA (1996) Bringing the 'community' into utilization models: how social networks link individuals to changing systems of care. Res Sociol Health Care 13:171–197

Pescosolido BA (2006) Of Pride and prejudice: the role of sociology and social networks in integrating the health sciences. J Health Soc Behav 47:189–208

Pescosolido BA, Rubin BA (2000) The web of group affiliations revisited: social life: postmodernism, and sociology. Am Sociol Rev 65:52–76

Quadagno J (2004) Why the United States has no health insurance: stakeholder mobilization against the welfare state, 1945–1996. J Health Soc Behav 45:25–44

Rogers A, Hassell K, Nocolaas G (1999) Demanding patients: analysing the use of primary care. Open University Press, Philadelphia

Ross CE, Mirowsky J (1995) Does employment affect health? J Health Soc Behav 36:230–243

Ross CE, Wu C-L (1996) Education, age, and the cumulative advantage in health. J Health Soc Behav 37:104–120

Ryder NB (1965) The cohort as a concept in the study of social change. Am Sociol Rev 30:843–861

Schaeper H, Falk S (2003) Employment trajectories of east and west German mothers compared: one nation – one pattern? In: Heinz WR, Marshall VW (eds) Social dynamics of the life course: transitions, institutions, and interrelations. Aldine de Gruyter, New York, pp 143–166

Scheff TJ (1966) Being mentally ill: a sociological theory. Aldine, Chicago

Scott R, Ruef M, Mendel P, Caronna C (2000) Institutional change and healthcare organizations: from professional dominance to managed care. University of Chicago Press, Chicago

Thoits P (2006) Personal agency in the stress process. J Health Soc Behav 47:309–323

Thoits PA, Hewitt LN (2001) Volunteer work and well-being. J Health Soc Behav 42:115–131

Thomas WI, Znaniecki F (1920) The Polish peasant in Europe and America, Volumes 1–2. Badger, Boston

Titma M, Tuma NB, Roosma K (2003) Education as a factor in intergenerational mobility in Soviet society. Eur Sociol Rev 19:281–297

Wakabayashi C, Donato KM (2006) Does caregiving increase poverty among women in later life? Evidence from the health and retirement survey. J Health Soc Behav 47:258–274

Waldron I, Jacobs JA (1988) Effects of labor force participation on women's health: new evidence from a longitudinal study. J Occup Med 30:977–983

Warner D, Hayward MD (2006) Early life origins of the race gap in men's mortality. J Health Soc Behav 47:209–226

Wheaton B (1990) Life transitions, role histories, and mental health. Am Sociol Rev 55:209–223

Wholey DR, Burns LR (2000) Tides of change: the evolution of managed care in the United States. In: Bird CE, Conrad P, Fremont AM (eds) Handbook of medical sociology, 5th edn. Prentice Hall, Upper Saddle River, NJ

Willson AE, Shuey KM, Elder GH Jr (2007) Cumulative advantage processes as mechanisms of inequality in life-course health. Am J Sociol 112:1886–1924

Yang Y (2007) Is old age depressing? Growth trajectories and cohort variations in late-life depression. J Health Soc Behav 48:16–32

Zhao X, Hou L (1999) Children of the cultural revolution: the state and the life course in the People's Republic of China. Am Sociol Rev 64:12–36

Chapter 24
The Complexities of Help-Seeking: Exploring Challenges Through a Social Network Perspective

Normand Carpentier and Paul Bernard

Complex Models in Health Sociology

By the end of the 1970s, the movement toward deinstitutionalizing mental health services had uncovered the complexity of developing a social model of care that would supplement, if not supplant, the traditional institutional model. The difficulties associated with the complexity of the social model of care are no less present today: some 30 years after the movement began, providing the right mix of community services and institutional care remains a delicate task (Thornicroft and Tansella 2004). Despite problems with the social model, however, the wave of deinstitutionalization of the psychiatric population in the 1970s was soon followed by an increase in community services for a second group: the growing population of elderly people. Ambulatory services for a great number of health problems were becoming less the exception than the norm and as time passed, it became evident that new treatments for chronic illnesses (serious psychiatric disabilities, cancer, Alzheimer-type dementia, etc.) and the emergence of a new biopsychosocial paradigm were leading researchers to consider several dimensions jointly rather than independently as they had done in the past. At the same time, the number of illnesses requiring long-term care was on the rise, and researchers began to analyze the help-seeking process more thoroughly, exploring such notions as community, networks of reciprocal obligations, and changes in values between successive generations (Mechanic 1989; Taylor and Bury 2007). This process led to the discovery of a serious mismatch: the public was reluctant to use the resources furnished by the medical community. This disparity between available resources and real needs was a major stumbling block in the attempt to create a social model of care. As a result, researchers came to question whether traditional healthcare models could cope with the changing reality of caring for chronic illness and whether they had sufficient explanatory power to bring new knowledge to a changing society (Pescosolido 1992; Silverstein et al. 2003). The response has been largely negative, making it necessary to develop complex models that consider such features of modern society as an ageing population, changing family structures, and the emergence of new kinds of solidarity, all of which have caused the State to redefine its role on an ongoing basis, especially in the light of globalization and fiscal pressures.

The new complex models of healthcare research thus developed have emerged in a number of fields, including population health (Berkman and Glass 2000; House et al. 1988), mental health (Pescosolido 1991, 1992, 1996; Rogler and Cortes 1993) and social gerontology (Litwak 1985; Messeri et al. 1993). While theoretical development is at different stages in different models, all

---

N. Carpentier (✉)
CSSS de Bordeaux-Cartierville-Saint-Laurent, 11822, avenue du Bois-de-Boulogne,
Montréal, QC, Canada H3W 2X6
e-mail: normand.carpentier@umontreal.ca

consider the concept of social networks to be fundamental. For this reason, we have chosen to focus on networks as a means to examine the four central dimensions of complex models: structure, culture, multilevel effects, and temporality. In her presentation of a new complex model, Pescosolido asks an intriguing question: *Is there, in fact, a discernable set of patterns, combinations of options, or strategies that individuals use during an illness episode? And, if so, are these patterns socially organized* (Pescosolido 1992, p. 1115). This striking hypothesis evokes individuals' decision-making capacities, the concept of agency, and the idea that social behaviour can be attributed to various organizational structures, all of which are central issues in social network theory.

Working from this perspective, this chapter has two objectives. First, we discuss why the architects of complex models accord such great significance to the concept of networks and how researchers can address networks in a systematic manner. We recognize that network analysis is an inductive process founded on observations from the field. Accordingly, researchers who wish to work with the network approach must be careful to obtain empirical data that match the requirements for complex models, a far from simple task. For this reason, our second objective is to suggest relevant methods and identify the resources that scholars might use to answer the greater issue raised in this Handbook, with respect to our specific concern here: what if the sociology of health took social networks seriously? Our fundamental concern is how researchers can capitalize on the wealth of ideas and data offered by the network approach in order to better grasp social realities and develop innovative interventions and policies adapted to a social model of care. Because to take social networks seriously, we must pay attention to both conceptual and methodological considerations.

The first element to be considered in this endeavour might well be the relevance of social networks at the conceptual level. The growing complexity of modern society and the recent proliferation of different kinds of lifestyles have made it increasingly difficult to describe the social fabric in terms of traditional categories (Pescosolido and Rubin 2000; White 2008). In many circumstances, individual attributes are simply too imprecise to reflect today's empirical reality. While variable-centred studies can generate important information that helps to frame the subject under study, network tools are essential to defining the social and relational context, especially when individuals and families find unprecedented ways to cope with emerging health problems and to seek help. A network perspective, for example, helps modulate the personal characteristics of "divorced individuals" so as to reflect the process as well as the end result. Take the following examples: separated parents who maintain close ties in order to take care of a sick child; former spouses who form new families and develop extended supportive networks; previously married persons who experience social exclusion after they divorce. These examples show that questioning an individual on his or her marital status alone can only produce limited data. Previously rare arrangements have become more common and cannot be inferred from an individual's personal characteristics. Rather than asking yes/no questions, the conscientious researcher must determine the unique web of relationships for each actor and social group. While it is possible (and might be well-advised) to introduce measurements from population studies and network analyses into statistical equations, to truly take the idea of social networks seriously is to subscribe to a formalist paradigm (Simmel 1971); that is, a relational sociology in which the social world consists primarily of dynamic unfolding relationships (Emirbayer 1997).

If we take networks seriously at a conceptual level, we must take them seriously at the methodological level as well. This implies adopting procedures and research frameworks that sometimes diverge from conventional approaches. In this context, the network approach, which cannot be considered a theory proper, becomes an amalgam of tools and strategies that allows the researcher to take fuller account of the interactions, negotiations, and conflicts that occur between actors, both individually and collectively. Determining this web of relationships is far from simple (Marin and Hampton 2007). The identity of network actors, the cartography of their relationships, and details of the links between network members cannot be ascertained with a few standard questions. The task is further complicated by the fact that it is difficult to evaluate the amount of time necessary to build a network, because this varies according to each actor's perception of the extent and dynamics of his or her network. Nonetheless, reconstructing the network is essential: the research community is presently moving from traditional models that seek to identify the factors that predict the use of services to complex models that aim to analyze the processes that lead to care pathways and determine their impact on health (Allen et al. 2004; Jones et al. 2009; Morgan et al. 2004). Social relations play a central role in this analysis.

The production of knowledge at this scale is admittedly still in the early stages and much research remains exploratory. Inspired by a few lead authors, however, the academic community has demonstrated considerable enthusiasm for projects that use a network perspective, and numerous researchers continue to apply themselves to perfecting indicators and developing theory (Degenne and Forsé 2004; Scott 2000; Wasserman and Faust 1994; Snijders and Doreian 2010). But development in this domain has been uneven so far, and scholars who work on indicators or try to explain social phenomena have frequently used easy-to-reach samples and populations far removed from the normal challenges of daily life. The development of "whole network" techniques (i.e., networks with closed boundaries that more easily fit mathematical procedures) is thus further advanced than that of "egocentric network" techniques. In addition, a large body of work has been conducted on themes in which subjects' actions can be explained by instrumental or rational motivations, reflecting the assumption that actors are utility maximizers: this had led researchers away from in-depth analysis of the relationship between social structure, agency, and culture (Emirbayer and Goodwin 1994, p. 1428). As a result, social network research has largely ignored a number of challenging fields, including health care (among exceptions, see Jippes et al. 2010; Levy and Pescosolido 2002; Lewis et al. 2008). And indeed, problems with the field of health care can be daunting. Addressing the question of service use in a chronic care setting requires dealing with populations that are difficult to recruit. It also means using techniques adapted to egocentric networks and approaching networks of people living in intense situations in which social relationships can quickly become complicated.

If, despite these obstacles, we persist in taking the notion of networks seriously and giving life to the complex models recently proposed, we must agree to study social relationships in crisis situations where networks are often composed of ambiguous relationships that contain the seeds of both conflict and support. While some of these relationships may be stable, others must be frequently renegotiated. We must also recognize the omnipresence of symbolic dimensions (social representations) and the constant human and social dilemmas that families face, making it difficult for them to set clear objectives. Furthermore, we must arm ourselves with tools and concepts that allow us to understand change. Finally, we must remember that the network approach was developed through a close relationship between theoretical advances and empirical analysis; consequently, the feasibility of data gathering must be a key consideration in the research process. Later in this chapter, we illustrate possible analytical avenues in relation to this last point, using one of the current projects of our research team as an example. In this project, begun in 2003, we formed a cohort of 60 caregivers of persons with Alzheimer's disease, with whom we met at 18-month intervals. Basing our analyses on the social network approach, social representation theory, and life history techniques applied within a multilevel and temporal framework, we sought to bring a new perspective to a field that continues to be largely dominated by individualistic models and the logic of rational choice.

In the sections that follow, we address three dimensions of the complex model of health seeking, namely the notions of structure, culture, and temporality. The first section addresses the notion of network structure, including the egocentric notion of networks and multilevel effects. We then move to the representation approach before discussing the sequential action approach.

Network Structures: Linking Individuals and Organizations

From the social network perspective, social structure can be defined as the linkages between individual and collective social actors as summed through an empirically established regularity of transactions (Emirbayer 1997; Erickson 2004). This understanding of social structure contrasts markedly with the definition of Marx, Parsons, or Weber (see Smelser 1988).

At first glance, it might seem relatively simple to reconstruct the network of an individual, a group, or an organization. A number of name generators with precisely this function have been developed over the course of the last few years. But each generator provides only one view of social structure. While some generators are designed to identify extended linkages (active and/or potential, direct and/or indirect, weak and/or strong, formal and/or informal), others aim to recreate an individual's primary network, the smaller and more stable environment in which self-confidence and identity grow. From the very beginning then, the study of relationships confronts the researcher with a crucial decision: which questions and research direction will allow him/her to construct a network that reveals the greatest possible number of facets of the object of analysis? An individual's description of his/her networks can only generate an incomplete image of interactions: under no circumstances can we expect to obtain all the data needed to account for the infinite subtleties of an individual's links and social relationships, especially when s/he is under the trying circumstances of chronic illness.

For our research programme, "Social Networks, Social Representation Project" (SNSR), we chose to use a name generator based on supportive relationships. Six questions allowed us to identify actors likely to provide our respondents, the caregivers, with emotional, instrumental, counselling, or companionship support. Our experience with this option leads us to make two observations. First, we must begin the data-gathering process by establishing a relationship with our respondent, especially if we hope to follow him or her over several years. The interview must be enjoyable and it is unrealistic to expect to obtain extensive network measurements, especially if certain aspects of our questions make respondents uncomfortable. We have, for example, frequently found respondents unable to discuss reciprocity, conflict, or intensity in the relationships among network members identified by the name generator. And a respondent who is made uncomfortable during an interview will be little disposed to see us again, especially if the illness has progressed and if his or her anxiety has grown since our last meeting. For this reason, we must sometimes reconstruct the nature of a respondent's relationships less formally, for example, by using material from his or her narratives. Our second observation is that supportive relationships are more complex than they seem. Some degree of simple classification is possible – one actor provides emotional support while another provides advice – but support can also be symbolic, invisible, stigmatizing, or pathological (Martuccelli 2002). If we are to exploit the notion of networks more fully, we must not only identify the functions of each link described by the name generator, but also attempt to discern the dynamics of the various elements working together as well as any differences between cases, differences that stem from respondents' subjectivity.

In addition to reconstructing an actor's relationships, network analysis allows us to move from one level to another by applying principles of extending and superimposing links and aggregates. For instance, Markovsky (1987) made propositions to theoretically integrate processes that operate at different levels. Without repressing individual actors or robbing them of their unique characteristics, we aim to imbed them within groupings that interact with other groupings also composed of individuals. Historically, the network approach has found fertile ground in organizational studies, and several classical network studies have analyzed political agencies (see Knoke 2004). In the field of health care, a number of concepts related to governance, integrated services, and network policy have originated in variations of the network perspective. Nonetheless, Dowding (1995) has shown that most research either continues to use networks metaphorically or makes only partial use of data that would allow for structural analysis (but see Lewis et al. 2008 for innovative works). This difficulty in taking networks seriously is understandable and can be explained by the complexity of the methodology. The very first step, mapping the links between actors, is already complex. Following this step, however, researchers must also obtain information such as the frequency and means of contact, the methods used to transfer information, and the sinuous paths of decision-making; to do so, they must investigate the medical practices of individuals who are not used to divulging the information requested and have little interest in doing so (i.e., highly qualified medical staff). Furthermore, to the extent that these research procedures are used to generate reports of staff activities, it is not inconceivable that network analysis could jeopardize participants' confidentiality or even lead to management reprisals against staff. Several ethical obstacles to the study of organizations must therefore be overcome before we can expect participants to lower their resistance (Borgatti and Molina 2005).

Ethical issues aside, the very number of organizations now on hand to help the victims of chronic illness poses another challenge. The network approach is obviously a powerful means to understanding the internal logic of groups and the possible links between organizations with different ideologies and diverse practical orientations. But this field is as yet unexplored, especially when it comes to the interface between family, professional, community, and private systems. And yet, critical issues such as the balance between the supply and demand of services and the continuity of care hinge on the ways that those systems connect.

Drawing on Pescosolido's *Multi-Level Network Model* (1996) and Martuccelli's work on social roles and the notion of respect (2002), we undertook an exploratory study of the social care interface in early-stage dementia (Carpentier et al. 2008b). The aim of our study was to understand the linkage process and the interaction between formal and informal systems of care as seen through four dimensions: professionals' care practices, the relationships between health professionals and caregivers and internal and external environments (the team's network and the organization's network, respectively). Our rationale was that individual health trajectories are complex and undoubtedly influenced by the nature and configuration of health services available in the community (Allen et al. 2004). But here again, difficulties quickly arose. We found it difficult to interpret the links between formal and informal networks: one respondent might feel strongly connected to the network with only a few contacts per year (but with attentive listening by a professional), while another might be in frequent contact with professionals and still feel abandoned. Apart from strongly institutionalized links, it was, in general, difficult to ascertain with any precision the nature and strength of links between any two actors, especially when tension or incompatible values jostled for place with norms of solidarity and obligation. These findings explain our conviction that links are complex and cannot be summarized using sundry measurements of frequency, duration, or intensity as perceived by the parties at play.

In summary, the fundamental idea behind the network approach is to consider several elements simultaneously: nodes (the actors), lines (the relationships), direct effects (breaking a link), secondary effects (a change in the status of a network member), and multilevel effects (a health organization moves to a location nearby). Considering several elements at the same time allows us to first graph actors' positions and then use inductive methods to glean how relationships are structured, how groupings occur, and whether actors are positioned so as to take advantage of certain resources or turn to alternative strategies. Completion of this analysis puts us in the position to identify social inequalities and understand the processes that lead to social exclusion. The data generated by these kinds of studies is thus invaluable to deepening our understanding of the help-seeking process and the care trajectory as complex models aspire to do. But much creativity in the field of health care remains to be developed before we can hope to exploit the concept of networks to its full potential.

Network Content: Actors' Social Representations

In the early days of network theory, theorists floated the idea that structure alone could explain the behaviour of groups or individuals (Brint 1992; Fuhse 2009). Since then, this hypothesis has been largely discarded, and scholars now agree that social phenomena like help-seeking processes are best explained when the symbolic and discursive dimensions of networks are taken into account. We should note that concepts related to symbolic dimensions have historically had little place in traditional service use models, principally because of the lack of explanatory power of cultural variables in multivariate analyses (Kasper 2000). Today's researchers must therefore look for ways to integrate the notion of culture into studies on service use in the spirit of a relational sociology that fits the network perspective put forward by the authors of complex models.

Three conditions appear necessary for this venture to succeed. First, instead of considering network content to consist of individual values and attitudes, we must conceptualize it as an ensemble of normatively driven communications, relationships, and transactions that may head in different directions at the same time (Emirbayer 1997). For this reason, under ideal conditions, one would meet several respondents for each network; if only one respondent is available, however, it would be essential to solicit his or her perceptions of the positions of the other network members. The second condition addresses the fact that the form and the content of networks seem to follow a double-edged principle. The first is the principle of relative autonomy between current structure and content, meaning that an individual's identity, values, and beliefs are based on his or her life experiences, events, and past relationships. The symbolic universe is much broader than the structure described by an actor at any given point in time. At the same time, it is not completely alien: hence, the second principle of the continuous and dynamic nature of the interaction between network structure and network content. According to this last principle, network links allow information and symbols to circulate and uphold an individual's cultural universe. Members of a dense and coherent network with defined objectives, for example, share a common culture because messages conveyed by strong links encounter few obstacles and reinforce group values. While the prevalence of this kind of network in contemporary society is open to debate, networks inarguably experience great difficulty when a network member becomes subject to chronic illness and must be cared for at home: numerous studies have demonstrated how networks become destabilized and tensions grow when network structures undergo change and families are confronted by different systems and alien values. A final condition for the successful integration of culture into studies on formal services use lies in the creation of a methodology that captures network change: it must distinguish the form of relationships from their content, while recognizing that these dimensions interact and influence each other over time.

Keeping these three conditions in mind, our team developed a strategy that uses a qualitative approach to capture the symbolic content of networks (Carpentier et al. 2008a). A qualitative approach is useful for uncovering meaning, grasping the extent of changes, and exploring the interplay between individual and collective dimensions. Our work takes place within a sociology of action framework: we hold that social phenomena result from direct interactions between social actors. This framework can be made to converge with the logic of social network analysis, even though some versions of the sociology of action view social norms as a main driver of action and structure as a secondary aspect. The norm-based approach is not without problems, not least because of the discrepancy between the norms expressed by social actors and their actual behaviour. In other words, it appears that action contexts are part of a complex universe that cannot be reduced to a few normative parameters; norms are actuated in constraining contexts.

It is in this context that we chose the social representation approach as a means to plumb the depths of network content. Our strategy composed four steps. The first was to construct a databank of concepts that covered some of the many elements that help form social representations. Because the literature on barriers to care covers a wide range of dimensions that could account for symbolic elements, we used an inventory of writings to identify 50 barriers to access to care: structural barriers (e.g., lack of access to trained physicians), relational barriers (e.g., conflict or lack of trust with professionals), cognitive barriers (e.g., normalization, denial), and cultural barriers (e.g., belief, norms, acculturation). Our second step was to identify the presence of those 50 barriers in the discourse of our interviewees, using content analysis. Our third step was to develop a conceptual model. As illustrated in Figure 24.1, our model is made up of six general concepts that comprise the 50 barriers referred to above. These 50 barriers cover the many facets that help form a respondent's social representations. In our study, the respondent is the caregiver of a person with chronic degenerative illness and is located at the centre of the model. The caregiver suggests a possible normative orientation for his or her network (which we could classify as collectivist, familiarist, or individualist), but content analysis reveals numerous other dimensions that influence the respondent's representation and impact his or her behaviour.

In the upper portion of our diagram, two dimensions refer to past experiences. *Social history* attests the quality of the relationship between the caregiver and his or her relative prior to the onset of disease. We consider a difficult or negative relationship to be a barrier to the use of services because relationship problems reduce interactions and negotiations between parties. The second dimension referring to past experiences consists in the caregiver's *experiences with assistance* in health problem situations. This concept is composed of three subgroups of elements: caregiver's past experiences with illness and health, his or her relationship with institutions (that is, his or her ideas about the responsibilities of institutions and attitude towards the healthcare system), and his or her perception of filial responsibilities and family values. At the centre of the model lie the *caregiver* and two categories of actors with whom the caregiver is in direct interaction. Caregivers report barriers such as acceptance or rejection of the disease by peers and tensions in relationships within the *informal system*, and facilitators such as medical referrals (each barrier has an opposite, that is to say, a facilitator). The next concept represented in the diagram is that of the *formal system*'s response to the needs expressed by the caregiver. Here, the different positions held by formal and informal actors help shape and transform the caregiver's representations. Finally, the *social context* shapes the larger process and environment in which the family is embedded.

Guided by this model of social representations, by our command of the literature, and by Pescosolido's model of service use (1992), we turned to the final step of our strategy, namely the interpretation of the influence of representations on the actor's behaviour. We wanted to accumulate sufficient information to construct what Geertz has termed a "thick" description of situations

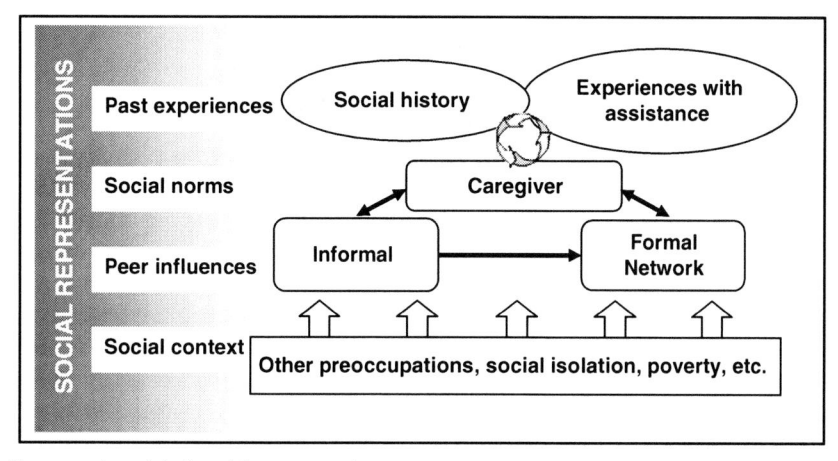

Fig. 24.1 Conceptual model of social representations

(1973), the best means of demonstrating the role of culture in social life. The structural approach of social representation theory allows the researcher to draw conclusions based on the frequency of occurrence of barriers as determined from the narrative material. Accordingly, we inserted all 50 barriers into a quadrant according to their frequency of occurrence, and in so doing produced a central system and three peripheral zones. Abric (1994) summed up the hypothesis of a central system as follows: "The organization of a representation presents a specific, particular modality: not only are the elements of the representation hierarchized but, what's more, all representations are organized around a central core comprising elements that give the representation its meaning" (p. 19). Accordingly, the central system presents the dimensions most frequently identified in the discourse and gives us an indication of recurring, common themes shared by the majority. The first zone of the peripheral system presents a starker contrast in elements and may provide the basis for intergroup differentiation. The second and third peripheral zones present dimensions that could relate to the past, could play a role in future, or could serve to personify life histories and provide an idea of singularities.

This approach is a promising way to account for network content because it fulfils all three conditions mentioned above: (1) acknowledgment of the different positions of network actors who interact with the respondent; (2) the principle of autonomy/dependence between structure and content; and (3) concern for the ever-changing nature of the symbolic universe. The model proposed here (Fig. 24.1) systematically identifies sources of influence that might help form an actor's social representations by acknowledging the importance of social actors who no longer belong to the network and by recognizing the daily, tangible links that influence an individual's representations and ultimately affect his or her behaviour. Performed for each wave of interviews, this analytical process not only reveals changes in barriers but also demonstrates how respondents' perceptions of the importance of those barriers change at different points in the care trajectory. Finally, with its use of central and peripheral zones, the model sheds light on the current debate on how individual status fits into culture. Let's take one example: the supposed uniformity of values among members of a given ethnic community. While a given ethnic group might have a certain degree of collective identity, different ethnic communities have similar values and attitudes. The central zone thus captures the fundamental representation to which all actors ascribe, regardless of ethnic status, social class, gender, or the structure of the social network. In contrast, the peripheral zones can capture differences that do not necessarily correspond to predefined social categories (we are currently examining this possibility). According to network theory, social representations vary according to structural parameters, even though individual characteristics like age, gender, and social class will always bear weight.

Sequence Analysis: Exploring Social Processes

Like structure and the symbolic universe, temporality is a fundamental dimension of complex models. In our examination of these dimensions thus far, we have made only indirect reference to the dynamics of situation. In order to meet theorists' ambitions, however, we must scrutinize the determinants of care pathways in greater detail, and this is where the researcher must choose an *action model* (Coleman 1986). Weber and Pareto are at the origins of the groundswell that produced one such model, the theory of rational choice. This theory has influenced traditional service use models to the extent that the "decision to seek care – and the choice of a specific provider – is often modelled using standard economic models such as those based on individuals maximizing their expected utility" (Shengelia et al. 2005, p. 98). According to this thinking, an individual instrumentally calculates the advantages and disadvantages of any given course of action and acts accordingly. She/he carefully sifts through available information and chooses the option that best meets his or her needs.

Rational choice holds that an individual's choice of alliances is strategic and opportunistic: people nurture relationships likely to further their interests.

Despite its popularity, the concept of rational choice has been contested by many social scientists. It seems particularly inappropriate in the case of chronic illness. As we have shown, the backdrop for decision-making in situations of chronic illness is largely made up of the interplay between network participants. Numerous cognitive, relational, and cultural barriers converge to create a complex system that constrains the actors' access to care. Far from witnessing rational actors working to maximize their profit, we observe mechanisms of decision-making in a context of multidimensional uncertainty. The unpredictable paths of chronic illness confront actors with a moral and emotional dilemma about the best course to follow: they are torn between the possibilities and frequently hesitate. Certain phases of the trajectory lend themselves well to rational choice, or even demand, but there is often no clear-cut best way to understand and handle the illness: actors must choose among a range of options that rest on contradictory assumptions. In these circumstances, any action or attempt at action impacts other players who subsequently reposition themselves in unforeseeable configurations because the lives of those involved are not insular but indeed interrelated. Furthermore, chronic illness often produces situations where precise objectives cannot be defined, where a single action can have multiple results, and where the serious nature of the consequences of many decisions requires the input of both central and peripheral care participants. Even after a decision has been made, uncontrollable events can call a chosen course of action into question at any time. In circumstances of chronic illness then, decisions can rarely be made on grounds of rationality: opposition and unforeseeable events are only too rife.

Once we reject rational action theory or at least question its relevance, the value of direct analysis of the process whereby an individual adapts his or her actions to the environment becomes apparent (Martuccelli 2005, p. 91). Over the past few years, studies have tended to address temporality with the concepts of careers, trajectories, or pathways, either by describing how an illness evolves through various stages or by enumerating the support resources sought at given points in time. Less frequent are studies that have looked at the social dynamics of the negotiations an actor must undertake in order to respond to the myriad phenomena encountered (Sørensen 1998).

A few researchers have nonetheless undertaken ambitious projects that attempt to evaluate the dynamics of change, for example, through narrative positivism (Abbott 1992), the creation of a "syntax" of social life (Abell 1987), or a formal approach for event sequence analyses (Heise 1991). This "return to the narrative" in the social sciences is part of a greater backlash against established analytical models and the purely quantitative treatment of data (see Bernard 1993, on causality). The new procedures use mixed methods and focus on the numerous challenges that face actors embedded within networks of relationships. The result has been a number of original studies (Stevenson and Greenberg 2000; Wiggins et al. 2007), many in the field of health care (Uehara 2001). Our team drew on these studies to develop a procedure to analyze action sequences (Carpentier and Ducharme 2005; Carpentier et al. 2010). Using a narrative approach and focusing our analysis on the concept of networks, we have attempted to identify the life events, negotiations, crisis episodes, and relationship structures that guide or hamper individuals in their search for and decisions to use formal, informal, or community care resources.

Figure 24.2 illustrates how narrative co-construction between the researcher and the narrator allows us to interpret action dynamics by looking at two networks at different points on the trajectory. Each interview solicits an "illness history" that allows us to analyze how the context of relationships has evolved since the last interview. Our first step is to evaluate the narrator's reflexive capacities. Symbolic interactionism holds that reflexivity is the process that accompanies action to the extent that actors can analyze the origins, procedures, and consequences of their actions. As Martuccelli has pointed out (2005), individuals constantly confront growing numbers of previously unencountered challenges and develop their reflexive abilities in consequence.

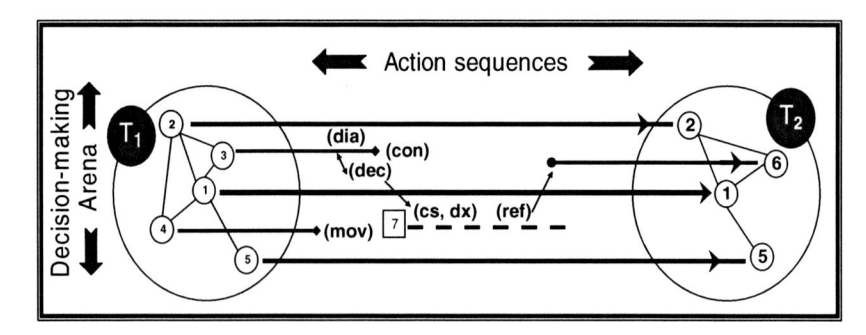

Fig. 24.2 Network transformation and action sequences

In affording us a personal interpretation of his or her life history, the narrator introduces us to the actors whom she/he considers to have participated in his or her decision-making process, either by blocking decisions or by facilitating them. Our diagram shows that five actors are active at T_1 and four are active at T_2 and that one of the actors at T_2 is new (two of the actors at T_1 having left the network). At this point, our goal is to explain the phenomenon of network change. This is not a novel endeavour: there exists a substantial body of literature on the structural principles that underlie transformation phenomena. Dense, closed networks, for example, are known to delay individual access to services, so that links with professionals do not emerge until later in the trajectory. There is also an extensive literature on symbolic elements: individualistic normative systems, for example, tend to cause families to disengage from their ill relative and delegate care to professional service providers, causing the network to include mostly nonfamily members. Our longitudinal procedure, however, uses the narrative approach and more direct observation to explore the general principles of network transformation. This allows us to be more precise in pinpointing mechanisms previously identified in the literature (and later to nuance them). Above all, it facilitates our simultaneous consideration of the structural (network) and cultural (social representation) dimensions of respondents' actions.

Figure 24.2 summarizes the action sequences thus: following a discussion (dia) with Actor 3, Narrator 1 decides (dec) to consult (cs) Doctor 7. This doctor makes a diagnosis (dx) before referring the family (ref) to Medical Specialist 6. During the same period, Actor 3 leaves the network because of conflict (con) over the narrator's interpretation of the illness and decisions about care. Actor 2, who was identified by the name generator as someone who provides emotional and instrumental support, does not participate in decisions during this period. Actor 4, who has been described as someone who provides companionship, moves (mov) to a new neighbourhood and the relationship ends. Actor 5 is a childhood friend and close confidant who is present at both T_1 and T_2. The narrator has informed us that Doctor 7, who had been consulted in the past, is present for some time but that ties are cut after the family is referred to a specialist. This illustration of action sequences is somewhat simpler than those we usually encounter. More frequent are sequences involving many kinds of actors, both those identified by the name generator and those who do not provide support but are named in the narrative. Sequence analysis also commonly reveals subgroupings of action sequences.

Our tool analyzes actions sequentially in order to show how events can influence a life course within the observation period. Our coding system for "action-sequence trajectories" uses over 120 kinds of events to create a "syntax," which, among other things, situates the first signs of dementia, the beginning of the caregiver role, the creation of new social relationships, the end of relationships, the assistance-seeking process, the breadth of family resources, conflict resolution, and other life events (suicide, hospitalization, loss of employment, etc.).

Our diagram starts by reducing the complexity of social life to the principal events identified by the narrator, and then allows us to analyze the help-seeking trajectory from two perspectives.

The first perspective focuses on the sequential nature of actions: the sometimes simultaneous succession of occurrences such as meetings with professionals, changes in states of being (deteriorating health, for example), and associated decisions and experiences. Successive interviews reveal actors disengaging, sometimes to return; families attempting again and again to obtain professional help; and periods of great tension that leave a mark on the mental and physical health of those providing care. Studying sequences of these events reveals the cumulative effect of the many dimensions that mould the course of the care trajectory. The second perspective we use to analyze the help-seeking process focuses on the "decision-making arena" (see Fig. 24.2), that is, the pool of actors among whom the action takes place. This arena can be limited to members of the respondent's support network but sometimes expands to include other actors and consequently accommodate new solutions that emerge as the illness evolves. The decision-making arena angle provides another view of trajectories and perhaps also a means of capturing weak ties. Weak ties are a central concept in network theory and theories of help-seeking processes. They are a singularly effective means of accessing other networks and they help to diversify information and increase the use of resources (Granovetter 1983). Identifying weak ties is a long and complicated process that has little place in interviews with actors grappling with serious, chronic difficulties, but life histories can be used to overcome these obstacles. Take, for example, the storey of a cousin who works in a hospital and informs the family about a specialized clinic, or the brief chat with a social worker at a neighbourhood party that starts the caregiver on a vast help-seeking mission. Both encounters provide useful information about the social elements that underlie the strategies of actors and their ability to interact with public organizations. Our preliminary results suggest that a range of weak ties is important to the first steps of the help-seeking process, but that a minimum of supportive actors is also necessary to retain links to formal resources. We suspect that while links with the outside world are never easy, continued dialogue with the informal network could be the factor that helps actors adjust their expectations and values so that a satisfactory relationship with formal resources can take place. It is interesting that in our study of caregivers to people with Alzheimer's disease, few support actors seemed to take part in important decision-making; it is as if caregivers seek to protect the inner core of their networks, perhaps in anticipation of difficulties to come.

To summarize, we believe that care trajectories for chronic illnesses are a social construction that involves a large number of players; these actors observe each other and either create forums for constructive decision-making or elect not to cooperate. Because the information available to actors at any given point in time is always fragmented and open to interpretation, frequent misunderstandings, disagreements, and missed appointments are inevitable. In circumstances where actors have multiple goals, and especially in cases where the consequences of an action will not be known until years later, the model of the rational actor who assesses his or her choices and acts accordingly does not fit a complex and evolving reality.

Conclusion

The main goal of this chapter has been to present the contribution of a network approach to the construction of complex models of help-seeking in cases of serious degenerative illness. Our approach follows the tenets of relational sociology (Emirbayer 1997; White 2008), which, while little used, seems singularly apt at providing insight into care trajectories. Much of today's research is dominated by surveys or experimental methods that abide by the biomedical paradigm or the framework of evidence-based medicine (Bond and Corner 2001; Dean 2004; Mykhalovskiy and Weir 2004). The network approach differs significantly from these methods by drawing on the teachings of the social sciences, stressing complexity, and attempting to integrate elements as disparate as individual subjectivity and wider contexts. By examining the dynamics of social actors with different statuses and a plurality of interests, this approach can be uncomfortable to elites whose interests tend to lie with the status quo (Learmonth 2003).

This chapter has attempted to ascertain the challenges inherent in this research approach and suggest ways of meeting them. Our examples draw largely on our own experiences; other teams have adopted other solutions. Using social networks as their main concept, authors have launched a range of innovative studies. Some examine the linkage process between clients and healthcare organizations (Jinnett et al. 2002) or evaluate community-based healthcare coalitions using game theory (Ford et al. 2004); others assess neighbourhood effects on health interventions (Chiu and West 2007), propose new ways for programmes evaluation (Eisenberg and Swanson 1996), or seek to deepen our understanding of governance (Maturo 2004). This growing body of research nonetheless frequently neglects to draw on a comprehensive conceptual model, and complex models have led to only a small number of research programmes so far. It is our hope that complex models will not remain mere references for a few specialized projects, but will instead inspire a new generation of researchers to initiate original studies bringing fresh solutions to complex social situations.

Current interest in the direct observation of social relationships, whether performed on a small or a large scale, is making it more possible than ever to see how interactions affect the care trajectory. By moving away from a purely metaphorical interpretation of the concepts of trajectories, support networks, and the interface between services, complex models can provide us with a new perspective on interventions and on the links to and between organizations. That this perspective has become invaluable is evidenced by the growth in the number of assistance services with sometimes contradictory ideologies and practices and the concomitant threat of a scramble for resources offered by community, private, and public organizations. While individual variables are not sufficient to explain the phenomena at hand, it is clear that social status will always be a key factor. Even then, network analysis discerns the compensatory strategies adopted by disadvantaged families and identifies means of entry into social networks that are closed or resistant to outside assistance. In other words, it is entirely possible that careful observation of the social practices and solutions adopted by actors within their particular social and cultural context can lead to more appropriate interventions.

We must nonetheless proceed prudently in our interpretation of trajectories, for the three angles of analysis presented here (structure, culture, and dynamics) have a number of limitations. With respect to networks, for example, we can never be sure of the validity of the construct that results from the use of a given name generator. When we ask someone about his or her support ties, what do we actually obtain? How does the respondent treat complexity, particularly when a tie involves elements of tension or conflict? How does she/he regard new acquaintances, broken friendships, hasty reconstitutions, or separations, be they temporary or caused by profound disagreement? Is the respondent capable of identifying latent support ties that can be mobilized if needed? Can we hope to obtain valid data in line with theoretical expectations? Our analyses so far have demonstrated good validity for our network constructs (Carpentier and Ducharme 2007), but we cannot deny that reported social relations are never more than a reflection of an actor's representations at a given point on the trajectory. Our treatment of social representations also raises questions. To what extent, for example, do representations guide respondents' behaviours? Representations are likely to provide orientation, but only to the extent that they precede behaviour and guide future action. To complete the picture, representations can have other functions as well (Abric 1994): an identity-forming function, where respondents identify with a group or a culture, or a justificatory function, where actors use representations *a posteriori* to justify their choices and maintain consistency between their actions and their words. And finally, what about action sequences? Much of the material that we use to build trajectories relies on respondents' recollection: we can never be sure that the histories thus reconstructed will really reflect the facts. The actual number of doctor's visits, the true impact of a certain discussion with a friend, whether or not a conflict was the real cause for the end of a relationship: these are examples of questions that will always remain. Still, after analyzing network data, social representations, and sequences of events in depth and over a long period of time, we think that we can draw a global portrait that, while imperfect, provides us with a relatively consistent image of the trajectories analyzed.

But the network concept is more than a powerful approach for the exploration of notions of structure, culture, and temporality: it also promotes the integration of theory and empirical research. Despite the jargon about interaction and social relationships and the resulting emphasis on collaboration, network theorists and researchers have tended to work in silos. This is regrettable, because the separation of the theoretical and empirical worlds does nothing to help the social sciences flourish in the field of health care. In fact, the more coherent, concrete, and action-oriented focus of the biomedical paradigm helps explain that paradigm's popularity. At the same time, however, the research programme of the biomedical model has increasingly engaged in quasi-routine activities that use standardized instruments and rote statistical procedures and may well hamper innovation. In contrast, the social science approach proposes an innovative analysis of social actors (both individual and collective) and leaves room for a range of research methods, promising a wealth of discovery in the process.

In closing, we may ask ourselves whether the procedures laid out in this chapter have brought us any closer to meeting the goals of the theorists of complex models and answering Pescosolido's (1992) question about the socially organized patterns that undergird the help-seeking process. But we can only answer after completing research programmes that cover the entire trajectory of care, use different research frameworks, and study various kinds of populations. At the very least, the network approach complements the data generated by traditional approaches and allows us to diversify our research questions. And a new look at service use problems is nothing short of essential, for two reasons. First, families are evolving and new kinds of solidarity have surfaced that we do not yet comprehend. Second, the healthcare system is straining to resolve a host of problems: the lack of compassion in the provision of care, an outdated technocracy, management techniques that are out of step with the social model of care, and an inability to control costs (Pescosolido and Kronenfeld 1995). A new generation of research will have to address emerging dilemmas in contemporary societies: individuals are both more autonomous and more vulnerable than they were in the past, and the environment in which they live is more difficult to master. New research programmes will have to generate plausible and original explanations about social phenomena and create new guidelines for interventions and the elaboration of social policy in the field of health care. The network project, if taken seriously, can help us reach this goal.

Acknowledgements This research was supported by *Le Fonds de Recherche en Santé du Québec* (FRSQ, reference no.8308). We would like to extend our gratitude to Jennifer Petrela for her editorial assistance and support.

References

Abbott A (1992) From causes to events: notes on narrative positivism. Sociol Methods Res 20:428–455
Abell P (1987) The syntax of social life: the theory and method of comparative narratives. Clarendon Press, Oxford
Abric J-C (1994) Les représentations sociales: Aspects théoriques. In: Abric J-C (ed) Pratiques Sociales et Représentations. PUF, Paris, pp 11–36
Allen D, Griffiths L, Lyne P (2004) Understanding complex trajectories in health and social care provision. Sociol Health Illn 26:1008–1030
Berkman LF, Glass T (2000) Social integration, social networks, social support, and health. In: Berkman LF, Kawachi I (eds) Social epidemiology. Oxford University Press, New York, pp 137–173
Bernard P (1993) Cause perdue? Le pouvoir heuristique de l'analyse causale. Sociol Soc XXV:171–189
Bond J, Corner L (2001) Researching dementia: are there unique methodological challenges for health services research. Aging Soc 21:95–116
Borgatti SP, Molina J-L (2005) Toward ethical guidelines for network research in organizations. Soc Networks 27:107–117

Brint S (1992) Hidden meanings: cultural content and context in harrison white's structural sociology. Sociol Theory 10:194–208

Carpentier N, Ducharme F (2005) Support network transformations in the first stages of the Caregiver's career. Qual Health Res 15(3):289–311

Carpentier N, Ducharme F (2007) Social network data validity: the example of the social network of caregivers of older persons with Alzheimer-type dementia. Can J Aging 26(suppl 1):103–116

Carpentier N, Ducharme F, Kergoat M-J, Bergman H (2008a) Barriers to care and social representations early in the career of caregivers of persons with Alzheimer's disease. Res Aging 30:334–357

Carpentier N, Pomey MP, Contreras R, Olazabal I (2008b) Social care interface in early-stage dementia: practitioners' perspectives on the links between formal and informal networks. J Aging Health 20(6):710–738

Carpentier N, Bernard P, Grenier A, Guberman N (2010) Using the life course perspective to study the entry into the illness trajectory: the perspective of caregivers of people with Alzheimer's disease. Soc Sci Med 70:1501–1508

Chiu LF, West RM (2007) Health intervention in social context: understanding social networks and neighbourhood. Soc Sci Med 65:1915–1927

Coleman JS (1986) Social theory, social research, and a theory of action. Am J Sociol 91:1309–1335

Dean K (2004) The role of methods in maintaining orthodox beliefs in health research. Soc Sci Med 58:675–685

Degenne A, Forsé M (2004) Les réseaux sociaux, 2nd edn. Armand Colin, Paris

Dowding K (1995) Model or metaphor? a critical review of the policy network approach. Polit Stud 43(1):136–158

Eisenberg M, Swanson N (1996) Organizational network analysis as a tool for program evaluation. Eval Health Prof 19(4):488–507

Emirbayer M (1997) Manifesto for a relational sociology. Am J Sociol 103(2):281–317

Emirbayer M, Goodwin J (1994) Network analysis, culture, and the problem of agency. Am J Sociol 99(6):1411–1454

Erickson B (2004) Social networks. In: Blau JR (ed) The Blackwell companion to sociology. Blackwell Publishing, Malden MA, pp 314–326

Ford EW, Wells R, Bailey B (2004) Sustainable network advantages: a game theoretic approach to community-based health care coalitions. Health Care Manage Rev 29(2):159–169

Fuhse JA (2009) The meaning structure of social networks. Sociol Theory 27:51–73

Geertz C (1973) The interpretation of cultures. Basic Books, New York

Granovetter M (1983) The strength of weak ties: a network theory revisited. Sociol Theory 1:201–233

Heise D (1991) Event structure analysis: a qualitative model of quantitative research. In: Fielding N, Lee R (eds) Using computers in qualitative research. Sage, Newbury Park, CA, pp 136–163

House JS, Umberson D, Landis KR (1988) Structures and processes of social support. Annu Rev Sociol 14:293–318

Jinnett K, Coulter I, Koegel P (2002) Cases, contexts and care: the need for grounded network analysis. In: Levy JA, Pescosolido BA (eds) Social networks and health, vol 8. Elsevier Science, Amsterdam, pp 101–110

Jippes E, Achterkamp MC, Brand PLP, Kiewiet DJ, Jan Pols J, van Engelen JML (2010) Disseminating educational innovations in health care practice: training versus social networks. Soc Sci Med 70:1509–1517

Jones IR, Ahmed N, Catty J, McLaren S, Rose D, Wykes T, Burn T (2009) Illness careers and continuity of care in mental health services: a qualitative study of service users and careers. Soc Sci Med 69:632–639

Kasper JD (2000) Health-care utilization and barriers to health care. In: Albrecht GL, Fitzpatrick R, Scrimshaw SC (eds) Handbook of social studies in health and medicine. Sage, London, pp 323–338

Knoke D (2004) Networks and organization. In: Blau JR (ed) The Blackwell companion to sociology. Blackwell, Malden, MA, pp 327–341

Learmonth M (2003) Making health services management research critical: a review and a suggestion. Sociol Health Illn 25(1):93–119

Levy JA, Pescosolido BA (2002) Advances in medical sociology, vol 8. Elsevier, Amsterdam

Lewis JM, Baeza JI, Alexander D (2008) Partnerships in primary care in Australia: network structure, dynamics and sustainability. Soc Sci Med 67:280–291

Litwak E (1985) Helping the elderly: the complementary roles of informal networks and formal systems. Guilford Press, New York

Marin A, Hampton KN (2007) Simplifying the personal network name generator: alternatives to traditional multiple and single name generators. Field methods 19:163–193

Markovsky B (1987) Toward multilevel sociological theories: simulations of actor and network effects. Sociol Theory 5:101–117

Martuccelli D (2002) Grammaires du l'Individu. Gallimard, Paris

Martuccelli D (2005) La Consistance du Social: Une sociologie pour la Modernité. PUR, Rennes

Maturo A (2004) Network governance as a response to risk society dilemmas: a proposal from the sociology of health. Topoi 23(2):195–202

Mechanic DM (1989) Health care and the elderly. Am Acad Pol Soc Sci 503:89–98

Messeri P, Silverstein M, Litwak E (1993) Choosing optimal support groups: a review and reformulation. J Health Soc Behav 34:122–137

Morgan C, Mallett R, Hutchinson G, Leff J (2004) Negative pathways to psychiatric care and ethnicity: the bridge between social science and psychiatry. Soc Sci Med 58:739–752

Mykhalovskiy E, Weir L (2004) The problem of evidence-based medicine: directions for social science. Soc Sci Med 59:1059–1069

Pescosolido BA (1991) Illness careers and network ties: a conceptual model of utilization and compliance. In: Albrecht G, Levy J (eds) Advances in medical sociology, vol 2. JAI Press, Greenwich, CT, pp 161–184

Pescosolido BA (1992) Beyond rational choice: the social dynamics of how people seek help. Am J Sociol 97(4):1096–1138

Pescosolido BA (1996) Bringing the "community" into utilization models: how social networks link individuals to changing systems of care. Res Sociol Health Care 13A:171–197

Pescosolido BA, Kronenfeld JJ (1995) Health, illness and healing in an uncertain era: challenges from and for medical sociology. J Health Soc Behav 36(Special Issue):5–33

Pescosolido BA, Rubin BA (2000) The web of group affiliations revisited: social life, postmodernism, and sociology. Am Sociol Rev 65:52–76

Rogler LH, Cortes DE (1993) Help-seeking pathways: a unifying concept in mental health care. Am J Psychiatry 150(4):554–561

Scott J (2000) Social network analysis: a handbook, 2nd edn. Sage, London

Shengelia B, Tandon A, Adams OB, Murray CJL (2005) Access, utilization, quality, and effective coverage: an integrated conceptual framework and measurement strategy. Soc Sci Med 61:97–109

Silverstein M, Bergtson VL, Litwak E (2003) Theoretical approaches to problems of families, aging, and social support in the context of modernization. In: Biggs S, Lowenstein A, Hendricks J (eds) The need for theory: critical approaches to social gerontology. Baywood, Amityville, NY, pp 181–198

Simmel G (1971) Group expansion and the development of individuality. In: Levine DN (ed) Georg Simmel on individuality and social form. University of Chicago Press, Chicago, IL

Smelser NJ (1988) Social structure. In: Smelser NJ (ed) Handbook of sociology. Sage, Newbury Park, CA, pp 103–129

Snijders TAB, Doreian P (2010) Introduction to the special issue on network dynamics. Soc Netw 32:1–3

Sørensen AB (1998) Theoritical mechanisms and the empirical study of social processes. In: Hedström P, Swedberg R (eds) Social mechanisms: an analytical approach to social theory. Cambridge University Press, Cambridge, pp 238–266

Stevenson WB, Greenberg D (2000) Agency and social networks: strategies of action in a social structure of position, opposition, and opportunity. Adm Sci Q 45(4):651–678

Taylor D, Bury M (2007) Chronic illness, expert patients and care transition. Sociol Health Illn 29:27–45

Thornicroft G, Tansella M (2004) Components of a modern mental health service: a pragmatic balance of community and hospital care: overview of systematic evidence. Br J Psychiatry 185:283–290

Uehara ES (2001) Understanding the dynamics of illness and help-seeking: event-structure analysis and a Cambodian–American narrative of 'spirit invasion'. Soc Sci Med 52(4):519–536

Wasserman S, Faust K (1994) Social network analysis: methods and applications. Cambridge University Press, Cambridge

White HC (2008) Identity and control: how social formations emerge, 2nd edn. Princeton University Press, Princeton

Wiggins R, Erzberger C, Hyde M, Higgs P, Blane D (2007) Optimal matching analysis using ideal types to describe the lifecourse: an illustration of how histories of work, partnerships and housing relate to quality of life in early old age. Int J Soc Res Methodol 10(4):259–278

Part VII
Connecting the Individual and the Body

Chapter 25
Bodies in Context: Potential Avenues of Inquiry for the Sociology of Chronic Illness and Disability Within a New Policy Era

Caroline Sanders and Anne Rogers

Introduction

The first decade of the twenty-first century is indeed a critical moment to reflect on the past and potential new avenues of inquiry focussed on chronic conditions. The recent re-shaping of policy and service delivery regarding chronic conditions across Western democracies provides both an old and new set of salient issues for sociologists to consider. Policy changes have occurred largely in response to demographic changes and concerns regarding the current and future burden of ageing, chronic disease and disability. The perceived economic implications of this "burden of chronic disease" has prompted the development and implementation of state-sponsored interventions to enhance self-care across international settings.

In attempting to look back and forward in sketching out a possible future for the sociology of chronic conditions, the themes we cover in this chapter overlap with other sections in this book. In thinking of the social experience of living with and managing a chronic condition in the twenty-first century, connections are readily apparent with *the body*, *communities*, as well as *cultural and health care systems*. This chapter will briefly reflect back on previous sociological work on chronic conditions, to highlight salient theoretical domains focussed on *biography*, *narrative* and *embodiment* evident in exploring key themes including *disruption*, *uncertainty* and *adaptation*. We also address a central area of debate reflected within previous sociological work on chronicity, that is, the relative importance of agency and structure in shaping experience and management. There are strong arguments for a dialectical approach that addresses both agency and structure, and importantly, the spaces in between, including policy and organisation regarding health and social care. The main areas requiring new avenues for critical sociological research are outlined more fully below with attention focussed on psychological determinism reflected within chronic disease management (CDM) policies and the need for a sociological focus on motivation associated with illness management. We also focus on the domains of contested knowledge and technological support for those with chronic conditions from the beginning to the end of illness trajectories. A final section of the chapter addresses theoretical and methodological directions for future research, arguing that a productive and critical approach can be achieved by drawing imaginatively on aspects of structural and post-structural sociology, including notions of "habitus," "therapeutic landscapes," and "social networks."

C. Sanders (✉)
Primary Care, Health Sciences, University of Manchester,
Williamson Bldg., Oxford Rd., Manchester, M13 9PL, UK
e-mail: caroline.sanders@manchester.ac.uk

Reflecting Back on the Sociology of Chronic Illness

One of the major contributions of medical sociology has been to draw attention to the ways in which the vast majority of health work takes place outside of the formal health care system (Stacey 1988). Early studies were informed by concerns about a clinical iceberg of symptoms lying undetected within communities due to unmet treatment needs (Last 1963). Sociologists turning attention specifically to chronic illness highlighted how people were adept at utilising existing social resources in managing and adapting to illness within a social context, often because there was limited help available from professional medicine (Bury 1997). Within this body of knowledge, self-care and self-management have been evident in the analysis of the impact of illness and the reactions to it.

Chronic Illness Experiences: Biography and Narrative

A focus on the notion of biography has illuminated the tendency for people to reflect on the trajectory of their lives in order to maintain a coherent sense of "self." Reflections on biographical pasts including reactions to personal crises and turning points provide insights into the way individuals construct their lives (Johnson 1976). Early sociological studies demonstrated that the onset of chronic illness often represents such a personal crisis characterised by *biographical disruption* (Bury 1982; Robinson 1988; Williams 1984) and *uncertainty* (Weiner 1975; Comaroff and Maguire 1981). In other words, people's lives were found to be disrupted and dominated by attempts to manage the ongoing uncertainty often associated with chronic illness. Such disruption was represented as a dramatic break with the usual trajectory of a person's biography, viewed as undermining their self-identity, their sense of security and their social relationships (Bury 1982; Conrad 1987; Corbin and Strauss 1987; Williams 1984). Bury conceptualised "biographical disruption" as the "kind of experience where the structures of everyday life and the forms of knowledge which underpin them are disrupted" (Bury 1982, p. 169).

In examining the meaning of symptoms, and the biographical impact of illness, Bury drew a helpful distinction between "meaning as consequence" and "meaning as significance" (Bury 1988). He used these terms to distinguish between the meaning of chronic illness concerning the problems created for the individual by activity restriction and social disadvantage (meaning as consequence); and the significance and connotations that conditions carry (meaning as significance). In other words, *meaning as consequence* is derived from the impact of symptoms at the practical and social level of daily life.[1] *Meaning as significance* refers to the symbolic significance of illness in a cultural context. It is important to acknowledge that the significance people attribute to their symptoms also stems from wider societal perceptions that influence the connotations and imagery associated with illness. Studies of chronic illnesses such as epilepsy and colitis highlighted the stigma associated with fitting and incontinence in a society that places great importance on bodily control (e.g., Scambler 1989; Kelly 1992).

Previous research on the experience of chronic illness illustrated the way in which self, identity and the social milieus are intimately related (Nettleton 1995:89). This is because how we are able to present ourselves to the outside world (our identity) impacts on our private sense of self. Cathy Charmaz (1983) described the impairment of such presentation by illness as a "loss of self" in a study where respondents reported how they constantly scrutinised encounters with others for hints of discreditation and negative reflections. She found that respondents became sensitive to the intentions and meanings of others and began to read statements and the actions of others in new, self-discrediting

---

[1] Physical impairment is obviously important in this respect, reflecting concerns with embodiment that have been picked up more fully in subsequent work.

ways. In consequence, they often became less capable of maintaining relationships, experiencing ever increasing degrees of social isolation. Other studies highlighted the interactional effects of uncertain illness trajectories that tested the limits afforded by close personal relationships, especially with family members (Bury 1988; Robinson 1988; Scambler and Hopkins 1988).

To demonstrate the significance of biography is to demonstrate the significance of a "story" about oneself, and for this reason, the "narrative" expression of illness experience has been repeatedly referred to in research on chronic illness (e.g., Kelly and Dickinson 1997; Williams 1984). Previous research has outlined the purpose of actively formulating and *reconstructing* (Williams 1984) or *re-casting* (Corbin and Strauss 1991) biographical narratives to make sense of illness experiences and to reconcile the past with the present. More recently, sociologists have drawn attention to the significance of perceptions about the future in exploring temporal aspects of narrative accounts (Faircloth et al. 2004b). Recent work has sought to extend and posit alternatives to the notion of "biographical disruption." Carricaburu and Pierret proposed the concept of "biographical reinforcement" as a more appropriate representation of experiences of men who are HIV-positive (Carricaburu and Pierret 1995). Concepts of biographical "continuity" (Williams 2000) or "flow" (Faircloth et al. 2004a) have been utilised to depict a notion of "normal" illness. For example, in the context of older age, people might present illness and disability (in the case of stroke) as a normal part of ageing (Pound et al. 1998) or as both normal and disruptive within single accounts (Sanders et al. 2002).

The Social and Cultural Significance of the Body

Over the past 2 decades, there has been an increased critical interest in the social and cultural significance of the body (e.g., Featherstone et al. 1991; Shilling 1993; Turner 1992), which has extended to include the study of chronic illness and disability (e.g., Kelly and Field 1996; Turner 2001; Williams 1996a, b, 1999; Frank 1991, 1995), ageing (Featherstone and Hepworth 1990), emotions and pain (e.g., Leder 1984b; Scarry 1985; Scheper-Hughes and Lock 1987; Williams and Bendelow 1998). The point has repeatedly been made that Western biomedicine is based on assumptions rooted in Cartesian dualism between the mind and body, whereby disease is present in the body and remains distinct from the mind (Leder 1984a). The physical reality of illness has tended to be categorised diametrically as either a naturalistic entity that legitimately belongs to the realms of medicine or biology or as something socially constructed via discourse (Kelly and Field 1996). A distinction has also been made between foundationalist approaches that accept the organic foundation of the body and anti-foundationalism that coincides with a social constructionist perspective (Turner 1992, 2001). These authors advocate a theoretical approach to the body that bridges this divide and can accept biological facts in addition to the social. Kelly and Field argue that the bodily experiences of pain in terms of the physical restrictions and discomforts have been neglected – a significant oversight because it is precisely these bodily experiences that have greatest weight in shaping interpretations and the attribution of meaning (Kelly and Field 1996).

The overlaps between themes of *embodiment*, *biography* and *the self* are obvious because bodily experiences (such as symptoms of illness) are part of our biographical make-up and our sense of self. As Williams points out, meanings born out of the significance and consequences of illness (as presented by Bury 1988) "have the notion of embodied experience at their centre, but rather than attempting to define functional incapacity or activity restriction in biomedical terms, they explore the ramifications of the experience from the point of view of the person affected" (Williams 1996a, p. 198). Williams also presents narrative reconstruction as an attempt to repair ruptures between body, self and society (Williams 1984). The links between biography and the self with the body and social identity in chronic illness experience are evident in the ascribed importance of body control and image for social representation and interaction in Goffman's work on Stigma (Goffman 1971).

These features were theoretically elaborated by Corbin and Strauss who describe three major dimensions of biography referred to as the BBC chain comprising: Biography (time past, present, future in which conceptions of self are imbedded); the Body (as a means of interacting with the world, self and others); and Conception of self identity (where the body becomes the medium through which we form our self-identity) (Corbin and Strauss 1987). Others exemplified the significance of embodiment in research showing how stigma is associated with bodily symptoms linked to feelings of shame, embarrassment and fear (e.g., Kelly 1992; Nijhof 1995; Scambler and Hopkins 1988), or where people attempt to disguise problems caused by physical functioning (Weiner 1975; Williams and Barlow 1998). Thus, bodily appearance and function have been perceived as central to the mobilisation of social identity (Turner 2001).

Adaptation

Coping, *strategy* and *style* are linked concepts used to articulate the processes of adaptation for those with chronic illness and disability. Coping refers to the cognitive and emotional mechanisms that "spill over" into the strategies that people adopt in managing the problems associated with their condition (Bury 1997, p. 131). "Coping" is a sense of coherence, which individuals maintain in the face of their condition (for example, preserving an impression of "normality" to the outside world) and the mobilisation of resources and the maintenance of normal activities and relationships (family, friends and occupations) in the face of an altered situation (Bury 1982). People adopt emotional and cognitive mechanisms as a means of recovering a sense of self-worth in response to biographical disruption, a process referred to by Corbin and Strauss as "comeback" (Corbin and Strauss 1991). The term "strategy" is used to focus on the resources and sources of support available to individuals in a wider social context and what they do to mobilise them in order to minimise problems in everyday life (Locker 1983). Strategies may be cognitive, physical or both. For example, those with chronic conditions often talk about mental and physical "pacing" to make life manageable (Williams 1993b; Weiner 1975). In contrast, "Style" is apparent in different narrative representations of illness experience within *interactional* contexts. Such styles develop as a means of preserving or re-forming personal identity and are symbolic means by which people present the "self" in social life (Radley and Green 1987). These styles may be classified, for example, as *comic*, *heroic* or *tragic* (Kelly and Dickinson 1997). This highlights the performance and moral aspects of storytelling about illness (Bury 2001; Williams 1993a).

In looking back, previous research has lent transparency to the complexities associated with identities, experience and management of illness and disability. Detailed qualitative studies have emerged from within interpretative sociology, declaring varied affinities to symbolic interactionism and phenomenology and often adopting a version of the grounded theory approach to provide insights into the minutiae of illness experience (Gerhardt 1989). Such research has highlighted the significance of embodiment within interactional and cultural contexts, highlighting the social experience of illness and the varied ways in which people manage illness for themselves. However, these self-care activities have traditionally been seen as having little to do with formal service provision, perceived instead as purposive action that stops at the outset of the consultation in which "proper" medicine takes over (Cunningham-Burley and Irvine1987). This picture of a "failure" of medicine to engage with the life worlds of patients encouraged a view in which living with chronic illness is conceptualised as a reactive flight into normalisation in which, over time, the patient becomes "free of medicine" (Rogers et al. 2007). While epidemiological studies indicated the ways in which people's own efforts were largely responsible for managing the large clinical iceberg of everyday symptoms experienced in the community, informal activity as a response to need has been largely ignored by health policy makers (Rogers et al. 1999). Over the last decade, this previous picture of lay self-care as an endeavour outside formal health care and beyond the influence of formal policy interventions has been radically challenged; this is illustrated by the many self-care interventions designed and implemented within Western democracies. This shifting terrain prompts the need for refining a sociological response that builds on the strengths of early work whilst engaging the changing face of health care policy for managing chronic conditions.

Engaging Policy: Exploring Motivation and Illness Management

Concerns about the economic implications of a perceived growing burden of ageing, chronic disease and disability within Western democracies have prompted extensive policy responses targeted at both *prevention* and *management* of chronic disease with the Chronic Care Model (CCM) leading the field (Barr 2003). Interventions flowing from this model have aimed to maximise self-care capacity, targeting the majority of the population with LTCs who have low-level needs for health interventions but who are considered to be at risk of greater need and dependency in the future. However, attempts to maximise self-care for those with high-level needs are also reflected in interventions targeted at both ends of the spectrum. For example, self-management training courses have incorporated an element on the subject of planning for end of life care, encouraging a greater degree of control and personal responsibility to plan for a time when people might be incapacitated and incapable of making choices regarding health care interventions (Sanders et al. 2008). At higher levels of need (requiring active monitoring of disease, medical and social case-management), telecare and telehealth interventions are being further utilised in order to maximise self-care capacity even when health service and social care requirements are considerable. By drawing on the collective bodies of sociological work that have emerged over recent decades, there is scope for sociologists to critically inform the design and evaluation of self-care interventions.

Self-care interventions that acknowledge patient expertise and capacity seem, on the face of things, to be an acknowledgment of sociological research that has traditionally highlighted these issues. However, critical evaluations demonstrate that such interventions are often divorced from social context and can be disrupting and disconnecting for patient experience and existing management practices (Wilson et al. 2007; Kennedy and Rogers 2001; Taylor and Bury 2007; Gately et al. 2007; Sanders et al. 2008). This suggests a need to build on the early work of sociologists focussed on *experience* from the patients' perspective and a need to give further attention to *management* (formal as well as informal) associated with the reorganisation of services for those with chronic conditions. The concept of "illness career" is particularly relevant to the issue of management as it has been prominent in efforts to convey the experience of illness over prolonged time-spans and especially the negotiation of pathways through professional services (Herzlich 1973; Pavalko et al. 2007).

The Limits of Psychological Determinism

The dominant etiological focus on risk factors associated with lifestyle and personal behaviour (e.g., smoking, lack of exercise and poor eating habits) has been used to shift responsibility from the state in support of government strategies that encourage adults to adopt healthier lifestyles mainly through educational interventions that focus on changing established "unhealthy" behaviour. Throughout the 1980s and the 1990s there was an extensive growth in the realm of "health promotion" and an accompanying moral discourse emphasising personal responsibility for the maintenance of good health and by implication for the occurrence of chronic disease. Better secondary prevention leading to reductions in mortality and the sequelae of chronic disease has been linked to better demand management and fiscal control of health services expenditure. The CCM highlights connections between health promotion and CDM, where interventions have been aimed at maximising the capacity of individuals to manage their own chronic condition as well as minimising risk of disease progression. This shifting terrain in CDM has been viewed to represent a "care transition" (Taylor and Bury 2007). It is this "care transition" that requires a critical sociological focus on motivation and the management of illness in order to move forward from the dependence on psychological and individualistic models of self-management interventions.

One of the most influential self-management interventions has been the Chronic Disease Self Management Programme (CDSMP) that was originally developed in the United States (Sobel et al. 2002) and has since been adapted and piloted in a number of countries around the world including China and the UK (Dongbo et al. 2003; Kennedy et al. 2007). The underlying philosophy of the CDSMP is that patients with different chronic diseases face similar self-management problems and disease-related tasks and that they can be educated to manage their conditions better, using fewer healthcare resources. Educational sessions within the programme cover a number of topics including: exercise; cognitive management techniques; nutrition, sleep; medications; emotion management; communication with health professionals; problem solving and decision-making. Courses such as the CDSMP have been predicated on outcomes relating to: changes in behaviour (the changing of diet, relaxation and "planned activity"); decreased utilisation of health services; and attitude (self-efficacy); or possessing better ability to "cope with symptoms." The capacity for change is seen to lie within the individual, leading to a focus on changes in behaviour and psychological outcomes. Psychological outcome measures such as "self-efficacy" (self-confidence specific to a behaviour; Bandura 1997) are viewed as being enhanced through a number of mechanisms, the most effective of which is "performance attainment" (i.e., actual experience of the success of actions), whilst depression and anxiety are viewed as impairing both self-efficacy beliefs and the ability to engage in behaviours that might increase self-efficacy. Other common psychological concepts used to evaluate the effectiveness of self-management programmes have been drawn from the health belief model tradition, which suggests two key factors – personal susceptibility and belief in the benefits of action – influence the likelihood of changing personal health action. A person must feel personally susceptible to a disease with serious or severe consequences and believe that the benefits of taking a particular course of action outweigh the perceived costs and barriers (Andersen and Keller 2002). The transtheoretical model of behaviour change (Prochaska et al. 1994) posits that people change behaviour through stages: pre-contemplation, contemplation, preparation, action and maintenance. The concept of "activation" comprises a broad range of elements that patients *need* in order to successfully manage a chronic illness: believing the patient role is important; having the confidence and knowledge necessary to take action; actually taking action to maintain and improve one's health; and staying the course even under stress (Hibbard et al. 2004). Similarly, Leventhal et al. (1998) have proposed a self-regulation model, which addresses the impact of emotion, the time course of the disease, and changes in the perception of threat over time on disease management. The patient is viewed as a problem solver able to assess the risk of the disease and identify what actions to take.

Techniques such as cognitive re-structuring and dedicated self-care education training have been attributed with beneficial outcomes in improving people's confidence to take care of themselves and engaging in shared decision-making with health professionals (Von Korff et al. 1997; Robinson et al. 2001; Bower 2002; Kennedy et al. 2004). Programmes such as the CDSMP (and EPP in the UK) are based on social cognitive and social learning theory in that the enhancement of self-efficacy is considered a mediator for change in health outcome.[2] Assumptions regarding cognitive strategies and actions of individuals conjure up notions of an "ideal type" of self-manager within discourse on

---

[2] The presence or absence of successful change as a result of the CDSMP is thought to be the result of the increased capacity of the individual following exposure to skills such as problem-solving, decision-making, resource utilisation, action planning, and partnership with health care providers.

patient change. Whilst policy makers might set goals that concur with such an ideal type, with interventions designed to move individuals from one stage to the next, it is unlikely that this normative view is a realistic picture of how people can and do behave. Notions of self-efficacy, self-image and self-worth are all constructs drawn from clinical traditions (i.e., clinical psychology and psychiatry) that have been driven by attempts to account for subjective distress. The "self" within this tradition is one viewed as being deficient or lacking in the properties to be a whole or fully functioning individual.

While self-management programmes are formulated in line with psychological theories, there is evidence that where change does occur, this does not necessarily follow the theoretical stages of change incorporated into models of health behaviour. More importantly, the use of models of psychological change may mask or detract from viewing change in relation to the complexities of patients' existing ways of behaving and responding to chronic illness. Within psychological theories of change, existing behaviour and activities in context are usually ignored or viewed as maladaptive requiring reform.[3]

Shifting Identities and Broader Social Influences in Chronic Disease Management

Theories predicated on changing individual beliefs are not designed to evaluate the everyday components of patient practices and strategies in a broader social context. Additionally, identifying aspects of interventions most likely to change behaviour via causal modelling may not be relevant to the priorities that individuals hold about managing a chronic condition. For example, symptom management may not be considered as important as preserving valued social roles, coherent identities and a "normal life" (Townsend et al. 2006). The tendency to attribute too much importance to the individual level of change at the expense of contextual variables, and the normative focus on how individuals "should" behave, fails to appreciate factors beyond individual control such as housing, hardship and discrimination (Bloor et al. 1992; Hodgins et al. 2006). An individual may be said to lack self-efficacy or have low self-esteem but may not have access to resources that are important mediators of favourable outcomes. By adopting self-efficacy as the primary mechanism of success in self-management interventions, models of the costly and "non-compliant" patient may be replaced by a subjective deficit model in which people are viewed as lacking the properties needed to be an appropriately functioning and independent individual.

Taylor and Bury (2007) observe the tensions between health policies presented as acknowledging the social determinants of chronic conditions and interventions based on individual models of behaviour change. The latter, they claim runs the risk "of "blaming the victims" rather than addressing the social factors more fundamentally responsible for their illnesses"(p. 32). Such a view echoes earlier debates about interventions implemented under the auspices of the "new public health" from the 1970s onwards (Brown and Piper 1995). Those supportive of collective approaches to health promotion argued that the focus on lifestyles and individualistic interventions based on "health persuasion techniques" (Beattie 1991) as a means of changing lifestyles and behaviour, were responsible for a victim-blaming ideology to the neglect of structural variables such as poverty (see also Blaxter 1983; Crawford 1977). Although, as Lupton states, it was "difficult to challenge because of

---

[3] The latter is evident in theories of 'planned action' (popular in health prevention but increasingly so in chronic illness) that are normative in assumptions about the desirability of changing one behaviour for another (e.g., smoking for non-smoking). Additionally, while such assumptions maybe appropriate regarding behaviour such as smoking, arguably this is less applicable to chronic illness given the variety of strategies drawn upon in coping or adjusting to illness.

its manifest benevolent goal of maintaining standards of health" (Lupton 1993). Beattie also examined the way health promotion could be used as a form of cultural control by imposing rules and constraints on people. However, whilst some critics of health promotion strategies perceived them to represent an extension of professional control, others pointed to paradoxical emancipatory dimension resulting from collective action: "There has been in recent health promotion simultaneously a marked tightening of the grip by powerful professionals and bureaucracies… and a vigorous opening up of consumer power and voluntary action…" (Beattie 1991, p. 187).

Contradictions have also been highlighted in analyses of state-sponsored self-management programmes (such as the EPP in the UK) where the notion of the "empowered patient" is noted as an ambiguous construct within professional discourse (Wilson 2001; Wilson et al. 2007). The potential for empowerment at a collective level has been seen to be rooted within the traditional ethos of the self-help movement that emerged from a critical stance against professionalism and an emphasis on consumers as managers of their own lives (Kendall and Rogers 2007). At the same time, the discourse of "empowerment" has been viewed as allowing an extension of professional expertise and adherence to the principles of clinical regimes into patients' everyday lives *and* allowing clinicians to withdraw from areas of patient need that are problematic to diagnose and manage (e.g., chronic symptoms such as pain and fatigue; Salmon 2000). This latter tension points to the blurring of boundaries between professionals and lay people in the area of chronic disease management, with the latter increasingly cast as reflexive consumers where the consumption process is actively bound with identity formation. The way in which self-identity is reflexively organised in response to social change is a recurring theme in contemporary sociology (Giddens 1991b; Lash and Friedman 1992). From this perspective, the paradigm of change in self-management can be viewed as part of a wider moral discourse on self-care within "late" or "post" modern societies promoting personal responsibility and self-government for all aspects of life including current and future health states. Ideas about the social significance of "self-governance" are important, and there are examples where related issues around embodiment, consumption and identity have been fruitfully explored within empirical work (Fox 2005; Fox and Ward 2006), to illustrate both conformity and resistance to dominant moral discourses. Others have also focussed on issues of embodiment and identity via narrative accounts of those with chronic and life-threatening illness. For example, Frank's view is that a greater equality between doctors and patients has occurred along with a decline in the mystique surrounding medicine, lending an empowering context for the expression of illness narratives. Narratives are viewed as an opportunity to reflexively reconstitute one's "self" and social relationships (Frank 1995, 1997; see also Charmaz 1995). However, these approaches have sometimes been criticised for being overly reflexive (Williams 1999) and optimistic (Bury 2001). Williams refers to them as "phenomenologically deep" because they retreat too far into the body and self and neglect the "material reality" of experience (Williams 1996a).

Oliver has pointed to the need for a political economy of disability and considers the way individualization of life within capitalist economies contributes to an ideology of individualised disability and the role of powerful groups such as the medical profession in reinforcing that individualism (Oliver 1990). While the focus of contemporary social theorists on self-identity and reflexive modernization potentially contributes to an ideology of individualism, examining the limits of self-determination and reflexivity can also provide a material critique of new economic forms and contemporary concerns with self-care (Webb 2004). May (1997) cautions against the de-politicisation implied by individualising vocabulary within contemporary social theory but states that the surrender of theories about motivation to the field of psychology is a serious problem within sociology. Rather, a strong sociological theory of motivation would enable us to account for the dynamic qualities of actors that propel the search for the authentic self, and that engender self-maximisation (p. 51). Such a focus is important to facilitate a sophisticated understanding of the limits and operationlisation of self-care and empowerment in practice. This is evident in the work of McDonald et al. (2007), who suggests that the emphasis placed on freedom and rationality by Giddens and other social theorists is too simplistic because of the multiple and contested nature of consumer identities. They describe varied consumption practices influencing identity work where there are conflicting ethical codes associated with a polarised rhetoric depicting patients as either "rational consumer" or "dependent patient." Respondents reflected a desire to be perceived as good citizens who adopt appropriate ways of acting (e.g., not using services unnecessarily) as opposed to the portrayal of the "bad citizen" who are unethical consumers of health care. However, participants also presented a sense of personal entitlement to services as well as a desire to be supportive of the needs of other members of society, alongside an acceptance of individual responsibility for health. McDonald et al. conclude that the government's promotion of particular health consumer identities can be seen as an attempt to disrupt, rather than rationalise certain existing relations by shifting responsibility from the state to the individual.

The social model of disability, along with more critical sociological approaches, has helped to foster a greater focus on political debate and citizenship. However, there is a need for sociological inquiry that considers the recognition of personal and bodily experience but within broader social, political, and organisational contexts. This is particularly important for shifting the focus away from individuals and their capacity to help themselves outside of formal health care, to a greater focus on interactional contexts in which health care is provided or negotiations about self-management take place, as well as the barriers to getting professional help when needed. Additionally, there is scope for sociologists to conduct more sophisticated research and analysis by engaging directly with clinical outcomes in studying disease management (Timmermans and Haas 2008). Timmermans and Haas highlight the seminal work of Parsons in drawing attention to the ways in which many conditions are open to therapeutic influence through motivational channels (p. 660). This latter observation adds weight to the argument that sociologists should take changes in the clinical markers of disease seriously when attempting to understand motivations for self-management at the interface with formal medical treatment and care. However, not all conditions have clear clinical markers of disease and we now extend the discussion to a focus on contested areas of knowledge regarding medically unexplained and hard to diagnose symptoms. We then consider the realm of ongoing change in the use of technological interventions to support illness management.

Exploring Evolving Domains of Knowledge and Technological Support from Beginning to End of Illness Trajectories

Additional areas for sociological research continue to arise with the emergence (and contestation) of new diagnostic categories (especially for medically unexplained chronic symptoms) and with the expansion of new technologies including the internet and telecare interventions that have become evermore a feature of CDM at the start of the twenty-first century. Such changes require sociologists to engage further with notions of expertise between professionals and non-professionals and the collective action associated with specific health movements. Whereas the concept of "illness career" has often been drawn upon to reflect personal journeys through the long-term management of a chronic condition, we increasingly need to focus on collective issues in the experience and management of chronic conditions. For example, collective support has emerged in response to the sharing of personal journeys between those with rare, medically contested conditions or mental health problems and via the disability movement. Contestations and expansions in arenas of knowledge and technology also require engagement with sociological work within the domain of Science and Technology Studies (STS) to study the translation of new technologies such as telehealth and telecare into areas of practice in the management of chronic conditions. Moreover, discussions about the appropriate use of technologies for those with end stage chronic conditions indicate that if we are to take seriously the illness trajectories of those with chronic conditions, then we need also engage further with a focus on the management of illness at the end of life.

Contested Knowledge and the Shifting Diagnostic Terrain for Chronic Symptoms

A shifting diagnostic terrain marked by an increase in new categories of medically unexplained illnesses presents the opportunity for extending sociological enquiry to considering conditions such as Chronic Fatigue Syndrome (CFS) and Myalgic Encephalitis (ME). This brings important issues to the fore, particularly at the beginning of illness trajectories where people often struggle to gain legitimate recognition for their illness.

An important distinction has traditionally been made that lay people "experience" illness, whilst doctors "diagnose" and treat disease (Eisenberg 1977), and attention has been drawn to an esoteric body of knowledge that preserves social distance between lay people and medical doctors, whilst conveying authoritative status on clinicians (Freidson 1970). Others have highlighted the relational nature of medical knowledge, noting that professionals and non-professionals alike can have expert knowledge and that lay people are often active in the construction of biomedical knowledge. The latter is evident at the margins of medical knowledge where the organic basis of disease remains elusive, or when pathophysiological explanations are contested. For example, Arksey studied the case of Repetitive Strain Injury (RSI) (Arksey 1994) and demonstrates the way in which "marginal actors can exploit their technical competence" in order to legitimate their illness experience:

> As their illness continued, many RSI victims became better informed about the disorder than their treating physician: they appropriated medical knowledge and terminology, and could distinguish and make judgments between the various theories of causation. For their part, sympathetic practitioners acknowledged their patients' subjective perceptions and annexed this lay expertise to further their own knowledge and understanding (1994, p. 455).

This study demonstrates that patients can be viewed as beating the experts at their own game by adopting a scientific approach in order to legitimate their illness. Similarly, people often appropriate medical narratives (referring to biomedical explanations), and in the process choose between conflicting scripts in negotiation with various medical practitioners (Seale 1996, p. 154). As Hess observes, there has been a marked shift from an unchallenged epistemic authority of professional medicine to a more complex field and an emerging "public shaping of science" with greater legiticimacy placed in social movements and lay advocacy organisations (Hess 2004).

As earlier sociological work has demonstrated, the issue as to whether disease is perceived as something subjective or objective is important because the objectification of disease can be a powerful cultural resource to individuals with chronic illness serving as a means of reifying disease, which in turn provides legitimisation and sanctioning of the behaviour of those who are "ill" (Bury 1982). Diagnosis of a chronic condition can bring a sense of relief in uncovering a legitimate reason for symptoms and is thus central in the sufferers' search for an adequate narrative that gives meaning to personal experience (Seale 1996). The diagnosis of an illness where people experience chronic pain provides a special form of relief, providing the bases from which people cope better with their perceived future (Hellstrom 2001).

A focus on contemporary lifestyles, self-governance and identity also draws attention to a blurring of boundaries between lifestyle choices and conditions designated as chronic. For example, Fox and Ward studied internet discussion forums based on three case studies: a pro-anorexia site, a site discussing purchase and use of the drug *Viagra* to improve sexual function, and a site focussed on the use of weight loss drugs for the treatment of obesity (Fox and Ward 2006). This study demonstrates varying degrees of conformity and resistance to notions of an "expert patient" that also reflects conformity or resistance to an illness identity. In the case of the pro-anorexia site, there was strong resistance to a predominant discourse representing anorexia as a medical condition requiring psychiatric management. Rather, members of the "pro-ana" forum promoted an idea of anorexia as a lifestyle choice, giving advice for those aspiring to be successfully anorexic. Conversely, the site discussing the use of weight loss drugs illustrated a strong conformity to biomedical narratives defining obesity as a medical condition.

Recent work on contested knowledge and the boundaries between chronicity and lifestyle highlight a need to focus on the interactional contexts in which contested knowledge is worked through in practice and the ramifications for care pathways followed (or not) by those with chronic symptoms that are hard to diagnose. While some have highlighted the traditional clinical emphasis on establishing certainty and "theoretical coherence" (e.g., Atkinson 1984; Pinder 1992; Salmon 2000), others have illustrated the flexibility of doctors in primary care prepared to advocate alternative treatments even if such treatments were perceived to be beyond their perception of biomedical rationality (May and Sirur 1998). However, tensions and conflict between doctors and patients regarding subjective and objective interpretations of sickness arise when there is difficulty establishing certainty and coherence in the management of chronic conditions that are hard to diagnose (May et al. 2004). Doctors' accounts of their management of musculoskeletal conditions and other hard-to-diagnose symptoms demonstrated that "models of illness were contested as patients tended to deploy an organic model of pathology, and doctors a psychosocial one." Such dissonance implies that many patients are often left feeling unsupported by formal healthcare and need to turn to other sources of support suggesting the relevance of inquiry of outside sources of support that come, for example, from new social movements (e.g., Brown 2004), or the use of informal networks to acquire or exchange new information (Lambert and Rose 1996). In this respect, recent studies have focussed on how people with rare and unexplained symptoms or those with conditions that might be highly stigmatised turn to the internet as a source of information and support (Barker 2008; Berger 2005; Mendelson 2003; Weisberger 2004).

Information and Assistive Technologies for Supporting Chronically Ill and Disabled People

The internet has been considered to be valuable for enabling people to seek out support and information, especially for those who may otherwise be isolated and unable to access other forms of support. However, there has also been concern expressed regarding a "digital divide" between the "information rich" and "information poor" with potential for the internet to increase social inequalities (Drentea and Moren-Cross 2005). A growing number of studies have reported on how use can vary according to factors such as age, gender and social class (Seale et al. 2006; Seale 2006a, b). Nettleton et al, point out that the reality of everyday internet use across social groups is much more complex than represented by views of a digital divide, indicating the need for further investigation regarding the potential use of the internet to support those living with chronic conditions (Nettleton et al. 2004). Examples demonstrate awareness of potential inequalities leading to the design of interventions to support internet use for those with chronic conditions targeted at disadvantaged groups as a means of enhancing self-care (Lindsay et al. 2007).

The complex arena of internet use that is ever expanding requires us to look further at how ideas about "informed" or "expert patients" are worked out within this changing era of e-scaped medicine. Some researchers have sought to illustrate the enactment of such roles as part of the reflexivity in contemporary social life. As Kivits found, people often use the internet to seek a different type of information based on everyday and "experiential" knowledge rather than medical expertise (Kivits 2007). However, findings also reflected a paradox of "reflexive" consumption associated with internet use, where it was simultaneously viewed as enabling greater choice to support informed decision-making while creating greater uncertainty due to the number of alternatives. The overwhelming number of choices available can be a source of greater insecurity and uncertainty in the context of societal pressures to demonstrate personal responsibility (Bauman 2000). Contrary to some assumptions, the reflexive use of the internet does not necessarily lead to a challenge to medical expertise even where dissatisfaction with medical advice had initially led people to seek information on the internet. Kivits (2007) found evidence of both displacement and replacement of trust towards medical professionals as patients using the internet were confronted with choices they find hard to navigate (see also, Nettleton et al. 2004). Similarly, Barker found online discussions within a support group for Fibromyalgia Syndrome simultaneously challenged the expertise of physicians and encouraged the expansion of medicine's jurisdiction (Barker 2008). Sandaunet (2008) also found adherence to a biomedical explanatory model to be an important mediator in the dynamics of using an online self-help group for people with breast cancer. The work of Sandaunet draws attention to the need to consider factors such as "non-participation" and "withdrawal" from using internet support groups in attempting to understand the role of such fora, highlighting that the common perception of them as arenas for successful coping can also be a barrier for their use.

Beyond informal use of the internet, there is a need to study further the ever changing provision of assistive and communication technologies to support the care of people with chronic conditions within community settings currently advocated by policy makers (Department of Health 2005, 2006). These technologies are increasingly being deployed to support the management of chronic conditions, but little is known about the impact and integration of such technologies with existing forms of support. Studies indicate that the capacity for specific technologies to promote independence and enhanced self-management is complex – fostering greater independence on the one hand while simultaneously inducing greater dependence on the other. Lehoux et al., who studied four technological health care interventions at home (IV antibiotic therapy, parenteral nutrition, peritoneal dialysis and oxygen therapy), found that patients were ambivalent about the benefits and drawbacks of technology, but experiences were intimately interwoven with the nature of the disease and with the patients' personal life trajectory (Lehoux et al. 2004). A number of studies also highlight that acceptability of assistive technologies is dependent on whether the device is perceived to support or undermine a sense of identity (Gitlin et al. 1998), views about perceived need (McCreadie and Tinker 2005), and the impact of surveillance on autonomy (Percival and Hanson 2006).

Nicolini (2006) discusses how telemedicine presupposes and entails significant changes in work processes that affect the relationships and practices of health care professionals such as the delegation of medical tasks to non-medical personnel and artefacts and the tendency of telemedicine to modify the existing geography within the health care environment. However, the delegation of medical tasks to machines can entail additional work for patients in areas previously unfamiliar (e.g., diagnosis). Such extension of work for patients can be highly valued as a source of new opportunities to complete aspects of illness work that were previously impossible, but technologies can also compound disruptive experiences as patients attempt to fit technologies into their existing management practices and daily lives (Gately et al. 2008; Oudshoorn 2008). Existing research has documented the impact on doctor–patient interactions with a sense of alienation arising from the use of teleconsultations and problems with doctor-patient interaction (Harrison et al. 2006). The changing nature of professional–patient interaction has also been found to be problematic for professionals who perceived the loss of interpersonal cues associated with teleconsultations to have a detrimental impact on management of mental health problems (May et al. 2001). All of these issues indicate the need to evaluate the implementation of new assistive technologies within the context of personal life trajectories as well as within the interactional settings where formal care pathways are followed – both can be conceptualised as key aspects of illness careers.

Theoretical, Conceptual and Methodological Considerations for Future Research

Having outlined some key topics requiring further research that are already emerging in current literature, we now turn to promising theoretical and conceptual frameworks that might usefully be drawn upon to facilitate new work. At times, the commentary on the subject of chronic illness and disability has been polarised with a tendency to subscribe to one of the two camps: disability theorists have been criticised for adopting an "over-socialised" perspective; versus medical sociologists who have been criticised for adopting an overly individualised perspective. Critical reflections on these diametric approaches suggest the need for some middle ground with the capacity to bridge the divide between agency and structure. At the methodological level, there has been calls to move beyond the predominant reliance on "one off interviews" that characterises much of early medical sociology research in this field, calling instead for longitudinal studies drawing upon multiple interviews and mixed qualitative methods including observational work in keeping with ethnographic approaches (Conrad 1990; Lawton 2003). More recently, reflections on theoretical contributions to the sociology of the body has been extended to consider the specific importance of biology and a *sociology of disease* for studying the dialectical relationships between social life and disease (Timmermans and Haas 2008). Timmermans and Haas question why sociologists have often failed to relate important "biomarkers" (e.g., blood sugar levels, cortisol levels) to studies of illness experience. They consider the great potential for future research that relates readily available health outcomes to ethnographic research on illness experiences, especially for illuminating inequalities in disease management. This section considers some particular promising domains of sociological inquiry that have been applied to the various aspects of social life and can inform new avenues of inquiry regarding chronic illness, disability and the management of LTCs.

Habitus, Therapeutic Landscapes and Social Networks

The sociology of chronic illness has in early work drawn extensively on a tradition of symbolic interactionism that has sometimes been criticised for failing to adequately address the broader social influences and resources impacting on experience and ability to manage chronic conditions. The changing policy environment and institutional arrangements for ministering healthcare, as well as the harnessing of technology for managing chronic conditions, point to the need to consider resources and interactions within and between multiple social domains. Three concepts are, we suggest, salient to developing and extending previous work, while bridging the divide between agency and structure. These are *habitus, therapeutic landscapes* and *social networks*. A sociological understanding of the management of chronic conditions can benefit from a perspective that draws on notions of deeply ingrained schemas and habits which Bourdieu referred to as *habitus* – the cyclical manner in which experience and action (individual and collective) are both structured by the sediments of previous experiences/ actions and themselves leave a "sediment," which will structure future experiences and action.[4,5] For Bordieu, the body is the locus of distinguishing characteristics that signify an individual's social location and it is the means through which the appropriate strategies and practices are executed within a given field (Crossley 2001). Camic (1986) also describes how notions of "habit" are identifiable as an important background within the writings of Durkheim and Weber. He argues that sociological concerns with habit started to disappear early in the twentieth century and suggests the concept was a casualty of sociology's revolt against behaviourism. However, the concepts of habit and habitus seem important for researching motivations for self-care, as discussed earlier, and how such motivations are linked to wider social structures.

---

[4] Bordieu used the concept of *habitus* to represent structured sets of values and ways of thinking as well as cultural symbols that distinguish social position, preserving and reproducing inequalities via differential accumulation of social capital between groups. His ideas about social capital were greatly influenced by Marxism, but he developed ideas about *habitus* to serve as a theoretical bridge between subjective agency and objective position and distinguished between cultural and material capital. This placed him at the *'crossroads of two central highways'* in sociological thought, integrating structuralist perspectives of inequality with constructivist perspectives of agency (Field 2003).

[5] Field draws attention to the limitations of Bordieu's work in failing to acknowledge that social capital can be detrimental and that less privileged individuals and groups might also find benefit from socialties.

Angus et al. (2005) have usefully drawn upon the concept of habitus in an empirical study exploring the significance of the home for understanding the experience of long-term home care. They found that deteriorating health and the accompanying mobility limitations altered the manner in which care recipients could engage in these relations. The disrupted concordance between care recipients' bodies and the objective conditions provided by the material spaces of the home signified altered or changing social placement. For example, assistive devices were regarded as symbols or distinctions of an unwelcome shift to a *habitus* of dependency or disability, whilst economic resources limited the logics and delivery of home care. Constraints and changes regarding forms of care available to clients associated with policy decisions resulted in impoverishment of cultural capital that altered the experience of the home. The impact of such constraints was inequitable because some participants were able to pay for private services that had previously been provided with public funds (Angus et al. 2005). This piece of work connects with important themes from previous research in considering the importance of embodiment in relation to impairment as well as the mundane aspects of the everyday management of illness. However, it also accounts for structural and material context that is in turn influenced by policy contexts and how these mediate bodily experience.

Bordieu also associates *habitus* with "generative structures" and a corresponding focus on interaction and social change. These ideas have been drawn upon via the concept of therapeutic landscapes to explore "changing places, settings, situations, locales and milieus that encompass the physical, psychological and social environments associated with treatment or healing" (Williams 1999; cited in Wilton and DeVerteuil 2006, p. 650). The focus of therapeutic landscapes is on locally specific studies, inequality and exclusion, which in turn can also be on obstacles and barriers to therapy and healing (Wilton and DeVerteuil 2006; Wilton 2006). For example, Wilton and DeVerteuil focus on alcohol recovery programmes as part of a therapeutic landscape and the way in which alcoholism has been defined as a loss of control or a "disease of the will." They claim "this rises interesting questions about the ways in which "recovery landscapes" work to re-establish control over individual conduct, and can therefore be understood as sites of governmentality" (p. 650). These ideas are relevant to CDM policy and interventions because these can be perceived as the social foundation upon which new environments for supporting self-management and case-management occur. Exposure to new interventions and organisational features of care bring about a process of comparison by patients with established regimens and give rise to reflection, internal contestation and the expression of (or resistance to) new practices. This also applies to health care practitioners, who have established schemas and patterns regarding the way they manage patients with chronic conditions (e.g., May et al. 2003a).

The work of Bordieu has also been highly influential within sociological research focussed on social networks and social capital largely through his theorising on the role of "cultural capital" in structuring inequalities. There has been some attention focussed on how social networks and social capital serve to support health as well as creating inequalities in the genesis of illness (Berkman et al. 2000). However, to date, there has been limited conceptual and empirical work on social networks and social capital focussed specifically on chronic illness and disability (Sanders and Rogers 2008). Previous research has established that network ties are known to advantage those who are already "rich" in terms of social capital, whereas other ties (or lack of them) serve to disadvantage those who are already lacking social capital. Social network research has been adept at exploring the impact of social exclusion on the body in creating illness inequalities, but the ability to form and maintain social ties may be the result of health, illness and disability problems, not simply factors implicated in their cause (Pescosolido 2001, p. 484). In considering the political and economic ramifications of contemporary changes in provision of healthcare for those with chronic conditions, the issue of inequalities should loom large on the agenda for sociologists focussed on chronicity.

Social network research has been particularly influential in highlighting the importance of place of residence in the creation of various social inequalities (Fischer 1982; MacDonald et al. 2005; Warr 2005).

Such work has often focussed on changes in urban environments that are linked to socioeconomic status and particularly how areas of urban decay are associated with deprivation (Cattell 2001). Others have focussed on the impact of socioeconomic decline in rural areas, or have contrasted communities living in deprived areas versus those in affluent areas to examine differentials in social capital generation (e.g., see Bagnall et al. 2003 on educational disparities). In relation to health, Dolan (2007) describe how the capacity to develop and access social capital via social networks demonstrates how deindustrialization and economic change, as well as material deprivation and perceived disinvestment in local communities, has impacted on capacity for building supportive health-enhancing relationships with other members of the community. The role of "place" in relation to inequalities in the experience and management of chronic illness and disability has to date been under-researched and warrants further investigation in attempting to investigate therapeutic landscapes. Consideration of the interface between organisational and informal networks at local level is particularly important. For example, the interface between organisational and informal networks for self-care support is illustrated in studies of community pharmacies located in rural versus inner city deprived areas where different levels of engagement and receipt of advice are evident. In rural pharmacies, the nature of contact and support was more integrated with other community networks, whereas barriers to such integration within urban-deprived settings stemmed from perceived locality threat (Rogers et al. 1998).

Social networks that might support or inhibit the management of LTCs within specific settings warrant further investigation. Many have commented on the importance of social relationships for managing LTCs with the family located as the primary resource for managing the impact of such conditions (Gallant 2003). However, the nature of reciprocal and trusting relations amongst neighbours within community settings (Bulmer 1986; Li et al. 2005) could be a focus for future work on illness experience and management, given the implications for self-management capacity. Network theorists have commented on the significance of specific forms of relationships such as friendships and the distinctions between friends and acquaintances associated with contemporary social changes (Allan 1996; Fischer 1982; Pahl 2000). "Naturally" occurring informal relationships have been regarded as a source of social support and resource that can be harnessed for supporting the management of chronic conditions or even more formally as part of health care interventions in the form of "lay helpers" or "be-friending" programmes. The potential value of the latter is implied from evidence of the substitutive use of professional networks as a means of accessing social support. For example, loneliness has been significantly associated with frequency of consultation with general practitioners in British primary care (Ellaway et al. 1999) and identified as a driver for recruitment to guided self-management programmes run by formal health service organisations (Kennedy et al. 2005). Similarly, the notion of "fringe work" refers to activities carried out by professionals in substitution for wider social support resources where they are lacking. Such activities are perceived as shaping reciprocal and trusting relationships between professional and non-professional client (De la Cuesta 1993). In addition to such "substitution," the more formal ties that connect individuals with chronic conditions to forms of professional and organisational support are important for studying changing systems of care within community settings (Pescosolido 1996). Pescosolido (2001) provides a useful model to study the "network episodes" associated with the management of chronic conditions that necessarily involves movement across multiple care settings. At the heart of Pescosolido's Multi-Level Network Model lies the idea that the "social structure," which influences health and illness behaviour and outcomes, is "the operation of professional, organisational, and community network ties" (Pescosolido 1996, p. 176). A further focus on network ties in addition to greater consideration of *habitus* offers potential to enhance understanding of the management of illness across multiple settings to take account of patients' own self-management practices in dynamic relation to experiences of managed care.

The focus on "networks" as a means of studying social relations has evolved in a distinct way within STS via Actor Network Theory (ANT) that adopts a strong relativist stance. However, there has been very little dialogue between this approach and the mainstream approach of Social Network

Analysis except some acknowledgement of common anthropological roots (Knox et al. 2006). However, May and colleagues (May et al. 2003; May and Ellis 2001; May et al. 2001, 2006) have successfully drawn upon theoretical, conceptual and empirical insights emerging from ANT to study the social relations that have a significant impact on shaping the trajectory of how telecare interventions come to be adopted or rejected within the context of existing organisation of care and caring relationships (May et al. 2003). More recently, the work of May and colleagues has resulted in the development of a distinct model to evaluate the implementation, embedding and integration of new practices and technologies into routine care. The model focuses on the nature of work associated with interventions within interactional contexts (May et al. 2009), offering a new framework for researching the implications of technological interventions currently being extensively deployed to support chronic disease management.

Conclusions

This chapter has reflected on the past and potential future development of the sociology of chronic illness within a changing societal, organisational, and policy climate. This requires new directions in sociological research to engage with and critically investigate the impact and response to new interventions. We have argued that a critical sociological perspective on "motivation" is important and represents an extension of wider sociological concerns with contemporary cultural changes associated with a rise of psychological discourses (Hazleden 2003) and the "demystification" of science within a period of "reflexive modernization," whereby lay people increasingly have the opportunity to reflect and act upon scientific knowledge, and in turn experts must reflect upon and act upon this lay response (Beck 1992; Giddens 1991a). Domains of contested knowledge and the extended application of technologies to support CDM are relevant areas for further sociological inquiry, especially at critical junctures in illness trajectories (e.g., those regarding the management of diagnosis and death). A focus on contested knowledge taps into interests with reflexivity in social life and a perceived collapsing of boundaries of expertise between professionals and non-professionals. In the case of technologies, there are particular debates regarding the potential value of the internet for supporting self-care and needs for technological interventions that might prolong life or enable people with high level needs to remain independent at home.

We can respond to the above issues by drawing on the rich theoretical and empirical work that has already been conducted by medical sociologists focussed on chronic illness and disability in the latter decades of the twentieth century. In this chapter, we have drawn attention to insights into the impact of chronic illness on constructions of biography and narrative as well as the forms of work (e.g., illness work and biographical work after Strauss) associated with the management of illness outside of formal health care (self-care) and the significance of the body in the experience of illness and disability. The concept of illness careers has been drawn upon to denote the temporal and cumulative nature of illness experience and particularly how this is shaped via interactions within health care organisations (Pavalko et al. 2007). This longitudinal view that enables a focus on transitions and key turning points in the *provision* as well as *experience* of care is now even more important in an era of rapidly changing interventions and services for those with chronic conditions.

We have argued that new directions for research can be productively followed by engaging with wider areas of sociological concern that enable us to make greater connections between individual social agents and the political and economic structures that constrain social action. The political economy of chronic illness and disability is important because as Albrecht and Bury argue, "… the stakes are high because of the size of the marketplace and the amount of money involved in dealing with the problem" (Albrecht and Bury 2001, p. 587). They also emphasise that decisions about the management of chronic illness and disability reflects how a society values human life and citizenship. A sociological focus on motivation is also important to research how identity and ideas about citizenship and entitlement are worked out in practice within the arena of healthcare provision for those with chronic conditions. This is especially important given contemporary policy changes designed to "enable" sustainable employment for those with chronic conditions, part of which entails rationing and withdrawing disability benefits (Meershoek et al. 2007; Salway et al. 2007).

Conceptual and empirical work emerging from a focus on habitus, therapeutic landscapes and social networks provide examples that readily connect with the salient issues outlined for future research on chronic illness and disability. Such examples demonstrate the importance of themes evident in early and more recent work on chronic illness, such as the importance of the minutiae of everyday life with a chronic condition, the significance of embodiment and the importance of material context. All of these themes are relevant to enhancing our future understanding of illness careers and current changes in policy and healthcare provision suggest the need to extend such themes more readily to organisational and policy contexts while also examining critically the implications of system changes for the experience and management of illness. A focus on *habitus, therapeutic landscapes* and *social networks*, we believe, will enable us to consider the dynamic impact of policy change in this new era of transition in chronic care.

References

Albrecht GL, Bury M (2001) The political economy of the disability marketplace. In: Albrecht GL, Seeelman KD, Bury M (eds) Handbook of disability studies. Sage, London, pp 585–609

Allan G (1996) Kinship and friendship in modern Britain. Oxford University Press, Oxford

Andersen S, Keller C (2002) Examination of the transtheoretical model in current smokers. West J Nurs Res 24(3):282–294

Angus J, Kontos P, Dyck I, McKeever P, Poland B (2005) The personal significance of home: habitus and the experience of receiving long-term home care. Sociol Health Illn 27(2):161–187

Arksey H (1994) Expert and lay participation in the construction of medical knowledge. Sociol Health Illn 16:448–468

Atkinson P (1984) Training for certainty. Soc Sci Med 19:949–956

Bagnall G, Longhurst B, Savage M (2003) Children, belonging and social capital: the PTA and middle class narratives of social involvement in the north-west of England. Sociol Res Online 8(4)

Bandura A (1997) Self-efficacy: The exercise of control. New York: Freeman

Barker KK (2008) Electronic support groups, patient-consumers, and medicalization: the case of contested illness. J Health Soc Behav 49(1):20

Barr VJ (2003) The expanded Chronic Care Model: an integration of concepts and strategies from population health promotion and the Chronic Care Model. Hosp Q 7(1):73–82

Bauman Z (2000) Liquid modernity. Polity Press, Cambridge

Beattie A (1991) Knowledge and control in health promotion: a test case for social policy and social theory. In: Gabe J, Calnan M, Bury M (eds) The sociology of the health service. Routledge, London

Beck U (1992) Risk society: towards a new modernity. Sage, London

Berger M (2005) Internet use and stigmatized illness. Soc Sci Med 61(8):1821–1827

Bower P (2002) Primary care mental health workers: models of working and evidence of effectiveness. Br J Gen Pract 52:926–933

Berkman LF, Glass T, Brissette I, Seeman TE (2000) From integration to health: Durkheim in the new millennium. Soc Sci Med 51:843–857

Blaxter M (1983) The causes of disease: women talking. Soc Sci Med 17(2):59–69

Bloor MJ, McKeganey NP, Finlay A, Barnard MA (1992) The inappropriateness of psycho-social models of risk behaviour for understanding HIV-related risk practices among Glasgow male prostitutes. AIDS Care 4(2):131–137

Brown P (2004) Embodied health movements: new approaches to social movements in health. Sociol Health Illn 26(1):50–80

Brown PA, Piper SM (1995) Empowerment or social control? Differing interpretations of psychology in health education. Health Educ J 54:115–123
Bulmer M (1986) Neighbours: the work of Philip Abrams. Cambridge University Press, Cambridge
Bury M (2001) Illness narratives: fact or fiction? Sociol Health Illn 23(3):263–285
Bury M (1982) Chronic illness as biographical disruption. Sociol Health Illn 4(2):165–182
Bury M (1997) Health and illness in a changing society. Routledge, London
Bury M (1988) Meaning at risk: the experience of Arthritis. In: Anderson NR (ed) Living with chronic illness. The experience of patients and their families. Unwin Hyman, London
Camic C (1986) The matter of habit. Am J Sociol 19(5):1039–1087
Carricaburu D, Pierret J (1995) From biographical disruption to biographical reinforcement: the case of HIV-positive men. Sociol Health Illn 17(1):65–88
Cattell V (2001) Poor people, poor places, and poor health: the mediating role of social networks and social capital. Soc Sci Med 52(10):1501–1516
Charmaz K (1995) The body, identity, and self. Sociol Q 36(4):657–680
Comaroff J, Maguire P (1981) Ambiguity and the search for meaning: childhood leukaemia in the modern clinical context. Soc Sci Med 158:115–123
Conrad P (1990) Qualitative research on chronic illness: a commentary on method and conceptual development. Soc Sci Med 30(11):1257–1263
Conrad P (1987) The experience of illness: recent and new directions. Res Sociol Health Care 6:1–31
Corbin J, Strauss AL (1991) Comeback: the process of overcoming disability. In: Albrecht GL, Levy JA (eds) Advances in medical sociology. JAI Press, Greenwich, CT, pp 137–159
Corbin J, Strauss AL (1987) Accompaniments of chronic illness: changes in body, self, biography, and biographical time. Res Sociol Health Care 6:249–281
Crawford R (1977) You are dangerous to your health. Int J Health Serv 7:663
Crossley N (2001) The phenomenological habitus and its construction. Theory Soc 30(1):81
Cunningham-Burley S, Irvine S (1987) And have you done anything so far? An examination of lay treatment of children's symptoms. Br Med J (Clin Res Ed) 295:700–702
De la Cuesta C (1993) Fringe work – peripheral work in health visiting. Sociol Health Illn 15(5):665–682
Department of Health (2005) Building telecare in England. London, Department of Health. Ref Type: Report
Department of Health (2006) Our health, our care, our say: a new direction for community services. London, The Stationary Office. Ref Type: Report
Dolan A (2007) That's just the cesspool where they dump all the trash: exploring working class men's perceptions and experiences of social capital and health. Health 11(4):475
Dongbo F, Hua F, McGowan P, Yi-e S, Lizhen Z, Huiqin Y, Jianguo M, Shitai Z, Yongming D, Zhihua W (2003) Implementation and quantitative evaluation of chronic disease self-management programme in Shanghai, China: randomized controlled trial. Bull World Health Organ 81(3):174–182
Drentea P, Moren-Cross JL (2005) Social capital and social support on the web: the case of an internet mother site. Sociol Health Illn 27(7):920–943
Eisenberg L (1977) Disease and illness: distinctions between professional and popular ideas of sickness. Cult Med Psychiatry 1:9–23
Ellaway A, Wood S, Macintyre S (1999) Someone to talk to? The role of loneliness as a factor in the frequency of GP consultations. Br J Gen Pract 49(442):363–367
Faircloth CA, Boylstein C, Rittman M, Young ME (2004a) Sudden illness and biographical flow in narratives of stroke recovery. Sociol Health Illn 26(2):242–261
Faircloth CA, Rittman M, Boylstein C, Young ME, Van Puymbroeck M (2004b) Energizing the ordinary: biographical work and the future in stroke recovery narratives. J Aging Stud 18:399–413
Featherstone M, Hepworth M (1990) Images of aging. In: Bond J, Coleman P (eds) Ageing in society: an introduction to social gerontology. Sage, London
Featherstone M, Hepworth M, Turner BS (1991) The body: social process and cultural theory. Sage, London
Field J (2003) Social capital. Routledge, Oxon
Fischer CS (1982) To dwell among friends. Personal networks in town and city. The University of Chicago Press, Chicago, IL
Fox N, Ward K (2006) Health identities: from expert patient to resisting consumer. Health 10(4):461–479
Fox NJ (2005) The 'expert patient': empowerment or medical dominance? The case of weight loss, pharmaceutical drugs and the Internet. Soc Sci Med 60(6):1299–1309
Frank AW (1991) At the will of the body – reflections on illness. Houghton Mifflin, New York
Frank AW (1995) The wounded storyteller, body, illness, and ethics. University of Chicago Press, Chicago, IL
Frank AW (1997) Illness as moral occasion: restoring agency to ill people. Health 1(2):131–148
Freidson E (1970) The profession of medicine. Dodd Mead, New York

Gallant MP (2003) The influence of social support on chronic illness self-management: a review and directions for research. Health Educ Behav 30(2):170–195

Gately C, Rogers A, Sanders C (2007) Re-thinking the relationship between long-term condition self-management education and the utilisation of health services, Soc Sci Med, 65:934–945

Gately C, Rogers A, Kirk S, McNally R (2008) Integration of devices into long-term condition management: a synthesis of qualitative studies. Chronic Illn 4:135–148

Gerhardt U (1989) Ideas about illness – an intellectual and political history of medical sociology. New York University Press, New York

Giddens A (1991a) Modernity and self-identity: self and society in the late modern age. Polity Press, Cambridge

Giddens A (1991b) The consequences of modernity. Polity, Cambridge

Gitlin LN, Luborsky MR, Schemm RL (1998) Emerging concerns of older stroke patients about assistive devices. Gerontologist 38(2):169–180

Goffman E (1971) The presentation of self in everyday life. Penquin Books, Harmondsworth

Harrison R, MacFarlane A, Murray E, Wallace P (2006) Patients' perceptions of joint teleconsultations: a qualitative evaluation. Health Expect 9(1):81–90

Hazleden R (2003) Love yourself: the relationship of the self with itself in contemporary relationship manuals. J Sociol 39(4)

Hellstrom C (2001) Affecting the future: chronic pain and perceived agency in a clinical setting. Time Soc 10(1):77–92

Herzlich C (1973) Health and illness: a social psychological analysis. Academic, London

Hess DJ (2004) Medical modernisation, scientific research fields and the epistemic politics of health social movements. Sociol Health Illn 26(6):695

Hibbard JH, Stockard J, Mahoney E, Tusler M (2004) Development of the Patient Activation Measure (PAM): conceptualizing and measuring activation in patients and consumers. Health Serv Res 39(4):1005–1026

Hodgins M, Millar M, Barry M (2006) ...it's all the same no matter how much fruit or vegetables or fresh air we get: Traveler women's perceptions of illness causation and health inequalities. Soc Sci Med 62(8):1978–1990

Johnson M (1976) That was your life: a biographical approach to later life. In: Munnichs JMA, Van Den Heuval WJA (eds) Dependency and interdependency in old age. Martinus Nijhoff, Hague

Kelly M (1992) Colitis. Tavistock, London

Kelly MP, Dickinson H (1997) The narrative self in autobiographical accounts of illness. Sociol Rev 42(2):254–278

Kelly MP, Field D (1996) Medical sociology, chronic illness and the body. Sociol Health Illn 18:241–257

Kendall E & Rogers A (2007) Exstinguishing the social?: state sponsored self-care policy and the Chronic Disease Self-management Programme, Disability & Society, 22(2):129–143

Kennedy A, Reeves D, Bower P, Lee V, Middleton E, Richardson G, Gardner C, Gately C, Rogers A (2007) The effectiveness and cost effectiveness of a national lay led self care support programme for patients with long-term conditions: a pragmatic randomised controlled trial. J Epidemiol Community Health 61:254–261

Kennedy AP, Rogers A, Gately C (2005) Assessing the introduction of the Expert Patients Programme into the NHS: A realistic evaluation of recruitment to a national lay led self care initiative, Primary Health Care Research and Development, 6:137–48

Kennedy A, Nelson E, Reeves D, Richardson G, Roberts C, Robinson A, Rogers A, Sculpher M, Thompson DG, the North-West Regional Gastrointestinal Research Group (2004) A randomised controlled trial to assess the effectiveness and cost of a patient orientated self management approach to chronic inflammatory bowel disease. Gut 53(11):1639–1645

Kennedy A, Rogers A (2001) Improving self-management skills: a whole systems approach. Br J Nurs 10(11): 734–737

Kivits J (2007) Researching the 'informed patient'. The case of online health information seekers. Inf Commun Soc 7(4):510–530

Knox H, Savage M, Harvey P (2006) Social networks and the study of relations: networks as method, metaphor and form. Econ Soc 35(1):113–140

Lambert H, Rose H (1996) Disembodied knowledge? Making sense of medical science. In: Irwin A, Wynne B (eds) Misunderstanding science? the public reconstruction of science and technology. Cambridge University Press, Cambridge, pp 65–83

Lash S, Friedman J (1992) Modernity and identity. Blackwell, Oxford

Last JM (1963) The Iceberg: "completing the clinical picture" in general practice. Lancet 282(7297):28–31

Lawton J (2003) Lay experiences of health and illness: past research and future agendas. Sociol Health Illn 25:23–40

Leder D (1984a) Medicine and paradigms of embodiment. J Med Philos 9:29–43

Leder D (1984b) Toward a phenomenology of pain. Rev Existential Psychiatry 19:255–266

Lehoux P, Saint-Arnaud J, Richard L (2004) The use of technology at home: what patient manuals say and sell vs. what patients face and fear. Sociol Health Illn 26(5):617–644

Leventhal H, Leventhal EA, Contrada RJ (1998) Self-regulation, health, and behavior: a perceptual-cognitive approach. Psychol Health 13(4):717–733

Li Y, Pickles A, Savage M (2005) Social capital and social trust in Britain. Eur Sociol Rev 21(2):109–123

Lindsay S, Smith S, Bell F, Bellaby P (2007) Tackling the digital divide. Exploring the impact of ICT on managing heart conditions in a deprived area. Inf Communication Soc 10(1):95–114

Locker D (1983) Disability and disadvantage: the consequences of chronic illness. Tavistock, London

Lupton D (1993) Risk as moral danger: the social and political functions of risk discourse in public health. Int J Health Serv 23(425):435

MacDonald R, Shildrick T, Webster C, Simpson D (2005) Growing up in poor neighbourhoods: the significance of class and place in the extended transitions of 'socially excluded' young adults. Sociology 39(5):873–891

May C (1997) Degrees of freedom: reflexivity, self-identity and self-help. Self, Agency Soc 1(1):42–54

May C, Ellis NT (2001) When protocols fail: Technical evaluation, biomedical knowledge, and the social production of 'facts' about a telemedicine clinic. Soc Sci Med 53:989–1002

May C, Gask L, Atkinson T, Ellis N, Mair F, Esmail A (2001) Resisting and promoting new technologies in clinical practice: the case of telepsychiatry. Soc Sci Med 52:1889–1901

May C, Mort M, Williams T, Mair F, Gask L (2003) Health technology assessment in its local contexts: studies of telehealthcare. Soc Sci Med 57:697–710

May C, Allison G, Chapple A, Chew-Graham C, Rogers A, Roland M (2004) Framing the doctor-patient relationship in chronic illness: a comparative study of general practitioners' accounts, Sociol Health Illn, 26:135–158

May C, Rapley T, Moreira T, Finch T, Heaven B (2006) Technogovernance: evidence, subjectivity, and the clinical encounter in primary care medicine. Soc Sci Med 62:1022–1030

May C, Mair F, Finch T, MacFarlanne A, Dowrick C, Treweek S, Rapley T, Ballini L, Ong BN, Rogers A, Murray E, Elwyn G, Legare F, Gunn J, Montori VM (2009) Development of a theory of implementation and intergration: Normalization Process Theory, BMC Implementation Science, 4:29, doi: 10.1186/1748-5908-4-29

May C, Sirur D (1998) Art, science and placebo: incorporating homeopathy in general practice. Sociol Health Illn 20(2):168–190

McCreadie C, Tinker A (2005) The acceptability of assistance technology to older people. Ageing Soc 1:91

McDonald R, Mead N, Cheraghi-Sohi S, Bower P, Walley D, Roland M (2007) Governing the ethical consumer: identity, choice and the primary care medical encounter. Sociol Health Illn 29(3):430–456

Meershoek A, Krumeich A, Vos R (2007) Judging without criteria? Sickness certification in Dutch disability schemes. Sociol Health Illn 29:497–514

Mendelson C (2003) Gentle hugs: Internet listservs as sources of support for women with lupus. Adv Nurs Sci 26(4):299–306

Nettleton S (1995) The sociology of health and illness. Polity, Cambridge

Nettleton S, Burrows R, O'Malley L, Watt I (2004) Health E-Types? An analysis of the everyday use of the internet for health. Inf Commun Soc 7(4):531–553

Nicolini D (2006) The work to make telemedicine work: a social and articulative view. Soc Sci Med 62(11):2754–2767

Nijhof G (1995) Disease as a problem of shame in public appearance. Sociol Health Illn 20:489–506

Oliver M (1990) The politics of disablement. St. Martin's, New York

Oudshoorn N (2008) Diagnosis at a distance: the invisible work of patients and healthcare professionals in cardiac telemonitoring technology. Sociol Health Illn 30(2):272

Pahl R (2000) On friendship. Polity, Cambridge

Pavalko EK, Harding CM, Pescosolido BA (2007) Mental illness careers in an era of change. Soc Probl 54(4):504–522

Percival J, Hanson J (2006) Big brother or brave new world? Telecare and its implications for older people's independence and social inclusion. Crit Soc Policy 26(4):888–909

Pescosolido BA (1996) Bringing the 'community' into utilization models: how social networks link individuals to changing systems of care. In: Kronenfeld JJ (ed) Research in the sociology of health care. JAI Press, Greenwich, CT, pp 171–198

Pescosolido BA (2001) "The role of social networks in the lives of persons with disabilities. In: Albrecht GL, Seelman KD, Bury M (eds) Handbook of disability studies. Sage, London, pp 468–489

Pinder R (1992) Coherence and incoherence: doctors' and patients' perspectives on the diagnosis of Parkinson's disease. Sociol Health Illn 14:1–22

Pound P, Compertz P, Ebrahim S (1998) Illness in the context of older age: the case of stroke. Sociol Health Illn 20(4):489–506

Prochaska J, Norcross JC, DiClemente CC (1994) Changing for good. Avon, New York

Radley A, Green R (1987) Illness adjustment: a methodology and conceptual framework. Sociol Health Illn 9(2):179–207

Robinson I (1988) Reconstructing lives: negotiating the meaning of multiple sclerosis. In: Anderson R, Bury M (eds) Living with chronic illness: the experience of patients and their families. Unwin Hyman, London, pp 43–67

Robinson A, Wilkin D, Thompson DG, Roberts C (2001) Guided self-management and patient-directed follow-up of ulcerative colitis: a randomised trial. Lancet 358(9286):976–981

Rogers A, Hassell K, Noyce P, Harris J (1998) Advice-giving in community pharmacy: variations between pharmacies in different locations. Health Place 4(4):365–373

Rogers A, Lee V, Kennedy A (2007) Continuity and change? Exploring reactions to a guided self-management intervention in a randomised controlled trial for IBS with reference to prior experience of managing a long term condition. Trials 8:6

Rogers A, Hassel K, Nicolaas G (1999) Demanding patients? Analysing the use of primary care. Open University, Buckingham

Salmon P (2000) Patients who present physical symptoms in the absence of physical pathology: a challenge to existing models of doctor-patient interaction. Patient Educ Couns 39(1):105–113

Salway S, Platt L, Harris K, Chowbey P (2007) Long-term conditions and disability living allowance: explaining ethnic differences and similarities in access. Sociol Health Illn 29:497–514

Sandaunet AG (2008) The challenge of fitting in: non-participation and withdrawal from an online self-help group for breast cancer patients. Sociol Health Illn 30(1):131

Sanders C, Donovan J, Dieppe P (2002) The significance and consequences of having painful and disabled joints in older age: co-existing accounts of normal and disrupted biographies. Sociol Health Illn 24(2):227–253

Sanders C, Rogers A (2008) Theorising inequalities in the experience and management of chronic illness: Bringing social networks and social capital back in (critically). Res Sociol Health Care 25:15–42

Sanders C, Rogers A, Gately C, Kennedy A (2008) Planning for end of life care within lay-led chronic illness self-management training: the significance of 'death awareness' and biographical context in participant accounts. Soc Sci Med 66:982–993

Scambler G (1989) Epilepsy. Routledge, London

Scambler G, Hopkins A (1988) Accomodating epilepsy in families. In: Anderson R, Bury M (eds) Living with Chronic Illness: The experience of patients and their families. Unwin Hyman, London, pp 156–176

Scarry E (1985) The body in pain – the making and unmaking of the World. Oxford University Press, Oxford

Scheper-Hughes N, Lock MM (1987) The mindful body: a prolegomenon to future work in medical anthropology. Med Anthropol Q 1(1):6–41

Seale C, Ziebland S, Charteris-Black J (2006) Gender, cancer experience and internet use: a comparative keyword analysis of interviews and online cancer support groups. Soc Sci Med 62(10):2577–2590

Seale C (1996) Pain and suffering. In: Davey B, Seale C (eds) Experiencing and explaining disease. Oxford University Press, Buckingham, pp 140–157

Seale C (2006a) Gender accommodation in online cancer support groups. Health 10(3):345

Seale C (2006b) Gender, cancer experience and internet use: a comparative keyword analysis of interviews and online cancer support groups. Soc Sci Med D 62(10):2577

Shilling C (1993) The body and social theory. Sage, London

Sobel DR, Lorig KR, Hobbs M (2002) Chronic disease self-management program: from development to dissemination. Perm J 6(2):15–22

Stacey M (1988) The sociology of health and healing. Unwin Hyman, London

Taylor D, Bury M (2007) Chronic illness, expert patients and care transition. Sociol Health Illn 29(1):27–45

Timmermans S, Haas S (2008) Towards a sociology of disease. Sociol Health Illn 30(5):659–676

Townsend A, Wyke S, Hunt K (2006) Self-managing and managing self: practical and moral dilemmas in accounts of living with chronic illness. Chronic Illn 2(3):185–194

Turner BS (2001) Disability and the sociology of the body. In: Albrecht GL, Seelman KD, Bury M (eds) Handbook of disability studies. Sage, London, pp 252–266

Turner BS (1992) Regulating bodies. Essays in medical sociology. Routledge, London

Von Korff M, Gruman J, Schaefer J, Curry S, Wagner E (1997) Collaborative management of chronic illness. Ann Intern Med 127(12):1097–1102

Warr DJ (2005) Social networks in a 'discredited' neighbourhood. J Sociol 41(3):285–308

Webb J (2004) Organizations, self-identities and the new economy. Sociology 38(4):719

Weiner C (1975) The burden of rheumatoid arthritis: tolerating the uncertainty. Soc Sci Med 9:97–104

Weisberger C (2004) Turning to the internet for help on sensitive medical problems. A qualitative study of the construction of a sleep disorder through online interaction. Inf Communication Soc 7(4):554–574

Wilton R & De Verteuil G (2006) Spaces of sobriety/sites of power: examining social model alcohol recovery programs as therapeutic landscapes, Soc Sci Med, 63(3):649–661

Williams B, Barlow J (1998) Falling out with my shadow. Lay perceptions of the body in the context of arthritis. In: Nettleton S, Watson J (eds) The body in everyday life. Routledge, London, pp 124–141

Williams G (1993a) Chronic illness and the pursuit of virtue in everyday life. In: Radley A (ed) Worlds of illness: biographical and cultural perspectives on health and disease. Routledge, London, pp 92–108

Williams G (1996a) Representing disability: some questions of phenomonology and politics. In: Barnes C, Mercer G (eds) Exploring the divide: illness and disability. The Disability Press, Leeds, pp 194–212

Williams G (1984) The genesis of chronic illness: narrative re-construction. Sociol Health Illn 6(2):175–200

Williams SJ (1999) Is anybody there? Critical realism, chronic illness and the disability debate. Sociol Health Illn 21(6):797–819

Williams SJ (1996b) Medical sociology, chronic illness and the body: a rejoinder to Michael Kelly and David Field. Sociol Health Illn 18:699–709

Williams S (2000) Chronic illness as biographical disruption or biographical disruption as chronic illness? Reflections on a core concept. Sociol Health Illn 22(1):40–67

Williams S (1993b) Chronic respiratory disorder. Routledge, London

Williams S, Bendelow G (1998) In search of the 'missing body': pain, suffering and the (post)modern condition. In: Scambler G, Higgs P (eds) Modernity, medicine and health. Medical sociology towards 2000. Routledge, London, pp 125–146

Wilson PM (2001) A policy analysis of the Expert Patient in the United Kingdom: self-care as an expression of pastoral power? Health Soc Care Community 9(3):134–142

Wilson PM, Kendall S, Brooks F (2007) The expert patients programme: a paradox of patient empowerment and medical dominance. Health Soc Care Community 15(5):426–438

Wilton R (2006) Spaces of sobriety/sites of power: examining social model alcohol recovery programs as therapeutic landscapes. Soc Sci Med 63(3):649–661

Chapter 26
Identity and Illness

Kathryn J. Lively and Carrie L. Smith

Introduction

Over the last several decades, sociological interest in and research on the relationship between illness and identity has flourished. Unlike disease, which refers primarily to physical pathology, illness generally refers to lived experience (Kleinman et al. 1978).[1] The foci of this research have been twofold: an examination of the public self (an individual's identity as perceived by others) and the private self (an individual's identity as perceived by oneself) and how the two interact with and affect each other (Kelly and Millward 2004). Yet, the commonality among the majority of studies focusing on illness and identity is that researchers have usually treated identity as a function of illness – that is, how one's identity forms or changes as a result of contracting a particular disease or condition. This approach has been represented most successfully by those sociologists who view illness as an identity disruption (e.g., see Charmaz 1993; Karp 1996) and those interested in the relationship among identity, stigma, and illness (e.g., see Link 1987; Link et al. 1991). Recent studies have focused on how individuals strive to maintain their sense of self in spite of illness. Hinojosa et al. (2008), for example, find that veterans who had suffered a stroke were able to maintain a continuous sense of self by drawing upon their religious beliefs and cultural expectations of aging. Likewise, Sanders et al. (2002) find that while people with osteoarthritis do talk about the disruptive effects of the condition on their daily lives, they still manage to view these symptoms as part of their normal lives.

While the field of identity and illness has progressed much beyond the Parsonian framework of the sick role (1951), it has done so, predominantly, with the inclusion of vague insights from symbolic interaction, rather than the incorporation of social psychological theories of identity. In this chapter, we identify new directions of scholarly inquiry in the area of identity and illness through the integration of existing social psychological conceptualizations of identity, identity formation, and identity disconfirmation/verification. Specifically, we highlight the potential contributions of identity theory (generally defined) before discussing in depth three variants: structural symbolic interaction, affect control theory, and identity control theory.

---

[1]Although the majority of work in this area focuses on diagnosed physical pathologies, some also document the lived experience of individuals whose conditions are still contested. For instance, Barker (2002) examines how self-help literature helps those diagnosed with Fibromyalgia syndrome (FMS) to construct a coherent illness identity. Fibromyalgia, as well as other forms of chronic pain, are particularly difficult for those who have it in that the symptoms associated with the condition are invisible or have no organic cause. In their study of individuals with facial pain, Lennon et al. (1989) point out that because pain cannot be explained biomedically, those who suffer from it are often stigmatized.

K.J. Lively (✉)
Department of Sociology, Dartmouth College, 6104 Silsby, Rm. 1034, Hanover, New Hampshire 03755, USA
e-mail: kathryn.j.lively@dartmouth.edu

We begin with a brief description of the general trends in identity and health research thus far. We then turn our attention to a set of social psychological theories of identity that have remained all but invisible within the broader discussion of identity and illness and illustrate how these theories have the potential to open up new avenues of research. In contrast to the dominant focus on the negative impacts of illness on the individual (Horwitz 2002), we posit that integrating these theories can provide valuable insight into the development of positive illness identities as well as the ways in which identity may have the ability to ameliorate the negative impact of disease.

We conclude by pointing to new methodological approaches that could be used in future work on identity and illness. Up to this point, most work in this area is qualitative and, in particular, has relied primarily on patients' narratives as a source of data (Bell 2000; Conrad 1990; Pierret 2003). We argue that the inclusion of social psychological theories of identity not only has the potential to open up new theoretical directions, but also methodological directions through the incorporation of complementary – if not alternative – methodologies, such as surveys, experiments, and computer simulations.

General Themes and Frameworks in the Field of Identity and Illness

The Effect of Illness on Identity

It is widely acknowledged that studies of identity and illness had their genesis in Parsons' (1951) theory of the sick role (e.g., see Lawton 2003), which hypothesizes that patients assume a set of rights and obligations that determine behavior once they have been diagnosed with a medical condition. Based on the assumption that illness is a form of dysfunction, Parsons argued that patients should be released from the obligations of other social roles and not held accountable for their actions in order to facilitate their return to health and reintegration into society. In return for these concessions, patients are expected to seek out and cooperate with competent medical professionals. This approach assumes that illness is a temporary condition and that patients desire to be healed.

Later generations of scholars have critiqued Parsons' (1951) theory for, among other things, neglecting the experiences of those with chronic illnesses (e.g., see Crossley 1998; Radley 1994) and for its overly deterministic nature (e.g., see Pierret 2003; Turner 1995). Additionally, given his view of illness as a form of deviance, Parsons has further been criticized for neglecting to incorporate the physical body and its impacts on the illness experience. It is difficult to avoid the reality that illness often brings with it physical aches and pains and limitations, and these physicalities surely impact the individual's sense of self, which is derived, in large part, from the reactions – real or perceived – of others (e.g., see Kelly and Field 1996). For our purposes, the most severe – and warranted – criticism is that with its focus on the "outsider perspective" (Lawton 2003), Parsons failed to acknowledge that patients have agency in constructing their illness experiences and identities and do not simply conform to what physicians, and the larger society, demands of them. In response, many researchers have sought to recover the individual's voice; and, as a result, much of this research draws upon qualitative narratives. As mentioned earlier, these studies also generally focus on the negative impacts of illness, and posit identity changes *in response* to illness.

A good illustration of this approach is Charmaz's (1983) seminal work on how individuals with chronic illnesses experience a "loss of self." She points out that those with chronic illnesses often face several negative reactions and life situations – from experiencing increased social isolation to being discredited by others. In dealing with these negative reactions and life situations, people's various identities and sense of self may collide with one another, such that a loss of self in one area of their lives might result in a loss of self in another area. Someone who is diagnosed with colon cancer, for example, may no longer be able to fulfill her role as CEO, forcing her to take a temporary, if not permanent, leave of absence. While Charmaz demonstrates that people do have agency in constructing their identities during illness – that is, how people begin to redefine what it means to be a parent or a spouse, while still dealing with their afflictions – her focus is overwhelmingly on how they do so *after* they become ill.

Charmaz's (1983) study, based on 73 in-depth interviews with 57 chronically ill individuals living with diseases ranging from diabetes to multiple sclerosis, remains one of the most cited studies in the field of identity and illness and exemplifies the general methodological approach of focusing on patients' narratives and giving voice to their day-to-day experiences. The value of utilizing qualitative narratives is that researchers are able to better ascertain how individuals define what their illnesses mean, and how they create meaning out of their illness experiences. Charmaz finds that with the exception of those whose physical conditions had improved, her respondents often used a language of loss and constraint to describe their illness experiences. For instance, a man undergoing kidney dialysis stated that he felt "less than human" (p. 173) while an elderly woman felt "badly about being dependent" (p. 188).

Many studies in this genre (e.g., Charmaz 1993; Gordon 1995; Karp 1996; Weitz 1991) draw almost exclusively from traditional symbolic interaction (Blumer 1969; Mead 1934). In one of the earliest statements of symbolic interactionist thought, Mead (1934) posited a reciprocal relationship between self and society – a relationship that has been mirrored in health scholars' discussions of the private and public self. Mead argued that self shapes society, and vice versa, just as more modern scholars argue for the reciprocal relationship between the public and private selves (e.g., see Kelly and Millward 2004). In his discussion of the self-concept, Rosenberg (1981) argued that the self (that is, the private self) is a product of society, as well as a social force (also see Callero 2003).

In addition to positing a social self, symbolic interaction also assumes that meaning is central to human life (McLeod and Lively 2007). This basic tenet asserts that meaning shapes not only how individuals interpret particular events, others, and their environments, but also themselves (Heise 2002; Smith-Lovin and Heise 1988). These interpretations, in turn, color how individuals respond to events and situations, regardless of the objective reality of the event itself (Charmaz 1980, 1993). In her study on cancer survivor support groups, for instance, Westphal (2004) found that individuals with cancer were encouraged by group leaders and other support group members to adopt specific preferred meanings regarding their current situation. Here, in routine interactions with similar others (Thoits et al. 2000), individuals were urged to view their conditions as acute (instead of chronic) and to see chemotherapy as a necessary evil in their "battle" against disease (instead of as a poison that made them tired, nauseous, and irritable). Although always within the rhetoric of support or "best interests," members were typically sanctioned when entertaining or promoting beliefs that undermined those that the group deemed desirable.

As the above suggests, one of the most enduring insights of symbolic interaction is that meaning – much like the self – is not static. Instead, meaning is expected to change over time as individuals develop new understandings of their situations (Blumer 1969). New understandings may result from the changing nature of a situation or event (as in the diagnosis of a debilitating or stigmatized disease or condition) or from self-reflection (Callero 2003). They may also arise out of social interactions with real or imagined others (as in getting to know or learning about other people who may share similar life circumstances). As individuals garner more information from the social world, their meaning of themselves may either be reaffirmed or altered, as may their view of the world around them. Further, because the meaning attached to the self tends to structure one's world view, individuals who see themselves in particular ways are also likely to view their illness or condition in ways that correspond to those self-definitions.[2]

---

[2] Additionally, meanings may also be linked to circumstances that extend beyond the immediate definition of the situation – that is, meanings may also be shaped by broader historical and cultural settings where "unarticulated assumptions about the nature of the person have their origins" (Callero 2003, p. 121).

One well-known example that illustrates the general tenets of symbolic interaction is that of the American Cancer Society's adoption of the term survivor, as opposed to victim. According to this new rhetoric, individuals are expected to see themselves and other cancer patients as potential survivors, and to take a more proactive stance towards their treatment regimens and their overall health. As noted previously, compared to those who see themselves as potential victims or sufferers, potential survivors are expected to develop new meanings about their illness, their treatment, their doctors, and their likelihood of survival that are consistent with their survivor identities (Westphal 2004). However, not all individuals adopt the identity of "survivor." In her study of women who were treated for breast cancer, Kaiser (2008) found that while some women adopt the identity of "survivor," others rejected it because it did not cohere with their illness experience. For some, the threat of a possible recurrence was powerful, while some felt that their illness experience had not been severe enough to warrant their adopting the "survivor" identity.

As the above examples suggest, the idea that individuals strive for cognitive consistency underlies much of symbolic interactionist thought. Cognitive consistency theory posits that individuals are motivated to act in ways, and have thoughts, values, and beliefs, that are consistent with their sense of self (Heise 1979; Stryker 1980). When someone fails to achieve the desired consistency – either in terms of their situation, behaviors, thoughts, attitudes, or beliefs – they experience some form of cognitive dissonance that often manifests itself as an emotional reaction (most typically, distress). According to this perspective, individuals who experience cognitive and/or emotional dissonance will enact behavioral and/or cognitive changes in order to bring their situations, behaviors, thoughts, attitudes, and beliefs back in line with their fundamental sense of self, even if it means surrendering a valued identity (e.g., see Charmaz 1983; Elson 2003; Gordon 1995).

One of the strengths of traditional symbolic interaction (Blumer 1969) as a perspective and a methodology is that it allows researchers to capture the rich complexity of lived experience. Drawing almost exclusively on narrative accounts, symbolic interaction allows scholars to tap into individuals' perceptions, thoughts, and feelings, while taking into account the uniqueness of their particular situation. Indeed, as we pointed out earlier, the majority of studies on identity and illness have privileged patients' narratives, providing us with rich, ethnographic data that highlights patients' voices and perspectives (Bell 2000; Conrad 1990; Pierret 2003). However, while narratives and in-depth interviews may be the best methods to capture and describe the nuances of lived experience, they do not necessarily lend themselves to prediction, or even replication. Indeed, one of the long-standing criticisms of traditional symbolic interaction (Blumer 1969) is its assumption that the social world and, hence, the self, is always in a state of flux or negotiation (Stryker 1980). Such an approach fails to account for the relative stability of society or the self over time, or even across a variety of situations (a point to which we return later).

The Interplay of Illness and Identity (Stigma and Labeling Theory)

One of the more developed lines of inquiry within the study of identity and illness is the internalization of stigma associated with having a particular condition. However, unlike the aforementioned studies – which assume that identity is a *function* of illness – scholarship on stigma posits a more explicitly reciprocal relationship between the two. In other words, while scholars focusing on the impact of illness and identity generally argue that illness may result in a stigma that affects one's sense of self (Karp 1996), those examining the relationships among stigma, illness, and identity argue that having a stigmatized identity may *also* result in compensatory behaviors that can influence subsequent health outcomes (Link 1987).

Although the concept has been used in a variety of ways, Goffman (1963) defined stigma as a socially discrediting blemish that may be of the body, of the character, or tribal in nature (e.g., race or ethnicity). Given the general processes of socialization (Mead 1934), most individuals within a society are raised with similar beliefs and attitudes regarding the types of conditions or characteristics that are likely to result in stigma. This is one reason why individuals holding a stigmatized characteristic or trait are likely to have the same beliefs and attitudes towards that trait (and therefore themselves) as those who do not have the trait.

Although all individuals may have some potentially stigmatizing characteristics (or engage in stigmatizing behavior), they will not necessarily be stigmatized until they have been labeled as such. A person with epilepsy, for example, may pass as "normal" until he has a seizure that is witnessed by someone who has the power to label him as such (e.g., a physician, a teacher, or a police officer). Once labeled, however, his status as "an epileptic" is made public and is routinely confirmed vis-à-vis interactions with others, as well as through daily limitations placed on behavior (e.g., the inability to drive a car).[3,4]

While the example above refers to primary deviance (that is, the behavior that gets one labeled to begin with), labeling theory also attempts to explain secondary deviance – that is, the additional deviance people continue to engage in once they have been labeled (Lemert 1999).[5] In this sense, labeling theory views identity not only as a result of the internalization of stigma, but also as a social force that has the ability to influence subsequent feelings, beliefs, and behaviors – both for those who are labeled and those around them (see also Britt and Heise 2000; Taylor 1995).

The labeling process works similarly with individuals who struggle with issues pertaining to mental illness, particularly for those who have been labeled formally. According to the modified labeling theory of mental illness (Link 1987; Link et al. 1989), the negative consequences of psychiatric treatment are rooted in cultural definitions of the "mentally ill." When an individual is diagnosed with a mental illness, cultural ideas about the mentally ill (e.g., incompetent or dangerous) become personally relevant and are transformed into expectations that others will devalue and discriminate against that person (Kroska and Harkness 2006). These negative expectations are associated with such undesirable outcomes as unemployment, low earnings, and feelings of demoralization, even after controlling for differences in psychiatric diagnoses (Link 1987). Further, these expectations are believed to promote behaviors aimed at preventing negative reactions: concealing treatment history, withdrawing from social interaction, and/or educating others about mental illness. Ironically, but perhaps unsurprisingly, both withdrawal and educating others are also linked to additional negative outcomes. The former restricts social networks (Link et al. 1989) and is related positively to both demoralization and unemployment (Link et al. 1991), and the latter increases the positive relationship between stigma beliefs (that is, beliefs that mental patients will suffer discrimination and be devalued) and demoralization (Link et al. 1991). Mirroring predictions from

---

[3] Note that the term epileptic is a social identity, rather than a condition. Scholars have argued that epilepsy is a deeply discrediting condition because it meets more than one of Goffman's (1963) characteristics of stigma. Other physical health conditions that are socially discrediting include HIV/AIDS (Fife and Wright 2000), eating disorders (e.g., see Rich 2006), and disability (e.g., see Rose 2006). Again, like epilepsy, each of these conditions contains multiple elements of stigma; specifically, each involves not only the individual's body, but also, in the minds of many, their character.

[4] Also see Schneider and Conrad's (1983) study on individuals with epilepsy.

[5] Secondary deviance is explained primarily in two ways. First, once individuals have been labeled as deviant, most – if not all – of their behaviors are viewed as a manifestation of their deviance. For instance, if individuals have been labeled as having depression, all of their behavior is interpreted to be a result of their mental state. Second, once individuals have been labeled as deviant, they may respond to what they perceive as others' reactions to them in ways that either inadvertently or intentionally reaffirms their stigmatized identity (Lemert 1999).

classic labeling theory, mental patients' expectation of rejection seems to set in motion a series of actions and reactions that fulfill their original fears.[6,7]

Focusing less on those who have been labeled by others, Thoits (1985), too, builds upon traditional labeling theory by elaborating the process of *self*-labeling (also see Taylor 1995). In an attempt to explain why people voluntarily seek counseling (psychiatric or otherwise) in spite of its potential to lead to stigmatization, Thoits (1985) focused her attention on the experience of emotional deviance. Feelings of emotional deviance are likely to occur when individuals become aware (or are made aware) that they are violating emotion norms – that is, norms that tell us what we should feel or how we should express emotions in a particular situation (Hochschild 1979). According to Thoits (1985), self-labeling takes place when individuals come to see themselves as feeling (or expressing) emotion in ways that are not consistent with widely held cultural norms about emotions and seek professional assistance to bring their emotions back in line with cultural expectations.

Notably, individuals who seek out less restrictive forms of treatment voluntarily are less likely to be stigmatized than those who are institutionalized against their will. Thoits (1985) attributes the lesser stigmatization of seeking counseling in outpatient settings to the growing utilization of private counselors throughout the general population. Despite the widespread use of individual counseling, however, there remains a lingering stigma associated with certain types of psychiatric disorders as well as psychiatric treatments that may or may not involve the use of psychotropic drugs (Benkert et al. 1997).

Taken together, studies focusing on stigma, identity, and illness are much better at documenting the reciprocal relationship that exists between identity and illness than those that simply examine the effect of illness on identity. While illness does, indeed, affect identity, the internalization of a stigmatized identity can, in turn, lead individuals to make choices or to engage in behaviors that may subsequently affect health and other health-related outcomes (e.g., see Reidpath et al. 2005). However, where these studies advance our understanding of the relationship between identity and illness, they, too, concentrate only on the negative effects of illness on identity. This pejorative focus may be understandable, however, given their interest in *stigmatizing* diseases and conditions that are, by definition, undesirable.[8] Moreover, while scholars have assumed a more reciprocal relationship between illness and identity once the stigma has occurred, scholars working in this area have failed to address how an individual's identity prior to the illness – or the labeling itself – can play a significant part in how that stigma and/or illness is experienced, negotiated, and acted upon.

The Effect of Identity on Illness

Although the majority of studies have focused on how illness affects identity, this is not to say that scholars have completely ignored how identity has the capacity to affect one's health or experience of disease. In his classic study on biographical disruption, for instance, Bury (1982) finds that those diagnosed with rheumatoid arthritis carefully select specific events in their earlier biographies to

---

[6] Elsewhere, Link and Phelan have identified stigma as a *fundamental cause* (2001) for mental health disorders.

[7] Despite the strength of this approach – as well as its intuitive appeal – recent narrative accounts of diagnosis suggest that some seem to experience their conditions as *improving* upon being labeled. In a personal memoir describing his experience with Asperger's Disease, John Robinson (2007) reports that instead of internalizing the stigma associated with the label, he was reassured by having gained a greater understanding of the thing he had been plagued by – unbeknownst to him – since childhood. His experience with Asperger's – a developmental disorder that leads to social and communicative difficulties – matches those of individuals who suffer from chronic pain and other "invisible" conditions who seek diagnosis as a means of legitimizing their experiences to the outside world.

[8] Recently, however, social movement scholars have noted that social movement organizations have become more skilled at recasting potentially stigmatized – or otherwise damaged – identities in a more positive light in order to better effect social change (Britt and Heise 2000; Taylor and Van Willigen 1996).

help make meaning out of their illness experience. For instance, one woman recounted her belief that her troubles with rheumatoid arthritis began with her then 7 year-old son's emergency appendectomy. The stress of that incident, she posited, might have triggered the illness. However, Bury does not theorize a more integrated concept of identity, choosing instead to focus almost entirely on the impact of particular events (also see Richardson et al. 2006; Wilson 2007). Building upon Bury's work, Williams (1984) proposed the concept of "narrative reconstruction." In studying how people make sense of their illness, Williams finds that not only do people focus on specific events in their earlier biographies, but they weave elaborate and concise narratives incorporating these events. He argues that these narratives help to reconcile the past and the present for the individual experiencing the illness. While Williams provides a more holistic theorization of how individuals make sense of their illness by drawing upon the pre-illness past, like Bury, he primarily focuses on the impact of specific events and does not examine how pre-illness identity might play a part (also see Alaszewski et al. 2006; Hallowell et al. 2006).

Some scholars – most typically affiliated with departments of psychology or schools of public health – have also begun to address the so-called "buffering" effects of identity. Specifically, they address how a strong identity might help mitigate the impact of illness. For instance, in their study of African–American men, Wester et al. (2006) find that particular aspects of racial identity attitudes helped to mediate the relationship between gender role conflict and psychological distress. Other studies have also examined how racial and/or ethnic identities play a role in mediating the impact of racial/ethnic discrimination on individuals' health (e.g., see Brown and Wallace 2001; Gee et al. 2007). Many of these studies, however, limit their conceptualization of self to the use of personality markers, such as mastery, self-esteem, or self-efficacy, as proxies for identity (e.g., Ohm and Aronson 2006; Tijerina 2006). While these approaches provide valuable insight into the protective nature of particular aspects of identity on the experience of illness, such one-dimensional measures tap into a limited and static understanding of the self (McLeod and Lively 2007). Moreover, these variable-based measures imply that the self is something inherent to the individual and, therefore, asocial – assumptions that are at odds with insights gained from social psychological theories. Just as the first group of studies fails to address the independent effects of identity on health, this third group fails to consider the social, dynamic, and interdependent aspects of the self that may ameliorate or exacerbate the experience of illness.

To summarize, the extant literature in this area has generally taken three approaches toward the study of identity and illness: focusing on the ways in which illness affects identity, the interplay between the two, and, somewhat less successfully, how identity has the ability to influence one's experience of disease and other debilitating conditions. With the exception of those studies based on the modified labeling theory of mental illness (Link 1987), the majority of this work has drawn only on vague insights from symbolic interaction, largely eschewing more developed social psychological theories of identity, which posit a more dynamic, proactive, social self that may lead individuals to make different choices regarding their health and illness and, subsequently, to different health outcomes. In the following sections, we will introduce identity theory (Stryker and Burke 2000), in more general terms, before turning our attention to three related, yet distinct theoretical perspectives: structural symbolic interaction (Stryker 1980), affect control theory (Heise 1979), and identity control theory (Burke 1991). Despite their similarities, each of these theories offers unique contributions that may further enrich our understanding of the relationship between identity and health.

Identity Theory

One of the strengths of symbolic interaction is its ability to capture the dynamic nature not only of reality, but also of the self. In contrast, many people (both sociologists and laypersons) tend to view the self as enduring or stable. In an attempt to explain this contradiction, various forms of identity theory were developed. Generally speaking, identity theory (Stryker and Burke 2000) focuses on how social structure influences individuals' identities and behaviors, as well as the role that individuals play in sustaining both the social structure and the normative order in which they are embedded. From this perspective, actors develop their identities from the social positions or roles they occupy within the social structure. Eventually, they come to derive meanings and normative behavior from these roles.

Social psychologists differentiate between different types of identities. Within sociology, the most common of these are "role identities," although some scholars also study "social identities" (Hogg 2003) and "person identities" (Stets and Burke 1996).[9] A role identity is the set of self-meanings an individual internalizes from his or her position within the larger social structure (McCall and Simmons 1978). Individuals derive meaning about the self and their surroundings – as well as behavior – by adopting role positions. As such, these positions shape the self in important ways and also serve to tie the individual to the very social structure from which the social roles originated.

Keeping this general framework of identity theory in mind, we now turn to three specific theories: structural symbolic interaction, affect control theory, and identity control theory. We argue that insights from these theories have the potential to open up new theoretical and methodological directions in the field of identity and illness. In the following discussion, we provide an elementary introduction to each of these perspectives and explicate their usefulness to the study of health and well-being.

Structural Symbolic Interaction

As noted above, structural symbolic interaction posits that the self stems largely from the larger social structure in which one is embedded, drawing our attention to the ways in which individuals' positions within the social structure impact behavior. According to this perspective, the self is made up primarily from the combination of role identities that the individual holds. Although there are several hundred social roles available to any given person at any given time (Heise 2006), Stryker (1980) argues that one's sense of self is typically comprised of a much smaller set of social roles or role identities. Indeed, the handful of role identities to which individuals are most strongly committed and are most salient make up one's identity hierarchy. Those identities at the top of the hierarchy are the ones to which the individual is most highly committed. Commitment, in this sense, refers to the number of social relations that one would lose if he were to abandon or lose a particular social role. Saliency refers to one's affective attachment (or the emotional rewards) that one has to a particular role. Saliency, for the most part, is believed to stem from commitment (Callero 1985; Stryker 1980). If a worker decides to exit the work role by seeking disability, for example, it may be more difficult if she believes that doing so will also risk her role of wife or, if she is her children's primary financial provider, her role as breadwinner. If the majority of her friendships are also dependent upon her role as worker, the decision may be even more difficult, for she runs the risk not only of losing the emotionally satisfying relationships with her husband and her children, but also with her peer group (also see Ebaugh 1988).

---

[9]"Social identities" refer to identities that are derived from group membership (e.g., female or Asian–American), whereas "person identities" refer to personal characteristics or attributes that describe a particular person *across* social roles (e.g., intelligent, compassionate, competitive). Indeed, Affect Control Theory (Heise 1979) treats "person identities" as attributes that have the ability to moderate role identities, instead of as identities in their own right.

According to Stryker (1980), individuals tend to hold some role identities in higher esteem than others. A role identity that is deeply embedded in one's social networks – that is, there are many relationships dependent upon one's occupancy – and has some degree of emotional payoff is likely to be more salient than those roles that are not deeply embedded or emotionally rewarding. Structural symbolic interaction assumes that individuals are especially motivated to act in ways that maintain their most highly committed and salient social roles. Given that social roles can be thought of as a bundled set of rights and obligations that exist between role partners (Heiss 1981; Stryker and Statham 1985), actors are expected to act in accordance with their rights and obligations. If they fail to do so, they can expect to be sanctioned by their role partner(s). When individuals are no longer able to meet the demands of the role, they may voluntarily leave the role or, at the very least, reduce its importance to their sense of self.[10]

When a role identity is particularly salient, Stryker (1980) suggests that individuals may find themselves engaging in the behavior associated with the identity even in situations where it is not appropriate. They may also purposely seek out events where they can enact that role without social sanction, as well as seek out people who support that role. For example, someone who is wedded to his patient identity may immerse himself in traditional treatments or seek out friends who are supportive, if not sympathetic, to his plight and distance himself from those who are not (Charmaz 1980).[11]

Additionally, however, individuals may eschew roles associated with their condition altogether, putting their energy into maintaining an identity – or identities – that have little to do with being a patient. It may also be that potential patients (or potential incumbents of the patient role) may choose to concentrate their energies on identities that have very little to do with illness. For example, someone who suffers from chronic lower back pain may not be highly committed to his role as a pain sufferer, although he may suffer a tremendous amount of pain on a daily basis. Instead, he may be more committed to his roles as *attorney*, *father*, or *athlete* – all of which may be fundamentally at odds with the patient role. Further, if *athlete* is his most salient role (in terms of emotional payoff), he may eschew the rights and obligations of the patient role – or the sick role – in lieu of those associated with the more favored role of athlete. That is, he may seek out health care providers (e.g., a chiropractor versus a surgeon) who promote exercise versus bed rest. Indeed, numerous studies reveal that patients tend to seek out, *and cooperate with* health care providers who, in some way or another, tell them what they want to hear (Lock and Kaufert 1998; Steinberg and Baxter 1998). However, when it is no longer possible for him to fulfill his role-related obligations, he may have no choice but to rearrange or otherwise alter his identity hierarchy.

Despite the flexibility of structural symbolic interaction and its ability to predict behavior across a broad spectrum of individuals, this approach has remained virtually invisible among those who study the relationship between health and identity. Indeed, to date, the most influential discussion

---

[10] In his account of his journey toward becoming a quadriplegic, anthropologist Robert Murphy (1990) discusses how his condition affected his ability to conduct fieldwork. As he pointed out, anthropologists garner status and prestige through their field work. In an effort to maintain some status within his chosen field, he turned to writing anthropology textbooks, even though he knew that such an activity was relatively devalued within his discipline.

[11] Recently psychologists have also become more interested in identity hierarchies, as they seem to operate like cognitive schemas. Self-schemas refer to cognitive filters that develop in the brain over time which affect the ways in which individuals attend to, store, and retrieve – in this case – self-referential information (Kilstrom and Cantor 1984; Markus 1977; also see Linville and Carlston 1994). To the degree that identity hierarchies operate similar to schemas, it may also be that individuals who hold an illness identity that is maintained within their significant social networks are more likely to notice, attend to, and remember information, encounters, and incidents that support their view of themselves and of their situation (Morgan and Schwalbe 1990). This suggests that someone for whom the illness identity is particularly salient may pay more attention to his or her aches and pains than those for whom the identity is not particularly salient. This is not to say that individuals willfully choose to process some information and ignore others; rather, their identity provides filters that operate at a more subconscious level.

of social roles in the health literature comes *not* from structural symbolic interaction, per se, but rather role theory and structural functionalism. Similar to structural symbolic interaction, role theory – the theory on which the sick-role (Parsons 1951) is based – assumes that individual behavior is largely dependent upon individuals' social roles, their role sets, and their role repertoires. Simply put, role theory assumes that once you are in a role, your behavior is, for the most part, determined by that role. Unlike structural symbolic interaction, however, role theory fails to explain how or why individuals adhere to particular roles and not others. Nor does it adequately explain variability *within* similar roles, or why it is that people tend to act similarly *across* varying roles.[12]

In an attempt to bridge the fluidity of symbolic interaction and the rigidity of role theory, Stryker and Statham (1985) have argued that structural symbolic interaction is based on the notion of role-making, as opposed to role-taking. According to this perspective, role-making refers to the give and take that exists between any given set of role-partners in a particular social interaction or network that explains the wide variability in the performance of particular social roles. For instance, some patients may be more involved in their treatment than others, allowing – or causing – their health care provider to be less authoritarian, just as some doctors may be emotionally engaged, thereby encouraging a more personal relationship with their patients. Alternately, some physicians may stay firmly behind the wall of affective neutrality, encouraging their clients to be less engaged in the establishment of care.

Taking a slightly different approach to explain the variability with which people approach, adopt, or enact certain roles, Callero (1994) argues that roles should be conceptualized not only as a set of rights and obligations that determine individual behavior (Merton 1957), but also as resources that individuals *seek to acquire* for their anticipated benefits. From this perspective, roles can be thought of as resources that individuals actively pursue in order to obtain access to symbolic, cultural, social, and material capital (Callero 1994; also see McLeod and Lively 2003). When an individual adopts – or maintains – a role such as patient, for example, she not only benefits from the increased access to resources associated with the role (e.g., the sympathy or releases from certain obligations, such as employment or domestic labor, associated with being ill), but she also acquires access to the others associated with the role. The social connections attached to roles grant individuals access to information networks that could potentially benefit them through material, emotional, cultural, or symbolic gains – thus acting as another means through which an individual may increase one's human capital. When individuals self-select into particular roles in order to achieve certain benefits or to avoid potential costs, they are, in a sense, exercising their own personal control and power (also see Callero 2003). Thus, roles are not only utilized to define the self, guide behavior, and buffer against life stress, but also to achieve desired ends (Callero 1994). In the context of identity and illness, this means that while the objective realities of individuals who experience the same disease may be similar, their subjective experiences (i.e., illness) may be different depending on the roles they chose to enact and maintain throughout their illness.[13] Unfortunately, however, this assertion remains virtually untested among those studying identity and illness.

To date, most studies of identity and health take their starting point from when the individual can no longer work around his or her condition or disease and is already in the position of having to

---

[12]Another insight that can be gleaned from these theories is the importance of considering actors' social networks. To date, scholars have become increasingly interested in the role that one's social networks have on a variety of health related behaviors, including the utilization of health care services (Pescosolido 1996, 2006), agreement to genetic testing and other forms of screenings (Husaini et al. 2001; Levy-Storms and Wallace 2003), and adherence to treatment regimens (Westphal 2004). According to a more network centered perspective, our social networks help influence our understanding of a particular situation; subsequently these understandings also affect future behaviors.

[13]While we recognize that some diseases are debilitating and may, to some degree, act as master statuses (Hughes 1945), there remain individuals who chose to invest in other role identities despite overwhelming odds. For instance, in a recent study of mothers who have HIV/AIDS, Wilson (2007) found that her respondents continue to cling to the mother identity and emphasize their need to survive and protect their children. Typically, however, individuals who are able to maintain alternate roles in the face of devastating illnesses or physical conditions tend to have considerable economic, cultural, and social capital at their disposal.

abandon emotionally salient and committed roles such a breadwinner or coach (Bury 1982; Charmaz 1980; Karp 1996; Williams 1984). Indeed, these are the experiences on which numerous narrative studies and patient memoirs are based. Before individuals reach this point, however, they may make decisions that are based less on their physical conditions and more on their subjective identities and desires. These decisions *may or may not* affect their eventual health outcomes. Given that this supposition has yet to be empirically tested, it may be worthwhile to examine individuals' identity hierarchies at the time of diagnosis, track how these hierarchies change, and how they affect individuals' decision making processes regarding their condition over time.

To conclude, structural symbolic interaction and recent conceptualizations of social roles have the potential to open up new theoretical directions for those studying identity and illness. In taking account of individuals' pre-existing identities, we are further able to examine the differential ways in which individuals handle and make decisions about their health. Further, incorporating insights from structural symbolic interaction also helps locate the contexts in which individuals use pre-existing identities to help alleviate the negative impacts of illness.

Affect Control Theory

Moving away from the notion of identity hierarchies, affect control theory (Heise 1979, 2006) focuses on the internal and behavioral processes an individual undertakes in regulating and maintaining an identity (also see Burke and Cast 1997). Unlike other theories of identity, which are primarily cognitive, affect control theory relies largely on sentiment structures to predict behavior. Sentiments, according to Heise (2006), are culturally shared affective meanings that individuals hold regarding elements of the social world. Specifically, affect control theorists are interested in the relationship between the *fundamental sentiments* that individuals hold generally and the *transient sentiments* that arise in situated interaction – that is, during a particular encounter between social actors.

Generally speaking, affect control theory is based on the premise that individuals are motivated to act in ways that keep their transient sentiments in line with their fundamental sentiments. When transient and fundamental sentiments are at odds, individuals are expected to act in ways that bring them closer together. According to Heise (2006), when individuals are *able* to confirm sentiments about their current identity, they are in essence actualizing their sense of self. When they are *unable* to confirm sentiments about their current identity, however, they experience inauthenticity that they resolve by enacting compensating identities or reframing the situation cognitively.[14]

Based on dozens of cross-cultural studies of affective meaning (Osgood et al. 1975), affect control theory assumes that the sentiments of people everywhere vary along the three dimensions of meaning: Evaluation, Potency, and Activity.[15] The theory also assumes that people who share a culture also

---

[14] In experimental settings, individuals are more likely to alter behavior – or their meaning of a behavior – before attempting to alter (or redefine) their own social identity or the identity of their interaction partner (Nelson 2006).

[15] Sentiments are measured through disaggregating the elements of social interactions – that is, role identities, behaviors, attributes, emotions, and settings – into three fundamental dimensions of affective meaning: Evaluation (how good or bad something is), Potency (how powerful or powerless), and Activation (how lively or quiet). These three aspects are usually referred to as EPA; and most affect control theorists assign them values ranging from approximately 4.0 to −4.0. As these values suggest, the three aspects of sentiments – Evaluation, Potency, and Activity – are matters of degree: E, P, and A values can be greater or less, in either a positive or negative direction. For example, *physician* has an EPA of 2.01, 1.67, −0.10, whereas a *nurse* has an EPA of 1.65, 0.93, 0.34, and a *patient*, 0.90, −0.69, −1.05, which suggests – not surprisingly – that in any given interaction, individuals who see themselves as patients are more likely to listen to or obey physicians than they are to adhere to the demands of nurses, whom they view as relatively less good and less powerful.

share sentiments about interactional elements within that culture, such as role identities, behaviors, settings, emotions, and attributes. In the USA, for example, Americans tend to view children as being fundamentally very good (in terms of Evaluation), fairly weak (in terms of Potency), and fairly active (in terms of Activation). However, in a situation when a child does something bad (such as kicking an infant, who is *also* viewed as very good, fairly weak, and fairly active), we construct a transient sentiment regarding that particular child, based on the combination of his identity as a child, his (very bad and fairly powerful) behavior, the equally good, weak, and active identity of the infant, and the setting in which the interaction occurred.[16]

The *difference* between one's fundamental sentiments that comprise the interaction and the transient sentiments that a particular interaction produces is referred to as deflection. Affect control theory, like symbolic interaction, assumes that individuals are motivated to confirm their fundamental sentiments and, thus, to minimize deflection. When deflection cannot be reduced through behavior alone (that is, the offending child cries, thus signaling remorse for his action and reducing his power in the situation in such a way that compensates for his previous powerful action against the infant) elements of the situation may have to be redefined (that is, the *child* is relabeled as a *delinquent* or the *kick* is redefined as an *accident* or as *playing*). A delinquent who kicks an infant or a child who plays with an infant seems much more likely an occurrence.

In addition to maintaining their own fundamental identities, affect control theory also assumes that people are also similarly motivated to maintain the identities of their interaction partners (Heise 2006). In other words, when interaction partners' identities are disconfirmed, actors are expected to act in ways to reset the balance. In the medical context, for example, this suggests that patients who view physicians as very good, very powerful, and somewhat inactive should act in ways that confirm their sentiments regarding the physician identity – meaning that they would be more likely to seek out medical attention and obey directives. Patients who view physicians with less esteem, however, would probably be less likely to seek out or adhere to medical advice because they are – even if only at the subconscious level – confirming their sentiments regarding the "negative," and potentially "powerless" and "inactive" identity of their health care provider who they may view as either a *quack*, or in the case of a younger physician, an *upstart*. According to affect control theory, it would not be unexpected for actors to disagree with, disparage, or ignore those whose identities are viewed as significantly worse, weaker, and less active than their own. From this perspective, knowing how different populations view physicians may help us to understand why some patients comply with physicians' orders, while others do not. It may also help to predict patients' reactions to different types of health care providers, given that different types of providers tend to be viewed differently (e.g., *competent healer* versus *new-age quack*).

Further, affect control theory has a predictive capacity that moves beyond other theories of identity. In order to specify the mathematical underpinning of the theory, Heise and colleagues have developed a computer simulation program, INTERACT, that allows researchers to simulate social interactions by entering in discrete elements of a social interaction (and their concomitant EPA values) and combining them to create transient sentiments. Using the EPA structures as data and the mathematical models that have been derived from affect control theory (Heise 1979, 2006;

---

[16] Although affect control theory assumes that the majority of sentiments within a culture are commonly shared, scholars have nonetheless documented some subcultural variations. Most subcultural differences in sentiments exist as a result of differences in identities or behaviors that are associated with one group and not another (Heise 2006). For example, Smith-Lovin and Douglass (1992) reported that members of a liberal gay church had more positive meanings attached to identities such as homosexual and behaviors such as sodomy than members of a fundamentalist church. Heise (2006) argues that 80 percent of people's affective sentiments come from the influence that the dominant culture wields, and the remaining percentage stems from personal experiences. Smith and colleagues (Smith and Francis 2005; Smith et al. 2001) have also found subtle, yet significant variations in the sentiment structures of Japanese and US samples.

Smith-Lovin 1987, 1990; Smith-Lovin and Heise 1988), INTERACT allows researchers to model interactions, not only from the perspective of the first actor (who may see herself as a *competent physician* who is in the act of *instructing* an *uninformed patient*), but also from the perspective of the second actor (who may see the situation from an entirely different perspective: *insensitive know-it-all talks down to competent professional*.)[17] INTERACT, as well as Affect Control Theory, reminds us of the importance of considering the perspectives of both (or all) actors within a given situation. Because of their differential perceptions, the actions that one actor may take in order to reduce deflection may be at odds with the prescribed steps of their interaction partner. That individuals may have different definitions of situations, which may result in incongruous behaviors, is not new; indeed, it is the stuff from which television sit-coms are born. While the mismatch of meaning can be humorous in a comedic setting, it can be disastrous in a medical context.

To date, there have only been a handful of studies that have applied insights from affect control theory towards the study of health and identity. Although all these speak of issues of mental illness, they have implications for physical health as well. Drawing on the experience of individuals entering into social support and grief management for those who were recently divorced or widowed, Francis (1997) found that support group leaders changed participants' emotional responses to loss by altering their underlying social identities. For instance, when individuals came in distraught over their divorce, the group leader would attempt to lower the member's evaluation of their spouse in terms of their relative goodness, powerfulness, and activation. They would also attempt to increase the relative goodness of the member. Similarly, widows or widowers – especially caregivers – who believed that they had failed their spouse, were encouraged to see the spouse's behavior (e.g., dying) as intentional, thereby reframing their death as a choice to leave or as a form of abandonment. By viewing the spouse's behavior as conscious and, therefore, significantly more negative, more powerful, and more active, the aggrieved spouse was able to see him or herself, as well as the deceased, in a different light. The transformation of identities (that arose predominantly from the reconceptualization of the behavior) positioned surviving spouses to deal more effectively with not only their guilt, but also their grief.[18]

Focusing more on sentiment structures than the transformation of social identities, Kroska and Harkness (2006) introduced the concept of stigma sentiments in order to test Link's modified labeling theory of mental illness (see earlier discussion). Stigma sentiments are the culturally held sentiments regarding individuals with mental illness. Based on surveys from four distinct populations that tapped not only into stigma sentiments, but also self-appraisals ("myself as I really am") and reflected self-appraisals ("myself as others see me"), Kroska and Harkness (2006) found that the self-appraisals and reflected self-appraisals of the mentally ill patients were closer to that of role identity of *person with mental illness* than those of non-patients.[19] Further, mentally ill patients' self-appraisals and reflected self-appraisals were also more positively associated with those of three other negative and potentially stigmatizing identities (e.g., *loser, outcast*, and *reject*) than non-patients. These findings are consistent with the modified labeling theory of mental illness (Link 1987), in that they, too, suggest that patients who have been diagnosed with mental illness do indeed come to see the negatives associated with mental illness as self-relevant.

---

[17] In order to use INTERACT, available at http://www.indiana.edu/~socpsy/ACT/interact.htm, one must put all interactions into the format of actor-behavior-object. Using advanced settings, the researcher can also choose personal attributes (e.g., opinionated, lazy, friendly), as well as the settings in which the interaction is likely to occur (e.g., a hospital, a clinic, a bar).

[18] Perhaps not surprisingly, individuals who attended the grief support group for widows and widowers were less inclined to accept a blatant negative reconceptualization of their deceased spouse's identity than those individuals who had lost a spouse to abandonment or divorce.

[19] The non-patient samples included both network members of the mentally ill as well as college students from a nearby state university.

Although one could argue that their findings merely replicate Link's (1987) already well-documented results, Kroska and Harkness (2006) argue that stigma sentiments may, in fact, be a superior measure of mental health stigma than the stigma beliefs (Link 1987). Unlike stigma beliefs, which are based on a relatively lengthy scale of historically and socially contextualized statements that may capture the assumptions of mental health researchers rather than the actual experiences of patients (e.g., "Most people would willingly accept a former mental patient as a close friend"; Link 1987), stigma sentiments are historically and socially context-free. They are also easier to collect – requiring only three simple ratings along the dimensions of Evaluation, Potency, and Activation – and are both highly comparable and reliable across cultures.

Although stigma sentiments have only been recently introduced to the study of mental health, they provide an intriguing opportunity for health researchers to understand how the onset and progression of disease may influence the effects of illness on various aspects of identity – particularly self-appraisals and reflected self-appraisals. Given Kroska and Harkness' (2006) purpose of testing modified labeling theory, it is not surprising that they failed to also address how these new (or altered) self-meanings may also impact individual choices related to disease, if not subsequent outcomes. Drawing on insight from affect control theory – that is, that individuals tend to create events that confirm their sentiments (Heise 2006) – it is likely that behaviors and outcomes will be affectively consistent with self-meanings. To date, however, there has been very little, if any, data collected on such a phenomena. Future studies would do well to collect self-appraisals from patients or those laboring under various diseases or conditions and – at least in the case of stigmatized conditions – self-*reflected* appraisals. Not only could researchers examine differences between patients and non-patients, following Kroska and Harkness (2006), but they could also follow changes in patients' self-meanings over time.

Identity Control Theory

Despite considerable overlap with ideas from structural symbolic interaction (Stryker 1980), affect control theory (Heise 1979, 2006; Smith-Lovin and Heise 1988), and identity theory more generally (Thoits 1983, 1986), identity control theory focuses on the more internal – as opposed to the behavioral – processes an individual undertakes in regulating and maintaining an identity (Burke 2005). In the identity control model, an individual controls her perception of the situational meanings via a feedback loop in which she strives to match situational inputs (i.e., how she perceives herself in the situation) with her identity standard (the set of meanings she holds for a particular identity, such as wife, student, or employee). Unlike affect control theory, which relies on fundamental sentiments held in common at the cultural level, identity control theory relies on identity standards that are collected directly from the individuals being studied. The goal of the identity control process is to bring the situational inputs into alignment with the identity standard (Burke and Cast 1997). Much like individuals who perceive an incongruence between fundamental sentiments and events are expected to alter one or more elements of the interaction in order to reduce deflection (Heise 1979, 2006), individuals who perceive an incongruence between situational inputs and their identity standards are expected to alter their behavior and/or perceptions until congruence between the situational inputs and the identity standard are achieved.[20]

---

[20] As do other theories of identity (Heise 1979, 2006; Stryker 1980), identity control posits that if an individual's restorative strategies fail to produce a correspondence between situational input and the identity standard, the identity standard itself may change (Burke and Cast 1997).

Scholars interested in health have not capitalized on identity control theory as much as they have on the other theories outlined above. Granberg's (2006) recent scholarship on sustained weight loss may represent the most successful application of identity control theory, at least in conjunction with the theory of possible selves (Markus and Nurius 1986; Markus and Ruvolo 1989) and narrative psychology. Specifically, she examined how individuals who experience significant and planned weight loss negotiate this self-imposed challenge to self and identity. Granberg's (2006) work extends the scope of identity control theory in important and significant ways. First, "possible selves" do not refer to whom individuals see themselves as currently, but rather how they could *possibly* be at some future time. According to Markus and Nurius (1986), the theory of possible selves focuses on gaps between who we are and who we might be, and links such discrepancies *directly* to the pursuit of self-relevant goals (Markus and Ruvolo 1989). In Granberg's study, many of the respondents' possible selves were based on what they thought their lives would be like upon reaching their weight loss goal or, in some cases, being found sexually attractive or buying a certain sized dress.

Second, prior to Granberg's (2006) study, identity theories have been considered to be most relevant to formal social roles, such as patient, invalid, doctor, etc., and to processes that promote stability and coherence in individuals' self-concepts. Therefore, identity theory has typically *not* been used to explore informal roles (or physical conditions), nor has it been applied to instances of self change. Unlike traditional applications of identity control theory that focus almost entirely on formal social roles and stability (Burke and Cast 1997), Granberg's work reveals that informal roles, such as "fat" or "thin," when invoked in social interactions, also influence thoughts, behaviors, and strategies. Moreover, they not only inform individuals' choices about maintenance, but they also motivate decisions and behaviors regarding continued self-change.

Third, Granberg shows that individuals' narratives about obesity, like those used in earlier accounts of identity and more formal illness (e.g., Bury 1982; Charmaz 1993), refer to stories used by individuals to relate their experiences in such a way that they incorporate an additional message or moral story (Orbuch 1997). They are also an important means through which the excitement generated by the hoped-for possible selves or the disappointment resulting from a failure of self-verification can be made comprehensible not only to the self, but also to others (Granberg 2006; also see Bruner 2002; Gergan 1994; Hyden 1997).[21]

In melding these three theoretical traditions, Granberg (2006) suggests that identifying the processes through which people resolve unmet expectations (about what they thought their lives would be like post-weight loss) can explain the very high rates of failure of weight loss as well as informing theoretical understandings of identity formation and maintenance. For instance, while individuals who are dissatisfied with their weight loss may be more inclined to gain the weight back, the successful "losers" in Granberg's study tended to either engage in behavioral strategies (e.g., exercise more or lower their goal weight) or reframe their desired self (e.g., from being sexy to being healthy).[22]

While her focus is on issues of obesity and weight loss, Granberg's (2006) observations may have implications for other forms of disease or other health-related conditions, especially since possible selves can incorporate any domain of self-conception, such as role identities (e.g., victim), personal attributes (e.g., disabled), or physical characteristics (e.g., obesity). Moreover, although

---

[21] Insights such as these may also be useful in furthering our understanding of other forms of self-change that involves the physical self – that is, the body (for recent examples, see Davis 1995; Gagne and Tewksbury 1999; Phelan and Hunt 1998; Preves 2001).

[22] Although obesity has not been fully accepted as a disease in the traditional sense, it is a physical condition that undoubtedly impacts health and contributes to other diseases, such as diabetes, hypertension, high-blood pressure, bulimia, etc. Gaining insight into the cognitive barriers to weight-loss, then, has important implications for a variety of health related dilemmas.

Granberg's (2006) analysis dealt only with possible selves that are positive, possible selves can also be negative (e.g., invalid) or represent conditions that individuals would prefer to avoid (e.g., incontinence). Future research in this area would do well to address how individuals use identity control processes when facing a wider array of health challenges that may, or may not, lead to the genesis of negative, or deteriorating, possible selves.

Conclusion

In this chapter, we have argued that a more thorough inclusion of social psychological theories of identity has the potential to remedy current oversights in the field of identity and illness. In particular, by taking into account people's identities before they become ill, we can examine how existing identities may not only shape individuals' subjective experience of their illnesses, but also their choices, behaviors, and, potentially, their outcomes. Although identity theories such as those we have discussed here have been used in a variety of contexts, from predicting blood donations (Callero 1985) to trial sentencing (Robinson et al. 1994), only rarely have they been incorporated into studies relating to illness (for exceptions, see Francis 1997; Granberg 2006; Kroska and Harkness 2006).

Structural symbolic interaction, affect control theory, and identity control theory all operate on the premise that individuals are motivated to protect (or maintain) their fundamental sense of self (but see Granberg 2006). For Stryker (1980), this means maintaining the role identities to which they are highly committed and find the most salient. For Heise (1979) and Burke (1991), however, it means creating (or perceiving) events that match their senses of self. While scholars have examined how illness impacts an individual's identity, we argue that fully incorporating these theories can contribute towards a more sophisticated and nuanced theory of the relationship between identity and illness. Furthermore, we believe that incorporating the theoretical insights from social psychological theories of identity would also assist researchers and possibly practitioners in understanding why it is that some seem more willing to succumb to disease, while others do not.

As noted previously, structural symbolic interaction (Stryker 1980) reminds us that individuals are motivated to maintain highly valued identities. When applied to medical research this suggests that those studying the relationship between identity and illness might benefit from paying closer attention to individuals' preferred social identities prior to and immediately following a diagnosis, as well as during treatment and, if applicable, throughout recovery. Because one's social role identities are closely tied to affect, cognition, and behavior, it is likely that individuals' outcomes may vary by the degree to which they embrace or reject the patient role, either surrendering or retaining other valued social roles in the process.

Similarly, affect control theory (Heise 1979, 2006) suggests that individuals are motivated to maintain their fundamental affective sentiments regarding their sense of self, others, and even settings where situated interactions are likely to occur. When individuals' fundamental sentiments are not matched by situated interactions, they may engage in behavioral or cognitive strategies to rectify these discrepancies as a means to avoid dissonant feelings. Again, when applied to the study of health and illness, it is possible that some groups of individuals may have different fundamental sentiments about what it means to be a patient, an invalid, or a physician. Additionally, they may also differ in terms of their understanding of hospitals and the type of activities that are likely to occur there. Taken together, these insights suggest that a more nuanced understanding of individuals' sentiments regarding social roles, behaviors, and settings within the medical context might shed light on why certain types of people may be more or less likely to seek out, receive, and adhere to medical care. Further, affect control theorists have also shown how important it is to truly understand and consider individuals' definition of the situation in the course of situated interactions (see Robinson et al. 1994). If scholars had access to such definitions, they would be better positioned to not only understand an individual's choices and motivations, but also to predict behaviors and develop successful interventions (again, see Francis 1997).

Finally, identity control theory (Burke 2005) also argues that individuals are motivated to maintain their preferred self-identities. Drawing on these insights, as well as Markus and Nurius' (1986) discussion of possible selves, Granberg (2006) showed that individuals are not only motivated to maintain their preferred self-identities as they are now, but also to reach identities that they may imagine in their future. Although Granberg's study is limited to positive possible selves, it stands to reason that some individuals may also be motivated to avoid negative possible selves. A postmenopausal cancer survivor, for example, may avoid taking prescribed hormone replacement drugs because of her fear of developing breast cancer, leaving herself open to a greater risk of heart disease and stroke. Insights like these would not only improve scholars' understanding of the decisions that individuals make, but could also lead to the development of important interventions within the field and practice of medicine.

Despite their roots in traditional symbolic interaction (Blumer 1969), the empirical applications of identity theory rely most commonly on quantitative methods. Indeed, part of Stryker's (1980) justification for a more structural perspective on identity was to move scholars away from traditional symbolic interaction's reliance on qualitative data and shift them towards survey methods that would result in more efficient data collection and greater replicability and generalizability. Notably, the two control theories (Heise 1979; Burke 1991) tend to utilize an even broader range of methodologies that includes not only ethnography and surveys, but also computer simulations and experiments. While we are by no means proposing to supplant qualitative methods, we argue that the introduction of complementary methods and data sources to the study of illness and identity would better allow scholars to not only ascertain the generalizability of their findings, but also more readily link their work to broader questions within sociology. For instance, by quantifying the insights garnered from narrative accounts or other forms of ethnographic research (e.g., creating identity hierarchies, collecting affective sentiments, etc.), researchers would be better positioned to understand the ways in which individuals' self meanings – particularly those associated with health, illness, and well-being – may be influenced by the larger social structures in which they are embedded. Indeed, drawing on insights from social structure and personality (see McLeod and Lively 2003 for a recent review) – and from social stratification more generally – it may be that potential shifts in individuals' identities that may arise from, or perhaps even buffer, an illness or other debilitating condition, are affected by broader factors such as race, class, gender, or sexuality. They may also be influenced by the social characteristics of friends, families, schools, or even neighborhoods. Further, the use of more highly structured data, in conjunction with the rich details that only narrative methods can provide, may also grant scholars the ability to more easily make comparisons not only between groups, but also *within* groups. It may also allow researchers to more efficiently and effectively track changes over time. Such strategies have the potential not only to deepen our appreciation of the effects of illness on identity *and vice versa*, but also to promote an inherently more sociological approach towards the study of identity and illness.

The authors would like to thank Brian Powell, Sean Smith, and Michael Yacavone for their assistance and support throughout this project. This draft was supported, in part, by the Rockefeller Center for Public Policy at Dartmouth College and the Faculty Grants Committee at Millersville University.

References

Alaszewski A, Alaszewski H, Potter J (2006) Risk, uncertainty, and life threatening trauma: analysing stroke survivor's accounts of life after stroke. Qual Soc Res 7:1–16
Barker K (2002) Self-help literature and the making of an identity illness: the case of Fibromyalgia Syndrome (FMS). Soc Probl 49:279–300
Bell SE (2000) Experiencing illness in/and narrative. In: Bird CE, Conrad P, Fremont AM (eds) Handbook of medical sociology, 5th edn. Prentice Hall, Upper Saddle River, NJ, pp 184–199

Benkert O et al (1997) Public opinion on psychotropic drugs: an analysis of factors influencing acceptance or rejection. J Nerv Ment Dis 185:151–158

Blumer H (1969) Symbolic interaction: perspective and method. Prentice-Hall, Englewood Cliffs, NJ

Britt L, Heise DR (2000) From shame to pride in identity politics. In: Stryker S, Owens TJ, White RW (eds) Self, identity, and social movements. University of Minnesota Press, Minneapolis, MN, pp 22–268

Brown TN, Wallace JM Jr (2001) Race-related correlates of young adults' subjective well-being. Soc Indic Res 53:97–117

Bruner J (2002) Making stories: law, literature, and life. Farrar, Straus, and Giroux, New York

Burke PJ (1991) Identity processes and social stress. Am Sociol Rev 56:836–849

Burke PJ (2005) Identities and addiction. Unpublished paper presented at the Kettil Bruun Society 31st Annual Symposium Didactic at the University of California, Riverside. Riverside, CA

Burke PJ, Cast AD (1997) Stability and change in the gender identities of newly married couples. Soc Psychol Q 67:5–15

Bury M (1982) Chronic illness as biographical disruption. Sociol Health Illn 4:167–182

Callero P (1985) Role-identity salience. Soc Psychol Q 48:203–215

Callero P (1994) From role-playing to role using: understanding role as resource. Soc Psychol Q 57:228–243

Callero P (2003) The sociology of the self. Annu Rev Sociol 29:115–33

Charmaz K (1980) The social construction of self-pity in the chronically ill. Stud Symbolic Interact 3:123–145

Charmaz K (1983) Loss of self: a fundamental form of suffering in the chronically ill. Sociol Health Illn 5:168–195

Charmaz K (1993) Good days, bad days: the self in chronic illness and time. Rutgers University Press, New Brunswick, NJ

Conrad P (1990) Qualitative research on chronic illness: a commentary on method and conceptual development. Soc Sci Med 30:1257–1263

Crossley M (1998) 'Sick role' or 'empowerment'? The ambiguities of life with an HIV positive diagnosis. Sociol Health Illn 20:507–531

Davis K (1995) Reshaping the female body: the dilemma of cosmetic surgery. Routledge, New York

Ebaugh HRF (1988) Becoming an ex: the process of role exit. University of Chicago Press, Chicago, IL

Elson J (2003) Am i still a woman?: hysterectomy and gender identity. Temple University Press, Philadelphia, PA

Fife BL, Wright ER (2000) The dimensionality of stigma: a comparison of its impact on the self of persons with HIV/AIDS and cancer. J Health Soc Behav 41:50–67

Francis L (1997) Ideology and interpersonal emotion management: redefining identity in two support groups. Soc Psychol Q 60:153–171

Gagne P, Tewksbury R (1999) Knowledge and power, body and self: an analysis of knowledge systems and the transgendered self. Sociol Q 40:59–83

Gee GC, Delva J, Takeuchi DT (2007) Relationships between self-reported unfair treatment and prescription medication use, illicit drug use, and alcohol dependence among Filipino Americans. Am J Public Health 5:933–940

Gergen KJ (1994) Realities and relationships: surroundings in social construction. Harvard University Press, Cambridge, MA

Goffman E (1963) Stigma: notes on the management of a spoiled identity. Prentice Hall, Englewood Cliffs, NJ

Gordon DF (1995) Testicular cancer and masculinity. In: Sabo D, Gordon DF (eds) Men's health and illness: gender, power, and the body. Sage, Thousand Oaks, CA, pp 246–265

Granberg E (2006) 'Is this all there is?' Possible selves, self-change, and weight loss. Soc Psychol Q 69:109–126

Hallowell N, Arden-Jones A, Eeles R, Foster C, Lucassen A, Moynihan C, Watson M (2006) Guilt, blame and responsibility: men's understanding of their role in the transmission of BRCA1/2 mutations within their family. Sociol Health Illn 28:969–988

Heise DR (1979) Understanding events: affect and the construction of social action. Cambridge University Press, New York

Heise DR (2002) Understanding social interaction with affect control theory. In: Berger J, Zelrich M Jr (eds) New directions in sociological theory: growth of contemporary theories. Rowman and Littlefield, Lanham, MD, pp 17–40

Heise DR (2006) Expressive order: confirming sentiments in social actions. Springer, New York

Heiss J (1981) Social roles. In: Rosenberg M, Turner RH (eds) Social psychology: sociological perspectives. Basic Books, New York, pp 94–132

Hinojosa R, Boylstein C, Rittman M, Hinojosa MS, Faircloth CA (2008) Constructions of continuity after stroke. Symbolic Interact 31:205–224

Hochschild AR (1979) Emotion work, feeling rules, and social structure. Am J Sociol 85:551–575

Hogg MA (2003) Social identity. In: Leary MR, Tangney JP (eds) Handbook of self and identity. Guilford Press, New York, pp 462–479

Horwitz AV (2002) Outcomes in the sociology of mental health and illness: where have we been and where are we going? J Health Soc Behav 43:143–151

Hughes EC (1945) Dilemmas and contradictions of status. Am J Sociol 50:353–359

Husaini BA, Sherkat DE, Bragg R, Levine R, Emerson JS, Mentes CM, Cain VA (2001) Predictors of breast cancer screening in a panel study of African–American women. Women Health 34:35–51

Hyden L-C (1997) Illness and narrative. Sociol Health Illn 19:48–69

Kaiser K (2008) The meaning of the survivor identity for women with breast cancer. Soc Sci Med 67:79–87

Karp D (1996) Speaking of sadness: depression, disconnection, and the meanings of illness. Oxford University Press, New York

Kelly MP, Field D (1996) Medical sociology, chronic illness and the body. Sociol Health Illn 18:241–257

Kelly MP, Millward LM (2004) Identity and illness. In: Kelleher D, Leavey G (eds) Identity and illness. Routledge, London, pp 1–18

Kilstrom JF, Cantor N (1984) Mental representations of the self. In: Berkowitz L (ed) Advances in experimental social psychology. Academic, New York, pp 2–48

Kleinman A, Eisenberg L, Good B (1978) Culture, illness, and care: clinical lessons from anthropologic and cross-cultural research. Ann Intern Med 88:251–258

Kroska A, Harkness SK (2006) Stigma sentiments and self-meanings: exploring the modified labeling theory of mental illness. Soc Psychol Q 69:325–348

Lawton J (2003) Lay experiences of health and illness: past research and future agendas. Sociol Health Illn 25:23–40

Lemert EM (1999) Primary and secondary deviance. In: Traub SH, Little CB (eds) Theories of deviance, 5th edn. State University of New York at Cortland Press, Cortland, NY, pp 385–389

Lennon MC, Link BG, Marbach JJ, Dohrenwend BP (1989) The stigma of chronic facial pain and its impact on social relationships. Soc Probl 36:117–134

Levy-Storms L, Wallace SP (2003) Use of mammography screening among older Samoan women in Los Angeles county: a diffusion network approach. Soc Sci Med 57:987–1000

Link BG (1987) Understanding labeling effects in the area of mental disorders: an assessment of the effects of expectations of rejection. Am Sociol Rev 52:96–112

Link BG, Phelan J (2001) Conceptualizing stigma. Annu Rev Sociol 27:363–385

Link BG, Cullen FT, Struening E, Shrout PE, Dohrenwend BP (1989) A modified labeling theory approach to mental disorders: an empirical assessment. Am Sociol Rev 53:400–23

Link BG, Mirotznik J, Cullen FT (1991) The effectiveness of stigma coping orientations: can negative consequences of mental illness labeling be avoided? J Health Soc Behav 32:302–320

Linville P, Carlston DE (1994) Social cognition of the self. In: Devine PG, Hamilton DL, Ostrom TM (eds) Social cognition: impact on social psychology. Academic Press, New York, pp 144–193

Lock M, Kaufert P (eds) (1998) Pragmatic women and body politics. Cambridge University Press, Cambridge

Markus H (1977) Self-schemata and processing information about the self. J Pers Soc Psychol 52:63–78

Markus H, Nurius P (1986) Possible selves. Am Psychol 41:954–961

Markus H, Ruvolo A (1989) Possible selves: personalized representations of goals. In: Pervin LA (ed) Goal concepts in personality and social psychology. Erlbaum, Hillsdale, NJ, pp 211–41

McCall GR, Simmons JL (1978) Identities and interaction: an examination of human associations in everyday life. Free Press, New York

McLeod JD, Lively KJ (2003) Social structure and personality. In: DeLamater J (ed) Handbook of social psychology. Kluwer, New York, pp 77–102

McLeod JD, Lively KJ (2007) Social psychology and stress research. In: Avison W, McLeod J, Pescosolido BA (eds) Mental health: social mirror. Springer, New York, pp 275–303

Mead GH (1934) Mind, self, and society. University of Chicago Press, Chicago, IL

Merton RK (1957) Social theory and social structure. Free Press of Glencoe, New York, revised and enlarged edition

Morgan DL, Schwalbe ML (1990) Mind and self in society: linking social structure and social cognition. Soc Psychol Q 53:148–164

Murphy RF (1990) The body silent: the different world of the disabled. W.W. Norton, New York

Nelson SM (2006) Redefining a bizarre situation: relative concept stability in affect control theory. Soc Psychol Q 69:215–234

Ohm R, Aaronson LS (2006) Symptom perception and adherence to asthma controller medications. J Nurs Scholarsh 38:292–297

Orbuch TL (1997) People's accounts count: the sociology of accounts. Annu Rev Sociol 23:455–78

Osgood CE, May William H, Miron MS (1975) Cross cultural universals of affective meaning. University of Illinois Press, Urbana, IL

Parsons T (1951) The social system. Free Press, Glencoe, IL

Pescosolido B (1996) Bringing 'community' into utilization models: how social networks link individuals to changing systems of care. Res Sociol Health Care 13:171–197

Pescosolido B (2006) Of pride and prejudice: the role of sociology and social networks in integrating the health sciences. J Health Soc Behav 47:189–208
Phelan MP, Hunt SA (1998) Prison gang members' tattoos as identity work: the visual communication of moral careers. Symbolic Interact 21:277–98
Pierret J (2003) The illness experience: state of knowledge and perspectives for research. Sociol Health Illn 25:4–22
Preves SE (2001) Seeing the intersexed: an analysis of sociocultural responses to intersexuality. Signs 27:523–56
Radley A (1994) Making sense of illness: the social psychology of health and disease. Sage, London
Reidpath DD, Chan KY, Gifford SM, Allotey P (2005) 'He hath the French Pox': stigma, social value, and social exclusion. Sociol Health Illn 27:468–489
Rich E (2006) Anorexic dis(connection): managing anorexia as an illness and an identity. Sociol Health Illn 28:284–305
Richardson JC, Ong BN, Sims J (2006) Is chronic widespread pain biographically disruptive? Soc Sci Med 63:1573–1585
Robinson JE (2007) Look me in the eye: my life with Asperger's. Crown, New York
Robinson DT, Smith-Lovin L, Tsoudis O (1994) Heinous crime or unfortunate accident? The effects of remorse on responses to mock criminal confessions. Soc Forces 73:175–190
Rose G (2006) A genealogy of the disabled identity in relation to work and sexuality. Disabil Soc 21:499–512
Rosenberg M (1981) The self-concept: social product and social force. In: Rosenberg M, Turner RH (eds) Social psychology: sociological perspectives. Basic Books, New York, pp 593–624
Sanders C, Donovan J, Dieppe P (2002) The significance and consequences of having painful and disabled joints in older age: co-existing accounts of normal and disrupted biographies. Sociol Health Illn 24:227–253
Schneider JW, Conrad P (1983) Having epilepsy: the experience and control of illness. Temple University Press, Philadelphia, PA
Smith HW, Francis LE (2005) Social vs. self-directed events among Japanese and Americans. Soc Forces 84:821–30
Smith HW, Matsuno T, Ike S (2001) The affective basis of attributional processes among Japanese and Americans. Soc Psychol Q 64:180–94
Smith-Lovin L (1987) Impressions from events. J Math Sociol 13:35–70
Smith-Lovin L (1990) Emotion as the confirmation and disconfirmation of identity: an affect control theory model. In: Kemper TD (ed) Research agendas in the sociology of emotion. State University of New York Press, Albany, NY, pp 238–270
Smith-Lovin L, Douglass W (1992) An affect control analysis of two religious subcultures. In: Gecas V, Franks DD (eds) Social perspectives on emotions, vol 1. JAI Press, Greenwich CT, pp 217–248
Smith-Lovin L, Heise DR (1988) Analyzing social interaction: advances in affect control theory. Gordon and Breach, New York
Steinberg CR, Baxter RJ (1998) Accountable communities: how norms and values affect health system change. Health Aff 17:149–158
Stets J, Burke PJ (1996) Gender, control, and interaction. Soc Psychol Q 67:155–71
Stryker S (1980) Symbolic interaction: a social structural version. Benjamin Cummings, Menlo Park, CA
Stryker S, Burke PJ (2000) The past, present, and future of identity theory. Soc Psychol Q 63:284–97
Stryker S, Statham A (1985) Symbolic interaction and role theory. In: Lindzey G, Aronson E (eds) Handbook of social psychology, vol 1. Random House, New York, pp 311–378
Taylor V (1995) Self-labeling and women's mental health: postpartum illness and the reconstruction of motherhood. Sociol Focus 28:23–47
Taylor V, Van Willigen M (1996) Women's self-help and the reconstruction of gender: the postpartum support and breast cancer movements. Mobilization 1:123–142
Thoits PA (1983) Multiple identities and psychological well-being: a reformulation and test of the social isolation hypothesis. Am Sociol Rev 48:174–187
Thoits PA (1985) Self-labeling processes in mental illness: the role of emotional deviance. Am J Sociol 91:221–249
Thoits PA (1986) Multiple identities: examining gender and marital status differences in distress. Am Sociol Rev 51:259–272
Thoits PA, Hohmann AA, Harvey MR, Fletcher B (2000) Similar-other support for men undergoing coronary artery bypass surgery. Health Psychol 19:264–273
Tijerina MS (2006) Psychosocial factors affecting mexican-american women's adherence with hemodialysis treatment. Soc Work Health Care 1:57–74
Turner BS (1995) Medical power and social knowledge, 2nd edn. Sage, London
Weitz R (1991) Life with AIDS. Rutgers University Press, New Brunswick, NJ

Wester SR, Vogel DL, Wei M, McClain R (2006) African American men, gender role conflict, and psychological distress: the role of racial identity. J Couns Dev 84:419–429
Westphal L (2004) Cancer support groups as subcultural phenomenon. Vanderbilt University, Nashville, TN. Unpublished Dissertation
Williams G (1984) The genesis of chronic illness: narrative re-construction. Sociol Health Illn 6:175–200
Wilson S (2007) When you have children, you're obliged to live. Sociol Health Illn 29:610–629

Chapter 27
Learning to Love Animal (Models) (or) How (Not) to Study Genes as a Social Scientist

Dalton Conley

Introduction

In this chapter, I will argue that social science and genomics can be integrated – however, the way this marriage is currently occurring rests on spurious methods and assumptions and, as a result, will yield few lasting insights. However, recent advances in both econometrics and in developmental genomics provide scientists with a novel opportunity to understand how genes and (social) environment interact. To presage my argument: Key to any causal inference about genetically heterogeneous effects of social conditions is that either genetics be exogenously manipulated while environment is held constant (and measured properly), and/or that environmental variation is exogenous in nature – i.e. experimental or arising from a natural experiment of sorts. Further, allele selection should be motivated by findings from genetic experiments in (model) animal studies linked to orthologous human genes. Likewise, genetic associations found in human population studies should then be tested through knock-out and over-expression studies in model organisms. Finally, gene silencing can be a promising avenue of research in humans if careful thought is given to when and which cells are harvested for analysis.

A History of Lurking Variables and Simplistic Models

Studying genetic–environmental (GE) interactions has long been a goal of social scientists fond of expressing the dependence of genetic expression on social structure. However, how do we get from the sociological adage that "a gene for aggression lands you in prison if you're from the ghetto, but in the boardroom if you're to the manor born" to a serious empirical research program on the study of GE interactions? *Even if* we are only interested in "pure" environmental effects, how do we empirically deal with the lurking variable of "genotype" that can – and should – haunt our claims of environmental causality?

This is a particularly propitious time to investigate such GE interactions since the biological sciences may meet us halfway. Specifically, among molecular biologists there is increased interest in epigenetics (e.g., Wong et al. 2005; Krishnan and Nestler 2008) – that is, the conditions under which and mechanisms by which genes are regulated (i.e. highly expressed or not) in response to environmental

D. Conley (✉)
Center for Advanced Social Science Research, New York University, 295 Lafayette Street,
4th Floor, New York, NY, USA
e-mail: dc66@nyu.edu

conditions through various mechanisms such as methylation and acetylation of histones (the nuclear material from which DNA must be uncoiled to be accessed for transcription), micro-RNA mediated posttranscriptional regulation (whether messenger-RNA [mRNA] gets translated into a protein or not), and posttranslational modifications of those protein products themselves to make them active or inactive (usually through phosphorylation of specific residues [i.e. amino acids]).

From Twin Studies to Data Mining: Contributions and Limitations of Traditional Genetics

The subfield of psychology known as behavioral genetics (BG) has long proffered an answer to these challenges. Notable researchers such as Richard Plomin and David Rowe, as well as many others, have argued that by comparing social outcomes among genetically identical twins (i.e. monozygotic twins who share 100% of their nuclear genes) with those from fraternal twins (i.e. dizygotic twins who share, on average, 50% of their genes, just like singleton siblings), we can properly estimate the genetic, shared environmental, and nonshared environmental components of traits (see e.g., Plomin et al. 2001).

In the most naïve approach, genetic heritability is calculated as two times the difference between the intraclass correlations of identical and fraternal twins. However, more recently, much more complex structural models have been offered to account for various complications such as the fact that – as a result of assortative mating at the parental level – fraternal twins may share more than 50% of their genes. Likewise, the "equal environments" assumption has been relaxed. For the naïve calculation mentioned above, it is necessary to assume that the covariance between environment and genetics is zero. Put another way, the simple estimation of heritability requires the rather heroic assumption that identical twins experience the same degree of similarity in environment as do (same sex) fraternal twins. Newer models include an estimate of the degree to which environmental similarity varies with genetic likeness. However, these are just that: estimates – often based on questions about whether or not respondents were "dressed alike" growing up, whether they were viewed as similar as "two peas in a pod" and so on (see e.g., Lichtenstein et al. 1992; Rodgers et al. 1999; Rowe and Teachman 2001; Guo and Stearns 2002). Such questions are likely to capture only some of the ways that environmental similarity differs across identical and fraternal twin pairs, which is troubling since Goldberger (1979) has shown that depending on the GE covariance assumed, estimates of heritability can be driven wildly up or down.

Other more recent work has used adoptees to infer biological estimates of the heritability of social traits. For example, Sacerdote (2004) used a dataset of Korean adoptees in the United States where assignment to families was random to examine the intergenerational correlation on important socioeconomic indicators such as educational attainment and income; on behaviors such as drinking and smoking; and on anthropometric measures such as height and weight. The results were then contrasted to intergenerational correlations among biological families from other data sources as well as biological children within those same families (for the subsample that contained biological children). The results showed that – as might be expected – heritability for physical traits was considerably stronger in biologically intact families. Education (specifically probability of graduating from a 4-year college) and income were also much more strongly inherited by biological children. However, health-related behavioral inheritance was similar across the two groups.

Before we accept the putative inference that education and income are predominantly genetically transmitted (while smoking and drinking are culturally transmitted) we must question the external validity of the adoptee sample. While there was adequate variation within the recipient families of adoptees, *on observables*, and while they did not look terribly different on average from nonadopting US families, on observables, we know, *ipso facto*, that families who adopt are a distinct social group on unobservables – as are the adoptees themselves. For example, if socialization is weaker among adoptees who do not feel connected to their adoptive parents, the difference in heritability could be weaker by virtue of this fact, not the absence of genetic similarity. There are many other dynamics that could be at work as well, such as increased (or decreased) parental investment, halo effects or stigma and truncated genetic variability among adoptees (or adopters), which may work to bias estimates for this population in unpredictable ways. The only adoption study that would avoid such questions would be one in which adoptees were randomly selected from the newborn population and then randomly assigned to parents, with both groups blind to the treatment (i.e. not knowing whether they were adopted or not) – all while prenatal environment was held constant. In other words, it is an impossibility to reliably estimate genetic heritability using such an approach.

Other recent work uses differences in subpopulations as a proxy for environmental differences to examine genotype expression. This line of argument purports that certain groups, such as minorities or low SES individuals, may face environmental obstacles to their full genetic expression (i.e. level of phenotypic capacitance). For example, Guo and Stearns (2002) argue that the heritability of verbal IQ for respondents in the National Longitudinal Survey of Adolescent Health (AddHealth) is weaker when a parent is unemployed than when no parent is unemployed (42% vs. 54%). Similarly, in a multivariate context, they document a lower heritability of verbal IQ for African American adolescents as compared to their white counterparts (58% vs. 72%). However, ascribing this difference across racial groups to a "constraining" effect of the environment – while playing on the nurturist sympathies of the sociological community – is premature. It could be the case, for instance, that due to different degrees of assortative mating or fertility patterns, the degree of genotypic variation in IQ-related genes is lower among blacks and the unemployed (downwardly biasing heritability estimates), or that there is greater mean-regressive measurement error among siblings in these groups. While environment could constrain the "full" expression of genetic profiles, it could also be the case that the genetic profile itself is different within and between families facing different environments (i.e., African American and white families, or families with and without unemployed parents).

SNP Research: A (Small) Step Forward for Mankind

Most recently, genetic markers on specific loci – such as single point mutation polymorphisms (SNPs) – have seemed to offer hope for those interested in an explicit research program aimed at specifying and measuring gene-environment interactions for complex traits (what geneticists call Quantitative Traits). Polymorphisms are genetic variants that occur in at least 1% of the population. They could include base-pair substitutions – among one of the four nucleotides that make up our genetic code (G, guanine; C, cytosine; A, adenosine; and T, thymine) – that may affect the amino acid produced out of that codon (a triplet of nucleotides that determine which amino acid should come next when the messenger-RNA is translated into a protein) if the polymorphism is in an open reading frame (ORF) of a gene (i.e. the protein-related coding region) and is nonsynonymous; they may truncate the protein by causing the transcription machinery to stop there (by producing a stop codon); or they may do nothing (what are called silent or synonymous mutations) since multiple three-letter codes may result in the same amino acid being produced (though, perhaps at different efficiency levels, something called codon-bias). Hence, these nonlethal polymorphisms, which result from mutations, may present an opportunity to study how specific environments – social or biophysical – may result in different outcomes depending on an individual's genotype.

The basic logic is the following: A certain proportion of a population sample is found to have a variant of a particular allele. *If* this allele is shown to be randomly distributed across demographic subgroups (or, for example, *within* a particular subgroup such as an ethnic group), and, likewise, it is found to be associated with a specific social outcome or tendency (such as addictiveness, shyness, schizophrenia, to name a few) *within* that same population (or subgroup as the case may be), then researchers may try to look for specific environmental conditions which seem to magnify or mitigate its effect – such as family structures, parents' behavior or simply socioeconomic status. If allele variation is studied within families (i.e. across siblings) then it does indeed offer a potential way to measure specific genetic influences with some certainty. One would then compare the expression of that allele – as compared to the sibling without the polymorphism, for example – in families of various demographic or economic backgrounds. However, we must be cautious with this approach as well since rates of genetic linkage may be different among population subgroups. More on this issue below.]

The location of the genetic effect in specific places on the genome – combined with the lack of reliance on unknowable assumptions (in contrast to the twin approach's assumption of a specific GE covariance matrix for DZ and MZ twins) – is seen as a key step forward from earlier BG research. (Recent models also allow for genetic dominance – that is, nonlinear interactions between alleles.) However, since the object of study is typically just *one* allele, such analysis tells us little about the overall genetic heritability of an outcome. Secondly, even if it were found to vary across environmentally distinct populations (such as blacks and whites or the college educated versus those who did not acquire a high school degree) it is not altogether clear whether differential effects are due to a genetic-environmental interaction [as purported in the adolescent IQ example of Guo and Stearns (2002)] or a gene–gene interaction. It could be that the allele(s) are interacting not with differential social environments, but rather with other, nonrandomly distributed genes (even if the principal gene in question is indeed randomly distributed).

For example, a paper by Caspi et al. (2002) that has become a classic in this area of research claims to have uncovered a GE-interaction by comparing male children who have a particular functional polymorphism in the MAOA gene (monoamine oxidase A) – an enzyme which breaks down various neurotransmitters once they are chaperoned out of the synaptic cleft – with those who do not among a longitudinal sample of 1,037 white Australians followed from ages 3–26. Those individuals who showed a variable number tandem repeat (VNTR) in the promoter region of the gene (the area that precedes the actual coding portion but which is important to transcriptional activation and regulation) putatively transcribe (and by extension translate) MAOA at a lower rate than those without this polymorphism on their X-chromosome. In turn, MAOA activity as indicated by this genetic difference was interacted with degree of maltreatment the respondents experienced between the ages of 3 and 11 to predict an index of antisocial behavior that included four measures ranging from criminal convictions to antisocial personality disorder criteria of the DSM-IV. They argue that while there do exist other MAO genes that may compensate for deficiencies in MAOA (in particular MAOB), among children these are not yet fully expressed, thus making MAOA particularly important with respect to moderating the effect of maltreatment during early childhood.

Eight percent of the sample experienced severe maltreatment, 28% experienced "probable" maltreatment and 64% experienced no maltreatment. In a multiple regression context, the main effect of maltreatment level on the antisocial behavior index was significant, whereas the main effect of MAOA activity level was not, but an interaction effect between the two measures was statistically significant at the $\alpha=0.01$ level. They argue that this is a true genetic–environmental interaction effect since the MAOA genotypes were not significantly differently distributed across maltreatment levels – suggesting that this genotype did not itself influence exposure to maltreatment (i.e. the environment is not standing in for the genotype).

In a follow-up study (2003), they use the same cohort to examine the interaction of stressful life events with alleles of the serotonin transporter gene (5-HTT) linked promoter region (5-HTTLPR). Specifically, individuals who have a short 5′ (i.e. upstream) promoter may show more propensity than those with a long promoter toward depression. However, previous studies had come to conflicting results; namely many replications have failed to produce results claimed in earlier linkage studies. Some researchers had despaired that psychiatric and other behavioral phenotypes were controlled by so many quantitative trait genes that modeling genetic effects in a robust, direct way would not be possible and/or would account for little of the variation (see e.g., Hamer 2002). Caspi et al. (2003), instead argue that, rather than complicated gene–gene interactions, the muddle of results could be resulting from GE interactions. This muddle motivates their search for an interaction effect of stressful life events and 5-HTTLPR allele.

This is an autosomal gene – meaning that individuals of both sexes have two copies – so they compared individuals with the homozygous long genotypes and heterozygotes (long/short) to those who were homozygous for the short alleles. They found that for those in the subsample who had experienced no stressful life events between ages 21 and 26, there was no difference between the three genotypes in the propensity to depression. However, as the number of self-reported stressful life events increased, the genotypes diverged with respect to their likelihood of clinical depression at age 26. They interpret this as a GE interaction.

However, it could still be possible that what Caspi et al. were uncovering was actually a gene–gene interaction in both studies, because they did not have an exogenous source of environmental variation. In the latter case, those with the "at risk," short alleles were, in fact, more likely to report stressful events than those who had long alleles. We may conclude, then, that measured genotype did influence the measured environmental factor. The researchers try to get around this by reversing the time order: Measuring stressful life events between ages 21 and 26 and measuring depression at age 21 (i.e. prior). When they do this, they do not find the significant interaction they did in the "correctly" ordered model. However, it still may be the case that depression was induced by a gene–gene interaction since it may be an underlying unmeasured gene that causes the phenotype of "negative life events" to emerge in one's early 20s: Imagine a gene that causes excessive thrill-seeking and risk-taking, which, in turn, manifests as negative events during one's early adulthood. As for the MAOA interaction, we face the same issue: While measured maltreatment did not vary by MAOA status, it could very well have varied by other genes (present in the parents and potentially passed on to the children). Thus, it would not be the maltreatment that interacted with MAOA status but rather the underlying, unmeasured genotype, which, in combination with given MAOA alleles, causes both parents and offspring to act antisocially.

Linkage and Gene Networks: Additional Layers of Complexity

To complicate matters even further, absent genetic experiments that knock out or over-express specific genes, we can never be sure that the allele in question is what is causing any observed effect (irrespective of environmental interactions), thanks to the possibility of genetic linkage mentioned above. Genes are "shuffled" across the chromosomes of a parent during the recombination period of meiosis. (Meiosis results in the formation of the 1N gamete – i.e. the sperm or egg.) However, two alleles are more likely to stay paired together in a given gamete the closer they are to each other on the chromosome – hence the term linkage or linkage disequilibrium – since they are more likely to be found on the same pieces of DNA that are exchanged.

A helpful analogy is the shuffling of a deck of cards: It is more likely that cards right next to each other will not get separated in the shuffling process than it is for cards separated by a longer "distance." So even when we know that a given gene is associated with a quantitative trait, we cannot be 100% sure (absent genetic experiments on nonhumans) that the said gene is causally responsible. The best we can say is that that area of the genome is associated with the phenotype under study. If we allow for different degrees of genetic linkage of particular genes with other genes by population – then we cannot even plausibly say (for sure) that a given gene is responsible for the outcome in two different populations even if we observe the same marker–phenotype association (never mind GE interactions)! And indeed, microsatellites (groups of genetically-linked genes) have been shown to vary across conventionally defined population groups (such as our folk-racial categories). Further, the lengths of microsatellite repeats (also known as simple sequence repeats [SSRs]) of DNA base pair motifs are, in fact, one way that geneticists identify human population origins since such repeats are frequently occurring (i.e. the DNA replication machinery makes this sort of coding error more frequently than other types) and since they do not appear to be under any selective pressure (at least about which we know). (However, some recent work on dogs suggests that they may, in fact, face selection pressures, particularly when they occur in a coding region.) For the most part, these repeated sequences appear to be junk DNA in noncoding regions that produce neither protein products, nor peptides, nor other important forms of RNA such as micro-RNAs, transfer-RNAs or ribosomal-RNAs. However, they may influence the degree to which important parts of the genome (such as genes themselves) are separated – and thus linked or de-linked – during recombination. [As a side note, this also means that the assumption of a *complete* lack of selective pressure on such microsatellite repeats may be incorrect to the extent that they fall between genes (or other important DNA products) that interact with each other in functionally important ways].

The real rub is that, since we can plausibly postulate second-, third-, fourth-, and ultimately, Nth-order interactions across alleles, there simply would not be enough degrees of freedom in the approximately seven billion human beings currently occupying the planet to properly test a fully specified model ($21,000! = 9.58$ E $81648 > 7,000,000,000$). The discovery of about 21,000 genes – a figure much lower than originally hypothesized – is good news in that it is a tractable number of alleles for geneticists to study. However, the irony lies in the fact that, if this lowly number of genes explains the development of human beings in all their glorious forms, then gene–gene interactions are probably quite important. There is also a recent explosion of discoveries relating to the important role of micro-RNAs in affecting how messenger-RNAs are spliced (and therefore can produce multiple products) and whether they get translated at all (as well as increased interest in other non-protein products of DNA once considered "junk").

In fact, supporting the notional importance of gene–gene interactions (and offering a competing model to GE interactions) is recent genetics research that has shown that among the genes studied in humans (or other [model] organisms such as the fruit fly, *drosophila melanogaster*, or the nematode worm, *Caenorhabditis elegans*), the vast majority of known genes are linked in a single network component when measured by either protein–protein interactions, by regulatory relationships or by phenotypic covariation (as illustrated in Fig. 27.1, below, for the case of brewer's yeast [*S. cerevisiae*] or the human case in Fig. 27.2, below). This suggests that, indeed, one cannot conceptualize the perturbation of one gene as unrelated to the impact of other genes. Conversely, the embeddedness of this network suggests that genomic systems are highly redundant and robust and that other genes may be up- (or down-) regulated to compensate when a given gene is nonfunctional (or hypertrophic). For example, Isalan et al. (2008) have shown that even random rewiring of 598 promoter-gene relationships (one at a time) has little effect on phenotypic outcome or expression levels in *Escherichia coli* as compared to wild-type bacteria of the same initial strain (95%survivorship among altered organisms) – suggesting networks that are highly robust to failure.

Gene networks need not even be confined within a single organism. There are notable, well-characterized evolutionary processes of genetic transfer across organisms, such as retroviral infection and horizontal transfer. There are also many examples of symbiotic and competitive relationships where the interaction manifests at a proteomic level. One notable case is sexual competition and coevolution, where the myriad male accessory gland proteins that are transferred during mating (in species including *drosophila* and humans) interact with the genes/proteins in the female. And, of course, among humans there may be cross-organism genetic interaction that is behaviorally mediated. Of particular interest is detecting cases where ego's genotype is conditioned not by alter's phenotype, but rather by his/her genotype [such as depression emerging when two asymptomatic individuals both with short 5-HTT (the gene that encodes a serotonin transporter) alleles are paired together or when weight-gain is modulated by *leptin* polymorphisms in both members of a dyad].

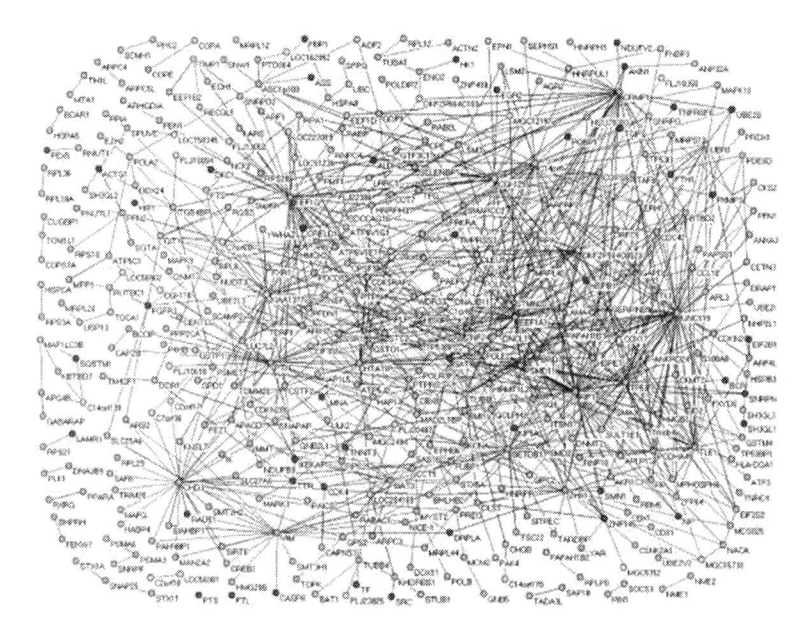

27 Learning to Love Animal (Models) (or) How (Not) to Study Genes as a Social Scientist

Fig. 27.1 Protein–Protein network in *S. cerevisiae* (Brewer's Yeast). 78 percent of the sampled proteome is linked in a single network component. Source: Jeong, Mason, Barabási and Oltvai (2001)

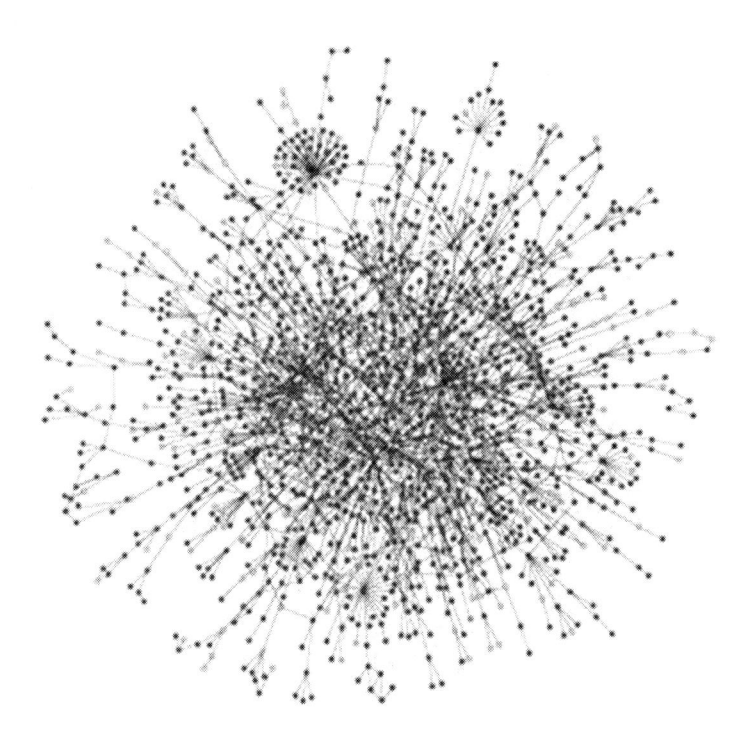

Fig. 27.2 Protein–Protein network humans. 87 percent of the proteome is linked in the single network component. Source: Stelzi et al. (2005)

Such a network view of (socio-) genomics calls into question simple one-gene causal models of genetic effects where multiple pathways may be affected by a change in that one gene.

By way of example, some polymorphisms in the dopamine receptor allele DRD4 have been linked to attention deficit hyperactivity disorder (ADHD) in humans through associational study (Brookes et al. 2006) and by virtue of experimental studies in animals. DRD4 is a g-coupled protein receptor that forms part of a signaling pathway in neurons in certain brain circuits responsible for pleasure. (The activated conformation of the receptor inhibits the activity of the enzyme adenylyl cyclase, which, in turn, lowers the concentration of cyclic AMP, an important intracellular signaling molecule.)

However, DRD4 is not only expressed in the central nervous system. A quick check on the National Cancer Institute's EST meta-database shows that DRD4 is also expressed in the kidney, in various components of the eye (including the lens), and in ovarian tumors. His list, of course, is incomplete and will inevitably grow longer and longer the more the gene is studied. These multiple expressions, therefore, call into question any claim that polymorphisms in this gene are causing ADHD through a specific pathway in the brain. Similarly, any second-order effects of DRD4-related ADHD on other outcomes as well as putative environmental interactions with DRD4 or gene–gene interactions may be under-identified due to the fact that DRD4 may be having other, unobserved effects on phenotype through its actions in the kidneys or eyes (or elsewhere). In other words, if DRD4 was observed to lead to ADHD and, in turn, that ADHD was associated with poor academic outcomes only in students who are in classrooms with more than 25 students, we could not be sure if it was genetically-caused ADHD that was interacting with class size through a brain-behavior mechanism or whether larger classes merely placed these students further from the blackboard and that a DRD4 effect on eyesight was responsible for poorer academic performance. Or worse yet, perhaps the associated ADHD diagnosis itself was attributable to the eyesight effect that led to a lack of concentration in school. In other words, by virtue of its multiple occasions of expression, *multiple* causal pathways are possible, throwing into jeopardy a social scientist's claims.

Conversely, running DRD4 through a web-interface (described later) that searches for similar genes yields a total of 172 homologous genes in the human species alone, including dopamine receptors (see Fig. 27.3).

Obtaining such results suggests – but by no means proves – that DRD4 might be "redundant" in the human body. Indeed, its change through mutation to a shorter version is nonlethal (hence our ability to study human variation). Perhaps one of these other 172 genes is over-expressed to

dopamine receptor D4; D(2C) dopamine receptor [H... 532 0.0 gi|4502357 dopamine receptor D3 isoform a [Homo sapiens] 259 3e-68 gi|17986270 dopamine receptor D2 isoform short [Homo sapiens] 243 1e-64 gi|4503382 dopamine receptor D2 isoform long [Homo sapiens] 234 6e-62 gi|15718670 alpha-2A-adrenergic receptor; alpha-2AAR subtyp... 207 1e-53 gi|4501987 alpha-2C-adrenergic receptor; alpha2-AR-C4 [Homo... 207 1e-53 gi|4501906 alpha-2B-adrenergic receptor; alpha-2-adrenergic... 206 3e-53 gi|4504521 5-hydroxytryptamine (serotonin) receptor 1A [Hom... 185 5e-48 gi|16445398 dopamine receptor D3 isoform c [Homo sapiens] 178 2e-43 gi|16445402 dopamine receptor D3 isoform e [Homo sapiens] 178 2e-43 gi|4557265 beta-1-adrenergic receptor [Homo sapiens] 169 3e-42 gi|4502727 adrenergic, beta-3-, receptor [Homo sapiens] 166 2e-41 gi|4504539 5-hydroxytryptamine (serotonin) receptor 2B [Hom... 156 3e-38 gi|6005762 histamine receptor H3; G protein-coupled recepto... 151 7e-37 gi|16415396 dopamine receptor D3 isoform b [Homo sapiens] 150 1e-36 gi|16445400 dopamine receptor D3 isoform d [Homo sapiens] 147 1e-35 gi|4502821 cholinergic receptor, muscarinic 4; muscarinic a... 146 7e-35 gi|4504533 5-hydroxytryptamine (serotonin) receptor 1B; 5-H... 146 7e-35 gi|4502815 cholinergic receptor, muscarinic 1; muscarinic a... 142 4e-34 gi|4501957 alpha-1D-adrenergic receptor; adrenergic, alpha-... 135 4e-32 gi|10834131 5-hydroxytryptamine (serotonin) receptor 7 isoform b; serot... 129 3e-30 gi|10880129 5-hydroxytryptamine receptor 7 isoform d; serot... 129 3e-30 gi|4504547 5-hydroxytryptamine receptor 7 isoform a; seroto... 129 3e-30 gi|10835175 5-hydroxytryptamine (serotonin) receptor 2A [Ho... 129 5e-30 gi|4502817 cholinergic receptor, muscarinic 2; muscarinic a... 127 1e-29 gi|4501959 alpha-1B-adrenergic receptor; adrenergic, alpha ... 126 3e-29 gi|15451761 alpha-1A-adrenergic receptor isoform 4; adrener... 123 2e-28 gi|15451759 alpha-1A-adrenergic receptor isoform 2; adrener... 123 2e-28 gi|15451757 alpha-1A-adrenergic receptor isoform 3; adrener... 123 2e-28 gi|4501961 alpha-1A-adrenergic receptor isoform 1; adrenerg... 123 2e-28 gi|4504541 5-hydroxytryptamine (serotonin) receptor 2C [Hom... 120 1e-27 gi|29727439 similar to 5-HT5B serotonin receptor [Homo sapi... 116 7e-27 gi|4503383 dopamine receptor D1 [Homo sapiens] 114 1e-25 gi|30150699 similar to D(1B) dopamine receptor (D(5) dopami... 114 1e-25 gi|4504545 5-hydroxytryptamine (serotonin) receptor 6 [Homo... 111 1e-24 gi|4503391 dopamine receptor D5; dopamine receptor D1B; D1b... 110 1e-24 gi|13236497 5-hydroxytryptamine (serotonin) receptor 5A [Ho... 110 2e-24 gi|4504537 5-hydroxytryptamine (serotonin) receptor 1E [Hom... 100 2e-21 gi|30148127 similar to D(1B) dopamine receptor (D(5) dopami... 99 7e-21 gi|4504535 5-hydroxytryptamine (serotonin) receptor 1D [Hom... 99 7e-21 gi|30148324 similar to D(1B) dopamine receptor (D(5) dopami... 97 2e-20 gi|13436406 histamine receptor H2; gastric receptor 1 [Homo... 96 5e-20 gi|10835137 5-hydroxytryptamine (serotonin) receptor 1F; 5-

Fig. 27.3 Homologous genes of DRD4 in *Homo sapiens*

compensate for a deficient DRD4 allele. Thus we face a similar problem of inference as with the expression data: Is any observed association with quantitative traits the direct result of DRD4 changes or the indirect affects of "compensation" in other parts of the genetic network?

What Is to Be Done? A Social Scientific Model for Genetic Research

Below I purport to offer a way out of this epistemological morass that involves isolating candidate genes not through associational studies, but through deployment of animal models, where genetic experimentation allows for causal inference with respect to specific genotype–phenotype relationships. Once candidate genes are identified in animal studies, these can then be linked to putative human genes that may play a similar role. Finally, the role of these genes can be studied in human population-based studies that have exogenous environmental variation.

Step 1: Deploy Animal Models

A potentially fruitful approach to identifying GE interactions may arise out of the deployment of animal models by bio-sociologists. Sociologists maintain a strangely ambivalent relationship to nonhuman animals. On the one hand, given the strong leftist leanings of many sociologists, pro-environment sentiment runs strong within the field. Central to the paradigm of environmentalism is the notion that humans do not occupy a privileged position within natural systems. This idea, of course, is not unique to environmental sociologists or even sociologists, but familiar to many humanists as well as natural scientists. Sociologists, however, occupy a uniquely paradoxical position within this group of scholars. This is due to the wholesale rejection by the mainstream of the discipline of animal models of social behavior. Having established ourselves in the early twentieth century as advocates of a science against the elemental, "reductionistic," naturalizing explanatory frameworks of the biological sciences, we have boxed ourselves into a corner by rejecting wholesale the notion that studies of other species may yield insight into human social phenomena.

This has, I argue, put us at an extreme disadvantage in an era when "model organisms" (to be defined below) are examined with increasingly powerful tools by biologists in order to illuminate generalizable phenomena about natural systems, innate and learned behavior; and even social life. By contemporary standards, a model organism is one in which the genome has been (largely) sequenced; where there is a short time between generations; where there is sexual reproduction; and for which a number of genetic tools that work for that organism (such as plasmid libraries, mutant lines and so on) have been developed. As mentioned above, current model organisms range from the nematode worm, (*Caenorhabditis elegans*) to the fruit fly (*Drosophila melanogaster*) to zebrafish (*Danio rerio*) to mice (*Mus musculus*). Each has advantages and disadvantages. For example, in comparing *C. elegans* to *D. melanogaster*, the generation time is faster for the worm (4 days) as compared to the fly (10 days) but if one is interested in behavior, the worm is perhaps too simple a system to study. Mice, as compared to flies, are, of course, mammals with nervous systems much closer to our own, but who have a much longer generation time and higher cost to maintain – not to mention fewer mutant lines that have been obtained as of yet. That is, though the mouse genome has been sequenced, less is known about the characteristics (i.e. expression patterns, protein structures, and so on) of mice genes as compared to those of the fruit fly.

The main advantage of using animals lies in the ability of the researcher to experimentally manipulate environmental and social conditions to study their epigenetic consequences while simultaneously being able to manipulate the genetic background of the creatures using knock-outs (vectors that disable expression of a particular gene) or hybrids (that allow for the expression of exogenous genes from other species within a given organism or the over-expression of certain endogenous genes under specific conditions of the scientist's design and choosing). The experimental approach of "bench science" genetics provides such great power in narrowing down molecular, causal pathways linking social or behavioral variation to outcomes that the tradeoff with concerns about the external validity of such results to human biosocial systems is more than adequately compensated for, in my opinion, at least. This holds true, I would purport, when the genes under study have clear orthologs in *Homo sapiens* (though even if they do not, such knowledge may provide a useful general understanding of the way social and genetic systems are linked that may still be informative).

The basic idea is the following: Use a particular genetic strain that has been well-characterized in a given model organism with respect to a specific behavior to identify specific genetic pathways that accentuate (or repress) the observed phenotype using adequate negative and positive controls. Once a gene of interest has been identified and well-understood (and putative gene-environment interactions have been tested), the researcher would then use the Basic Local Alignment Sequence Tool (BLAST – http://blast.ncbi.nlm.nih.gov/Blast.cgi) to find an orthologous gene in humans (see Fig. 27.4, below). BLAST identifies statistically significant similarities between a given genetic sequence and a database of sequences for a particular species. If the gene is highly conserved across taxa (and thus, putatively important), then there should be a well-matched homolog in the human species. This gene then provides a good starting point for looking at potential associations with behavioral outcomes.

Current behaviorally-related genes that have been isolated in model organisms such as *Drosophila melanogaster* include *dunce* (learning); *rutabaga* (memory); *fruitless* (courtship and aggression in males). This is, of course, a small sample of a rapidly growing list of genes in model organisms ranging from *C. elegans* to mice and rats that have been linked to behaviors that have clear human analogs. To be fair to Caspi et al. as well as others, the genes that they explored (notably 5-HTT and MAOA) were not targeted thanks to data mining exercises but rather as a result of animal studies as suggested above. However, a number of counter examples can be found where associational fishing expeditions have led to more tenuous findings that have not withstood the rigors of replication.

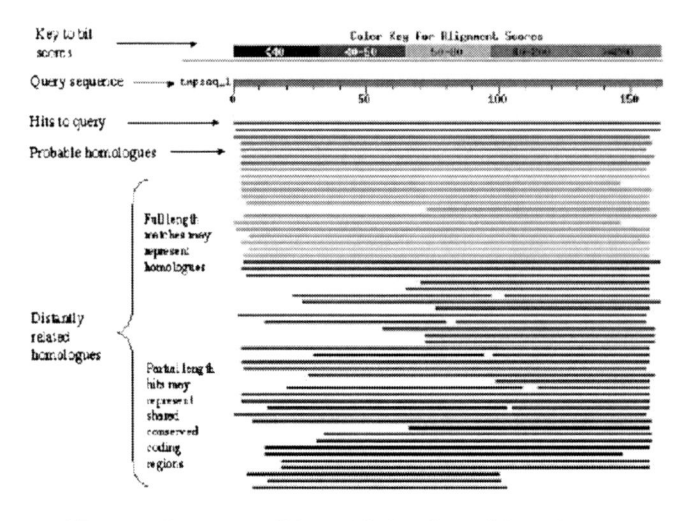

Fig. 27.4 Legend to BLAST output. Source: http://blast.ncbi.nlm.nih.gov/Blast.cgi

One notable example can be found in the so-called "gay gene." Hamer et al. (1993) published an article in *Science* showing an association between a microsatellite on the X-chromosome (called Xq28) and homosexuality in men. The conclusion rested on the greater propensity of gay brothers to share genetic markers at this locus as well as pedigree analysis that showed a greater likelihood of gay men to have other gay male relatives on their maternal side (since the X that males receive always comes from their mother). Later work (see, Rice et al. 1999) failed to replicate the findings among a similar sample of Canadian brothers and a heated debate ensued. Hamer et al.'s study is among the better of the associational studies given its pedigree-based analysis, but like many others in the field it relies on a small, nonrepresentative sample and purports to explain a complicated phenotype: *stated* sexual orientation. I underline "stated" for a reason: Even if the results could be routinely replicated, it may be the case that the Xq28 locus is associated with willingness to reveal homosexuality to survey takers rather than to homosexuality itself, given its sometimes stigmatizing status in North American culture.

Step 2: Apply to Human Population Data and Add Exogenous Environmental Variation

Once human candidate gene markers have been deduced from experimental results in animal studies (in contrast to the typical association studies currently used by human population geneticists), the study of these genes in human social life can proceed. Below, I am going to argue that it is, in fact, possible to obtain empirically robust estimates of genetic environmental interaction effects. That is, differences in genetic expression depending on social environment that cannot be attributed to genetic or environmental factors alone.

However, the strategy needed to parameterize such effects relies on the proper estimation of truly exogenous, causal *environmental* effects. Once an exogenous source of environmental variation has been identified, then it is possible to look for differential treatment effects based on genotypical characteristics – polymorphisms, haplotypes (groups of polymorphisms that cluster uniquely together) and the like – that vary randomly within a given subpopulation (family, ethnic group and so on). So, in short, the first task at hand for the sociologist who desires to show environmental–genetic interactions is the same task facing all sociologists who seek to rule out genetic (or other unobserved) factors when assessing causal, environmental effects.

Once we have an exogenous source of variation in, let us say, schooling, then we can identify an interaction effect between years of schooling and some genetic marker in looking at outcomes such as income, criminality, shyness and so on. Let us take the example of Lleras-Muney (2005): She estimated the mortality returns to an additional year of high school by focusing on educational variation generated by changes in compulsory schooling laws during the first half of the twentieth century. These changes in state laws generate an exogenous change in the environmental characteristics of schooling because they affected everyone, regardless of genetic makeup or other characteristics. If she had enjoyed access to genetic information in her sample (which she did not, having used the U.S. Census as her data source), she would have been able to interact instrumented years of schooling (predicted based on these exogenous law changes and individual-level characteristics) with a given genetic marker when estimating the mortality effects of schooling (assuming the genetic marker was not significantly associated with education and was randomly distributed across existing population divisions – such as race and SES). In this way, she would have been able to tell if certain genetic profiles receive larger health benefits from additional schooling than other genotypes. Of course, hopefully one would begin such a project with a theory about why the expression of a given gene (that is, the causal pathway from gene to protein to outcome) would vary based on an environmental characteristic like education – rather than just going in with a fishing net to troll for associations. (Multiple hypothesis testing – with so many potential genetic loci of study – is of major concern here. Luckily, biologists have elaborated on the Bonferroni correction to produce a series of ways to approach the problem of false positives; see e.g., Thornton and Jensen 2007).

In sum, in order to investigate GE interactions, we need some source of exogeneity on the environmental side as a lever for estimation (as well as evidence that the marker is not significantly associated with plausible subgroups in our sample or statistical controls for such possible associations). Until such time that we can exogenously affect genotype through genetic manipulation or through a natural experiment that results in genetic variation (such as genetic drift of some measurable sort or monozygotic twin differences in mitochondrial DNA), but which does not affect environmental influence (fat chance), exogenous environmental variation is our only hope to identify a GE interaction in a human population.

There are a number of ways that economists have pioneered to get closer to causal estimates. First, there are instrumental variable (IV) strategies (also called 2-Stage Least Squares), which use a source of exogenous variation (i.e. the instrument, Z) to predict the covariate of interest (X), and then use the predicted covariate (X^*) to model the outcome. [For a general review see Angrist and Krueger (2001) or Winship and Morgan (1999).] A particularly notable example of instrumental variable estimation is provided by Angrist (1989) who estimated the effect of military service during the Vietnam War period on subsequent earnings, using the draft lottery as a source of exogenous variation in veteran status. Another example is provided by Conley and Glauber (2006) who estimate effects of sibship size on parental educational investment, using the sex mix of the first two children born into a family to instrument whether parents have a third child. The sex of a child depends on the random segregation of X and Y chromosomes in the paternal gametes and U.S. parents are more likely to have a third child if the first two are of the same sex. Exploiting this exogenous shock on sibship size, we assess the causal effect of an additional child on private school attendance and academic performance. More recently, economists have deployed regression discontinuity (RD) designs (see e.g., van der Klaauw 2002, on the effects of financial aid on college enrollment decisions or Lee 2008 on the power of Congressional incumbency on subsequent vote share), where researchers compare subjects that fall just on either side of an otherwise arbitrary cut-off point – such as those who score a few points above or below an admissions test. And then, of course, there is actual experimentation in which researchers determine what sorts of conditions subjects are exposed to (see, for example, research on the randomized housing program, Moving to Opportunity; Katz et al. 2001). In any of these cases, if genetic information were available for respondents, then researchers could have estimated GE interactions – because they had properly estimated the "E" part in a way that we could be sure was uncorrelated with G. (Alas, currently, the only large-scale nationally representative survey with genetic information is the National Longitudinal Survey of Adolescent Health.) Another benefit of having genetic information is that researchers can demonstrate that a given genetic trait is not correlated with the presumed exogenous variation (e.g., the instrument or the randomized experiment) and that it is randomly distributed across at least measurable social categories. The major problem with the natural experiment approach, however, is that IV and RD approaches typically require huge sample sizes since they are inefficient estimation strategies. These are precisely the data sources – Social Security records, Census samples, to name a couple – that are not likely to have genetic information. But there are other forms of putatively exogenous variation in social conditions that require smaller sample sizes. One such example is provided by the work of Strully (2009) who examined the health effects of job loss by comparing the impact of plausibly exogenous employment shocks (such as plant closings) to outcomes resulting from putatively endogenous sources of unemployment (such as dismissal for cause) using the Panel Study of Income Dynamics (PSID). If Strully had enjoyed access to genetic markers within the PSID she may have been able to estimate a GE interaction with some confidence using her approach, even given the relatively small sample size (~1,500 persons).

Some researchers have taken a converse approach: Using randomization of genotype to study the effect of a phenotype. One illustration of this approach is provided by Ding et al. (2006), who use sibling fixed-effects to identify "random" genetic variation within families and thereby hold parental genotype, as well as shared environment, constant. (They, correctly, examine animal-identified genes – the same ones Caspi et al. use plus two dopamine receptor alleles DRD4 and DRD2 and the dopamine transporter gene DAT1.) Indeed, they do find effects of some of the genes of interest on behavioral phenotypes [such as depression and Attention Deficit Hyperactivity Disorder (ADHD), as well as obesity]; however, they then push the data too far. They assert that these randomized genes can be used as instrumental variables (Z) in order to predict such behavioral outcomes (X) and, in turn, instrumented behavior (X*) can be used to generate unbiased estimates of the effects of child behavioral health on schooling outcomes. Of course, while the genes-as-instruments meet the first qualification of a valid instrument; that Z predicts X strongly enough (otherwise known as the weak instrument test), they fail the second requirement, the exclusion restriction (namely that Z has no effect on Y net of X). In other words, for genes to be used as IVs, they must not only be randomized within a population (such as between nonidentical twin siblings), they must have no other effect on the ultimate outcome of interest other than through their causal impact on the intermediary phenotype measured. Does DRD4 only affect school performance through the pathway of diagnosed ADHD? Of course not. ADHD is a complicated syndrome that involves lots of measurement errors and thus most likely reflects a whole host of other unmeasured traits. And even if ADHD were measured perfectly by the researchers, that's not to say that there would not be other effects of the genes in question on educational outcomes through any number of mechanisms ranging from memory to eyesight to stature – direct or indirect through the single-component gene network shown earlier.

Undoubtedly, there would be more opportunities for finding exogenous environmental variation once sociologists fully appreciate the importance of this necessary condition to their (even nongenetic) research endeavors. These opportunities may run the gamut from datasets that contain siblings or twins (such as PSID and AddHealth) that allow for within family difference approaches (but which do not capture all genetic and environmental differences, merely those constant in the family) to natural experiments such as roommate or classroom random assignment, draft lotteries, and so on to explicit experiments (such as the RAND health insurance study, the Negative Income Tax experiment, or myriad smaller scale studies with randomization to treatment and control groups). Ideally, one would want a randomized environment (in the form of a natural or unnatural experiment) *and* randomized genes in the form of sibling differences. However, unless there is a specific policy intervention or other sort of randomization that includes multiple, genetically related individuals from the same family and which randomizes within families, this is likely not possible. In lieu of sibling differences, the most important concern is environmental exogeneity and the best we can do for obtaining the pure effect of genotype is to control for demographic factors (such as ethnicity which, while a social/cultural category, is somewhat associated with different geographic population origins) that may be associated with particular markers, on the one hand, and behavioral phenotypes, on the other hand (see e.g., Knowler et al. 1988). That said, even with such a limitation, analysis such as those suggested above would greatly advance our understanding of GE interactions to a greater extent than a dozen more studies that lack plausible environmental exogeneity. A number of researchers are now deploying such an approach. One notable example uses college roommate random assignment to study GE interactions around college-related outcomes and behaviors such as binge drinking (Duncan and Guo 2009; Conley 2009).

Dead Man Walking

Polymorphic variation of DNA within protein coding regions (i.e. genes) is just one way that genetic expression can differ between individuals. Complex development of organisms requires the ability of that living system to up and down regulate gene transcription (and translation, not to mention protein modifications and localization) over the life course and/or in response to environmental stressors. For example, a number of classes of short RNAs (such as micro-RNAs) have been found that regulate gene fates posttranscriptionally. Likewise, transcription itself is controlled by a number of mechanisms including histone acetylation and DNA-methylation, epigenetic mechanisms that have garnered much recent attention.

If extended end-to-end and joined, the nuclear DNA located on the 23 chromosome pairs in each somatic human cell would stand six-feet tall. In order to compact it down to fit into the nucleus of the cell, it is tightly wound around positively charged proteins called histones (DNA is negatively charged). These histones have "tails" that stick out and to which can be added acetyl groups. When added, the DNA surrounding this area is unwound enough such that the transcriptional machinery (RNA polymerase and its associated components) can access the open reading frame. Thus, histone acetylation is a way to turn genes on and deacetylation is a way to turn genes off. Likewise, if a methyl group is attached to the DNA itself, then transcription is blocked (methyl groups can attach where a G follows a C – called a CpG, the p standing for the phosphate backbone linker between the two nucleotides). These mechanisms work sequentially, by opening up the chromatin (the DNA-histone complex); histone acetyltransferase (HAT) allows DNA to be demethylated and thus be ready for transcription.

Recent epigenetic studies have shown that these mechanisms of gene activation and deactivation are not only important in conducting the orchestra of cellular development and differentiation, but also allow organisms to react to environmental stressors and stimuli. For example, in a now-classic study Meaney and his colleagues (Caldji et al. 1998) showed that infant rats raised by mothers who licked (i.e. groomed) them at a significantly lower than average rate showed low transcriptional activation of the GR exon of the I_7 promoter gene in the hippocampus (an area of the brain related to memory and space among other functions). And this, in turn, resulted in similar behavior (i.e. low rates of offspring licking) in these rats when they became mothers themselves. This molecular and phenotypic effect persisted intergenerationally but could be interrupted through environmental intervention (i.e. adopting the pups out to high-licking mothers).

Of course, individual genes are switched on and off over the normal course of development as cells multiply and differentiate from stem cells to the myriad of cell types in the human body. Even in adulthood, in different cells and different times distinct sets of genes are transcriptionally active (or not). Thus, while it is easy to get the genome – which barring somatic mutations is relatively constant over the lifecourse – simply by obtaining any particular cell through a relatively noninvasive procedure [such as a buccal (i.e. cheek) swab], studying epigenomic programming is considerably more daunting. For example, as behavioral scientists, the cells about which we would want to know epigenetic status are most likely neurons in various regions of the brain. Obviously, these are not accessible to researchers of any discipline.

One recent line of research does show promise in understanding epigenetic programming, however: Studies of human corpse brains. If harvested within the first 24 h of death the methylation state of particular regions of DNA can be mapped by analysis with sodium bisulfite. This can tell us something about the level of transcriptional activity of that particular gene (or genes). In one recent study, for instance, McGowan et al. (2008) compare the methylation states of the ribosomal RNA (rRNA) promoters in hippocampus neurons of suicide victims (who had experienced childhood abuse or neglect) with decedents matched on postmortem interval, age and gender who experienced alternate forms of sudden death (and had no history of childhood abuse or neglect). Both groups showed equivalent genotypes in this promoter region. The hippocampus was selected since previous studies had shown that hippocampal volume is smaller in patients with a history of childhood trauma. Ribosomal RNA, in turn, is a "bottleneck" gene in that it is needed to translate all other genes (and thus may be related to total protein volume). The researchers found that methylation (and correspondingly, RNA expression) was depressed in the suicide group as compared to the treatment group. As a check, they showed that methylation was similar in the cerebellum (as a localization control) and genome-wide (as a molecular-level control).

Of course, one would appreciate more specific information than the authors have provided as to the histories and causes of death for the control group, since it could equally be the case that the cause of their demise had induced hypomethylation of this particular promoter region, though the previous anatomical studies showing reduced hippocampal volume among individuals who were abused or neglected in childhood probably mitigates this possibility. Postmortem analysis, then, may provide a fruitful way to analyze epigenetics in important regions in the brain – as long as the genes (and brain regions) under consideration are selected based on earlier experimental results (i.e. the animal models mentioned earlier). What the social scientist confronts, however, is the difficultly in selecting the control and "treatment" groups for comparison.

Again, here, as in the case of studying the interaction of environment with genetic markers mentioned above, the researcher is on safer ground if s/he selects a sorting criterion that is putatively exogenous. For example, one might compare limbic system-wide expression of the behaviorally related genes mentioned above (such as DRD2 and DAT1) by birth order (which is putatively exogenous), by draft lottery number, by sex mix of one's sibship, by participation in a randomized economic intervention or by any other form of environmental variation that the researcher can safely claim to predict epigenetic state (while not being predicted by the genetic or epigenetic state). (The limbic system is involved in pleasure and reward circuits; appropriate control regions of the brain would need to be investigated as also control regions of the genome.) Thus, whether the human object of inquiry is dead or alive, the same concerns about environmental exogeneity are at play if one is interested in understanding causal relations between the social environment and the genome.

Conclusion

As the preceding examples and discussion, I hope, have made clear, doing socio-genomics is difficult but not impossible. There is no reason why social scientists should be left out of the gold rush of analysis that is ensuing from the decoding of the human genome. However, if human population geneticists and social scientists continue to follow the tradition of Darwin – the observational ethologist – and pursue their analysis with little concern for complex, networked genomic pathways and little regard for exogenous sources of environmental (and/or genetic) variation, they may reinforce a pattern of fishing for gene-phenotype associations that may make headlines, only to be later called into question when attempts at replication come to different results. If, instead, bio-sociologists (and others) follow the lead of Mendel – the experimentalist – and build up deductively from solid studies that vary one thing at a time and include proper negative and positive controls, a rich and sturdy understanding of how the social world is influenced by (and influences) the molecular level of genes can be gained. It is a slower road to travel, but it leads to the promised land of durable knowledge.

References

Angrist JD (1989) Using the draft lottery to measure the effect of military service on civilian labor market outcomes. In: Ehrenberg R (ed) Research in labor economics, vol 10. JAI Press, Inc., Greenwich

Angrist JD, Krueger AB (2001) Instrumental variables and the search for identification: from supply and demand to natural experiments. J Econ Perspect 15(4):69–85

Brookes K et al (2006) The analysis of 51 genes in DSM-IV combined type attention deficit hyperactivity disorder: association signals in DRD4, DAT1, and 16 other genes. Mol Psychiatry 11:934–953

Caldji C, Tannenbaum B, Sharma S, Francis D, Plotsky PM, Meaney MJ (1998) Maternal care during infancy regulates the development of neural systems mediating the expression of fearfulness in the rat. Proc Natl Acad Sci U S A 95(9):5335–5340

Caspi A et al (2002) Role of genotype in the cycle of violence in maltreated children. Science 297:851–854

Caspi A et al (2003) Influence of life stress on depression: moderation by a polymorphism in the 5-HTT gene. Science 297:851–854

Conley D (2009) GE interactions in college social networks. Research in progress

Conley D, Glauber R (2006) Parental educational investment and children's academic risk: estimates of the impact of sibship size and birth order from exogenous variation in fertility. J Hum Resour 41(4):722–737

Ding W, Lehrer SF, Rosenquist JN, Audrain-McGovern J (2006) The impact of poor health on education: new evidence using genetic markers. NBER Working Papers 12304. National Bureau of Economic Research

Duncan GJ, Guo G (2009) Dopamine transporter genotype and freshman roommate assignment to a binge drinker. Research in progress

Goldberger AS (1979) Heritability. Economica 46(184):327–47

Guo G, Stearns E (2002) The social influences on the realization of genetic potential for intellectual development. Soc Forces 80(3):881–910

Hamer D (2002) Rethinking behavior genetics. Science 298(5591):71–72

Hamer DH, Hu S, Magnuson V, Hu N, Pattatucci A (1993) A linkage between DNA markers on the X chromosome and male sexual orientation. Science 261(5119):321–327

Isalan M et al (2008) Evolvability and hierarchy in rewired bacterial gene networks. Nature 452:840–845

Jeong H, Mason SP, Barabási A-L, Oltvai ZN (2001) Lethality and centrality in protein networks. Nature 411:41–42

Katz LF, Kling JR, Liebman JB (2001) Moving to opportunity in Boston: early results of a randomized mobility experiment. Q J Econ 116:607–654

Knowler WC, Williams RC, Pettit DJ, Steinberg AG (1988) GM3;5, 13, 14 and type 2 diabetes mellitus: an association in American Indians with genetic admixture. Am J Hum Genet 43:520–526

Krishnan V, Nestler EJ (2008) The molecular neurobiology of depression. Nature 455:894–902

Lee DS (2008) Randomized experiments from non-random selection in the U.S. house elections. J Econom 142:675–697

Lichtenstein P, Pedersen NL, McClearn GE (1992) The origins of individual differences in occupational status and educational level: a study of twins reared apart and together. Acta Sociol 35:13–31

Lleras-Muney A (2005) The relationship between education and adult mortality in the United States. Rev Econ Stud 72(1):189–221

McGowan PO, Sasaki A, Huang TCT, Unterberger A, Suderman M, Ernst C, Meany MJ, Turecki G, Szyf M (2008) Promoter-wide hypermethylation of the ribsomomal rna gene promoter in the suicide brain. PLoS One 3(5):1–10

Plomin R, DeFries JC, McClearn GE, McGuffin P (2001) Behavioral genetics, 4th edn. Worth Publishers, New York

Rice G, Anderson C, Risch N, Ebers G (1999) Male homosexuality: absence of linkage to microsatellite markers at Xq28. Science 284:665

Rodgers JL, Rowe DC, Buster M (1999) Nature, nurture and first sexual intercourse in the USA: fitting behavioural genetic models to NLSY kinship data. J Biosoc Sci 31:29–41

Rowe DC, Teachman J (2001) Behavioral genetic research designs and social policy studies. In: Thornton A (ed) The well-being of children and families: research and data needs. University of Michigan Press, Ann Arbor, pp 157–187

Sacerdote B (2004) What happens when we randomly assign children to families? NBER Working Paper No. 10894

Stelzl U, Worm U, Lalowski M, Haenig C, Brembeck F, Goehler H, Stroedicke M, Zenkner M, Schoenherr A, Koeppen S, Timm J, Mintzlaff S, Abraham C, Bock N, Kietzmann S, Goedde A, Toksöz E, Droege A, Krobitsch S, Korn B, Birchmeier W, Lehrach H, Wanker E (2005) A human protein–protein interaction network: a resource for annotating the proteome. Cell 122:957–968

Strully KW (2009) Job loss and health in the U.S. labor market. Demography 46(2):221–246

Thornton KR, Jensen JD (2007) Controlling the false-positive rate in multilocus genome scans for selection. Genetics 175:737–750

van der Klaauw W (2002) Estimating the effect of financial aid offers on college enrollment: a regression-discontinuity approach. Int Econ Rev 43:1249–1287

Winship C, Morgan S (1999) The estimation of causal effects from observational data. Annu Rev Sociol 25:659–706

Wong AH et al (2005) Phenotypic differences in genetically identical organisms: the epigenetic perspective. Hum Mol Genet 14(Review issue 1):R11–R18

Chapter 28
Taking the Medical Sciences Seriously: Why and How Medical Sociology Should Incorporate Diverse Disciplinary Perspectives

Brea L. Perry

> *"Failure of a science to invent or recognize a new paradigm, when one is needed, exacts the penalties of stagnation and inertia. Adoption of a new concept awakens a discipline to new potential."*
>
> Mervyn Susser (1998, p. 60)

Introduction

Over the past two decades, sociologists have increasingly begun to advocate the synthesis of sociological and biological approaches to health and illness (Mechanic and Aiken 1986; Cohen and Williamson 1991; Fremont and Bird 2000; Guo 2006; Schwartz 1999), and several recent reports from the National Research Council suggest that biomedical scientists also promote an integrative model (e.g., *From Neurons to Neighborhoods*; Shonkoff and Phillips 2000; *New Horizons in Health*; Singer and Ryff 2001; *Genes, Behavior, and the Social Environment*; Hernandez and Blazer 2006). Scholars from diverse disciplines now recognize the futility of the nature/nurture debate (Hernandez and Blazer 2006; Shonkoff and Phillips 2000), and instead assert that health outcomes are the result of complex interactions between social, psychological, and biological factors being mediated in the brain and body (Hamer 2002; Singer and Ryff 2001). Arguably, the twenty-first century holds the promise of a new kind of health science in which disciplinary boundaries are becoming increasingly blurred. Medical sociology is at a crossroads: On the one hand, we can continue to focus narrowly "on the connections of social conditions to single diseases via single mechanisms at single points in time (Link and Phelan 1995, p. 81)," a strategy which limits our ability to achieve a complete understanding of even those causal factors that are central to sociology. Alternatively, sociologists have the opportunity to contribute to a process of integration and collaboration in which the best theoretical and methodological approaches, irrespective of discipline, are brought to bear on the most pressing empirical questions and public health problems of our generation.

For medical sociologists, the challenge is how to participate in this synthesis without being coopted by the biomedical sciences. In its December 2007 issue, Science magazine named research on human genetic variation – most notably the discovery of genes associated with more than a dozen diseases, including diabetes, cancer, and heart disease – the scientific "breakthrough of the year" (Pennisi 2007). Moreover, advancements relating to genetic variation, sequencing, and behavior

B.L. Perry (✉)
Department of Sociology, University of Kentucky, 1527 Patterson Office Tower, Lexington, KY 40506, USA
e-mail: breaperry@uky.edu

have been given this top honor no less than four times since 2000, and have made multiple appearances on the top-10 list every year (Couzin 2002; Culotta and Pennisi 2005; Kennedy et al. 2003, 2004, 2006; Pennisi 2000, 2007). In fact, 2000 has been called "the year of the genomes," prompting one *Science* writer to note, "it might well be the breakthrough of the decade, perhaps even the century, for all its potential to alter our view of the world we live in (Pennisi 2000, p. 2220)." Indeed, the scientific community and the public at large are enamored with the potential of genomics and other biomedical research to provide a cure for the nation's most lethal diseases, reverse the effects of aging, and unlock the mysteries of the immune system (Pennisi 2007).

Given the enormous power and prestige of biomedical research and the institution of medicine more broadly, why and how should medical sociologists contribute to the study of disease processes in the twenty-first century and beyond? This chapter first presents an introduction to the integrative perspective of health and illness, and proposes that dominant ideologies within the discipline have stymied empirical assessments of such models by medical sociologists. Next, the chapter highlights three key physiological systems in which social and biological processes have been shown to interact in ways that critically shape health outcomes. The chapter then identifies professional and institutional barriers that pose challenges for individual researchers interested in engaging in integrative research. Finally, this chapter suggests directions for future research that are informed by theoretical and methodological advances in the medical sciences, and perhaps represent sociology's best chances for occupying a central role in cutting-edge medical science in the future.

The Complexity of Disease Processes: An Integrative Model of Health and Illness

The sequence of biological, psychological, and social events and conditions that both precede illness and determine its course and consequences has been given multiple names in the social sciences, including "career" (Parsons 1951; Pescosolido 1991), "pathway" (Singer and Ryff 2001), and "trajectory" (Corbin and Strauss 1988). Though this terminology may evoke an orderly, linear progression to a single endpoint, in reality disease processes are characterized by countless convoluted and interacting pathways that may culminate in any of a number of physical, emotional, or behavioral manifestations. The complexity of disease processes derives in part from the seemingly endless possibilities for interaction between physiological systems and the multiple levels at which social factors might impact health outcomes – including macro social processes related to culture and social systems, social networks and interaction, and individual social-psychological or other micro-level processes.

Social scientists have developed a number of taxonomies to manage these complexities, dividing the "environment" into a series of mutually-influencing levels that shape health outcomes. The ecological perspective (Belsky 1980; Bronfenbrenner 1979; Cicchetti and Toth 1997), for example, identifies four levels represented by concentric circles: The outermost circle, the macrosystem, includes social norms as well as cultural beliefs and values; the exosystem refers to social structures and institutions such as education, employment, the media, and the community; the microsystem captures the influence of personal social networks, group memberships, and home, school, and work environments; and finally, the innermost circle, the ontological system, represents the individual's social, cognitive, and psychological competencies, including self-esteem, coping strategies, interpersonal skills, and intelligence. These different levels of the environment interact not only with each other, but also with physiological properties and processes like genetic predisposition, neurochemical functioning, and hormonal activity in the brain and body. Since these biological systems are less familiar to sociologists than the four levels of the environment, they are reviewed in more detail later in this chapter.

In order to illustrate the complex nature of disease processes, it is useful to examine a fairly well-understood case in which multiple pathways link one social condition (stress) to one health outcome (infectious disease). Cohen and Williamson (1991) identify mechanisms through which stress predisposes individuals to the onset of new infections and influences the severity and duration of an existing infection. In this model, stress can affect immunity by innervating the Central Nervous System directly, or by triggering the release of hormones that result in changes in immune system function. In addition, stress may lead to negative health behaviors such as smoking, drinking, and poor diet, which in turn suppress the immune system, making individuals more susceptible to pathogens and less effective at fighting infection. Stressful conditions might also compel individuals to seek support from members of the social network, increasing exposure to infectious viruses and bacteria. Finally, stress can also affect the likelihood that individuals who believe they are ill seek medical treatment, influencing the course and prognosis of the illness.

These etiological processes become exponentially more complicated when you consider that there are innumerable social antecedents to stress, many different types of stressors (e.g., chronic daily stressors, stressful life events, current and past stressors, etc.), and a multitude of outcomes linked to exposure to stressful conditions (Aneshensel 1999; Cohen and Williamson 1991; Pearlin et al. 1981; Pearlin 1999; Wheaton 1999). In short, any one health outcome has many determinants and any one determinant might have many outcomes, and all of these interact in complex ways at multiple levels, from cells to social structure.

Boundary Work and Ideological Speedbumps in the Twentieth Century

Sociologists and epidemiologists have developed numerous metaphors and models [see, for example, the "web of causation" in MacMahon et al. (1960); the "ecosocial framework" in Krieger 1994; "ecoepidemiology" in Susser 1998; and the Network Episode Model III in Pescosolido 2006] to illustrate the complex and overlapping nature of pathways to illness. Models of "multiple causation" encourage the consideration of relationships between variables at the levels of society, group, individual, and intra-individual. However, despite their enormous potential, empirical assessments of these interactive models are all but anomalous. I argue that sociologists' participation in integrative research has been limited, in part, by two key ideologies that have narrowed the scope of medical sociology in the latter half of the twentieth century. These are (1) the focus on so-called "distal" causes of disease and (2) the emphasis on the social experience of illness.

The idea of fundamental social causes of disease was developed in response to "risk factor" epidemiology, with its exclusionary focus on the identification of individual-level causes and interventions. The predominant view of disease etiology for much of the twentieth century held that "even knowledge of one small component may allow some degree of prevention since wherever the chain is broken, the disease will be prevented" (MacMahon et al. 1960, p. 18). As a result, the field of public health, in particular, long ignored broader social determinants of disease and other macro-level influences that are more distal in the so-called 'chain' of causation (Krieger 1994; Link and Phelan 1995).

In the 1990s, Link and Phelan (1995) argued that in concentrating on intervening mechanisms underlying relationships between macro-level social conditions and disease, health researchers were unwittingly overestimating the influence of individual-level determinants and underestimating the power of social structural position. They claimed that there exist certain fundamental social conditions (e.g., SES, gender, race, etc.) with relationships to disease that persist even as intervening and individual-level factors change or are eliminated. These fundamental causes endure because they involve access to power, money, social connectedness, information, and other resources that minimize the risk and consequences of disease. Hence, because one cannot escape the effects of these fundamental social conditions, our focus as medical sociologists should be on these.

Importantly, we are now discovering that, in the metaphor of a chain of causation, biological processes are both distal and proximal to disease outcomes, which renders this distinction and nomenclature essentially meaningless. On one hand, social conditions shape health outcomes through their impact on gene expression, organ function, hormonal activity, and other mechanisms at the cellular level that ultimately produce physical, emotional, and behavioral manifestations of disease. Thus, biological mechanisms occurring in the brain and body are among the most proximal in the development of physical and mental illness. On the other hand, recent studies suggest that powerful sociological determinants – including, for example, educational achievement (Guo and Stearns 2002), socioeconomic status (Pescosolido et al. 2008), marital status (Dick et al. 2006a), and even adherence to social norms (Udry 2000) – are influenced, in part, by heritable physiological and developmental processes. As these kinds of genetic predispositions are present at conception, and shape some of the fundamental social causes that Link and Phelan (1995) reference, biology is also among the most distal in the "chain" of causation.

Because social, psychological, and biological factors interact at every level of analysis, the "chain" metaphor and the distal/proximal distinction does not accurately convey the convoluted nature of disease processes, and may unintentionally facilitate complacency among medical sociologists. Arguments that advocate restricting theoretical or empirical focus to any one level, be it individual or social structural, run the risk of generating an incomplete or inaccurate understanding of health and illness. Although certain social and individual causes of disease may be "fundamental" in that they persist in a dynamic system, researchers in any discipline have yet to identify a risk factor with a one-to-one relationship to health outcomes. The degree and even the direction of the impact of any one risk factor is inevitably contingent in part on social and biological conditions at different levels of analysis. While the minimalist, "black box" logic in health research might suffice if either biological or social processes had an independent or additive influence on health, a wealth of evidence suggests that interactions between biological and social factors critically shape disease outcomes (Freese et al. 2003; Krieger 1994). Hence, research that ignores either social-structural or individual-level mechanisms is likely to underestimate the influence of both. Additionally, from a public health standpoint, interventions that are interdisciplinary and multi-level have the best chance of being effective for biologically and socially diverse populations (Link and Phelan 1995).

Another ideology that may have contributed to the neglect of biological mechanisms by medical sociologists was best described by Sue Estroff (1981) in her seminal work on living with mental illness. Estroff noted that the etiology of mental disorder – a debate that was particularly contentious in the 1970s and 1980s – has no bearing on the utility of social sciences for studying mental illness. Whatever its cause, be it purely genetic/biological or purely social, people with mental illness still have to live in a social world. That is to say, individuals make sense of their illness in terms of cultural meanings and values, and must contend with stigmatization, the institution of medicine, and other structural and cultural constraints in their everyday lives (Estroff 1981).

Though there are many areas of medical sociology where it is relatively safe to continue without considering biology, such an endeavor is likely to provide unique insight into social processes and lead to new and interesting questions. Physical and psychological aspects of illness related to biological processes contribute to the ways in which others perceive ill individuals, and to the overall experience of illness. For example, Charmaz's (1991) groundbreaking work on living with chronic illness suggests that the physical progression of disease directly affects social integration and access to social resources, as well as matters of self and identity. Similarly, some biologically-influenced aspects of illness (visibility, controllability, threat to others, etc.) determine the magnitude of stigmatization, and therefore one's social and social psychological experiences (Crocker et al. 1998). Further, individuals' responses to these social experiences and relationships and their ability to cope with stigmatizing definitions of their illness depend in part on temperament and other heritable or biologically-influenced cognitive processes and patterns of interaction (Compas et al. 2004; Saudino 2005). While the experience of illness is, indeed, a reflection of one's social world, individuals must also cope with the biological realities of their own physical, cognitive, and psychological limitations. As for research looking at the ways in which social and biological constraints are interdependent, there is much work yet to be done.

The contention that the *social experience* of illness, on one hand, or the *fundamental social causes* of illness, on the other, are the most appropriate or fruitful areas of research for medical sociologists has had unintended consequences for the discipline. Though these strategies were apt responses to threats from within and outside the discipline, they have provided justification for an exclusive focus on one level or aspect of the disease process. Both arguments constitute boundary-work (Geiryn 1999) – an attempt to establish the legitimacy of medical sociology and a call to return to what sociologists know and do best. However, at the onset of an era of health research that will be marked by a breaking down of disciplinary boundaries, such isolationism is no longer appropriate. There is a need for medical sociology to communicate and evolve with the broader medical and scientific community, which requires a basic knowledge of biological systems involved in the social experience and causation of illness.

Points of Convergence: Interactions Between Biological and Social Systems

Research identifying pre-disease pathways requires an assessment of risk across multiple social and biological systems (Singer and Ryff 2001). The recognition by sociologists that disease pathways involve complex interactions is a critical, but insufficient, first step in building an interdisciplinary agenda (Freese and Powell 2003). In order to disentangle these complexities, we must incorporate relevant biological theories, concepts, and measures in our own research – an enterprise that is becoming more feasible with the advent of new methodologies and publicly-available datasets (Guo 2006; Freese et al. 2003; Pescosolido 2006). However, for sociologists untrained in the biological sciences, it is difficult to know where to begin. Conveniently, interactions between social and biological variables can largely be traced to three interrelated physiological mechanisms: (1) endocrine and nervous system activity; (2) neuroplasticity; and (3) gene-environment interactions.

Endocrine and Nervous System Activity: Conversations between Brain and Body

Bodily functions are regulated by a complex hierarchy of control and feedback systems (Fremont and Bird 2000). Both the endocrine and nervous systems are involved in transmitting information between the brain and the body. Because these systems are responsible for receiving sensory input from the social environment, integrating and interpreting it, and formulating a physiological response, they are a powerful mechanism in the link between social conditions and disease.

The role of the endocrine and nervous systems in the stress process has been well documented by sociologists as well as biomedical researchers (Aneshensel 1999; Cohen and Williamson 1991; Fremont and Bird 2000; Pearlin 1999; Wheaton 1999). The sympathetic nervous system and the Hypothalamic Pituitary Adrenal (HPA) axis control the release of epinephrine (adrenaline) and cortisol, respectively (Fremont and Bird 2000). During exposure to stress, the sympathetic nervous system and the HPA axis become overactive, increasing heart rate, muscle tone, and glucose and fatty acid levels. These physiological responses are associated with an elevated risk for many physical and mental health problems, including cardiovascular disease, ulcers, hypertension, depression, and anxiety (Fremont and Bird 2000; House et al. 1988). In addition, because the endocrine, immune, and nervous systems interact with one another, social stress can affect immune functioning, increasing or decreasing vulnerability to bacterial and viral infection as well as influencing allergic reaction and healing.

Research on endocrine and nervous system function has important implications for sociological theory in that it provides a potential underlying mechanism. For instance, because different kinds of social contact activate or suppress the secretion of stress hormones, the impact of stress on health outcomes is mediated in part by social conditions that exacerbate or attenuate its influence (e.g., the presence of social support "buffers" the effects of stressful life events; Bovard 1985; House et al. 1988; Pearlin 1999). In a similar vein, stressors having to do with social interaction consistently produce larger and longer lasting effects than other kinds of stressors (Brown and Harris 1978; Brown et al. (1977); Mueller 1980; Paykel 1978; Perry 2006). In short, understanding the physiological mechanisms driving sociological findings is essential for explaining the impact of social conditions on health. For example, research suggests that early and persistent poverty is more strongly correlated with children's mental health outcomes than transient poverty (McLeod and Shanahan 1993, 1996). This pattern may relate to biomedical research suggesting that severe and chronic exposure to stress, particularly in early childhood, permanently alters the physiological responses to additional stressors, such that the effects of destructive social circumstances build up over time (Fremont and Bird 2000; Rutter and Stroufe 2000). Social conditions, then, can shape biological processes in ways that critically determine individuals' subsequent health trajectories.

Neuroplasticity: The Brain that Changes Itself

In his best-seller, *The Brain That Changes Itself* (2007), psychiatrist Norman Doidge presents inspiring medical case histories – a blind man "learning" to see, a woman with mental retardation "curing" herself, and depression and anxiety "disappearing." According to Doidge, the physiological process generating these incredible results is neuroplasticity, or environmentally-induced changes in the functional or physical anatomy of the brain. Throughout the life course, but especially in infancy and early childhood, the brain is constantly forming new neural connections or circuits, strengthening or weakening existing ones, and removing those that are unused.

The maturation and maintenance of neural connections depends on patterned, species-specific neural activity and sensory input. Neurological growth is "experience-expectant," which is to say that it will not occur without exposure to particular stimuli at critical periods in development (Greenough and Black 1992). An infant's primary caregiving environment must be "safe, nurturing, predictable, (and) repetitive" in order for neurological development to proceed normally (Perry and Pollard 1998). The absence of certain universal stimuli – including social interactions involving touch, speech, and responsive gaze – can impede the formation of normal circuits (Grossman et al. 2003; Perry and Pollard 1998). In short, social conditions not only influence brain development, but are *critical components* of the process.

On the other hand, neuroplasticity that depends on individuals' unique experiences (versus those that are common to particular species and critical developmental periods) is referred to as experience-dependent (Greenough and Black 1992). This type of brain development reflects our ability to adapt to our environment, regardless of whether the adaptations are ultimately advantageous or disadvantageous. For example, neuroplasticity is responsible for recent therapeutic advances in brain and spinal cord injury (Dobkin 1993), prompting some to suggest that our brains engage in a kind of "neural Darwinism" (Edelman 1987). Conversely, we now know that prolonged exposure to psychosocial stressors significantly reduces the formation of new neural connections, and has neurodegenerative effects in the hippocampus (Post 1992). As a result, the brain becomes restructured in such a way that makes individuals vulnerable to spontaneous and increasingly frequent depressive episodes.

Until recently, the generation of new neurons was thought to be limited to prenatal development and early infancy. However, although aging is associated with decreasing neural responsivity to new information and injury (Tucker 1992), research now suggests that in some regions of the brain, new neurons are generated even in old age (Eriksson et al 1998; Grossman et al. 2003; Rice and Barone 2000). This has important implications for later-onset degenerative neurological disorders, such as Huntington's, Alzheimer's, and Parkinson's Disease. Exposure to enriching environments can induce neurogenesis in individuals with these degenerative disorders, slowing the progress of disease (Spires and Hannan 2005). Importantly, factors that increase neurogenesis in adulthood – including social interaction, cognitive stimulation, and physical activity – are structured by individuals' social conditions, including socio-economic status, race, and gender (Blau 1977; Link and Phelan 1995; Simmel 1955; Spires and Hannan 2005; Williams and Collins 1995).

Gene-Environment Interactions: Beyond the Nature/Nurture Debate

As the 2003 (Kennedy et al.) "breakthrough of the year" piece in *Science* suggests, "Data mining" – or the inductive process of identifying genes associated with particular disease outcomes – has recently benefited from an explosion in interest, funding, and new methodologies made possible by technological advances (Chanock et al. 2007). While this trend might initially be perceived as a threat to sociological explanations of disease etiology, geneticists have recently adopted, in theory if not in practice, a multifactorial model that acknowledges the critical role of environmental influence (Hamer 2002; Singer and Ryff 2001). It is now widely accepted that the majority of diseases, from schizophrenia to some cancers, are coded by sets of genes working together, and that the expression of these "polygenes" is dependent on interactions with social and other environmental conditions (Chakravarti and Little 2003; Portin and Alanen 1997; Singer and Ryff 2001). In fact, recent evidence suggests that even disorders once believed to be primarily genetic in origin can have significant environmental influences (i.e., the manifestation and severity of autistic-like behaviors, seizures, and attention deficits in individuals with fragile X syndrome, a recessive genetic trait, is dependent on the quality of the home environment; Dyer-Friedman et al. 2002; Hessl et al. 2001).

The integral relationship between genes and the environment is due to the molecular nature of DNA. Because genes are molecules, they are subject to regulation by intracellular factors (e.g., what molecules go in and out of a cell and at what rate), which are a reflection of the social and physical environments in which an individual functions (Singer and Ryff 2001). From the standpoint of natural selection, the plasticity of gene expression is necessary and advantageous because it allows organisms to adapt to changing environmental stimuli (e.g., climate, stress level, food availability, etc.).

There exist three conceptually-distinct approaches to the relationship between genes and the social environment (Dick et al. 2006a; Grossman et al. 2003; Pescosolido et al. 2008; Shanahan and Hofer 2005): First, social factors can trigger or suppress the expression of injurious genes (i.e., stressful life events trigger the onset of major depression in individuals with a high-risk genotype; Caspi et al. 2003; Kendler et al. 1995; conversely, family-based social support and religious upbringing reduce the likelihood of alcohol abuse and dependence among those at high genetic risk; Koopmans et al. 1999; Pescosolido et al. 2008). Second, genes can attenuate or exacerbate the effects of social stressors and negative life events (i.e., certain protective genotypes minimize the causal relationship between childhood maltreatment and adult antisocial behavior; Caspi et al. 2002). Finally, genetic factors can influence social processes that have implications for health outcomes (i.e., certain genotypes increase the likelihood of being stably married, which in turn shapes risk for substance abuse and other mental illnesses; Dick et al. 2006a). Because genes and social environments interact in these complex ways, any attempt to assert the relative contribution of either factor likely underestimates the influence of both.

Confronting Professional and Institutional Barriers to Integrative Research

As the above review would suggest, integrative studies are now becoming the vanguard of health research. However, professional norms and values, as well as the structure of academic and research institutions, continue to pose significant problems for the average researcher interested in this line of work. Despite the fact that most social and biomedical scientists recognize a need for integrative health research, few are willing to abandon their relatively narrow disciplinary foci (Pellmar and Eisenberg 2000). Integrative research, if done well, is believed to require mastery of two or more disciplines – a discouraging prospect given the time and resources involved in achieving expertise in one field (Freese et al. 2003). This belief may contribute to the perception that interdisciplinary research rarely maintains the depth and quality of intradisciplinary science. Researchers express fear of failing in their own disciplines, being lost in team efforts, and losing their professional identity (Pellmar and Eisenberg 2000). Hence, efforts to "homogenize" the health sciences (Pescosolido 2006) are likely to be met with substantial resistance.

In response to these challenges, Pescosolido (2006) advocates science that is *multi*disciplinary rather than *inter*disciplinary. For research efforts to be successfully integrated, disciplines need not abandon their unique perspective and specialized set of theoretical and methodological tools. In fact, to do so would be to cast aside decades of scientific progress. Rather, in the twenty-first century, professional training and socialization in the health sciences will require a deep understanding and appreciation of the value and limitations of one's own field, in conjunction with "regular and routine points of research contact and collaboration with other disciplines (Pescosolido 2006, p. 201)."

Unfortunately, the organization of research and academic institutions poses difficult challenges for those who wish to engage in collaboration with colleagues outside their own discipline (Pellmar and Eisenberg 2000). The presence of some system of academic departmentalization is virtually universal at colleges and universities, which inhibits intellectual debate and communication among scholars in diverse disciplines. Also, promotion and tenure processes often depend on publishing in journals that are discipline-specific and conducting research that is consistent with departmental goals and values (Pellmar and Eisenberg 2000). Moreover, funding agencies and peer reviewers rarely possess expertise in more than one discipline, which makes it difficult to fairly assess the merit of integrative research proposals and manuscripts.

In 2000, the Institute of Medicine issued a committee report that contains innovative suggestions for improving institutional structure in ways that would facilitate collaborative research (Pellmar and Eisenberg 2000). However, it contains little practical advice for individual researchers. Hence, many of us who recognize the urgent need for sociological input in integrative and collaborative projects face these professional and institutional barriers without guidelines for how to proceed or where best to make our mark.

Beyond Business as Usual: Directions for Future Research

The bottom line is this: medical sociologists can no longer treat biological systems as a black box. If we do, we are in danger of losing funding opportunities and being omitted from important committees, institutes, and initiatives that influence health-related clinical and policy decisions both nationally and globally (Freese et al. 2003). Given that most sociologists struggle to keep abreast of new research in their own field, how can we conduct research that is informed by cutting-edge insights, concepts, and methods employed in the medical sciences? In which areas of research are sociologists uniquely positioned to contribute?

Dynamic Developmental Models and the Life Course Perspective

Developmental psychopathology was among the first subfields to advocate a multi-level or multi-system model of illness. Perhaps as a function of having roots in developmental theory, much of today's integrative health research has adopted a dynamic, stage-dependent approach that is congruous with sociology's life course perspective. Both social context and biological processes evolve in relatively predictable ways as individuals progress through different periods of the life course, which renders this approach particularly well-suited for integrative analysis.

Thoughtful consideration of the particular social, psychological, and physical conditions that characterize each period of development provides invaluable insight into the dynamic interactions occurring between these different levels. As people transition from childhood to adolescence to young adulthood, they are increasingly able to choose their own social context, control their social mobility, and form attitudes and values that shape behavior (Shanahan et al. 2003). As a result, heritability may be stronger or weaker, or can have different implications, at each stage of the life course (Dick et al. 2006b; Shanahan et al. 2003). For example, the same variant of the gene GABRA2 confers risk for conduct disorder in childhood and adolescence, but is associated with an elevated risk for alcohol dependence beginning in young adulthood (Dick et al. 2006b). GABRA2 influences these mental health outcomes through a predisposition toward risk-taking and disinhibition, which manifests as conduct disorder or alcohol dependence at different developmental stages. Importantly, the authors note that the age at which GABRA2 is associated with the onset of alcohol dependence corresponds not only to laws regulating alcohol use, but also to a period in the life course when young people tend to move out of their childhood homes and begin to work or attend college. In short, the expression of the GABRA2 gene is dependent, in part, on opportunity structures, social context, and the level of social control in a given group.

In particular, medical sociologists would be well-served to study integrative disease processes in children and youth. Childhood is a crucial period of development for even adult-onset physical and mental disorders (Damon and Eisenberg 1998; Rutter and Stroufe 2000). Not only is the brain more plastic during youth (detriments experienced in childhood are difficult to overcome in adulthood for this reason), but it is during this period in the life course when personality, temperament, and lifelong patterns of interaction are set (Damon and Eisenberg 1998; Grossman et al. 2003; Rutter and Stroufe 2000). If we want to capture the effects of social variables on physical and mental health, we will capture these processes on a much grander scale in childhood.

Yet, it is critical to track the effects of childhood experiences into adulthood, and to compare the relative contribution of social factors to the etiology of early and late onset diseases and other health outcomes. As we have seen, social events and conditions can permanently alter gene expression, sympathetic nervous system response to stressors, and the maturation and maintenance of neural connections (Caspi et al. 2003; Fremont and Bird 2000; Grossman et al. 2003). Accordingly, the key to the strength and significance of relationships between social factors and health may lie in the intensity and duration of past exposure to social and environmental stress coupled with the ongoing availability of social support and other coping resources. We cannot begin to understand interactions between biological and social pathways to disease if we examine only one small slice of a person's experiences. We must trace the pathways from beginning to end, or as completely as is possible.

The Promise of a Social Networks Approach

Though social interaction is operationalized in myriad ways across the social and medical sciences – from civic participation to parenting style – the message is clear: Our connectedness to others, the availability of social network resources, and the quality of our social interactions are critical determinants of physical and mental health outcomes (See, for example, Cohen and Syme 1985; Mirowsky and Ross 1986; Pescosolido and Levy 2002). We know that "environmental effects" relating to social interaction and social network disruption consistently produce the largest and longest lasting effects on physical and mental health (Brown and Harris 1978; Brown et al. 1977; Fremont and Bird 2000; Mueller 1980; Perry 2006). In fact, in both animals and humans, the presence of a familiar member of the same species has been found to buffer the effects of naturally-occurring and experimentally-induced stress on a variety of psychological and physiological outcomes, including ulcers, hypertension, cardiovascular activity, arteriosclerosis, depression, and anxiety (House et al. 1988). Because the link between social interaction and health is so strong, some scholars have suggested that social networks may be the key to integrating the health sciences (Mueller 1980; Pescosolido 2006).

Social interaction influences health both directly and indirectly through various related mechanisms. Social contact stimulates the amygdala, which has multiple consequences for health through its role in the endocrine and nervous systems and in immune function (House et al. 1988). Social interaction also enhances the positive effects of restorative behaviors, such as sleep (Singer and Ryff 2001), and modifies gene expression (Caspi et al. 2003; Pescosolido et al. 2008). At the psychosocial level, emotional support provided by social relationships improves self-esteem and increases feelings of efficacy and control, thereby increasing well-being (Kessler and McLeod 1985). In addition, social networks transmit information, opinions, advice, and assistance with problem-solving that influences peoples' preventative health beliefs and behaviors like diet and exercise (Berkman and Breslow 1983; Horwitz 1977; House 1981; Wills 1985). Finally, social relationships have important effects on symptom recognition and patterns of utilization, including whether individuals seek treatment, what type of healers they consult, and whether they follow the recommendations of health services providers (Kadushin 1966; Pescosolido 2000; Wellman 2000). In short, social interaction shapes health outcomes at every stage in the disease process, from immune response to health care utilization.

Most importantly, a social network approach also bridges multiple levels of analysis, which is an essential quality in a unifying theory (Pescosolido 2006). An individual's psychological and biological competencies, limitations, tendencies, and predispositions embedded in social relationships provide a basis for network structures, upon which communities, social institutions, and cultures are built (Lin and Peek 1999). Social network theory sees individual-level cognitive and biological factors as critically tied to ongoing social relationships in the larger context of people's lives (Pescosolido 2000). Moreover, it allows both social and life scientists to operationalize abstract concepts like "community" or "society" by looking at the set of social interactions that occurs within these. Because networks have recently been used to describe phenomena at virtually every level of analysis, from cellular to organizational, across disciplines as diverse as neurology and public health, the perspective is broadly resonant (Pescosolido 2006; Weiner 1998). In short, the social network perspective is accessible to all, and enables researchers to examine intricate causal pathways between and among the most macro and micro-level variables (Wellman and Frank 1999).

The Interplay of Culture and Biology

One potential area of study to which sociologists have much to contribute is the interplay between biology and culture. It is widely acknowledged in medical sociology that culture constrains the perceptual, explanatory, and behavioral options that individuals have for responding to disease (Angel and Thoits 1987; Kleinman 1988). Individuals learn from their cultures vocabularies of health and illness which structure help-seeking options and limit the possibilities for the interpretation of physical and psychological states (Angel and Thoits 1987). However, what has been largely ignored by health researchers are the ways in which biological realities might constrain cultural aspects of health, illness, and healing.

Culture is socially constructed, with social norms, roles, and meanings emerging and being institutionalized through human interaction (Berger and Luckmann 1966; Peterson and Anand 2004; Turner 1992). Nonetheless, culture and meaning are constrained by the physical environment and other objective realities. In the culture of health and illness, this includes our bodies' physical characteristics, symptoms of disease, and various biological processes (Angel and Thoits 1987; Carpentier et al. 1999; Healy 1997; Kleinman 1988; Williams 2006). How we make sense of disease, the meanings and values that we attribute to health and illness, and our culturally proscribed illness behaviors (e.g., the sick role) are all dependent in part on objective features of the illness experience and other physical, cognitive, and emotional realities (Angel and Thoits 1987; Conrad 1987; Parsons 1951; Williams 2006).

A small amount of research in this vein is beginning to be carried out, but more is needed. For example, our cultural conceptions of depression and other mental illnesses have changed radically in the past 20 years, in large part because of the advent of effective pharmaceuticals and because of research identifying genetic and physiological components in the etiology of mental disorders (Healy 1997). These developments have deflected blame away from the individual, and have helped to ameliorate symptoms of mental illness. These insights into the biology of mental illness coupled with pharmaceutically-induced changes in the neurochemistry of diagnosed individuals have significantly reduced the stigma attached to mental illness, and have undoubtedly improved the community and social experiences of people with some disorders (Link et al. 1999; Martin et al. 2000, 2007; Mechanic et al. 1994; Pescosolido et al. 2000). Still, the American public attaches very different meanings to disorders like depression and schizophrenia, in part because of media representations that exaggerate dangerousness, disordered thought patterns, and other biologically-driven symptoms of psychopathology (Link et al. 1999).

Interestingly, as the public's knowledge and understanding of biological disease processes increases, the culture of illness and healing appears to change as well. For example, large public opinion studies suggest that peoples' beliefs about the etiology of mental illness (do they attribute disorders to more social/environmental causes like upbringing or to more biological causes like chemical imbalance or genetic defect) affect the labels that they attach to mental health problems and their desire for social distance from people with those disorders (Link et al. 1999; Martin et al. 2000, 2007; Mechanic et al. 1994; Pescosolido et al. 2000). Additionally, increasing public awareness of disease processes and their treatments has radically influenced consumer power and autonomy in American medicine (Light 1991; Mechanic 1996). The nature of the physician-patient relationship and indeed the profession of medicine as a whole is evolving as we become more informed consumers, have a greater tendency to self-diagnose, and even ask for medications by name (Light 1991; Mechanic 1996; Pescosolido et al. 2001). Similarly, in the professional sphere, medical research funded by drug companies influences physicians' understandings of disease categories and their etiology, which in turn affects clinicians' responses to complaints, their willingness to apply a diagnosis, and what diagnoses they apply (Healy 1997). Needless to say, the social construction of diagnosis, which depends in part on perceptions of biological mechanisms underlying disease, has far-reaching implications for sick people and their families (Brown 1995; Kleinman 1988; Mirowsky and Ross 1989).

This brief review highlights a few of the many ways that biological processes and the public's knowledge of them might constrain the culture of health, illness, and healing. Happily, an investigation of how cultural meanings, values, and behaviors are influenced by the objective realities of symptoms of disease and other physical and psychological experiences does not necessarily require an extensive knowledge of genetic or physiological mechanisms. In most cases, research of this kind only requires that we begin asking different questions that are informed by biomedical breakthroughs and attend to our cultural understandings of and responses to them.

The Physical Experience of Illness

In studying the social effects of illness, it may be useful to incorporate indicators of the physical experience (i.e., the nature or severity) of illness. There are fairly consistent patterns of pain, disability, behavior, and cognition associated with various diseases that can impact and interact with the social experiences of diagnosed persons, and it is important to take these into account.

Many variables that reflect the severity of disease are easily accessible, and may be suggestive of the degree to which biological processes are driving social outcomes. In mental illness, information such as the number of positive or negative symptoms, Global Assessment of Functioning (GAF), hospitalization history, medication regimen, the presence of comorbidity, and other factors often significantly shape social experiences. To the degree that relationship quality and function depend on the success of social interactions between individuals, behaviors associated with mental illness (e.g., symptoms) that impede mutual understanding and communication can disrupt social networks (Rosenberg 1984). For example, research indicates that the sexual and romantic experiences of people with serious mental illness are determined in part by the physical realities of sexual dysfunction, which patients tend to classify either as a symptom of their disorder or as a side-effect of their medication (Wright et al. 2007). Furthermore, the mechanisms underlying social network attrition in people with mental illness, including social rejection and strategic social withdrawal, are shaped, in part, by the number of positive and negative symptoms they experience and the acute or chronic status of the disorder (Perry 2005). In short, the nature and severity of one's psychological symptoms influence patterns of utilization and compliance, social structural outcomes (e.g., education, income, employment, marital status, residential stability), the function and structure of social networks, and so on.

This approach is relevant in cases of physical illness, as well. For instance, staging is used by physicians to assess the size and location of a patient's cancer and to note whether it has spread to other organs. A person with Stage I cancer is likely to have an entirely different illness experience than someone with Stage IV cancer (the most advanced stage). The stage of one's cancer determines prognosis and shapes treatment options, and is indicative of the level of pain and disability experienced by a patient. Stage is likely related to feelings of hopelessness and sense of control, the construction of self and identity, the fulfillment of social roles and expectations, and the nature of social interactions. Similarly, the type of cancer one has may involve feelings of attractiveness and self-worth (breast cancer), femininity or masculinity (ovarian and testicular cancer), or stigma and self-blame (lung cancer), and will thereby influence the illness experience (Kaiser 2006). Other indicators of the severity or nature of physical illness that might have social consequences are Type I versus Type II diabetes, variants of hepatitis, and the HIV/AIDS distinction. Because features of the physical experience of disease are likely to shape the social experience of illness, the inclusion of variables typically employed by the medical profession to describe disease is likely to inform our own research.

The Need for Thoughtful Methodology

Many sociologists prefer to study changes in sub-clinical health problems that are arguably more socially malleable than severe, clear-cut cases of disease. A literature search in *Sociological Abstracts* turns up significantly more hits for studies of depression than schizophrenia, for example. Continuous measures of sub-clinical health problems, like Rosenberg's Self-Esteem Scale or the Center for Epidemiological Studies Depression Scale (CES-D), have numerous advantages. Indeed, a notable strength of our discipline is that we question an arbitrary threshold for disease, which allows us to identify marginal and at-risk individuals, and acknowledge the socially constructed nature of science and medicine (Gieryn 1983; Horwitz and Wakefield 2007).

With regard to the CES-D and similar measures of psychological distress, statistical significance and substantive significance are not synonymous. At some point we must ask ourselves whether 1 or 2 more days per month of "feeling blue" (Radloff 1977) constitutes a meaningful difference in the lives of everyday people. Further, as argued by Horwitz and Wakefield (2007), the "symptoms" captured by the CES-D may simply reflect a normal grief reaction to social conditions such as divorce, unemployment, the death of a loved one, and even the typical ups and downs of adolescence. Because the criteria for applying a diagnosis of depression using the CES-D are far less rigorous than the DSM-IV, comparisons to a population with clinical depression are inappropriate. However, researchers using the CES-D often employ such terms as depression, psychological distress, disorder, and mental illness interchangeably, conflating the study of normal reactive sadness or distress with the study of actual psychiatric disorder (Horwitz and Wakefield 2007). In light of increasing calls for integrative research, we must be more thoughtful about our methodology and its implications (Mechanic 1989).

Several medical sociologists have advocated a return to the study of severe mental and physical illness (Cook and Wright 1995; Levine 1995). We cannot expect to be able to collaborate, communicate, and integrate with the biological sciences if we are studying marginal cases of vaguely-defined "psychological distress" in the general population, while they are confining their samples to clinical populations with severe disorder. Furthermore, decades of focus on mild or marginal cases means that we now know relatively little about social causation processes in what we have assumed to be largely biologically or genetically-driven diseases and disorders. Given recent findings on gene–environment interactions and neuroplasticity, it is likely that social conditions play a larger role in many health outcomes than we once assumed (Grossman et al. 2003).

In identifying interactions between biological mechanisms and features of the social environment, it may be necessary to study clinical populations. As noted previously, any given physical or mental health outcome might have countless determinants and any one determinant might have countless outcomes, and all of these can interact in complex ways. It is crucial that we begin constructing theories and models that are dynamic, multi-method, and multi-level, and that we develop more advanced statistical techniques to test these models (Mechanic 1989; Pescosolido and Kronenfeld 1995). It may be difficult to achieve significance in these kinds of complex models without examining populations in which disorder is prevalent and there is sufficient variation among cases. Unfortunately, this may mean ignoring marginal cases for now, but medical sociologists can return to these more refined pursuits when these methodologies have advanced and complicated relationships are better understood.

The Role of Medical Sociology: A Developmental Model Meets Social Constructionism

As mentioned previously, the field of developmental psychopathology was one of the first disciplines to prioritize the integration of social, psychological, and biological perspectives in health research. In principle, if not always in practice, the discipline is committed to a cutting-edge research agenda that investigates complex, interactional, and multi-level developmental pathways leading to mental illness. However, the weaknesses of developmental psychopathology correspond to the strengths of sociology. Just as our training forces us to "make due" with more simplistic measures of biological processes than are ideal, developmental psychopathologists tend to examine relatively crude measures of social context. Further, their "environment" is an amalgam of all cultural, social, geographical, physical, and chemical factors external to the individual that may play a role in disease pathways, and there is no conceptual or operational definition or unifying perspective that helps individual researchers distinguish among these different levels (Boyce et al. 1998).

Moreover, developmental psychopathology has tended to focus on micro-level social, and particularly familial, context (i.e., parental attachment, marital conflict, etc.) and psychological processes (i.e., coping mechanisms, temperament, etc.) to the detriment of more macro-level factors like cultural norms and values as well as social structures, institutions, and organizations (Jessor 1993). Finally, faced with the complex and layered nature of social life, research in developmental psychopathology that considers relationships between *two or more* levels (i.e., healthcare policy and mothers' prenatal care), contexts (i.e., family and school), or dimensions (i.e., parenting style and parents' mental health status) is virtually nonexistent (Boyce et al. 1998).

The discipline of medical sociology is uniquely situated to provide the theoretical, conceptual, and methodological tools that developmental psychopathologists and other integrative health researchers lack. As described above, integrative research is compatible with classic sociological theories of meaning and culture, stigma and labeling, the social construction of illness, and the illness experience, all of which are only strengthened by a thoughtful consideration of the role of biological and psychological processes. In addition, sociologists are adept at services research and studies of utilization and compliance, the profession of medicine, physician–patient interaction, and other clinical realities that developmental psychopathologists, not to mention biologists, ignore. Sociology also brings to the table the ability to look beyond individual-level or dyadic social interaction to the structural nature of social networks, neighborhood, communities, and organizations. Thus, if sociologists are not involved in collaborative research efforts, from theoretical conception through publication, not only scientific understanding but also advancements in health policy and practice will be stymied.

In order to demonstrate the utility of a sociological perspective, it is useful to examine an innovative, dynamic, multi-level model of the etiology of psychopathology proposed by Grossman et al. (2003). According to the authors, adult psychopathology is the culmination of a long sequence of neurodevelopmental insults of varying intensity. Stressful experiences early in the progression of mental illness may result in altered gene expression that modifies structural and functional characteristics of the brain and produces increasing vulnerability to future biological and environmental insults. Developmental psychologist C.H. Waddington (1957) developed the concept of canalization to describe how genetic and environmental influences interact to affect the developmental trajectory, and Grossman et al. (2003) recently modified the model to explain the etiology of psychopathology (See Fig. 28.1). "Normal"

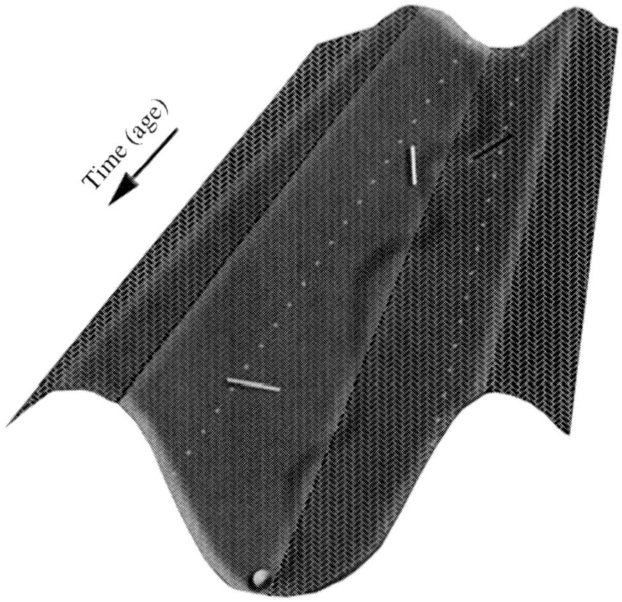

Fig. 28.1 View of Development, modified from C.H. Waddington's (1940; 1957) concept of canalization

development is represented by a groove in the lowest point of a valley on a long surface that models the normative developmental progression. The individual (the ball) begins at the top of the model, and progresses downward with age. At the top of the model (the early stages of development), the walls are less steep than at later points in development, which portrays the phenomenon that individuals become progressively more resilient and less mutable over time. Genetic and environmental conditions or events shape the development of the brain, which we now know is surprisingly plastic, even into adulthood. These conditions may either have a restorative effect (i.e., maternal warmth and intimacy) or might disrupt normative development (i.e., chronic poverty), leading the ball away from the center groove. If genetic and environmental conditions are strong enough, an individual might cross the threshold (the dotted line) into psychopathology (Grossman et al. 2003).

Mental illnesses are seen as developmental disorders whose manifestation represents a point along a continuum at which the impact of genetic and environmental disruptions surpasses a threshold for symptom expression. Early, minor signs of mental disorder observed in childhood are thought to be physical and cognitive phenotypic expressions of increasingly compromised brain organization, and are said to comprise the pre-psychosis prodromal state on the continuum from normality to full-blown psychiatric disorder. The presence of vulnerable neuronal circuits is purportedly largely masked until taxed by later developmental demands, as during adolescence. If either the circuitry or any of the processes involved in more complex brain adaptation or refinement of synaptic connectivity have been compromised in early development, the stress of adolescence may lead to the expression of psychotic symptoms (Grossman et al. 2003).

The canalization model (Grossman et al. 2003) has potential for integrating research efforts from multiple disciplines. However, certain biases related to the disciplinary perspective of the authors are evident. Most notably, the concept of a threshold of symptomatology is worthy of further consideration. Holistically, the model is visually and conceptually based on the idea that psychopathology is a continuum (hence, the slope). However, the threshold concept suggests that symptomatology is simply turned on and off. Although the underlying biology and brain organization is said to be continuous, the authors imply that one either clearly has the phenotypic disorder or does not.

One sociological perspective holds that the dotted line (or threshold) has no underlying biological determinants, but is instead a product of social construction. The threshold is simply the point at which behavior and cognitions are labeled "abnormal" by the individual, members of the social network, a mental health professional, and/or some other provider of medical or social services. The threshold likely varies cross-nationally, cross-culturally, historically, and across different subgroups within a population. Moreover, the effects of crossing the threshold, or being labeled, have their own implications for the course of disorder. Thus, the dotted line should be viewed as having its own impact on the developmental trajectory. A great deal of research has demonstrated that psychiatric labeling is associated with stigmatization that profoundly affects social psychological factors like self-esteem, self-efficacy, and hopelessness, as well as opportunities for employment, education, housing, and social relationships independent of the symptoms themselves (Link et al. 1989; Link and Phelan 1999). In fact, research suggests that treatment with anti-depressants has positive long-term effects on dendritic branching in the hippocampus, and can reverse stress-induced dendritic atrophy (Magarinos et al. 1999). However, despite the potential for anti-depressants to "cure" depression, it is often a chronic disorder characterized by multiple episodes over a lifetime. The self-fulfilling nature of labeling makes it very difficult for individuals to cross back over into normality, even after the underlying neurological disorder has been corrected or improved using psychotropic medications or other clinical interventions (cognitive-behavioral therapies, social skills training, and family therapy have been reported to have similar effects) that restore healthy neurochemical functioning.

The idea of a movable, socially constructed threshold can apply to physical illness as well. Although the diagnosis and labeling of physical illnesses are generally thought to be more objective than those of mental illnesses, several instances of the imposition of seemingly random thresholds in the practice of regular medicine readily come to mind. For instance, the distinction between infection with HIV (the virus that causes AIDS) and an actual diagnosis of AIDS comes down to nothing more than having a T-cell count (indicative of immune functioning) below 200, and two or more opportunistic infections. Although the criteria for an AIDS diagnosis are really somewhat arbitrary and contestable, they have very real implications for the progression of the disease because federal and insurance reimbursement, availability of certain drug treatments, and eligibility for social assistance depend on this distinction.

The apparent omission of social constructionism, which is widely accepted in at least some form by sociologists, from the canalization model is indicative of the need for disciplinary collaboration in theory and model development. One of the greatest strengths of sociologists is their willingness and ability to theorize complex and multifaceted relationships that often contradict taken-for-granted cultural, institutional, and professional beliefs as well as challenge the dominant, status quo organization of social life. It is imperative, then, that sociologists be involved in the development of theories of physical and mental illness trajectories *before* data is collected.

Scheff (1966) advocates developing theories that are the antithesis of other theories. The result, he claims, is the elimination of all of the problems of both theories, and the integration of the best parts of both. In order to integrate, however, scholars must have a good working knowledge of both perspectives. Thus, in the coming decades, the most successful and innovative work in the discipline of medical sociology will likely reflect at least a basic understanding of biomedical principles. Further, it will demonstrate a willingness to incorporate relevant biomedical advances (e.g., those involving biological systems that represent a "point of convergence," or intersection of social and biological mechanisms) into our own research. Work reviewed here suggests that the time to integrate the biological, psychological, and social approaches to health and illness is now. If integrative models are to benefit from our long tradition of social theory and research on health and medicine, medical sociologists must play a central role in their development.

References

Aneshensel CS (1999) Outcomes of the stress process. In: Horwitz AV, Scheid TL (eds) A handbook for the study of mental health. Cambridge University Press, New York, pp 211–27

Angel R, Thoits PA (1987) The impact of culture on the cognitive structure of illness. Cult Med Psychiatry 11:465–94

Belsky J (1980) Child maltreatment: an ecological integration. Am Psychol 35:320–35

Berger PL, Luckmann T (1966) The social construction of reality: a treatise in the sociology of knowledge. Anchor Books, Garden City, NY

Berkman LF, Breslow L (1983) Health and ways of living: the alameda county study. Oxford University Press, New York

Blau P (1977) A macrosociological theory of social structure. Am J Sociol 83:26–54

Bovard EW (1985) Brain mechanisms in effects of social support on viability. Perspect Behav Med 2:103–129

Boyce TW, Frank E, Jensen PS, Kessler RC, Nelson CA, Steinberg L, the MacArthur Foundation Research Network on Psycho-pathology and Development. (1998) Social context in developmental psychopathology: recommendations for future research from the MacArthur network on psychopathology and development. Dev Psychopathol 10:143–64

Bronfenbrenner U (1979) The ecology of human development: experiments by nature and design. Harvard University Press, Cambridge, MA

Brown P (1995) Naming and framing: the social construction of diagnosis and illness." J Health Soc Behav (Extra Issue):34–52

Brown G, Harris T (1978) The social origins of depression. Free Press, New York

Brown G, Harris T, Copeland JR (1977) Depression and loss. Br J Psychiatry 130:8–20

Carpentier N, Lesage A, White D (1999) Family influence on the first stages of the trajectory of patients diagnosed with severe psychiatric disorders. Fam Relat 48:397–403

Caspi A, McClay J, Moffitt TE, Mill J, Martin J, Craig IW, Taylor A, Poulton R (2002) Role of genotype in the cycle of violence in maltreated children. Science 297:851–854

Caspi A, Sugden K, Moffitt TE, Taylor A, Craig IW, Harrington HonaLee, McClay J, Mill J, Martin J, Braithwaite A, Poulton R (2003) Influence of life stress on depression: moderation by a polymorphism in the 5-htt gene. Science 301:386–9

Chakravarti A, Little P (2003) Nature, nurture, and human disease. Nature 421:412–14

Chanock SJ, Manolio T, Boehnke M, Boerwinkle E, Hunter D, Thomas G, Hirschhorn J, Abecasis G, Altshuler D, Bailey-Wilson J, Brooks L, Cardon L, Daly M, Donnelly P, Fraumeni JF, Freimer N, Gerhard D, Gunter C, Guttmacher A, Guyer M, Harris E, Hoh J, Robert Hoover C, Kong A, Merikangas K, Morton C, Palmer L, Phimister E, Rice J, Roberts J, Rotimi C, Tucker M, Vogan K, Wacholder S, Wijsman E, Winn D, Collins F (2007) Replicating genotype-phenotype associations. Nature 447:655–60

Charmaz K (1991) Good days, bad days: the self in chronic illness and time. Rutgers University Press, New Brunswick, NJ

Cicchetti D, Toth SL (1997) Transactional ecological systems in developmental psychopathology. In: Luthar SS, Burack JA, Cicchetti D, Weisz JR (eds) Developmental psychopathology: perspectives on adjustment, risk, and disorder. Cambridge University Press, Cambridge, MA, pp 317–49

Cohen S, Syme L (1985) Social support and health. Academic, New York

Cohen S, Williamson GM (1991) Stress and infectious disease in humans. Psychol Bull 109:5–24

Compas BE, Connor-Smith J, Jaser SS (2004) Temperament, stress reactivity, and coping: implications for depression in childhood and adolescence. J Clin Child Adolesc Psychol 33:21–31

Conrad P (1987) The experience of illness: recent and new directions. Res Sociol Health 6:1–31

Cook JA, Wright ER (1995) Medical sociology and the study of severe mental illness: reflections on past accomplishments and directions for future research. J Health Soc Behav (Extra Issue):95–114

Corbin J, Strauss A (1988) Unending work and care. Jossey Bass, San Francisco,CA

Couzin J (2002) Breakthrough of the year: small RNAs make big splash. Science 298:2296–97

Crocker JB, Major B, Steele C (1998) Social stigma. In: Gilbert DT, Fiske ST (eds) The handbook of social psychology, 2nd edn. Mcgraw-Hill, Boston, MA, pp 504–553

Culotta E, Pennisi E (2005) Breakthrough of the year: evolution in action. Science 310:1878–79

Damon W, Eisenberg N (1998) Handbook of child psychology: social emotional, and personality development, 5th edn. Wiley, New York

Dick DM, Agrawal A, Schuckit M, Bierut L, Hinrichs A, Fox L, Mullaney J, Cloninger C, Hesselbrock V, Jr JI, Nurnberger LA, Foroud T, Porjesz B, Edenberg H, Begleiter H (2006a) Marital status, alcohol dependence, and GABRA2: evidence for gene-environment correlation and interaction. J Stud Alcohol 67:185–94

Dick DM, Bierut L, Hinrichs A, Fox L, Bucholz K, Kramer J et al (2006b) The role of GABRA2 in risk for conduct disorder and alcohol and drug dependence across developmental stages. Behav Genet 36:577–590

Dobkin BH (1993) Neuroplasticity: key to recovery after central nervous system injury. West J Med 159:56–60

Doidge N (2007) The brain that changes itself. Viking Books, New York

Dyer-Friedman J, Glaser B, Hessl D, Johnston C, Huffman LC, Taylor A, Wisbeck J, Reiss A (2002) Genetic and environmental influences on the cognitive outcomes of children with fragile X syndrome. J Am Acad Child Adolesc Psychiatry 41:237–44

Edelman G (1987) Neural Darwinism. The theory of neuronal group selection. Basic Books, New York

Eriksson PS, Perfilieva E, Bjork-Eriksson T, Alborn AM, Nordborg C et al (1998) Neurogenesis in the adult human hippocampus. Nat Med 4:1313–17

Estroff S (1981) Making it crazy: an ethnography of psychiatric clients in an American community. University of California Press, Berkeley, CA

Freese J, Powell B (2003) Tilting at windmills: rethinking sociological responses to behavioral genetics. J Health Soc Behav 44:130–35

Freese J, Li Jui-Chung Allen, Wade LD (2003) The potential relevances of biology to social inquiry. Annu Rev Sociol 29:233–56

Fremont AM, Bird CE (2000) Social and psychological factors, physiological processes, and physical health. In: Bird C, Conrad P, Fremont A (eds) Handbook of medical sociology. Prentice-Hall, Upper Saddle River, NJ, pp 334–352

Geiryn T (1999) Cultural boundaries of science: credibility on the line. University of Chicago Press, Chicago, IL

Gieryn TF (1983) Boundary-work and the demarcation of science from non-science: strains and interests in professional ideologies of scientists. Am Sociol Rev 48:781–95

Greenough W, Black J (1992) Induction of brain structure by experience: substrate for cognitive development. In: Gunnar MR, Nelson CA (eds) Developmental behavioral neuroscience. Lawrence Erlbaum, Hillsdale, NJ, pp 155–200

Grossman AW, Churchill JD, McKinney BC, Kodish IM, Otte SL, Greenough WT (2003) Experience effects on brain development: possible contributions to psychopathology. J Child Psychol Psychiatry 44:33–63

Guo G (2006) The linking of sociology and biology. Soc Forces 85:145–150

Guo G, Stearns E (2002) The social influences on the realization of genetic potential for intellectual development. Soc Forces 80:881–910
Hamer D (2002) Rethinking behavior genetics. Science 298:71–72
Healy D (1997) The anti-depressant era. Harvard University Press, Cambridge, MA
Hernandez LM, Blazer DG (2006) Genes, behavior, and the social environment: moving beyond the nature/nurture debate. National Academy Press, Washington, DC
Hessl D, Dyer-Friedman J, Glaser B, Jacob Wisbeck R, Barajas G, Taylor A, Reiss AL (2001) The influence of environmental and genetic factors on behavior problems and autistic symptoms in boys and girls with fragile X syndrome. Pediatrics 108:88–97
Horwitz A (1977) Social networks and pathways to psychiatric treatment. Soc Forces 56:86–105
Horwitz A, Wakefield JC (2007) The loss of sadness: how psychiatry trans-formed normal sorrow into depressive disorder. Oxford University Press, New York
House JS (1981) Work stress and social support. Addison-Wesley, Reading, MA
House JS, Landis KR, Umberson D (1988) Social relationships and health. Science 241:40–45
Jessor R (1993) Successful adolescent development among youth in high risk settings. Am Psychol 48:117–26
Kadushin C (1966) The friends and supporters of psychotherapy: on social circles in urban life. Am Sociol Rev 31:786–802
Kaiser K (2006) Making sense of cancer: the impact of culture and social interaction on the self of the cancer survivor. PhD Dissertation, Indiana University
Kendler KS, Kessler RC, Walters E, MacLean C, Neale M, Heath A, Eaves L (1995) Stressful life events, genetic liability, and onset of an episode of major depression in women. Am J Psychiatry 152:833–42
Kennedy D, The News and Editorial Staffs (2003) Breakthrough of the year: the runners-up. Science 302:2039–45
Kennedy D, The News and Editorial Staffs (2004) Breakthrough of the year: the runners-up. Science 306:2013–2017
Kennedy D, The News and Editorial Staffs (2006) Breakthrough of the year: the runners-up. Science 314:1850–55
Kessler RC, McLeod JD (1985) Social support and psychological distress in community surveys. In: Cohen S, Syme SL (eds) Social support and health. Academic, New York, pp 19–40
Kleinman A (1988) Rethinking psychiatry: from cultural category to personal experience. The Free Press, New York
Koopmans JR, Slutske WS, van Baal GCM, Boomsma DI (1999) The influence of religion on alcohol use initiation: evidence for genotype x environment interaction. Behav Genet 29:445–53
Krieger N (1994) Epidemiology and the web of causation: has anyone seen the spider? Soc Sci Med 39:889–903
Levine S (1995) Time for creative integration in medical sociology. J Health Soc Behav (Extra Issue):1–4
Light DW (1991) Professionalism as a countervailing power. J Health Polit Policy Law 16:499–506
Lin N, Peek KM (1999) Social networks and mental health. In: Horwitz AV, Scheid T (eds) A handbook for the study of mental health. Cambridge University Press, New York, pp 241–258
Link BG, Phelan JC (1995) Social conditions as fundamental causes of disease. J Health Soc Behav (Extra Issue):80–94
Link BG, Phelan JC (1999) Labeling and stigma. In: Aneshensel CS, Phelan JC (eds) Handbook of the sociology of mental health. Kluwer, New York, pp 481–94
Link BG, Cullen FT, Struening E, Shrout P, Dohrenwend BP (1989) A modified labeling theory approach in the area of mental disorders: an empirical assessment. Am Sociol Rev 54:100–23
Link BG, Phelan Jo C, Bresnahan M, Stueve A, Pescosolido BA (1999) Public conceptions of mental illness: labels, causes, dangerousness, and social distance. Am J Public Health 89(9):1328–1333
MacMahon B, Pugh T, Ipsen J (1960) Epidemiologic methods. Little Brown, Boston, MA
Magarinos AM, Deslandes A, McEwen BS (1999) Effects of anti-depressants and benzodiazepine treatments on the dendritic structure of CA3 pyramidal neurons after chronic stress. Eur J Pharmacol 371:113–22
Martin JK, Pescosolido BA, Tuch SA (2000) Of fear and loathing: the role of "disturbing behavior", labels and causal attributions in shaping public attitudes toward people with mental illness. J Health Soc Behav 41:208–23
Martin JK, Pescosolido BA, Olafsdottir S (2007) The construction of fear: Americans' preferences for social distance from children and adolescents with mental health problems. J Health Soc Behav 48:50–67
McLeod JD, Shanahan MJ (1993) Poverty, parenting, and children's mental health. Am Sociol Rev 58:351–66
McLeod JD, Shanahan MJ (1996) Trajectories of poverty and children's mental health. J Health Soc Behav 37:207–20
Mechanic D (1989) Some tensions among theory, method, and substance. J Health Soc Behav 30:147–60
Mechanic D (1996) Changing medical organization and the erosion of trust. Milbank Q 74:171–189
Mechanic D, Aiken LH (1986) Applications of social science to clinical medicine and health policy. Rutgers University Press, New Brunswick, NJ
Mechanic D, McAlpine D, Rosenfield S, Davis D (1994) Effects of illness attribution and depression on the quality of life among persons with serious mental illness. Soc Sci Med 39:155–164
Mirowsky J, Ross CE (1986) Social patterns of distress. Annu Rev Sociol 12:23–45
Mirowsky J, Ross CE (1989) Psychiatric diagnosis as reified measurement. J Health Soc Behav 30:11–25

Mueller DP (1980) Social networks: a promising direction for research on the relationship of the social environment to psychiatric disorder. Soc Sci Med 14A:147–61
Parsons T (1951) The social system. The Free Press, Glencoe, IL
Paykel ES (1978) Contribution of life events to causation of psychiatric disorder. Psychol Med 8:245–53
Pearlin LI (1999) Stress and mental health: a conceptual overview. In: Horwitz AV, Scheid TL (eds) A handbook for the study of mental health. Cambridge University Press, Cambridge, p 676
Pearlin LI, Menaghan EG, Lieberman MA, Mullan JT (1981) The stress process. J Health Soc Behav 22:337–356
Pellmar TC, Eisenberg L (2000) Bridging disciplines in the brain, behavioral, and clinical sciences. Institute of Medicine Committee Report. National Academy Press, Washington DC
Pennisi E (2000) Breakthrough of the year: genomics comes of age. Science 290:2220–21
Pennisi E (2007) Breakthrough of the year: human genetic variation. Science 318:1843–43
Perry BL (2005) Disordered minds, disrupted relationships? Social network attrition in mental illness careers. Presented at the Society for the Study of Social Problems Annual Meetings, Philadelphia, PA
Perry BL (2006) Understanding social network disruption: the case of youth in foster care. Soc Probl 53:371–91
Perry BD, Pollard R (1998) Homeostasis, stress, trauma, and adaptation: a neuro-developmental view of childhood trauma. Child Adolesc Clin North Am 7:33–51
Pescosolido BA (1991) Illness careers and network ties: a conceptual model of utilization and compliance. Adv Med Sociol 2:161–84
Pescosolido B (2000) The role of social networks in the lives of persons with disabilities. In: Albrecht GL, Seelman KD, Bury M (eds) Handbook of disability studies. Sage, Thousand Oaks, CA, pp 468–89
Pescosolido BA (2006) Of pride and prejudice: the role of sociology and social networks in integrating the health sciences. J Health Soc Behav 47:189–208
Pescosolido BA, Kronenfeld JJ (1995) Health, illness, and healing in an uncertain era: challenges from and for medical sociology. J Health Soc Behav (Extra Issue):5–33
Pescosolido B, Levy J (2002) The role of social networks in health, illness, disease, and healing: the accepting present, the forgotten past, and the dangerous potential for a complacent future. Soc Netw Health 8:3–25
Pescosolido BA, Martin JK, Link BG, Kikuzawa S, Burgos G, Swindle R (2000) Americans' views of mental illness and health at century's end: continuity and change. Indiana Consortium for Mental Health Services Research, Bloomington, IN
Pescosolido BA, Tuch SA, Martin JK (2001) The profession of medicine and the public: examining Americans' changing confidence in physicians from the beginning of the 'health care crisis' to the era of health care reform. J Health Soc Behav 42:1–16
Pescosolido B, Perry BL, Scott Long J, Martin JK, Nurnberger JI Jr, Kramer J, Hesselbrock V (2008) Under the influence of genetics: how transdisciplinarity leads us to rethink social pathways to illness. Am J Sociol 114:S171–S201
Peterson RA, Anand N (2004) The production of culture perspective. Annu Rev Sociol 30:311–34
Portin P, Alanen YO (1997) A critical review of genetic studies of schizophrenia. Acta Psychiatr Scand 95:73–80
Post RM (1992) Transduction of psychosocial stress into the neurobiology of recurrent affective disorder. Am J Psychiatry 149:999–1010
Radloff LS (1977) The CES-D scale: a self-report depression scale for research in the general population. Appl Psychol Meas 1:385–401
Rice D, Barone S (2000) Critical periods of vulnerability for the developing nervous system: evidence from humans and animal models. Environ Health Perspect 108:511–33
Rosenberg M (1984) A symbolic interactionist view of psychosis. J Health Soc Behav 25:289–302
Rutter M, Stroufe LA (2000) Developmental psychopathology: concepts and challenges. Dev Psychopathol 12:265–96
Saudino KJ (2005) Behavioral genetics and child temperament. J Dev Behav Pediatr 26:214–23
Scheff T (1966) Being mentally ill: a sociological theory. Aldine, Chicago, IL
Schwartz S (1999) Biological approaches to psychiatric disorders. In: Horwitz AV, Scheid TL (eds) A handbook for the study of mental health. Cambridge University Press, Cambridge, pp 79–103
Shanahan MJ, Hofer SM (2005) Social context in gene-environment inter-actions: retrospect and prospect. J Gerontol B Psychol Sci Soc Sci 60:65–76
Shanahan MJ, Hofer SM, Shanahan L (2003) Biological models of behavior and the life course. In: Mortimer JT, Shanahan MJ (eds) Handbook of the life course. Plenum, New York, pp 597–622
Shonkoff JP, Phillips DA (2000) *From neurons to neighborhoods: the science of early childhood development.* Institute of Medicine Committee Report. National Academy Press, Washington DC
Simmel G (1955) Conflict and the web of group affiliations. Free Press, New York
Singer BH, Ryff CD (2001) New horizons in health: an integrative approach. National Academy Press, Washington DC
Spires TL, Hannan AJ (2005) Nature, nurture, and neurology: gene-environment interactions in neurodegenerative disease. FEBS J 272:2347–61

Susser M (1998) Does risk factor epidemiology put epidemiology at risk? Peering into the future. J Epidemiol Community Health 52:608–11

Tucker D (1992) Developing emotions and cortical networks. In: Gunnar MR, Nelson CA (eds) Developmental behavioral neuroscience. Lawrence Erlbaum, Hillsdale, NJ, pp 75–128

Turner BS (1992) Regulating bodies: essays in medical sociology. Routledge, New York

Udry JR (2000) Biological limits of gender construction. Am Sociol Rev 65:443–57

Waddington CH (1957) The strategy of the genes. MacMillan, New York

Weiner H (1998) Notes on an evolutionary medicine. Psychosom Med 60:510–520

Wellman B (2000) Partners in illness: who helps when you are sick? In: Kelner M, Wellman B, Pescosolido BA, Saks M (eds) Complementary and alternative medicine: challenge and change. Harwood Academic, Amsterdam, pp 143–162

Wellman B, Frank K (1999) Network capital in a multi-level world: getting support from personal communities. In: Lin N, Cook K, Bury R (eds) Social capital: theory and research. Aldine de Gruyter, Chicago, IL, pp 233–73

Wheaton B (1999) The nature of stressors. In: Horwitz A, Scheid TL (eds) A handbook for the study of mental health. Cambridge University Press, Cambridge, p 676

Williams SJ (2006) Medical sociology and the biological body: where are we now and where do we go from here? Health 10:5–30

Williams DR, Collins C (1995) U.S. socioeconomic and racial differences in health: patterns and explanations. Annu Rev Sociol 21:349–86

Wills TA (1985) Supportive functions of interpersonal relations. In: Cohen S, Syme L (eds) Social support and health. Academic, New York, pp 61–78

Wright ER, Wright D, Perry BL, Foote-Ardah CE (2007) Stigma and the sexual isolation of people with serious mental disorders. Soc Probl 54:73–93

Index

A
Academy Health, 275
Accreditation Council of Graduate Medical Education (ACGME), 208, 209, 239
Adult psychopathology, 556
Agency for Healthcare Research and Quality (AHRQ), 274, 275
Alzheimer's disease, 51–52
American Journal of Sociology, 7, 11
American Sociological Review, 11
American Universalism, 28
American with Disabilities Act (ADA), 160
Antisocial personality disorder (APD), 144
Attention deficit hyperactivity disorder (ADHD), 534

B
Bales' interaction process analysis, 327
Basic Local Alignment Sequence Tool (BLAST), 536
Behavioral genetics (BG), 528
Beveridge model, 102
Beyond Depression (Dowrick), 22
Biocapital, 183–184
Biocitizenship, 185
Bioeconomy, 183–184
Biomedicalization theory
  aging, 188
  biocapital and bioeconomy, 183–184
  biopolitical economy, 189–190
  biopower and biopolitics, 181
  critiques, 185–187
  definition, 177–179
  difference and enhancement, 189
  history, 179–181
  human cloning and stem cell research, 188
  life itself, 182–185
  optimization, 190
  origin, 176
  reproductive technology, 182
  risk studies, 188
  science and technology studies, 174
  technogovernance, 188
  technoluxe, 190
  weaponry and warefare, 190
Biopiracy, 184
Biopolitical economy, 177, 189–190
Bioprospecting, 184
Bismarck model, 102
Body mass index (BMI), 417
British health care policy
  clinical practice guidelines, 93
  hospital Trusts, 90–91
  National Health Service, 90, 93
  National Institute for Clinical Excellence, 93
  pay for performance, 92

C
Canadian healthcare system, 88
Canalization model, 557
Center for Epidemiological Studies Depression Scale (CES-D), 554
Chronic Care Model (CCM), 487
Chronic disease management (CDM), 483
Chronic Disease Self Management Programme (CDSMP), 488
Chronic Fatigue Syndrome (CFS), 492
Chronic illness and disability
  adaptation, 486–487
  biography and narrative
    biographical disruption, 484
    illness experiences, 485
  illness trajectories
    information and assistive technologies, 493–494
    shifting diagnostic terrain, 492–493
  motivation and illness management
    chronic disease management, 489–491
    psychological determinism, limits of, 487–489
  psychological determinism, 483
  social and cultural significance, 485–486
  state-sponsored interventions, 483
  theoretical and conceptual frameworks
    ethnographic approaches, 495
    self-management capacity, 497

Chronic illness and disability (*cont.*)
    social network research, 496
    symbolic interactionism, 495
    technological interventions, 498
Civic professionalism, 212
Classical labelling theory, 29
Clinical practice guidelines (CPGs), 92–93
Community core subsystem, 55–56
Complexity theory, 39
Conflict of interest (COI), 210
Constituency based movements, 300
Conversational diaries. *See* Conversational journals
Conversational journals, 431, 432, 444
Corporate healthcare systems, 318
Cumulative advantage/disadvantage theory (CAD), 453

D
Diagnostic and Statistical Manual (DSM), 383
Diagnostic-related groups (DRGs), 90–91
Diaries. *See* Conversational journals
Direct to consumer advertising (DTCA), 297
Doctor–patient interaction
    biopsychosocial approach, 325
    coding, 330
    consumerist relationship, 326, 328
    conversation analysis
        antibiotic prescription, 335
        diagnosis, 332–333
        interactional choices, 334–335
        multivariate analysis, 336
        perspective display sequence, 333
        primary care interaction, 332
        problem presentations, 334
        qualitative and quantitative analysis, 334
        sequence organization, 332–333
        symptoms only descriptions, 335
    gender-based communication patterns, 329
    medical discourse, 329
    microanalytic discourse approach, 328–329
    mutual model, 326
    paternalistic relationship, 326, 328
    patient-centered method, 325
    process analysis, 327–328
    sociological approach, 324–325
    three-function model, 325–326
DRGs. *See* Diagnostic-related groups
DTCA. *See* Direct to consumer advertising
Durkheimian theory, 53–54

E
Electronic health records (EHRs)
    barriers, 346
    benefits, 345–346
    objective, 345
Embodied health movements (EHM), 119, 300–301
Environmental breast cancer movement (EBCM)
    illness experience, 125–127
    lay-professional conflict, 127–128
Ethical biocapital, 183
Evidence based medicine (EBM), 206

F
Family and Medical Leave Act (FMLA), 239–240
Federal poverty line (FPL), 369
Fee-for-service payment system, 92
Flexner Report, 8
FMLA. *See* Family and Medical Leave Act
Fordist model, 314
Fundamental causality, SES-health relationship
    diabetes, 76
    differences in means, 70–71
    education, health behaviors, 73
    goal, 68
    habitus, 73–74
    health disparities, 68
    health paternalism, 77
    income inequality, 76
    institutional policy leverage, 78
    intelligence, 69
    macrosocial comparison, 75
    massively multiple mechanisms, 69
    material resources, 71–72
    meaning, 68
    metamechanism, 69
    negative association, 67
    public interventions, 77
    risk-factor research, 75
    smoking and obesity, 73
    social institutions, 74–75
    social resources, 71–72
    social shaping approach, 78
    spillovers, 72–73
    systematic asymmetry, 69
    technology and health policy, 77–78

G
Gendered health disparities
    biological differences, 417
    cross-sectional information, 425
    differential exposure and vulnerability, 417
    health damaging behaviors, 418
    health status, 411
    immigration
        demographic composition, 421
        female migrants, 420
        immigrant health, 419
        socioeconomic status, 420
    life course perspective
        aging process, 423
        biological and social risk factors, 422
        gender gap, 421
        longitudinal data sources, 423
    lifestyle activities, 417
    mental and physical health, 423–424
    mortality, 412–413
    physical health
        morbidity paradox, 413

Index 565

    self-rated health, 414
        US racial and ethnic populations, 415
    preventive health care, 418
    race/ethnicity, 419
    socioeconomic status, 418, 419
    stressors and social support networks, 418
    violence, 417
Genetic-environmental (GE) interactions, 527
Genetic linkage
    DRD4, 534
    gene–gene interactions, 532
    homologous genes, 534
    meiosis, 531
    protein–protein network, 533
Germany's health care system, 89–90

H

HCUP. *See* Healthcare Cost and Utilization project
Health advocacy organizations, 298–300
Health belief model (HBM), 44
Healthcare Cost and Utilization project (HCUP), 274
Health care systems
    cross-national variation, 104
    national welfare system, 102
    welfare state, 102–104
Health disparities
    of African Americans, 391
    African Black ancestry, 386
    of Afro-Caribbeans, 391
    of Black middle class
        educational attainment, 387
        health paradox, 388
        stratification, dimension of, 387, 388
    of Blacks and non-Hispanic Whites, 389–390
    Black–White gap, 383
    of Caribbeans, 386
    chronic health and mortality, 364
    communities, 370–371
    complex community-based designs, 377
    death rates, 383, 384
    DSM criteria, 383
    dual systems in operation
        domain interactions, 369
        SCF-HSD, 368
    ethnic and nativity heterogeneity, 400
    federal agencies, 386
    federal state and economic policy, 369–700
    hypersegregation, 386
    hypertension, 401
    individual level factors
        educational attainment, 375
        ethno-cultural populations, 375, 377
        health behavior, 376
        Medicaid beneficiaries, 375
        testable hypotheses, 376
    infant mortality, 385
    informal community system, 373
    mental disorders, 383, 384
    of non-Hispanic Whites, 384
    physiological changes, 400
    provider-client interactions, 374
    provider organizations, 371–372
    race and ethnicity, 363
    racial/ethnic groups, 389
    racism, 385
    SCF-HSD, 364
    SES-health gradient
        African Americans, 391–399
        Afro-Caribbeans, 394, 397, 400
    social inequality, 376
    social network
        Black middle class, 401
        healthy behaviors, 403
        low-income communities, 402
        NSAL, 405–406
        physical vulnerability, 403
    social processes, 386
    sociological and social science roots
        cumulative advantage, 365
        health care, nature of, 364
    transdisciplinary and translational
        research agendas, 377
    US Census Bureau, 386
Health information technology (HIT)
    definition, 344
    deprofessionalization, medicine, 352–354
    doctor–patient interaction, sociological study, 347
    electronic health record
        barriers, 346
        benefits, 345–346
        objectives, 345
    patient–provider relationship
        clinical interaction, 348
        confidentiality and security, 349
        information exchange, 349–350
        trust, 349
        verbal and nonverbal behaviors, 348
    personal data assistants, 346
    personal health record, 346–347
    social dynamics
        data processing, 352
        electronic health record, 350
        information collection, 351–352
        provider–patient interaction, 351
Health Insurance Portability and
        Accountability Act, 263
Health interventions
    AIDS
        blood test, 438
        misconceptions, 441–444
        official information, 440–441
        physical symptoms, 438
        sexual behaviors, 439
        tacit knowledge, 440
        VCT, 438
    classical ethnography, 431
    ethnographic journals, 433–434
        agency and action, 436–438
        incentives, 435
        journalists close networks, 434
        public health interview/survey, 433

Health interventions (*cont.*)
    semi-structured interviews, 433, 435
    social networks, 433
  hearsay ethnography, 432
  survey research, 431
Health maintenance organizations (HMOs), 370
Health Security Act, 276
Health social movements (HSMs), 184, 300
  constituency-based health movements, 119
  EBCM, 117
  ecosocial theory, 131–132
  EHM
    acting on science, 131
    interpreting science, 130
    long-term effects, chemicals, 131
    standards of proof, 130
    toxic ignorance, 131
    weight of evidence approach, 130
  environmental health, 118
  federal agencies, 118
  health access movements, 119
  illness experiences, 117
  medical institutions, 128–130
  medical sociology, 117
    empowerment, 121–123
    institutional political economy, 124–125
    medicalization and disempowerment, 123–124
  Occupational health and safety movements, 118
  typologies, 121
  women's health movement, 119
Hearsay ethnography
  AIDS
    diagnosis of, 441
    information, domestication of, 440–441
    misconceptions about, 441–444
    moral biography and, 439
    sexual behavior and, 440
    symptoms of, 438, 442, 443
  behavior change, 432
  condom, 434, 440, 443
  conversation, 438, 440, 442
  death, 434, 440
  fatalism, 442
  health knowledge, 431, 432
  HIV
    prevention strategies, 442, 443
    transmission probabilities, 442, 443
  journal; journalist (diary; diarist), 433–438
  meaning, 431
  networks, 434–436
  public
    conversation, 432
    culture, 432
    discourse (talk), 432
  research methods
    ethnography, 433, 436
    focus group, 437
    interview, 431, 433, 436, 437
    survey, 431, 433, 436
  social autopsies, 438, 441–443

Help-seeking process
  actors social representations, 470–472
  biopsychosocial paradigm, 465
  community-based healthcare coalitions, 476
  healthcare research, 465
  individuals and organizations, 468–469
  network analysis, 466
  quasi-routine activities, 477
  relational sociology, 466
  social processes
    decision-making, 473
    evidence-based medicine, 475
    narrative co-construction, 473
    network transformation and action sequences, 474
    rational choice, theory of, 472
    sequence analysis, 474
    successive interviews, 475
    traditional service use models, 472
  social relations, 467
  theoretical development, 465
Histone acetyltransferase (HAT), 540
HIT. *See* Health information technology
Hormone replacement therapy (HRT), 128
Human genome project, 7, 46
Hypothalamic Pituitary Adrenal (HPA), 547

I
Identity and illness
  affect control theory
    fundamental sentiments, 515
    INTERACT, 516–517
    interactional elements, 516
    internal and behavioral processes, 515
    predictive capacity, 516
    stigma sentiments, 517–518
    transient sentiments, 515, 516
  effects of
    biographic disruption, 510
    cancer patients, 508
    chronic illness, 506
    cognitive consistency, 508
    illness experiences, 507
    narrative reconstruction, 511
    negative reactions and life situations, 506
    pre-illness identity, 511
    qualitative narratives, 506
    reciprocal relationship, 507
    rights and obligations, 506
    social interactions, 507
    survivor identity, 508
    traditional symbolic interaction, 507
  methodological approaches, 506
  role identity, 512
  social psychological theories, 505
  social structure, 512
  stigma and labeling theory
    compensatory behaviors, 508
    emotional deviance, 510
    individual counseling, 510

Index 567

  internalization, 508
  negative expectations, 509
  self-labeling, 510
  structural symbolic interaction
    commitment, 512
    health care providers, 513
    individual behavior, 514
    individuals pre-existing identities, 515
    role identity, 513
    saliency, 512
    subjective experiences, 514
Identity control theory
  behavioral strategies, 519
  identity standards, 518
  self change, 519
  situational inputs, 518
Individual core subsystem, 55, 58–59
Institute of Medicine (IOM), 241–242
Institutional control, layering of
  criminalization, 140–141
  deviant behavior, 152
  institutional division of labor for deviance, 141
  medicalization, 140–141
  psychopathy
    cognitive theories, 147
    concept of evil, 150–152
    crimino-legal arenas, 148–150
    diagnosis, 145–146
    fear-conditioning deficit, 147
    neurocognitive theories, 147–148
    psychoanalytic models, 147
    structural abnormalities, 148
    treatment, 148
  social control, 142–143
  sociology, 153–154
Institutional logics and trust,
      US health care system
  American cultural preference, 258
  consumer protection laws, 265
  contract failure, 257–258
  for-profit logic, 260
  government failure, 257
  historical eras, 268
  macroinstitutional logics, 269
  market competition, 268
  nonprofit logic, 259
  organization types, 256
  private for-profit logic, 263–264
  private logic, 258–259
  private market failure, 257
  private nonprofit logics, 260–261
  public for-profit logic, 264–266
  public logic, 259
  public nonprofit logic, 262
  S-CHIP, 265
  universal health care, 266
  voluntary failure, 257–258
Institution and organization core subsystem, 55–57
IOM. *See* Institute of medicine

J
Journal of Health and Social Behavior, 11, 24–25
Journals. *See* Conversational journals

K
Kaiser permanente triangle, 311–312

L
Legal and mental health systems
  civil commitment proceedings, 161
  cooperation, 164
  court rulings and legislation, 160
  criminal mental patients, 161
  deviant behavior, 159
  diversion programs, 164–166
  due process rights, 161
  economic forces, 162–163
  involuntary hospitalizations, 161
  medication and psychotherapy, 160
  patient treatment rights, 161
  public deviance, 160
  social services, 167
  social welfare role, 160
  state mental hospitals, 162
  therapeutic jurisprudence, 166
  treatment, 160
Life course approaches
  agency within constraints, 456–458
  age-related trajectories, 453
  basic principles
    antecedents and life transitions, 451
    choices and decisions, 452
    historical events, 451–452
    human development and aging, 450
    interdependence, 451
  between-group inequality, 454
  CAD, 454
  cross-sectional/longitudinal data, 455
  cumulative advantage/disadvantage theory, 453
  European approaches, 452–453
  functional impairment, 453
  inequality mechanisms, 456
  intracohort inequality, 454
  long-term longitudinal analysis, 461
  long-term obesity, 454
  organizational and historical contexts, 458–460
  physical and mental health disparities, 453
  selective mortality, 456
  socioeconomic status, 455
  sociological imagination, 449

M
Madness Explained (Bentall), 22
Malawi, 431–433, 435, 437, 438, 441–444
Malawi Diffusion and Ideational Change project (MDICP), 433
Managed care organizations (MCOs), 95–96

Medical Expenditure Panel Survey (MEPS), 274
Medicalization
    challenges, 176
    demedicalization, 175–176
    economic health markets, 304
    imperialism, 174–175
    individual consumers, 291
    knowledge, 302–303
    markets and consumers, 175
    patients, clients, consumers, and health movements
        consumerism, 298
        definition, 294–295
        direct to consumer advertising, 297
        doctor–patient relationship, 304
        embodied health movements, 300–301
        free market system, 298
        health and medical care, 296–297
        market ideology, 298
        medical consumer, 295–296
        medical licensing, 297
        self-help and advocacy groups, 298–300
    political economic approach, 292
    professional dominance, 174–175
    risk trafficking, 176
    shifting engines and biomedicalization
        individuals and consumers, 294
        medical imperialism, 293
        micro and meso level approaches, 293
        professions and deviance, 292
        technoscientific biomedicine, 293
    social class and intersectionality, 301–302
    sociological literature, 291
Medical sociology
    biological and social factors, 546
    biological and social systems, 547
    biomedical scientists, 543
    boundary divisions, 11
    chain of causation, 545
    conceptualizing social life, 4
    connecting individual and body, 18
    cross-national analyses, 15
    culture and biology, 552–553
    decoding of disciplines, 10–11
    demise of training programs, 12
    developmental models, 551
    disease processes, 544–545
    endocrine and nervous system activity, 547–548
    epidemiology and outcomes, 6
    fundamental causes, 545
    gene-environment interactions, 549
    genetic predispositions, 546
    health and illness career, 17–18
    health outcomes, 543
    human genome project, 7
    integrative research, 545
    mental illness, 546
    metaphor of cultural cartography, 6
    methodologies, 554–555
    neuroplasticity, 548–549
    Obama's Health Care Plan, 9
    organizing by elevation, 14–15
    personal and cultural systems, 17
    physical experience of illness, 554
    professional and institutional barriers, 550
    profession and organizations, 16
    rethinking communities and landscapes, 13–14
    risk factor epidemiology, 545
    shortage of expertise, 13
    social autopsy, 12
    social constructionism
        adult psychopathology, 556
        anti-depressants, 557
        developmental psychopathology, 555
        genetic and environmental conditions, 556
        individual researchers, 555
        integrative research, 556
        mental illness, 555
        normative developmental progression, 557
        psychiatric labeling, 557
    social networks approach, 551–552
    social relationship in clinic, 16–17
    sociological determinants, 546
    sociological imagination, 5
    symptomatology, 557
    translational problem
        dissemination problem, 7
        failure of clinical trials, 8
        implementation problem, 7
        integration, 7
Medicine, family-friendly profession
    convenient care clinics, 243
    cultural and organizational factors, 231–233
    decline of, 249
    economic constraints, 233–235
    gender differences, 223
    individual male and female physicians
        breast-feeding, 244–245, 248
        child care responsibilities, 246
        coping strategies, 245–246
        education system, 248
        housekeeping and child care services, 247
        in-home nanny care, 247
        parenting and domestic challenges, 245
        physician mothers, 243–244
    institutional reforms, 223–234
    legal profession, 222
    part-time work, obstacles, 230–231
    physician mothers, 243–244
    practice consideration, 235–237
    primary care, 249–250
    professional commitment
        bureaucratization, 229
        community-based physicians, 228
        structural pressures, 230
    residents and 80-h-per-week rule
        American council on graduate medical, 238–239
        Family and Medical Leave Act, 239–240
        inadequate maternity leaves, 239
        IOM recommendations, 241–242

Index 569

occupational safety and health administration, 238
on-site child care program, 240
residency programs, 239–240
training programs, regulation of, 238
women physicians, 221–222
workaholics/overwork, 226–227
work-family balance, 221–222
workweek, 224–226
Mental health services, 296–297
Mental health system, 39–40
Mental illness, 24–25
MEPS. *See* Medical Expenditure Panel Survey
Mmonoamine oxidase A (MAOA gene), 530
Model program, 39–40
Mundane healthcare, therapeutic relationships and clinical encounter
   biographical disruption, 319
   chronic illness
      cognitive participation, 315
      coherence, 313–314
      collective action, 316
      division of labor, 314–315
      Fordist model, 314
      Kaiser permanente triangle, 311–312
      professional intermediaries, 315–316
      professional–patient relationship, 316
   corporate healthcare systems, 318
   decision-management technologies, 317
   evidence-based medicine, 317–318
   normalization process theory, 311
   Parson's analysis, 310
   reflexive monitoring, 318
   technogovernance, 317

N
National Center for Health Services Research (NCHSR), 273–274
National Center on Minority Health and Disparities (NCHMD), 281
National Health Service (NHS), 90–91
National Institute for Clinical Excellence (NICE), 93
National Study of American Life (NSAL), 389
Network-Episode Model, 365
Network episode model III-R
   complexity theory, 39
   core subsystems
      community, 54–55
      genes and proteins, 59
      individual, 55, 58–59
      institutional and organization systems, 55–57
      personal networks, 57–58
   Durkheimian theory, 53–54
   epigenetics, 46
   frameworks, 43–44
   geography and community, 46
   goal, 41
   health and illness career subsystem
      advantage, 49
      Alzheimer's disease, 50–51
      mental illness, 49–50
      substance use disorders, 49–50
   health belief model, 44
   human genome project, 46
   individual hospitalizations, 39–41
   mental health system, 39–40
   model program, 39–40
   origins and base, 44–46
   primary level subsystems, 47
   rational choice models, 43
   rational choice theory, 43–44
   Simmel's network conceptualization, 60
   social actor, 61
   social circles, 59–60
   social interactions, 42
   social organization strategy, 44
   social safety net, 62
   sociobehavioral model, 44
   transtheoretical model, 43–44
   vermont longitudinal study, 39, 41
   vermont state hospital, 40–41
NHS. *See* National Health Service
NICE. *See* National Institute for Clinical Excellence
Normalization process theory, 311, 320
Nostalgic professionalism, 208, 210
Nurse practitioners (NPs), 95

O
Occupational Safety and Health Administration (OSHA), 238
Office of Management and Budget (OMB), 386
On-site child care program, 240
Open reading frame (ORF), 529

P
Panel study of income dynamics (PSID), 538
Patients organizations, 184
Pay for performance (P4P), 92
PDS. *See* Perspective display sequence
Personal data assistants (PDAs), 346
Personal health record (PHR), 346–347
Personal networks core subsystem, 55–57
Perspective display sequence (PDS), 333
Primary care trusts (PCTs), 93
Private for-profit logic, 263–264
Private logic, 258–259
Private nonprofit logics, 260–261
Professional Dominance (Freidson), 204
Professionalism movement
   conflict of interest, 210
   corporatization, 205
   cultural divide, 201–202
   debate, 204–207
   evidence based medicine, 206
   lifestyle specialties, 213
   medicine, Parsons' analysis, 203–204

Professionalism movement (*cont.*)
   medicine's discourse, 209–210
   new professionalism literature, 211–212
   organized medicine
      accreditation council of graduate medical education, 208–209
      commercialism, 208
      corporate medicine, 207
      health care marketplace, 207
      nostalgic professionalism, 208
      Parsons' analysis, 213
      physicians' Charter, 208
      residency programs, 208–209
      U.S. stock market, 207
   sociology, 203, 212–214
Professionalism: The Third Wave (Freidson), 206
Profession of Medicine (Freidson), 205
Promissory capital, 183, 190
Psychiatry and sociology
   medicalisation of stigma, case study
      challenges for psychiatric profession, 31–32
      labelling (or societal reaction) theory, 29
      Stigma Campaign, 29–30
   mental disorder, 21–23
   pschoanalysis, case study, 32–33
   social psychiatry, case study
      American Universalism, 28
      collaboration, 23–24
      de-institutionalisation policy, 25
      mental illness, 24–25
      new-Kraepelin orthodoxy, 25
      pharmacological revolution, 25
      symbolic interactionism, 26
Psychoanalysis, 22, 32–33
Psychopathy
   APD markers, 144
   cognitive theories, 147
   concept of evil, 150–152
   crimino-legal arenas, 148–150
   diagnosis, 145–146
   fear-conditioning deficit, 147
   intraspecies predators, 143
   neurocognitive theories, 147–148
   personality disorder, 143
   psychoanalytic models, 147
   psychopathology, 145
   sociopaths, 143
   structural abnormalities, 148
   treatment, 148
Psychopathy Checklist-Revised (PCL-R), 143
Public for-profit logic, 264–266
Public logic, 259
Public nonprofit logic, 262

R
Race and gender, health disparities, 17
Rational choice models, 43
Rational choice theory (RCT), 43–44
Residency programs, 239–240

RIAS. *See* Roter interaction analysis system
Ribosomal RNA (rRNA), 540
Roter interaction analysis system (RIAS), 327–328

S
S. cerevisiae, 533
Self-help groups, 298–299
Semashko model, 102
Serotonin transporter gene linked promoter region (5-HTTLPR), 530
Single point mutation polymorphisms (SNIPs)
   MAOA activity, 530
   polymorphism, 529
Social organization strategy (SOS), 44
Social psychiatry
   collaboration, 23–24
   de-institutionalisation policy, 25
   mental illness, 24–25
   new-Kraepelin orthodoxy, 25
   pharmacological revolution, 25
   symbolic interactionism, 26
The Social Transformation of American Medicine (Starr), 207
Sociobehavioral model (SBM), 44
Socio-Cultural Framework for Health Service Disparities (SCF-HSD)
   cumulative disadvantage, 366
   inequities, 367
   life course and illness careers, 365–366
   race and ethnic differences, 366–367
Socioeconomic status (SES), 387
Socio-genomics
   environmental exogeneity, 541
   epigenetics, 527
   GE interactions, 527, 531
   genetic research
      animal models, deployment of, 535–537
      exogenous environmental variation, 537–539
   histones, 540
   methylation, 541
   ribsomal RNA, 541
   traditional genetics
      behavioral genetics, 528
      genetic linkage, 531–535
      intergenerational correlation, 528
      prenatal environment, 529
      SNIP research, 529–531
Special lay interest groups, 299
State child health insurance program (SCHIP), 272, 276
Stigma Campaign, 29–32
Stigma, medicalisation of
   challenges for psychiatric profession, 31–32
   labelling (or societal reaction) theory, 29
   Stigma Campaign, 29–30

T
Technogovernance, 188
Technoluxe, 190

Index

Telecare systems, 318
Three-function model, doctor–patient interaction, 325–326
Tissue economy, 183–184
Transtheoretical model (TTM), 43–44

U

US health care policy
    diagnostic-related groups, 90–91
    health policy research
        cost control, state/market, 86
        efficiency and equality, 86–87
        social rights and government responsibility, 87–88
    hospital Trusts, Britain, 90–91
    and medical sociology
        Academy Health, 275
        access to, 277
        agency for healthcare research and quality, 274–275
        Clinton health care plan, 276
        costs and expenditures, 277–278
        disparities and sociological interests, 281–282
        federal and state welfare programs, 272
        healthcare cost and utilization project, 274
        insurance coverage, 279–280
        market and bureaucratic reform approach, 275
        Medicaid, 272, 273
        medical expenditure panel survey, 274
        Medicare, 275–277
        Medicare drug benefit, 276
        National Center for Health Services Research, 273–274
        politics, 283–285
        public opinion research, 282–283
        quality, 280–281
        racial/ethnic disparities, 281
        state child health insurance program, 272, 276
        structural interest approach, 275
    National Health Service, Britain, 90–91
    poverty reduction, 96
    primary care
        managed care organizations, 95–96
        nurse practitioners, 95
        OECD countries, 95
    public and private funding
        Canadian healthcare system, 88–89
        Germany's health care system, 89–90
        government role, 88
        social insurance system, 89–90
    race and ethnicity, 96
    rationing, 94–95
    rewarding and guiding providers
        clinical autonomy, 91–92
        clinical practice guidelines, 92–93
        fee-for-service, 92
        government agency, 93
        Medicare fee schedule, 92
        National Institute for Clinical Excellence, 93
        pay for performance, 92
        primary care trusts, 93
    social discrimination, 96

V

Vermont Longitudinal Study (VLS), 39, 41
Vermont State Hospital (VSH), 40–41
Voluntary counseling and testing (VCT), 438

W

Welfare states
    Beveridge system, 103
    health care, 102, 107–108
    health inequalities, 103
    institutionalizing inequalities
        income inequality, 106
        individual-level health outcomes, 107
        market exchanges, 105
        meso-level health determinants, 106
        social cohesion, 106
        social organization, 105
    labor market, 102
    mental health policy, 103
    national culture, 108–110
    research agenda, 110–112
    social-democratic, 103
    stratification research, 104
    theories of, 104–105
Western Canada Wait List Project, 94
Women's health movement, 299–300